T0293651

# Cardiovascular Systems: Mathematical and Numerical Modeling

# Cardiovascular Systems: Mathematical and Numerical Modeling

Editor: Cameron Middleton

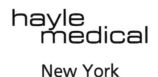

New York

Hayle Medical,
750 Third Avenue, 9th Floor,
New York, NY 10017, USA

Visit us on the World Wide Web at:
www.haylemedical.com

ISBN 978-1-64647-554-4 (Hardback)

**Cataloging-in-Publication Data**

Cardiovascular systems : mathematical and numerical modeling / edited by Cameron Middleton.
   p. cm.
Includes bibliographical references and index.
ISBN 978-1-64647-554-4
1. Cardiovascular system--Diseases. 2. Cardiovascular system--Mathematical models.
3. Cardiovascular system--Diseases--Mathematical models. 4. Cardiology. I. Middleton, Cameron.
RC667 .C375 2023
616.1--dc23

# Contents

# Preface

It is often said that books are a boon to mankind. They document every progress and pass on the knowledge from one generation to the other. They play a crucial role in our lives. Thus I was both excited and nervous while editing this book. I was pleased by the thought of being able to make a mark but I was also nervous to do it right because the future of students depends upon it. Hence, I took a few months to research further into the discipline, revise my knowledge and also explore some more aspects. Post this process, I begun with the editing of this book.

The cardiovascular system consists of the heart and a network of blood vessels. It is primarily involved in the distribution of nutrients and blood throughout the body, and the transportation of deoxygenated blood back to the lungs. Numerical simulation tools, mathematical models and algorithms can be used for the investigation of the human cardiovascular system. The mathematical and numerical modeling of the cardiovascular system encompasses the development of mathematical and computational models along with their efficient numerical solution, in-vivo and in-vitro validation, and filtering the data. It also involves identifying the parameters of mathematical models, devising optimal treatments and accounting for uncertainties. This book provides comprehensive insights on the mathematical modeling and numerical simulation of the human cardiovascular system. A number of latest researches have been included to keep the readers up-to-date with the global concepts in this area of study. This book aims to serve as a resource guide for students and experts alike and contribute to the growth of the discipline.

I thank my publisher with all my heart for considering me worthy of this unparalleled opportunity and for showing unwavering faith in my skills. I would also like to thank the editorial team who worked closely with me at every step and contributed immensely towards the successful completion of this book. Last but not the least, I wish to thank my friends and colleagues for their support.

**Editor**

# Validated Computational Model to Compute Re-Apposition Pressures for Treating Type-B Aortic Dissections

*Aashish Ahuja[1], Xiaomei Guo[1], Jillian N. Noblet[2], Joshua F. Krieger[2], Blayne Roeder[2], Stephan Haulon[3], Sean Chambers[2] and Ghassan S. Kassab[1]\**

[1] California Medical Innovations Institute, San Diego, CA, United States, [2] Cook Medical, Bloomington, IN, United States, [3] Aortic Center, Hôpital Marie Lannelongue, Université Paris Sud, Paris, France

**\*Correspondence:**
Ghassan S. Kassab
gkassab@calmi2.org

The use of endovascular treatment in the thoracic aorta has revolutionized the clinical approach for treating Stanford type B aortic dissection. The endograft procedure is a minimally invasive alternative to traditional surgery for the management of complicated type-B patients. The endograft is first deployed to exclude the proximal entry tear to redirect blood flow toward the true lumen and then a stent graft is used to push the intimal flap against the false lumen (FL) wall such that the aorta is reconstituted by sealing the FL. Although endovascular treatment has reduced the mortality rate in patients compared to those undergoing surgical repair, more than 30% of patients who were initially successfully treated require a new endovascular or surgical intervention in the aortic segments distal to the endograft. One reason for failure of the repair is persistent FL perfusion from distal entry tears. This creates a patent FL channel which can be associated with FL growth. Thus, it is necessary to develop stents that can promote full re-apposition of the flap leading to complete closure of the FL. In the current study, we determine the radial pressures required to re-appose the mid and distal ends of a dissected porcine thoracic aorta using a balloon catheter under static inflation pressure. The same analysis is simulated using finite element analysis (FEA) models by incorporating the hyperelastic properties of porcine aortic tissues. It is shown that the FEA models capture the change in the radial pressures required to re-appose the intimal flap as a function of pressure. The predictions from the simulation models match closely the results from the bench experiments. The use of validated computational models can support development of better stents by calculating the proper radial pressures required for complete re-apposition of the intimal flap.

Keywords: aortic dissection, bench tests, porcine aorta, finite element analysis, re-apposition pressure, simulation models

## INTRODUCTION

The incidence of aortic dissection (AD) in the United States is approximately 2,000 cases per year and early mortality is as high as 1% per hour if untreated (Vecht et al., 1980; Roberts, 1981). AD occurs when there is a tear in the intimal lining of the aorta, allowing blood to flow between the intimal and medial layers of the aorta. Complicated type-B acute AD is specifically defined as dissection associated with rupture, malperfusion syndromes, refractory pain, or rapid aortic expansion at onset or during hospital stay (Fattori et al., 2008). Currently, there are three modes of treating patients suffering from type-B acute AD: medical management, open surgery, or endovascular treatment. While medical management is suggested for patients who have uncomplicated dissections, open surgery or endovascular treatment is recommended for complicated dissections.

Recently, clinicians recommend the minimally invasive endovascular grafting procedure over open surgery for complicated type-B patients suffering from impending or actual complicated dissections because surgical methods have approximately a 13% higher mortality rate at 5-year follow-up as compared to endovascular grafting (Moulakakis et al., 2014). The endograft is first deployed to exclude the proximal entry tear to redirect blood flow toward the true lumen (TL) and then a stent or graft is used to push the intimal flap against the false lumen (FL) wall such that the aorta is reconstituted by sealing the FL. Although stent grafting has been largely successful in closing the initial entry tear (Kato et al., 2002; Song et al., 2006; Marcheix et al., 2008; Sayer et al., 2008; Alves et al., 2009; Manning et al., 2009; Czerny et al., 2010), patients may still undergo re-interventions in the form of multiple stent-grafts or open surgery due to ongoing complications (Thrumurthy et al., 2011; Fattori et al., 2013; Andersen et al., 2014; Faure et al., 2014). Aortic aneurysm is one of the complications that develops in the FL wall after successful endovascular treatments. The occurrence of aneurysm in patients with successful treatments is reported to be about 7% (Won et al., 2006)–20% (Lopera et al., 2003), which is likely attributed to perturbation of significant mechanical forces on the aorta (Kassab, 2006; Fortier et al., 2014). Moreover, a significant enlargement of the aortic diameter above the stent graft has been observed during deployment, which is important because this may reflect increased strain and stress on the aorta in the segments adjacent to the stent graft (Trimarchi and Eagle, 2016).

The observation of aortic aneurysm in the FL after the stent graft procedure illustrates the necessity of fine-tuning the procedure to minimize the risk for the patient of reintervention after the initial endovascular graft. Using a detailed and systematic biomechanical analysis of blood pressure in both the mid and distal regions of the TL, may lead to the design and use of proper endovascular grafts or bare metal stents which provides sufficient radial forces on the intimal flap to re-appose it against the FL wall. This may allow reconstitution of the aortic wall without imposing high mechanical stresses on the FL wall, leading to a decrease in secondary complications such as aortic aneurysm. The development of effective mechanical devices for endovascular grafting requires the use of computational techniques such as Finite Element Analysis (FEA) to analyze the structural interaction between the rigid stents (usually composed of Stainless steel or Nitinol alloy) and different tissue segments of the dissected aorta (i.e., intimal flap, FL wall, and true lumen [TL] wall). FEA has been used in the past to compute radial forces and improve stent designs being deployed for treatment of stenosed valves (Kumar and Mathew, 2010), atherosclerotic coronary arteries (Eshghi et al., 2011) and aortic aneurysms

(Arokiaraj et al., 2014). The present study utilized FEA utilized to develop a bench-validated computational model based on contact mechanics to quantify the radial pressures required to reconstitute the aorta from dissection and promote remodeling, without exerting undue strains on the vessel wall.

The purpose of this study is to provide a validated computational model of flap re-apposition which can be used as a benchmark for testing different therapies in a virtual setting. The proposed model aims to reduce the overall time and cost required to perform pre-clinical *in vivo* studies in porcine and expedite the development of better endovascular therapies for treating AD in humans. From the bench tests and computational simulations presented, it is observed that the radial pressure for re-apposition of intimal flap increases monotonically with increase in aortic pressure.

# MATERIALS AND METHODS

## Bench Experiments
### Aorta Preparation and Dissection
Five fresh thoracic aorta samples harvested from healthy porcine were prepared for bench tests by removing all connective tissue and ligating all branches using 2-0 sutures. Samples were stored at ~2°C until tested. Samples were not used for any testing prior to this research. Next, the porcine aorta was inverted exposing the intima and dissections were created ~6–8 cm from the left subclavian artery (LSA). The percent circumferential length of the entry tear, calculated as 100 × (circumference of the flap/circumference of the aorta), was approximately 50–60% of aorta circumference (Canchi et al., 2017). Dissections in healthy descending thoracic aorta represent the case of acute Type-B AD. Using a surgical blade, a cut was made in the inner lining of the aortic wall. The layers were separated using a surgical blade and advanced using fine-tip forceps to the desired axial length. The depth of incision for dissection was typically set between 30 and 50% of the wall thickness. A resulting intimal flap of about ~10–13 cm in length was created due to surgical dissection as shown in **Figure 1**. A reentry was then created, and the flap separated the TL from the FL of the aorta.

### Protocol for Bench Testing
After the dissection was created in the aorta sample, it was mounted on a customized static pressure fixture developed for this study as shown in **Figure 2**. In the setup, the pressure line was connected to stopcock valve which was attached on the other end with an axle as shown in left side of image. The stopcock on right was always closed and to prevent outflow of saline. A saline water reservoir was fed with a compressed air line at a specific pressure and as a result, the pressure line was filled with saline water. The saline solution was transmitted to the suspended aorta which inflated under the applied pressure. Prior to performing the bench test, a Cook CODA balloon catheter (CODA-2-9.0-35-100-32) was advanced into, either the mid (~6–8 cm from LSA) or distal (~11–14 cm from LSA) region of the TL, such that the entire balloon was contained within the dissection. The aorta was then pressurized to static

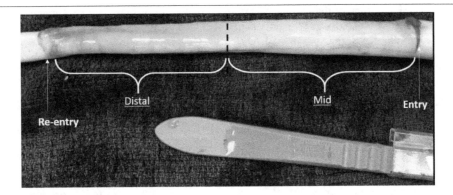

**FIGURE 1 |** An inverted aorta with an imposed dissection. An entry was initially created in the descending thoracic aorta and propagated using forceps to the distal region of the aorta where a pocket of re-entry was created. Tissue specimens from two regions (mid and distal) were extracted and tested on planar biaxial testing machine for material characterization.

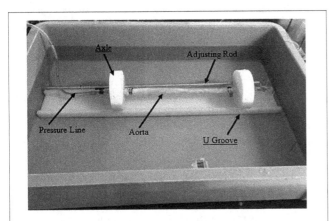

**FIGURE 2 |** Fixture and setup for conducting bench tests on dissected aorta.

pressures between 70 and 140 mmHg in increments of 10 mmHg. Higher aortic pressures simulated patients with hypertension, which is considered one of the primary risk factors for AD. For each of the sample pressure values, the balloon was inflated by filling it with water until the intimal flap re-apposed against the outer wall. The reconstitution of the aortic wall was confirmed via ultrasound imaging (Philips iE33) and the corresponding pressure for balloon inflation was recorded using pressure transducer. The pressure for re-apposition was calculated as the difference between balloon and static aorta pressure; i.e., $\Delta$ (Balloon-Aortic pressure). **Figure 3** shows the schematic of bench test.

## Finite Element Modeling of Dissected Aorta

### Tissue Materials

Aortic dissection splits a single aortic lumen into two lumens: FL and TL. As a result, material properties for the dissected layers (i.e., FL wall and intimal flap), in addition to the undissected TL wall, are required to develop fully informed FEA models. As demonstrated in Ahuja et al. (unpublished) the material characterization for the mid and distal regions of the dissected layers, FL wall, and intimal flap, were calculated first by, conducting planar biaxial testing on porcine tissue specimens and then, using a non-linear regression algorithm (Nelder-Mead optimization method; Nelder and Mead, 1965) to fit experimental data against a structural constitutive model (Gasser et al., 2006). Details of the material characterization of tissue samples including their measured experimental curves with model fitting are shown in Appendix 1.

The tissue components of the dissected aorta behave as a hyperelastic material. Since the intimal flap undergoes large bending stresses due to distension of the expansion member, different material properties are applied in the definition of both

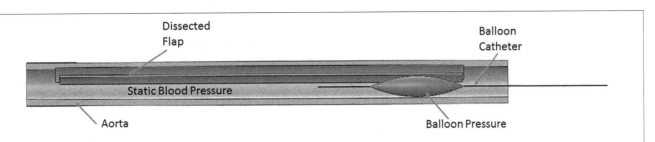

**FIGURE 3 |** Representation of the protocol followed during the bench test. A balloon catheter was inserted into the true lumen (TL). The balloon was inflated with water which applied bending forces to either the mid or distal region of the flap in the presence of static aortic pressure. The balloon pressure on re-apposition of flap was recorded using a pressure transducer.

mid and distal flap segments. Using each of the porcine aortas, we created five sets of parameters for mid flap segments and four sets of parameters for distal flap segments. Thus, a total of nine different flap geometries were created using computer aided design (CAD) software. One set of material definitions for descending thoracic TL wall, mid FL wall and distal FL wall were used throughout the simulations. **Table 1** gives the parameter estimates for the mid and distal flaps and **Table 2** gives the parameter values for the TL wall, Mid FL wall, and Distal FL wall.

## Pre-processing

Idealized models of a dissected aorta were prepared using Solidworks (v2017, Dassault Systemes) and simulated in Abaqus (v6.13.5, Dassault Systemes) using the Abaqus CAE (Complete Abaqus Environment) standard module. The 3D CAD geometry for the porcine aorta is shown in **Figure 4** which consisted of three layers; i.e., TL wall, FL wall and intimal flap. The circumferential length of the intimal flap was adjusted to be within 50–60% of the aortic circumferential length. A rigid expansion member was modeled within the TL of the dissected aorta to re-appose the intimal flap by expansion, which is analogous to the inflation of a balloon.

All the components of the model were meshed using hexahedral elements (C3D8RH), except the expansion member, which was meshed using linear shell elements (S4). The intimal flap underwent bending due to contact force being applied by the expansion member which was meshed with at least two rows of C3D8RH elements to avoid hourglass effects. Three contact interactions were established between the following: (1) the expansion member and intimal flap, (2) the expansion member and TL wall, and (3) the intimal flap and FL wall. The simulation

for re-apposition of the intimal flap was conducted over two steps to match the protocol followed for bench tests:

Step 1: Pressurize the dissected aorta to the required internal pressure (70–140 mmHg) (**Figure 5A**)

Step 2: While maintaining the aorta in a pressurized state (from Step 1), distend the expansion member and achieve full re-apposition of the intimal flap (**Figure 5B**).

Four boundary conditions (BCs) and one loading condition (LC) were applied:

BC 1: Constrained the z-deformation of vessel end faces.
BC 2: Constrained the nodes lying on YZ-plane passing through center of dissected aorta (X-symmetry).
BC 3: Constrained the nodes on faces containing flap, FL wall, and TL wall to move along the y-direction.
BC 4: Dilated the expansion member using specified displacement in Step 2.
LC 1: Pressurized the interior of the aorta by applying pressure to selected areas in Step 1.

A sensitivity analysis on mesh was performed to show that the results converged to the same solution with a refined mesh as well. A global element size of 0.3 mm for both the dissected aorta and expansion member was selected for all the samples and cases considered. The results for radial pressures at 100 mmHg converged to the same solution within an error of 2.5% compared to a refined mesh. Since the thicknesses of flaps varied between computational models, mesh sensitivity results from Distal Sample #1 are presented here. The global element size of 0.3 mm resulted in 69,126 hexahedral elements for the dissected aorta model. The radial pressures from this model only decreased by 1.7% when compared to a model with a global element size of 0.2 mm (233,655 hexahedral elements). Also, choosing the latter finer mesh size increased computational time by an average of 200% (from 0.63 h to 1.9 h) when solved on *San Diego Supercomputer Center's* (SDSC) workstation utilizing 24 cores (Towns et al., 2014).

## Post Processing

The contact pressure applied to the expansion member due to interaction with the intimal flap and TL wall was computed for all aortic pressures between 70 and 140 mmHg. The average of the contact pressure over all elements of the expansion member returned the radial pressure, which was calculated using a customized Python script. The radial pressures computed for each static aorta pressure was compared with re-apposition pressure obtained from bench experiments.

## RESULTS

### Re-apposition of Mid Flap Against the Mid FL Wall

Under this solution, the expansion member was distended to push the mid region of the intimal flap until it re-apposed

**TABLE 1 |** Parameter estimation for mid and distal flap.

| Pig # | Thickness (mm) | C10 (Pa) | k1 (Pa) | k2 | α (degrees) | κ |
|---|---|---|---|---|---|---|
| **Parameter estimation for mid flap** | | | | | | |
| 1 | 0.58 | 92,963 | 230,290 | 13.9 | 87.1 | 0.33 |
| 2 | 0.59 | 73,144 | 235,075 | 7.86 | 68.7 | 0.3 |
| 3 | 0.54 | 64,042 | 212,120 | 4.99 | 23.5 | 0.32 |
| 4 | 0.70 | 52,072 | 125,430 | 5.87 | 53.9 | 0.26 |
| 5 | 0.47 | 45,588 | 149,880 | 1.42 | 55.6 | 0.21 |
| **Parameter estimation for distal flap** | | | | | | |
| 1 | 0.4 | 103,140 | 61,969 | 4.1 | 62.4 | 0.1 |
| 2 | 0.34 | 171,740 | 661,830 | 8.05 | 86.5 | 0.3 |
| 3 | 0.43 | 78,686 | 239,090 | 3.18 | 89.9 | 0.3 |
| 4 | 0.29 | 63,554 | 77,013 | 4.76 | 83.4 | 0.11 |

**TABLE 2 |** Parameter estimation for TL wall, mid FL wall, and distal FL wall.

| | Parameter estimation for mid flap | | | | | |
|---|---|---|---|---|---|---|
| Region | Thickness (mm) | C10 (Pa) | k1 (Pa) | k2 | α (degrees) | κ |
| TL wall | 1.76 | 78,219 | 201,440 | 1.52 | 87.1 | 0.2 |
| Mid FL wall | 1.3 | 53,456 | 952,380 | 4.94 | 7.5 | 0.3 |
| Distal FL wall | 1.24 | 72,996 | 20,894 | 9.01 | 66.5 | 0 |

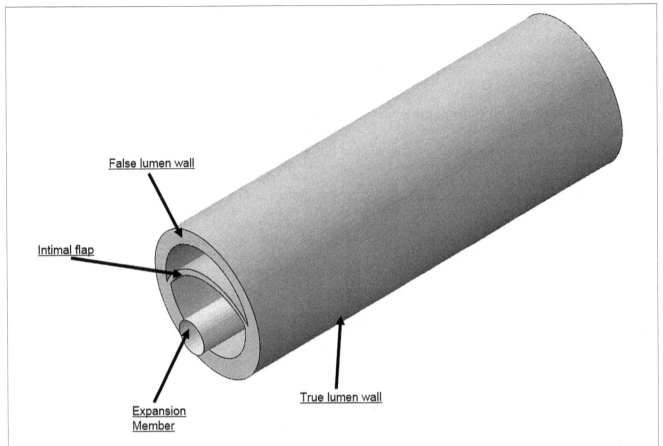

**FIGURE 4 |** Different geometries required to simulate aortic dissection are developed as 3D computer aided design (CAD) models and imported into finite element analysis (FEA) software.

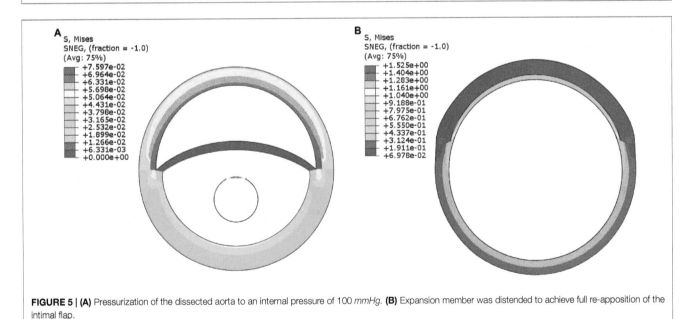

**FIGURE 5 | (A)** Pressurization of the dissected aorta to an internal pressure of 100 *mmHg*. **(B)** Expansion member was distended to achieve full re-apposition of the intimal flap.

completely against the mid FL wall. An increase in the diameter of the aorta was observed after re-apposition of intimal flap. During experiments, the static pressure was homogenously applied to the entire aorta vessel as well as to the expanding balloon. In the case of simulations, the aorta vessel was loaded with a pressure equal to that applied during bench testing, but the expansion member was unloaded. Hence, we define re-apposition pressure as $P_{re-app} = P_{balloon} - P_{aorta}$ in the experimental results, while for simulations we obtain this value, $P_{re-app}$ (simulation), directly from the pressure applied on the expansion member. The values of $\Delta$ (Balloon-Aortic pressure) with respect to static aortic pressures are shown in **Figures 6A,B**.

## Re-apposition of Distal Flap Against Distal FL Wall

Similarly, the expansion member was distended to push the distal region of the flap until it re-apposed completely against the distal FL wall. The radial pressures required for re-apposition were smaller than those required for re-apposition of mid flap. The results from bench tests and computational models are shown in **Figures 7A,B**, respectively.

## Change in Diameter of Aorta Due to Re-apposition

Results from the bench experiments showed an increase in the diameter of a dissected aorta with application of aortic pressure. Specifically, the diameter of the dissected aorta was affected by two parameters:

(1) An increase in pressure resulted in an overall increase in the diameter of the vessel
(2) An increase in diameter imposed additional tension on the flap which increased the net balloon pressure to re-appose the flap. This, in turn required a bigger balloon diameter to re-appose the flap completely against the wall.

The increase in the internal diameter of the aorta for all considered static pressures ( i.e., 70–140 mmHg), for distal and mid region is shown in **Figure 8**. The values for the diameter of the vessel after re-apposition were measured from ultrasound images. The images were captured at the start of each bench experiment (when balloon was completely crimped) and at the end of expansion (when flap was in complete contact with false

lumen wall). As an example, **Figure 9** shows the ultrasound images highlighting the expansion of CODA balloon under 80 mmHg aortic pressure. It should be noted that the diameter of the distal part of the aorta always had a smaller value than the mid region of the aorta, for all static pressures imposed during bench testing.

## Sensitivity Analysis

The flap, which is pre-stressed as part of the intact aorta, shortens after the dissection. It also undergoes large bending and stretching during the re-apposition process which also leads to further stiffening of the flap. Since the present study used material properties based on biaxial testing of different samples of intimal flap, sensitivity analyses were conducted on TL and FL walls for both mid and distal regions of the dissected aorta. It was observed that only the intimal flap largely influenced the radial pressures recorded during the re-apposition process. To conduct the sensitivity analysis, we varied the material properties of the distal FL wall, mid FL wall or TL(using Tables 2, 3, 5 from the Appendix). The material properties from Sample #1 were utilized for dissection components that are unchanged.

The simulations were executed for aortic pressures of 70, 100, and 140 mmHg. It was concluded that the radial pressures can be accurately predicted by varying material behavior of intimal flap while using only one set of TL and FL wall properties since the average results from Samples 2–5 are within 6 and 8% of the mid and distal computational results, respectively, observed for Sample #1. See **Figures 10A,B**.

## DISCUSSION

Since the introduction of thoracic endovascular aortic repair (TEVAR) in Dake et al. (1999), Mitchell et al. (1999), TEVAR has gained popularity over surgical repair for treating complicated Stanford Type B aortic dissections. Many studies have shown favorable short- and mid-term outcomes for Type B

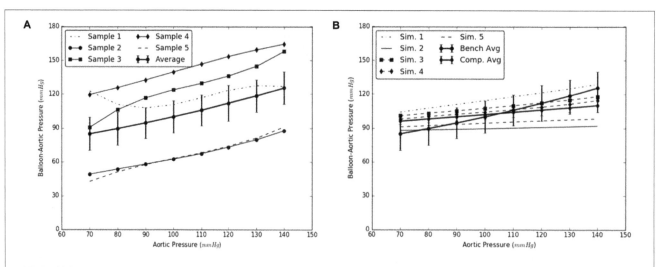

**FIGURE 6 | (A)** Bench test measurements for re-apposition of mid flap against the mid false lumen (FL) wall. **(B)** Computational measurements for re-apposition of mid flap and its comparison with bench results.

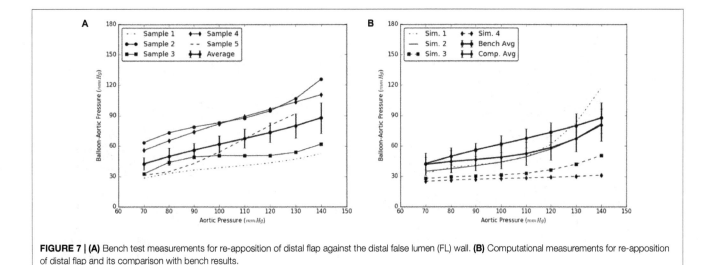

**FIGURE 7 | (A)** Bench test measurements for re-apposition of distal flap against the distal false lumen (FL) wall. **(B)** Computational measurements for re-apposition of distal flap and its comparison with bench results.

dissections using TEVAR. In mid-term and long-term follow-ups, however, distal stent-related complications including distal re-entry, pseudoaneurysm formation, and aneurysm formation are observed (Neuhauser et al., 2008; Thrumurthy et al., 2011). Studies have reported that the incidence of new re-entries at the proximal and distal ends of the stent graft, combined are 3.4% (out of 651 patients) (Dong et al., 2010). In a sub-cohort of 23 patients with re-entries (3.4% of the 651 patients), 25% (4 of 16) were at the proximal end of the stent graft and 28.6% (2 of 7) were at the distal ends of the stent graft, leading to a total mortality rate of 23.1% of the sub-cohort. Most of the stent-related complications were caused by conventional stent grafts which likely imposed abnormally high stresses and strains on the aortic wall. The present study utilized FEA to develop a bench-validated computational model which quantified the exact radial pressures required to re-appose the flap after dissection. This will allow proper stents and grafts sizing, while avoiding oversizing to prevent undue strains and stresses on the aorta which can lead to retrograde dissection (Leshnower et al., 2013), in-folding, and graft occlusion (Kasirajan et al., 2012).

The use of this validated computational models can expedite the development of novel stents and therapies in treating aortic dissection. The model presented in this study uses a well-informed but idealized computer model of dissection in porcine, which captures the balloon pressures that are required to re-appose the intimal flap in reconstituting the aorta lumen. We developed two sets of models, one for mid dissections and one for and distal dissections, and presented results for radial pressures under static aortic pressures. From our plots in **Figure 6**, we observed that the computational models captured the bench results for all pressures, 70–140 mmHg. This included physiological blood pressures (mean pressure ~90 mmHg) as well as high blood pressures. A small standard error (2.8 – 6.1 mmHg) between results from computational models and bench test measurements was observed and the slope for average curve was small. The radial pressures applied to stent grafts for re-apposition increased slowly in the case of mid region. Overall for distal region shown in **Figure 7**, the radial pressures

required for re-apposition were lower than those observed in mid region, but also increased slowly. There were two reasons for lower radial pressure values: (1) The distal aorta had a smaller diameter as compared to mid aorta and thus the balloon or expansion member required less distension to re-appose the intimal flap, and (2) The distal flap underwent lower circumferential stretch as compared to mid flap and was hence, more compliant at those stretch values (Ahuja et al. unpublished). Finally, the average results from bench experiments were within the range for computational outputs for both mid and distal regions.

As the aortic pressure increased, we simultaneously saw an increase in the resultant diameter of the vessel following the re-apposition of intimal flap. The resulting diameters for both, mid and distal regions, increased monotonically and followed the same trend for all pressures, 70–140 mmHg. These curves, shown in **Figure 8**, had large slopes for pressures ≤110 mmHg, but became more horizontal at greater pressures. This behavior

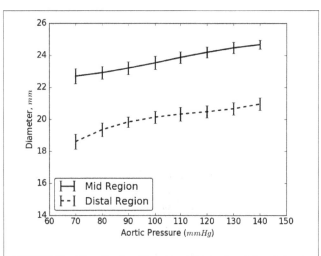

**FIGURE 8 |** Resulting diameter of the mid and distal region of dissected aorta on complete re-apposition of intimal flap.

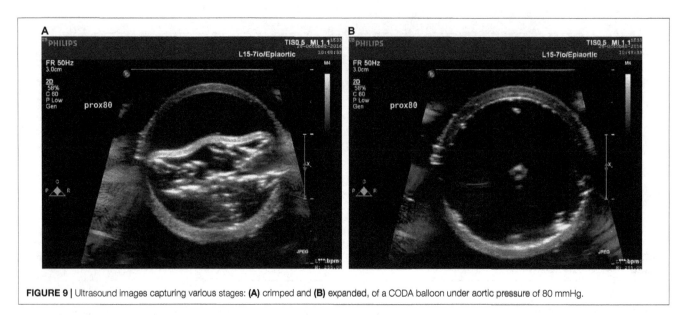

**FIGURE 9 |** Ultrasound images capturing various stages: **(A)** crimped and **(B)** expanded, of a CODA balloon under aortic pressure of 80 mmHg.

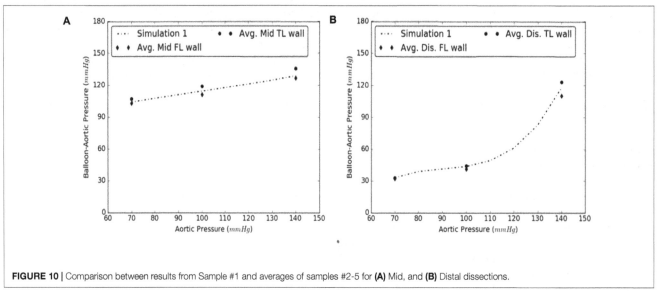

**FIGURE 10 |** Comparison between results from Sample #1 and averages of samples #2-5 for **(A)** Mid, and **(B)** Distal dissections.

may be attributed to the presence of collagen fibers which became uncrimped and lead to stiffening of tissues at higher pressures. The fibers may have reduced the rate of dilation of the aorta and hence smaller changes were observed in the diameters at higher pressures.

## Limitations

The computational model for re-apposition considered an informed geometrically idealized model to validate the results from bench experiments. Further, we used different samples for bench and computational studies. A more accurate computational model based on one-to-one true geometry of the aorta would have generated results that correlated closer with those obtained from bench tests. An accurate model could be reconstructed from echocardiography by acquiring high resolution cross-sectional images for the entire aorta with a thickness of around 1 mm/slice (Ohbuchi and Fuchs, 1991).

Despite the geometric idealization, our current model predictions were in very good agreement with the bench data.

Furthermore, current simulations considered balloon inflation through displacement boundary conditions. Realistic approaches for inflation of the balloon could be found in the literature (e.g., De Beule et al., 2008; Martin and Boyle, 2013; Schiavone and Zhao, 2015). Our current study relied on static aortic pressure to quantify the radial pressures required to re-appose the flap. In future models, we could correlate our computational results with *in vivo* studies using a better representation of folded balloon inflation, experiencing the dynamic conditions of aortic blood flow and pressure. In bench testing, we manually created dissections by first, initiating a tear and then using a surgical blade to advance the tear into a flap. This method leads to generation of a straight linear flap. *In vivo* dissections have shown the intimal flap to rotate inside the aorta as it progresses from the thoracic aorta to abdominal aorta (i.e., spiral dissections)

(Armstrong et al., 1996). Also, the occurrence of dissection may lead to creation of multiple re-entries along the length of the intimal flap (Criado, 2011). These complicated dissections have been known to increase the difficulty of the implementation of endovascular therapy and can result in a patent FL (Qing et al., 2016). Future computational models should include multiple re-entry sites and dissection anatomies with rotated flaps to follow clinical observations. The present analysis serves as a foundation for future more realistic refinements of aortic dissection models.

## AUTHOR CONTRIBUTIONS

AA is the first author of this research and contributed to this manuscript extensively. XG created dissections manually in the porcine samples, prepared them for bench testing, and assisted AA in conducting bench tests. JN prepared the tissue specimens and supervised the planar biaxial testing according to the protocol and assisted AA with the biomechanical characterization of tissues. JK provided expert insight into the material behavior of tissues and assisted with the calibration and functioning of bench testing machine. SH provided clinical inputs to the paper and contributed extensively to the section "Introduction" as well as in steering the objectives of this study. JN, BR, SC, and GK contributed to critical sections of the paper, the protocol, managing resources for bench tests and computational studies, and approving results for preparation of manuscripts.

## ACKNOWLEDGMENTS

This work used the Extreme Science and Engineering Discovery Environment (XSEDE), which is supported by National Science Foundation grant number ACI-1548562. This work used the Extreme Science and Engineering Discovery Environment (XSEDE) Comet supercomputer located at San Diego Supercomputer Center through allocation Charge # TG-MCB170015.

## REFERENCES

Alves, C. M. R., da Fonseca, J. H. P., de Souza, J. A. M., Kim, H. C., Esher, G., and Buffolo, E. (2009). Endovascular treatment of type B aortic dissection: the challenge of late success. *Ann. Thorac. Surg.* 87, 1360–1365. doi: 10.1016/j.athoracsur.2009.02.050

Andersen, N. D., Keenan, J. E., Ganapathi, A. M., Gaca, J. G., McCann, R. L., and Hughes, G. C. (2014). Current management and outcome of chronic type B aortic dissection: results with open and endovascular repair since the advent of thoracic endografting. *Ann. Cardiothorac. Surg.* 3, 264–274. doi: 10.3978/j.issn.2225-319X.2014.05.07

Armstrong, W. F., Bach, D. S., Carey, L., Chen, T., Donovan, C., Falcone, R. A., et al. (1996). Spectrum of acute dissection of the ascending aorta: a transesophageal echocardiographic study. *J. Am. Soc. Echocardiogr.* 9, 646–656. doi: 10.1016/S0894-7317(96)90060-7

Arokiaraj, M. C., De Santis, G., De Beule, M., and Palacios, I. F. (2014). Finite element modeling of a novel self-expanding endovascular stent method in treatment of aortic aneurysms. *Sci. Rep.* 4:3630. doi: 10.1038/srep03630

Canchi, S., Guo, X., Phillips, M., Berwick, Z., Kratzberg, J., Krieger, J. F., et al. (2017). Role of re-entry tears on the dynamics of type B dissection flap. *Ann. Biomed. Eng.* 46, 186–196. doi: 10.1007/s10439-017-1940-3

Criado, F. J. (2011). Aortic dissection: a 250-year perspective. *Tex. Heart Inst. J.* 38, 694–700.

Czerny, M., Roedler, S., Fakhimi, S., Sodeck, G., Funovics, M., Dumfarth, J., et al. (2010). Midterm results of thoracic endovascular aortic repair in patients with aneurysms involving the descending aorta originating from chronic type B dissections. *Ann. Thorac. Surg.* 90, 90–94. doi: 10.1016/j.athoracsur.2010.04.001

Dake, M. D., Kato, N., Mitchell, R. S., Semba, C. P., Razavi, M. K., Shimono, T., et al. (1999). Endovascular stent–graft placement for the treatment of acute aortic dissection. *N. Engl. J. Med.* 340, 1546–1552. doi: 10.1056/NEJM199905203402004

De Beule, M., Mortier, P., Carlier, S. G., Verhegghe, B., Van Impe, R., and Verdonck, P. (2008). Realistic finite element-based stent design: the impact of balloon folding. *J. Biomech.* 41, 383–389. doi: 10.1016/j.jbiomech.2007.08.014

Leshnower, B. G., Szeto, W. Y., Pochettino, A., Desai, N. D., Moeller, P. J., Nathan, D. P., et al. (2013). Thoracic endografting reduces morbidity and remodels the thoracic aorta in DeBakey III aneurysms. *Ann. Thorac. Surg.* 95, 914–921. doi: 10.1016/j.athoracsur.2012.09.053

Lopera, J., Patiño, J. H., Urbina, C., García, G., Alvarez, L. G., Upegui, L., et al. (2003). Endovascular treatment of complicated type-B aortic dissection with stent-grafts: midterm results. *J. Vasc. Interv. Radiol.* 14, 195–203. doi: 10.1097/01.RVI.0000058321.82956.76

Dong, Z., Fu, W., Wang, Y., Wang, C., Yan, Z., Guo, D., et al. (2010). Stent graft-induced new entry after endovascular repair for Stanford type B aortic dissection. *J. Vasc. Surg.* 52, 1450–1457. doi: 10.1016/j.jvs.2010.05.121

Eshghi, N., Hojjati, M. H., Imani, M., and Goudarzi, A. M. (2011). Finite element analysis of mechanical behaviors of coronary stent. *Procedia Eng.* 10, 3056–3061. doi: 10.1016/j.proeng.2011.04.506

Fattori, R., Montgomery, D., Lovato, L., Kische, S., Di Eusanio, M., Ince, H., et al. (2013). Survival after endovascular therapy in patients with type B aortic dissection: a report from the international registry of acute aortic dissection (IRAD). *JACC Cardiovasc. Interv.* 6, 876–882. doi: 10.1016/j.jcin.2013.05.003

Fattori, R., Tsai, T. T., Myrmel, T., Evangelista, A., Cooper, J. V., Trimarchi, S., et al. (2008). Complicated acute type B dissection: is surgery still the best option?: a report from the international registry of acute aortic dissection. *JACC Cardiovasc. Interv.* 1, 395–402. doi: 10.1016/j.jcin.2008.04.009

Faure, E. M., Canaud, L., Agostini, C., Shaub, R., Böge, G., Marty-ané, C., et al. (2014). Reintervention after thoracic endovascular aortic repair of complicated aortic dissection. *J. Vasc. Surg.* 59, 327–333. doi: 10.1016/j.jvs.2013.08.089

Fortier, A., Gullapalli, V., and Mirshams, R. A. (2014). Review of biomechanical studies of arteries and their effect on stent performance. *IJC Heart Vessels* 4, 12–18. doi: 10.1016/j.ijchv.2014.04.007

Gasser, T. C., Ogden, R. W., and Holzapfel, G. A. (2006). Hyperelastic modelling of arterial layers with distributed collagen fibre orientations. *J. R. Soc. interface* 3, 15–35. doi: 10.1098/rsif.2005.0073

Kasirajan, K., Dake, M. D., Lumsden, A., Bavaria, J., and Makaroun, M. S. (2012). Incidence and outcomes after infolding or collapse of thoracic stent grafts. *J. Vasc. Surg.* 55, 652–658. doi: 10.1016/j.jvs.2011.09.079

Kassab, G. S. (2006). Biomechanics of the cardiovascular system: the aorta as an illustratory example. *J. R. Soc. Interface* 3, 719–740. doi: 10.1098/rsif.2006.0138

Kato, N., Shimono, T., Hirano, T., Suzuki, T., Ishida, M., Sakuma, H., et al. (2002). Midterm results of stent-graft repair of acute and chronic aortic dissection with descending tear: the complication-specific approach. *J. Thorac. Cardiovasc. Surg.* 124, 306–312. doi: 10.1067/mtc.2002.122302

Kumar, G. V. P., and Mathew, L. (2010). Effects of design parameters on the radial force of percutaneous aortic valve stents. *Cardiovasc. Revasc. Med.* 11, 101–104. doi: 10.1016/j.carrev.2009.04.005

aortic dissection: implications for management. *Eur. J. Vasc. Endovasc. Surg.* 36, 522–529. doi: 10.1016/j.ejvs.2008.06.023

Schiavone, A., and Zhao, L. G. (2015). A study of balloon type, system constraint and artery constitutive model used in finite element simulation of stent deployment. *Mech. Adv. Mater. Mod. Process.* 1:1. doi: 10.1186/s40759-014-0002-x

Manning, B. J., Dias, N., Ohrlander, T., Malina, M., Sonesson, B., Resch, T., et al. (2009). Endovascular treatment for chronic type B dissection: limitations of short stent-grafts revealed at midterm follow-up. *J. Endovasc. Ther.* 16, 590–597. doi: 10.1583/09-2717.1

Marcheix, B., Rousseau, H., Bongard, V., Heijmen, R. H., Nienaber, C. A., Ehrlich, M., et al. (2008). Stent grafting of dissected descending aorta in patients with Marfan's syndrome. mid-term results. *JACC Cardiovasc. Interv.* 1, 673–680. doi: 10.1016/j.jcin.2008.10.005

Martin, D., and Boyle, F. (2013). Finite element analysis of balloon-expandable coronary stent deployment: influence of angioplasty balloon configuration. *Int. J. Numer. Methods Biomed. Eng.* 29, 1161–1175. doi: 10.1002/cnm. 2557

Mitchell, R. S., Miller, D. C., Dake, M. D., Semba, C. P., Moore, K. A., and Sakai, T. (1999). Thoracic aortic aneurysm repair with an endovascular stent graft: the first generation. *Ann. Thorac. Surg.* 67, 1971–1974. doi: 10.1016/ S0003-4975(99)00436-1

Moulakakis, K. G., Mylonas, S. N., Dalainas, I., Kakisis, J., Kotsis, T., and Liapis, C. D. (2014). Management of complicated and uncomplicated acute type B dissection. A systematic review and meta-analysis. *Ann. Cardiothorac. Surg.* 3, 234–246. doi: 10.3978/j.issn.2225-319X.2014.05.08

Nelder, J. A., and Mead, R. (1965). A simplex method for function minimization. *Comput. J.* 7, 308–313. doi: 10.1093/comjnl/7.4.308

Neuhauser, B., Greiner, A., Jaschke, W., Chemelli, A., and Fraedrich, G. (2008). Serious complications following endovascular thoracic aortic stent-graft repair for type B dissection. *Eur. J. Cardiothorac. Surg.* 1, 58–63. doi: 10.1016/j.ejcts. 2007.10.010

Ohbuchi, R., and Fuchs, H. (1991). "Incremental volume rendereing algorithm for interactive 3D ultrasound imaging," in *Information Processing in Medical Imaging*, eds A. C. F. Colchester, D. J. Hawkes (Berlin: Springer), 486–500.

Qing, K. X., Chan, Y. C., Ting, A. C. W., and Cheng, S. W. K. (2016). Persistent intraluminal pressure after endovascular stent grafting for type B aortic dissection. *Eur. J. Vasc. Endovasc. Surg.* 51, 656–663. doi: 10.1016/j.ejvs.2016. 01.006

Roberts, W. C. (1981). Aortic dissection: anatomy, consequences, and causes. *Am. Heart J* 101, 195–214. doi: 10.1016/0002-8703(81)90666-9

Sayer, D., Bratby, M., Brooks, M., Loftus, I., Morgan, R., and Thompson, M. (2008). Aortic morphology following endovascular repair of acute and chronic type B

Song, T. K., Donayre, C. E., Walot, I., Kopchok, G. E., Litwinski, R. A., Lippmann, M., et al. (2006). Endograft exclusion of acute and chronic descending thoracic aortic dissections. *J. Vasc. Surg.* 43, 247–258. doi: 10.1016/ j.jvs.2005.10.065

Thrumurthy, S. G., Karthikesalingam, A., Patterson, B. O., Holt, P. J. E., Hinchliffe, R. J., Loftus, I. M., et al. (2011). A systematic review of mid-term outcomes of thoracic endovascular repair (TEVAR) of chronic type B aortic dissection. *Eur. J. Vasc. Endovasc. Surg.* 42, 632–647. doi: 10.1016/j.ejvs.2011. 08.009

Towns, J., Cockerill, T., Dahan, M., Foster, I., Gaither, K., Grimshaw, A., et al. (2014). XSEDE: accelerating scientific discovery. *Comput. Sci. Eng.* 16, 62–74. doi: 10.1109/MCSE.2014.80

Trimarchi, S., and Eagle, K. A. (2016). Thoracic endovascular aortic repair in acute and chronic type B aortic dissection. *JACC Cardiovasc. Interv.* 9, 192–194. doi: 10.1016/j.jcin.2015.11.033

Vecht, R. J., Besterman, E. M., Bromley, L. L., Eastcott, H. H., and Kenyon, J. R. (1980). Acute dissection of aorta: long-term review and management. *Lancet* 1, 109–111. doi: 10.1016/S0140-6736(80)90601-7

Won, J. Y., Suh, S. H., Ko, H. K., Lee, K. H., Shim, W. H., Chang, B. C., et al. (2006). Problems encountered during and after stent-graft treatment of aortic dissection. *J. Vasc. Interv. Radiol.* 17, 271–281. doi: 10.1097/01.RVI.0000195141. 98163.30

# 2

# Role of Coronary Myogenic Response in Pressure-Flow Autoregulation in Swine: A Meta-Analysis With Coronary Flow Modeling

*Gregory M. Dick, Ravi Namani, Bhavesh Patel and Ghassan S. Kassab* *

*California Medical Innovations Institute, San Diego, CA, United States*

**\*Correspondence:**
*Ghassan S. Kassab*
*gkassab@calmi2.org*

Myogenic responses (pressure-dependent contractions) of coronary arterioles play a role in autoregulation (relatively constant flow vs. pressure). Publications on myogenic reactivity in swine coronaries vary in caliber, analysis, and degree of responsiveness. Further, data on myogenic responses and autoregulation in swine have not been completely compiled, compared, and modeled. Thus, it has been difficult to understand these physiological phenomena. Our purpose was to: (a) analyze myogenic data with standard criteria; (b) assign results to diameter categories defined by morphometry; and (c) use our novel multiscale flow model to determine the extent to which *ex vivo* myogenic reactivity can explain autoregulation *in vivo*. When myogenic responses from the literature are an input for our model, the predicted coronary autoregulation approaches *in vivo* observations. More complete and appropriate data are now available to investigate the regulation of coronary blood flow in swine, a highly relevant model for human physiology and disease.

Keywords: arteriole, microcirculation, smooth muscle, myography, coronary blood flow

## INTRODUCTION

Myogenic reactivity can be described as the mechanism underlying the Bayliss effect (Bayliss, 1902). That is, when blood pressure is elevated, arteries distend, and the smooth muscle cells in the vascular wall respond by contracting. Autoregulation is the phenomenon where coronary blood flow remains relatively constant over a wide range of perfusion pressures (Mosher et al., 1964). The Hagen-Poiseuille relationship predicts that—in the absence of other changes—when the pressure gradient increases, flow should increase. This is because flow is directly related to the pressure gradient and to the 4th power of the vessel radius, while inversely related to blood viscosity and vessel length. Thus, one reasonable assumption to explain this autoregulatory behavior is that vessels of the coronary tree actively adjust their diameter as pressure is varied. The mechanism by which coronary resistance vessels alter their diameter in response to pressure changes is the myogenic response. We aim to synthesize the relevant existing data for coronary myogenic responses and autoregulation in a single species: swine. There are, of course, many studies from other species and they are extremely important because of the mechanistic insights provided. One of the most complete data sets is available from swine, however, and these animals are invaluable experimental models because of similarities with humans in coronary anatomy, physiology, and disease (Suzuki et al., 2011; Lelovas et al., 2014).

## Myogenic Responses

The myogenic response is generally thought of as vasoconstriction in response to increased intraluminal pressure, but reducing pressure also elicits vasodilation (**Figure 1**). The myogenic response is typically studied *ex vivo* using pressure myography methods. Small arteries and arterioles are dissected from living tissue, bathed in physiological solutions at body temperature, cannulated, connected to a pressure source, and imaged to determine the inner diameter as the distending internal pressure is varied with no flow. The vascular myogenic response and its mechanisms have been the subject of many studies and reviews (Davis, 2012; Hill and Meininger, 2012). From a teleological perspective, myogenic responses may represent the efforts of a blood vessel to minimize the stress on its wall. This is because, according to the law of Laplace, mean wall stress is directly proportional to the product of pressure and radius, while inversely related to wall thickness. Thus, if blood pressure were to increase, elevated vascular wall tension could be mitigated by an arteriole actively decreasing its radius and/or thickening its wall. Further, myogenic responses could provide a certain degree of constriction at normal intraluminal pressures (i.e., give the vessel a basal, intrinsic, or spontaneous tone from which to deviate). This would allow coronary vascular diameter, and thus resistance, to change in either direction through the action of vasodilator and vasoconstrictor influences such as metabolic demands, neural activity, and paracrine stimuli

(Duncker and Bache, 2008; Tune, 2014; Goodwill et al., 2017). This idea of intrinsic tone in a coronary arteriole is an important one, because flow is related to diameter in a power-law manner. Thus, very small adjustments in coronary arteriolar diameter in either direction have substantial effects on myocardial blood flow.

The first study of coronary myogenic reactivity in swine (or any species, for that matter) was published in 1988, demonstrating what has come to be considered classic coronary myogenic responsiveness (Kuo et al., 1988; **Figure 2**). The PubMed engine was used to search the MEDLINE database for published studies focusing on myogenic responses in swine coronary small arteries and arterioles. Using the search terms swine, coronary, and myogenic returned 54 publications. A total of 11 relevant studies are identified in **Table 1**. Between 1988 and 1991, Kuo et al. published three seminal papers describing fundamental properties of the myogenic response in swine coronary arterioles. First, the myogenic responsiveness of subepicardial arterioles exceeded that of similarly sized subendocardial arterioles; i.e., a transmural gradient of myogenic reactivity exists in the swine heart (Kuo et al., 1988). Second, myogenic responses were similar in swine coronary arterioles with and without functional endothelium, indicating that the behavior is inherent to the smooth muscle (Kuo et al., 1990a). Third, pressure (causing myogenic vasoconstriction) and flow (producing endothelium-dependent vasodilation; Kuo et al., 1990b) interact to determine the resulting vascular tone in swine coronary arterioles with intact endothelium (Kuo et al., 1991). In the ensuing years, several other groups published studies documenting how the myogenic responses of swine coronary arterioles were impacted by exercise, clinical

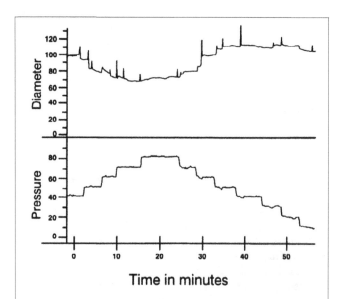

**FIGURE 1 |** Example of myogenic reactivity in a swine coronary arteriole. Muller et al. demonstrated how coronary arteriolar diameter (in μm; **top**) changed as transmural pressure (in mmHg; **bottom**) was varied (Muller et al., 1993; reproduced with permission). As distending pressure was increased from 40 to 80 mmHg in 10 mmHg increments, the steady-state diameter decreased. When transmural pressure was reduced from 80 mmHg, diameter increased.

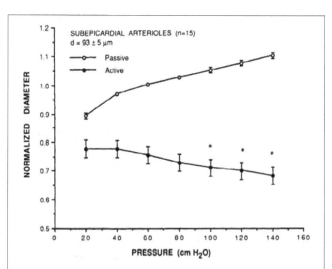

**FIGURE 2 |** Prototypical description of coronary myogenic reactivity. Kuo et al. showed the pressure-diameter relationship of swine coronary arterioles (Kuo et al., 1988; reprinted with permission). The active curve was observed under control conditions, while the passive curve was measured in the presence of 100 μM sodium nitroprusside, a source of the vasodilator nitric oxide. Diameters are normalized to the passive diameter at 60 cmH$_2$O (44.1 mmHg). Asterisks indicate an active diameter significantly different from that at 60 cmH$_2$O.

**TABLE 1 |** Characteristics of swine and their arterioles in 11 previous studies of coronary myogenic reactivity.

| References | Variety | Gender | Weight (kg) | Age (mo.)[b] | Layer[c] | Territory[d] | Diameter[e] |
|---|---|---|---|---|---|---|---|
| Kuo et al., 1988 | Domestic | M, F | 10 | 1-2 | Epi and Endo | LAD and LCx | 134 and 136[f] |
| Kuo et al., 1990a | Domestic | M, F | 10[a] | 1-2 | Epi | LAD and LCx | 91[f] |
| Kuo et al., 1991 | Domestic | M, F | 11-22[a] | 1.5-2.5 | Epi | LAD and LCx | 85[f] |
| Muller et al., 1993 | Yucatan | F | 25-40 | 6[+] | Epi | LV wall | 124-129 |
| Rajagopalan et al., 1995 | Domestic | M, F | 10 | 1-2 | Epi | LAD | 188 |
| Wang et al., 1995 | Domestic | M, F | 19-23 | 2-3 | Epi | LCx | 150 |
| Wang et al., 1997 | Domestic | M, F | 20-25 | 2-3 | Epi | LAD | 168 |
| Tofukuji et al., 1997a | Domestic | M, F | 20-25 | 2-3 | Epi | LAD | 141 |
| Tofukuji et al., 1997b | Domestic | M, F | 20-25 | 2-3 | Epi | LAD | 138 |
| Liao and Kuo, 1997 | Domestic | M, F | 16-30[a] | 2-3 | Epi | LAD and LCx | 254, 164, 99, and 64[f] |
| Sorop et al., 2008 | Domestic | M, F | 66 | 4[+] | Endo | LAD and LCx | 229 |

[a]Weight estimated from growth charts using age provided.
[b]Approximate age estimated from weight using growth chart. Plus sign (+) signifies that age may be greater than indicated number of months.
[c]Indicates whether vessels were from subepicardium (Epi) or subendocardium (Endo).
[d]Left anterior descending (LAD) artery, left circumflex (LCx) artery, left ventricular (LV) wall.
[e]Passive inner diameter @ 80 mmHg (μm).
[f]Average of passive diameters at 73.5 and 88.2 mmHg.

interventions, or cardiovascular disease. For instance, Muller et al. demonstrated that endurance exercise training increased the myogenic reactivity of coronary arterioles from swine (Muller et al., 1993), while Sellke and colleagues documented the deleterious effects of coronary bypass and cardioplegia on the myogenic reactivity of swine coronary arterioles (Wang et al., 1995). Most recently, Sorop et al. demonstrated that myogenic responses were blunted downstream of a chronic coronary occlusion in swine (Sorop et al., 2008).

## Coronary Autoregulation

Given a constant myocardial oxygen demand, perfusion can remain relatively constant over a considerable pressure range (Mosher et al., 1964). One idea is that this coronary autoregulation may be mediated, at least in part, through pressure-induced changes in the diameter of coronary vessels (Johnson, 1980, 1986; Hoffman and Spaan, 1990). In other words, coronary vascular resistance changes as pressure is varied to maintain a relatively constant myocardial blood flow. An example of coronary pressure-flow autoregulation is shown in **Figure 3**. PubMed was used to search the MEDLINE database to find studies that focused on coronary pressure-flow autoregulation in swine. Many references (>300 each) were returned when performing searches with the terms porcine, coronary, and autoregulation or swine, coronary, and autoregulation. Ten pertinent pressure-flow autoregulation studies were identified (**Table 2**). Some show the control (active or autoregulated) response while others show the passive (or maximally dilated) response. A few studies show both behaviors. An example of coronary pressure-flow autoregulation in swine is shown in **Figure 4**.

Whether myogenic responses play a role in coronary pressure-flow autoregulation was debated in the past (Dole, 1987; Feigl, 1989). This debate centered on three points: (a) the myogenic response of isolated coronary arterioles had not yet been

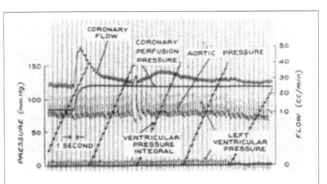

**FIGURE 3 |** A representative tracing of coronary pressure-flow autoregulation in a dog from the classic study of Mosher et al. (1964; reproduced with permission). Note that as coronary perfusion pressure is suddenly increased from 82 to 110 mmHg, coronary blood flow transiently increases, but then rapidly returns toward its previous level.

observed; (b) indirect assessments of myogenic behavior (e.g., hyperemic responses following brief coronary occlusions) were equivocal due to the overriding effects of metabolism; and (c) there had not been a direct assessment of coronary myogenic behavior *in vivo* (e.g., with intravital microscopy in the beating heart). Most of these issues have been addressed, as the myogenic responses of isolated coronary are now widely recognized and intravital microscopy studies of arterioles *in vivo* have been completed. Intravital microscopy shows that coronary arterioles dilate as pressure is reduced (Chilian and Layne, 1990; Kanatsuka et al., 1990; Merkus et al., 2001), but experiments with increased pressures are lacking. The scarcity of data with increasing pressure is likely because it is more practical to reduce coronary pressure without altering myocardial oxygen demand. It should be recognized that there are other mechanisms which contribute to coronary pressure-flow autoregulation (e.g., by metabolic and endothelial influences), but coronary myogenic responses are widely believed to be fundamental to the phenomenon.

**TABLE 2 |** Studies of coronary pressure-flow relationships in swine.

| References | Variety | Gender | Weight (kg) | Age (mo.)[a] | Territory[b] | Autoregulated? | Dilated? |
|---|---|---|---|---|---|---|---|
| Pantely et al., 1985 | Domestic | NS | 29-55 | 3-6 | LAD | Yes | Yes |
| Johnson et al., 1988 | Domestic | M, F | 26-45 | 2.5-4 | LCx | Yes | Yes |
| Schulz et al., 1991 | Domestic | NS | 20-45 | 2.5-4 | LAD | Yes | No |
| McFalls et al., 1991 | Domestic | M, F | 24-42 | 2.5-4 | LAD | Yes | Yes |
| Chilian, 1991 | Domestic | M, F | 7-15 | 1-2 | LAD and LCx | No | Yes |
| Guth et al., 1991 | Göttingen | M, F | 25-35 | 3-6 | RCA[c] | Yes | No |
| Duncker et al., 1992 | Domestic | M, F | 25-45 | 2.5-4 | LAD | No | Yes |
| Shnier et al., 1994 | Domestic | NS | 40-50 | 5-6 | LAD | Yes | No |
| Berwick et al., 2012 | Ossabaw | NS | 30-60 | 3-6 | LAD | Yes | No |
| Schampaert et al., 2013 | Domestic | NS | NS | NS | LAD and LCx[d] | No | Yes |

NS, Not specified.
[a]Approximate age estimated from weight using growth chart.
[b]Left anterior descending (LAD), left circumflex (LCx), and right coronary (RCA) artery.
[c]In addition to the right ventricle, the RCA perfuses the interventricular septum. Only the septal data were included for analysis here.
[d]Total coronary blood flow was multiplied by 68.3% to estimate left ventricular perfusion (Feigl et al., 1990).

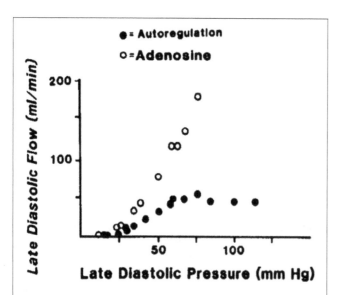

**FIGURE 4 |** An example of coronary pressure-flow autoregulation in swine (Pantely et al., 1985; reprinted with permission). Flow in the LAD artery was measured in an open-chest, anesthetized pig. An inflatable perivascular occluder was used to constrict the artery while pressure and flow distal to the occlusion was measured. This was done before (autoregulation) and after intracoronary infusion of the vasodilator adenosine.

Three groups have successfully modeled coronary pressure-flow autoregulation by including a myogenic mechanism. Liao and Kuo (1997) generated a model that qualitatively reproduced the coronary pressure-flow relationship observed in Langendorff-perfused hearts (Ueeda et al., 1992). The model of Cornelissen and colleagues incorporated a network of vessels with diameter-dependent myogenic responses and generated theoretical pressure-flow curves with prominent autoregulation (Cornelissen et al., 2000, 2002). Most recently, Namani et al. provided an integrative model of coronary flow based on a realistic anatomy, active and passive flow determinants, and

myogenic reactivity data (Namani et al., 2018). While important mechanistic insights were provided by these studies, a limitation of the previous modeling efforts is that they relied upon data from dissimilar species and/or *ex vivo* active autoregulation data (i.e., isolated hearts in which coronary flow typically exceeds values seen *in vivo*). All modeling studies were informed by myogenic responses from swine coronary arterioles, but none considered the coronary pressure-flow relationship in swine (**Table 2**; **Figure 4**).

Eliminating as many potential species- and method-related discrepancies from the input data sets for coronary myogenic responses and pressure-flow autoregulation may improve model output. Our meta-analysis has the following three goals. First, we analyzed previous studies of swine coronary myogenic responses with standard criteria. Particularly, we aimed to simplify inter-study comparisons by converting all units (to μm and mmHg) and applying a single method of presentation and analysis. Second, we assigned results to diameter categories defined by the morphometry of Kassab et al. (1993). This should facilitate comparisons between studies, as myogenic behavior is reported to be diameter-dependent (Liao and Kuo, 1997). Third, we compiled studies of coronary pressure-flow autoregulation from swine, then used myogenic responsiveness in porcine coronary arterioles to compute the pressure-flow autoregulation profile and compare it to what has been observed in the same species.

## COLLECTING AND ANALYZING EXISTING DATA

It was necessary to extract data from original reports (**Tables 1, 2**) for our analysis. This was achieved by obtaining Portable Document Files and analyzing digital images of the figures with WebPlotDigitizer (https://automeris.io/WebPlotDigitizer by Ankit Rohatgi, Austin, TX). Arteries and arterioles of different calibers were assigned to specific categories in a modified Strahler scheme based on morphometric data from the swine coronary circulation provided by Kassab et al. (1993). In this anatomical framework, the capillary is considered order 0. Upstream vessels are numbered sequentially. For the left anterior descending (LAD) artery perfusion territory, arterial segments range from 9.2 μm (order 1; the precapillary arteriole) to 3.2 mm (order 11; at the origin) (Kassab et al., 1993). In the myocardial region supplied by the left circumflex (LCx) artery, there are 10 arterial branch orders upstream of the capillary ranging from 9.2 μm to 2.6 mm (Kassab et al., 1993). Branches were assigned to orders based on their passive inner diameter at 80 mmHg; therefore, data from the studies of myogenic reactivity were sorted according to the same characteristic. Diameter category boundaries (rounded to the nearest 0.1 μm with no overlap) were using Equations (1, 2):

$$D_{min} = (D_{(n)} - SD_{(n)} + D_{(n-1)} + SD_{(n-1)})/2 \quad (1)$$

$$D_{max} = (D_{(n+1)} - SD_{(n+1)} + D_{(n)} + SD_{(n)})/2 \quad (2)$$

$D_{min}$ and $D_{max}$ are minimum and maximum diameters for a category, D is diameter, SD is the standard deviation, and (n) represents an order with its downstream (n − 1) and upstream (n + 1) neighbors. The order numbering scheme is shown in **Figure 5**.

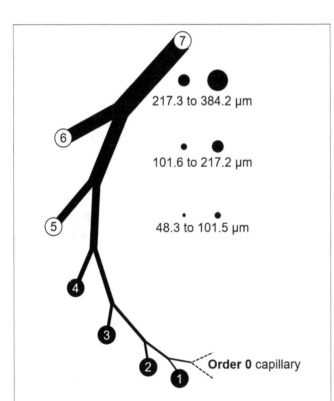

**FIGURE 5 |** Branch order patterns and availability of myogenic reactivity data from swine. The cartoon shows branches from the capillary (order 0) to order 7. The circles and numbers to the right represent the relative sizes and exact diameters of vessels in orders 5, 6, and 7 of the LAD perfusion territory. Equivalent diameter ranges for those same orders in the LCx territory would be 52.1 to 101.7, 101.8 to 202.6, and 202.7 to 363.8 μm. Published data for myogenic reactivity in swine coronary arterioles are available for orders 5–7.

The passive vessel radius ($R_p$) is a sigmoidal function of the intraluminal pressure ($\Delta P$; Equation 3; Young et al., 2012).

$$R_p(\Delta P) = B_p + \frac{A_p - B_p}{\pi}\left[\frac{\pi}{2} + arctan\left(\frac{\Delta P - \phi_p}{C_p}\right)\right] \quad (3)$$

$A_p$ and $B_p$ are the maximum and minimum vessel radii, $\phi_p$, is the pressure corresponding to the mean vessel radius, and $C_p$ is the pressure bandwidth for the transition in radius from $A_p$ to $B_p$. Radius in the active myogenic response ($R_m$) is also a sigmoidal function of the intraluminal pressure (Equation 4).

$$\Delta R_m(\Delta \bar{P}) = \frac{\rho_m}{\pi}\left[\frac{\pi}{2} - arctan\left(\left[\frac{\Delta \bar{P} - \phi_m}{C_m}\right]^{2m}\right)\right] \quad (4)$$

The four model parameters are: (1) the maximum decrease in vessel radius (or the peak amplitude), $\rho_m$; (2) $\phi_m$ is the transvascular pressure at which the vessel radius decreases by $\rho_m$ (the pressure at peak amplitude); (3) the pressure bandwidth of the vessel radius change is $C_m$ (Namani et al., 2018); (4) and the exponent, $m$, is assumed to be 2.0 (Young et al., 2012). The literature (**Table 1**) provides pressure-diameter relationships for swine coronary arterioles for vessel orders 5–7 only. This is likely for technical reasons, as the tiny arterioles of order 4 (<48.3 μm) and below are challenging to cannulate and it would be difficult to image the lumen of the thicker walled vessels of order 8 (>384.2 μm) and above. To model flow control in the entire coronary tree, however, active constitutive properties are needed for vessels above and below orders 5–7. Thus, some assumptions and simplifications were introduced. Based on the weak or absent myogenic responses in vessels above order 7 (Nakayama et al., 1988; Liao and Kuo, 1997), these vessels were considered to have only passive properties in the model. Because capillaries (order 0) lack smooth muscle, these vessels were also considered to have only passive responses. Myogenic parameters for vessel orders 1–4 were extrapolated from the extracted myogenic parameters of vessels order 5–7. The longitudinal distribution of the myogenic parameters was fit with a three-parameter Weibull distribution function (Equation 5).

$$\begin{bmatrix} \rho_m \\ \phi_m \\ C_m \end{bmatrix} = \left\{ C\left(\frac{R}{a}\right)^{b-1} e^{-\left(\frac{R}{a}\right)^b} \right\} \quad (5)$$

The Weibull distribution defines the myogenic response as a function of the vessel cast radius and serves as an input to the flow analysis in the coronary tree (Namani et al., 2018). Subepicardial and subendocardial vessels of the same order may have different myogenic responses (Kuo et al., 1988), which could affect the longitudinal distribution of myogenic parameters transmurally. The available data are predominantly from subepicardial vessels, whereas only two data sets are available for subendocardial vessels; therefore, there will be greater uncertainty in myogenic properties of vessels from this region.

To understand the effect of the myogenic response on coronary pressure-flow autoregulation, the flow regulation model was simulated with and without active myogenic responses in trees from the subepicardium and subendocardium. Trees were composed of 400 vessels to minimize computational effort. When active myogenic responses were removed, the vessels were given a basal tone (i.e., a degree of constriction that is independent of the transvascular pressure). The tone described here is meant to be of the same nature as myogenic contractions. That is, the tone is inherent to the smooth muscle itself (i.e., it is myogenic and not due to extrinsic factors), but does not vary with pressure. The prescribed basal tone (15%; an indicator of viable arterioles in *ex vivo* experiments Muller et al., 1993) was made uniform in all vessel orders (1–7) of the subtree to simplify the simulation.

## COMPILING AND INTEGRATING THE EXISTING DATA

Pressure-diameter data from the 11 previous studies cover orders 5, 6, and 7. Data from subepicardial vessels span all three orders, while data from subendocardial vessels are available for only orders 6 and 7. There is some variability in the pressure ranges and units (e.g., $cmH_2O$ vs. mmHg) used to describe the results in the studies of **Table 1**. Further, pressure-diameter relationships from those studies are expressed differently (e.g., a percentage of the maximum diameter vs. µm). Thus, the data were extracted, converted to standard units of µm vs. mmHg, and assigned to the appropriate branch order and myocardial layer. Then those data were fit with Equations (3) (passive curve) and (4) (active myogenic response). Data are not available for the diameters of coronary arterioles at pressures greater than 100 mmHg, but data for coronary autoregulation extend past that pressure; therefore, pressure-diameter curves were extrapolated using the following logic. First, pressure-diameter data at higher pressures are available from mesenteric and femoral arterioles and can be used as a guide (Carlson and Secomb, 2005). These data show that the myogenic diameter converges with the passive vessel diameter at high transvascular pressures (100–200 mmHg). Second, Young et al. found that extrapolation of the myogenic pressure-diameter relationship beyond 100 mmHg is reasonable (Young et al., 2012). Third, Hamza et al. measured the passive pressure-diameter relationship of larger coronary vessels up to 150 mmHg and found a typical sigmoidal shape (Hamza et al., 2003). It is important to point out, however, that there are no data available to indicate whether the pressure-diameter relationships of isolated arterioles are reflective of *in situ* properties. Thus, our assumptions may need to be revisited. Example curve fits are shown in **Figure 6**. These curve fits were sampled in 20 mmHg increments from 0 to 120 mmHg to obtain data suitable for calculating mean (with standard error, where possible) pressure-diameter relationships in each available vessel order of the subepicardium and subendocardium (**Figure 7**). These pressure-diameter relationships are referred to as the "composite," as they represent the average of responses available from the literature.

Our literature search identified 10 studies of coronary pressure-flow autoregulation in swine (**Table 2**). Eight were *in vivo* studies (Pantely et al., 1985; Johnson et al., 1988; Guth et al., 1991; McFalls et al., 1991; Schulz et al., 1991; Duncker et al.,

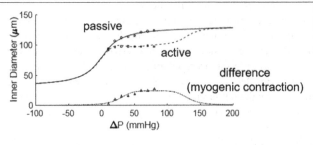

**FIGURE 6** | Fitting the active and passive pressure-diameter relationships with Equations (3, 4). The data were obtained from the study of Muller et al. (1993).

1992; Shnier et al., 1994; Berwick et al., 2012), while two were *ex vivo* studies of isolated, blood-perfused swine hearts (Chilian, 1991; Schampaert et al., 2013). There were seven studies that provided active autoregulatory data (all of those were *in vivo* studies; see **Table 2** for "Yes" in the "Autoregulated" column). Four of the eight *in vivo* studies provided pressure-flow data from vasodilated hearts (passive responses; see **Table 2** for "Yes" in the "Dilated" column). Both *ex vivo* studies were sources of data for the pressure-flow relationship in the vasodilated (passive) coronary circulation only. Data were extracted from the studies, flows converted to ml/min/g (where necessary), and curve fitted. To determine flow per gram of myocardium, we estimated heart weight from body weight. In swine, the heart weight to body weight ratio is the same as humans (5 g/kg; Lelovas et al., 2014). To determine the weight of a particular perfusion territory (e.g., LCx or LAD), data from canine hearts were used (Feigl et al., 1990), as no similar data exist for swine. Feigl's analysis indicates that the LCx perfusion area is 39.0% of heart weight, while that of the LAD zone is 29.3%. For the active (autoregulated) response, data were fit with a third order polynomial (cubic; Equation 6) and the goodness of fit had $R^2$ values between 0.94 and 0.99.

$$f(x) = ax^3 + bx^2 + cx + d \qquad (6)$$

For the passive (vasodilated) response, data were fit with a second order polynomial (quadratic; Equation 7) and the goodness of fit had $R^2$ values above 0.98.

$$f(x) = ax^2 + bx + c \qquad (7)$$

Curve fits of data obtained from studies in **Table 2** were sampled at 20 mmHg intervals from 20 to 140 mmHg to obtain data suitable for creating composite group data with means and standard errors (**Figure 8**).

## DATA ANALYSIS

The active myogenic parameters obtained from the 11 data sets that were fit with Equation (4) are listed in **Table 3**. Among the three myogenic parameters the highest certainty is in $\rho_m$ (peak amplitude), while the least certainty resides in the parameter $\phi_m$ (pressure at $\rho_m$). There is high uncertainty in fitting $\phi_m$, as many of the data sets do not have vessel diameters beyond pressures

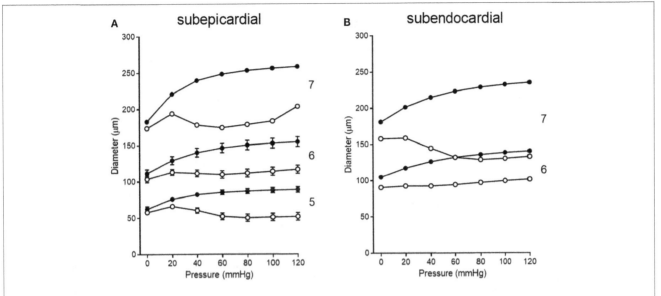

**FIGURE 7 |** Composite pressure-diameter relationships for all studies of swine coronary arterioles listed in **Table 1**. Filled symbols represent the passive curves, while open symbols represent the active myogenic responses. Order numbers are given to the right of each data set. In the subepicardium **(A)**, data are available from order 7 (1 study), order 6 (9 studies), and order 5 (3 studies). For subendocardial vessels **(B)**, data are available for orders 7 and 6 (1 study each).

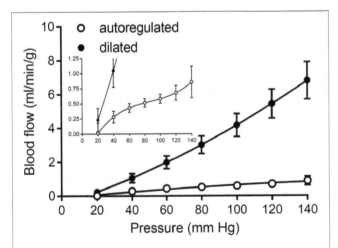

**FIGURE 8 |** Composite of coronary pressure-flow autoregulation in swine. Open symbols represent the actively autoregulated response (Pantely et al., 1985; Johnson et al., 1988; Guth et al., 1991; McFalls et al., 1991; Schulz et al., 1991; Shnier et al., 1994; Berwick et al., 2012). Closed symbols are the pressure-flow relationship in the vasodilated coronary circulation (Pantely et al., 1985; Johnson et al., 1988; Chilian, 1991; McFalls et al., 1991; Duncker et al., 1992; Schampaert et al., 2013). The inset contains the same data, but with a magnified y-axis to appreciate the shape of the active autoregulation curve.

**TABLE 3 |** Myogenic parameters of arterioles sorted by layer and order.

| Layer | Order | $\rho_m$ (μm) | $\phi_m$ (mmHg) | $C_m$ (mmHg) |
|---|---|---|---|---|
| Subepicardium | 5 | 33.6 ± 8.4 | 91.8 ± 19.4 | 63.0 ± 5.1 |
| | 6 | 40.2 ± 18.7 | 96.9 ± 8.5 | 73.1 ± 26.7 |
| | 7 | 74.1 | 77.3 | 51.3 |
| Subendocardium | 6 | 38.9 | 103.0 | 92.6 |
| | 7 | 102.3 | 120.0 | 93.7 |

The maximum decrease in radius is $\rho_m$, while the pressure at which radius decreases by $\rho_m$ is $\phi_m$. The pressure bandwidth of changes in radius is $C_m$.

$\rho_m$, $\phi_m$, and $C_m$, are model inputs to the coronary flow analysis. Among the three parameters, the myogenic amplitude, $\rho_m$, is a sensitive indicator of the strength of the reactivity for a given vessel order. Due to the limited data in the subendocardium (only two data points), statistical analysis could not be performed for transmural differences in myogenic parameters. Further, the Weibull fit of subepicardial data have a greater uncertainty than the fit of the epicardial vessels, hence the transmural differences in myogenic parameters should be interpreted cautiously. However, the myogenic amplitude, $\rho_m$, in vessel order 7 is 38% higher in subendocardium than subepicardium. Finding greater myogenic reactivity in subendocardial vessels of the same order contrasts with conclusions made by Kuo et al. (1988). This is not entirely surprising; however, as Sorop et al. documented very prominent myogenic reactivity in arterioles form the subendocardium (Sorop et al., 2008; **Figure 7B**, order 7).

We simulated coronary autoregulation with various flow control mechanisms in place (**Figures 10, 11**). To do so, we used our recently developed model that considers realistic anatomy and integrated passive and active determinants of flow (Namani

of 100 mmHg. During the curve fit, if $\varphi_m$ and $C_m$ (pressure bandwith) exceeded the maximum pressure in the data, it was truncated at that pressure.

The longitudinal distribution of myogenic parameters as a function of the vessel cast radius is shown in **Figure 9**. A Weibull fit was used to determine the distribution of parameters of vessels from the subepicardium (top panel) and subendocardium (bottom panel). The distributions of these myogenic parameters,

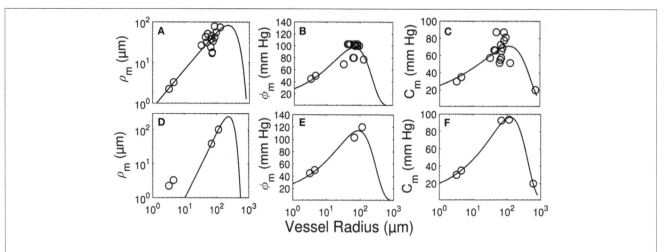

**FIGURE 9 |** Longitudinal distribution of the myogenic parameters of coronary arterioles. Results are shown for vessels from the subepicardial (top row; **A-C**) and subendocardial (bottom row; **D-F**) layers. The left column (**A,D**) displays the maximum decrease in vessel radius, $\rho_m$. The middle column (**B,E**) shows $\varphi_m$, the transvascular pressure at which the vessel radius decreases by $\rho_m$. The right column (**C,F**) displays the pressure bandwidth of changes in radius, $C_m$.

et al., 2018). It has been proposed that physical myocardial-vessel interactions (MVI) are important in coronary flow regulation and heterogeneity (DeFily and Chilian, 1995). Our previous modeling indicates that the combined effects of cavity-induced extracellular pressure and shortening-induced intramyocyte pressure are a good reflection of intramyocardial pressure and MVI (Algranati et al., 2010). Thus, flow regulation by MVI was included in our current model. Network flow is influenced by various regulatory mechanisms and transmural location (**Figure 10**). Flow was lowest with myogenic regulation only, whereas flow was highest in the passive state. Adding shear stress-dependent effects increased flow over myogenic regulation alone, but adding metabolic mechanisms increased flow almost maximally (**Figure 10**). Flow is not autoregulated in the simulations of **Figure 10**. In our model, it is optimization of metabolism and the presence of myogenic responses that provides predicted flow resembling autoregulation (**Figure 11**). In all simulations, three control mechanism were always present: (1) metabolism (at varying levels); (2) shear; and (3) MVI. In contrast, and most importantly, simulations were run with and without myogenic reactivity, as it was our goal to determine how myogenic responses contribute to coronary pressure-flow autoregulation. When myogenic reactivity was included, the model inputs were the composite pressure-diameter relationships obtained from our analysis of the literature (**Figure 7**). When myogenic reactivity was removed from the simulations, it was replaced by a constant, pressure-independent tone of 15%. The autoregulation model predicts different pressure-flow patterns in the subendocardial and subepicardial layers of the heart (**Figure 11**; compare **Figures 11A,C**). Further, the autoregulation model predicts substantial changes in the pressure-flow relationship within a layer when myogenic reactivity is absent (**Figure 11**; compare **Figures 11A,B** and **Figures 11C,D**).

When the autoregulatory profiles of the subendocardium and subepicardium are compared, a major difference is noted. The predicted autoregulatory range in the subendocardium is greater than that in the subepicardium. Specifically, when myogenic responses are included in the simulation, the perfusion pressure range for appreciable autoregulation in the subendocardium is approximately 75–135 mmHg (**Figure 11C**). In contrast, in the subepicardium, when myogenic reactivity is included in the simulation, the pressure range for appreciable autoregulation is approximately 75–120 mmHg (**Figure 11A**). When myogenic reactivity is eliminated from the simulations, the pressure range for appreciable autoregulation considerably reduced in both layers of the myocardium. That is, autoregulatory pressure ranges in both layers are reduced to approximately 75–105 mmHg (**Figures 11B,D**). Thus, the myogenic response has a significant influence in regulating flow at higher perfusion pressures, as active myogenic contractions reduce flow at higher pressures and extend the autoregulatory range. The removal of myogenic responses caused the flow-perfusion curve to approach that of a passive vessel tree, demonstrating the uncoupling of myogenic regulation from flow and metabolic regulation.

To determine how well the model prediction agrees with *in vivo* coronary pressure-flow autoregulation, we compared the simulation data in **Figures 11A,C** to the composite data of **Figure 8**. This analysis had two parts and is shown in **Figure 12**. In the first part of the comparison, both the model and composite autoregulation curves were normalized to their own respective flow values at a pressure of 90 mmHg (simulation data from the subendocardial and subepicardial layers were averaged for this comparison; **Figure 12A**). The composite and predicted curves are quite similar in shape, but the zero-flow pressure from the simulation is right shifted approximately 25 mmHg compared to the composite data. For the second half of the analysis, closed loop autoregulatory gain was calculated for active curves from both the model and the composite data (**Figure 12B**). Gain was calculated using Equation (8)

$$1 - [(\Delta F/F_i)/(\Delta P/P_i)] \qquad (8)$$

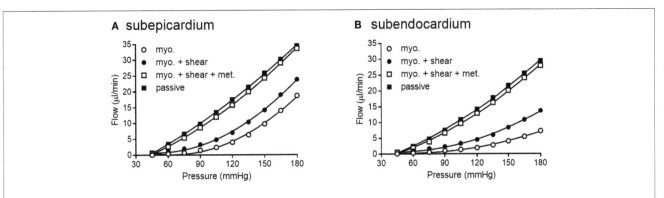

**FIGURE 10 |** Network flow is influenced by regulatory mechanisms. **(A,B)** show flow for subepicardial and subendocardial networks, respectively. The lowest curve is flow in the presence of myogenic regulation only. The highest curve is flow in the passive state. Adding shear stress-dependent effects to the model increases flow some, but adding metabolic mechanisms brings the flow curve close to that in the passive state.

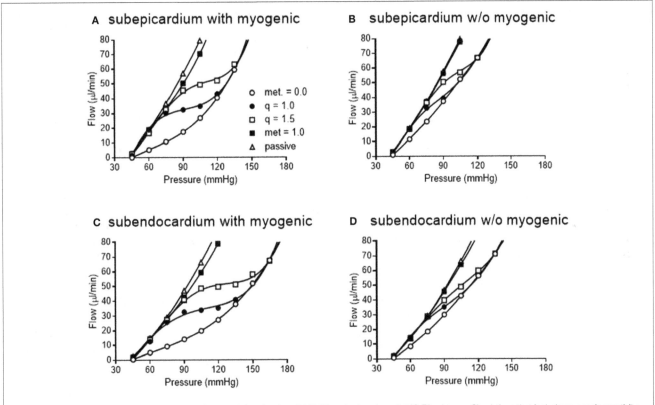

**FIGURE 11 |** Simulated pressure-flow autoregulation curves in subepicardial **(A,B)** and subendocardial **(C,D)** subtrees. Simulations that include myogenic reactivity are in **(A,C)**. Simulations that do not consider myogenic reactivity are in **(B,D)** (vessels do have 15% tone that is independent of pressure).

Where F is flow at pressure P, $F_i$ and $P_i$ are initial flow and pressure, $\Delta F$ is $F_i - F$, and $\Delta P$ is $P_i - P$. Positive gain values indicate active autoregulatory behavior (i.e., vasoconstriction as pressure is increased), negative gain values indicate vasodilation, while a gain of 1 is perfect autoregulation. Peak autoregulatory gains are similar (approximately 0.5 in both the simulated and actual data); however, the peak pressure for autoregulation from the simulation is right-shifted from the composite *in vivo* data by approximately 15 mmHg (**Figure 12B**). Further, the effective

range of autoregulation predicted by the model appears to about half of that observed in the composite *in vivo* data (approximately 30 vs. 60 mmHg; **Figure 12B**).

## SUMMARY, CONCLUSIONS, AND PERSPECTIVES

Direct comparisons of coronary pressure-diameter relationships and coronary blood flow in the same species are lacking. Because

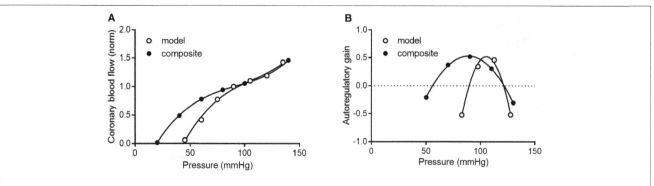

**FIGURE 12 |** Comparison of composite and simulated coronary pressure-flow autoregulation. **(A)** shows normalized coronary pressure-flow curves for the composite data of **Figure 8** and the averaged subendocardial and subepicardial data from simulations in **Figures 11A,C**. Data were normalized to their respective flow at 90 mmHg. **(B)** contains a comparison of autoregulatory gains calculated by Equation (8).

data exist on both coronary myogenic reactivity (**Table 1** and **Figure 7**) and coronary pressure-flow autoregulation in swine (**Table 2** and **Figure 8**), we performed a meta-analysis with three parts. First, we analyzed 11 prior studies of myogenic responsiveness in swine coronary arterioles with standard criteria (converting diameters and pressures to μm and mmHg, respectively; **Figure 7**). Second, we used morphometry to sort the myogenic responses to diameter-defined categories (**Figure 7**). Third, the pressure-diameter relationships of coronary arterioles were used as an input to our recently developed integrative model of coronary blood flow regulation (Namani et al., 2018). This allowed us to compare simulated coronary pressure-flow autoregulation results to *in vivo* blood flow measurements (**Figures 8**, **11**, **12**). Our study shows that the composite myogenic reactivity of swine coronary arterioles fits with simulated pressure-flow autoregulation in the same species in a qualitative and quantitative manner. Specifically, while some differences exist (e.g., the zero-flow pressure and the pressure range of coronary autoregulation), our model simulations produce pressure-flow curves that have the same general shape and slope as what is observed from *in vivo* experiments (**Figure 12A**). Importantly, the magnitude of autoregulatory gain in simulations and composite data show excellent agreement (**Figure 12B**).

No data exist regarding myogenic responses in swine coronary arterioles of orders 1, 2, 3, or 4. These vessels all have inner diameters less than 48 μm and present methodological challenges using standard pressure myography techniques. This could possibly be remedied by using techniques developed for studying isolated nephrons (Burg perfusion; Burg et al., 1966) and successfully used to study very small arterioles (down to 12 μm) from other vascular beds (Duling et al., 1981). An advantage of Burg perfusion equipment is that can remove the necessary manual manipulation required to cannulate and secure small vessels. No data exist regarding myogenic responses in swine coronary arterioles of order 8 or larger. These vessels have thicker walls and it is difficult to image the lumen using conventional pressure myography methods.

Existing data on myogenic reactivity in swine coronary arterioles (**Table 1**) have been collected, analyzed, presented in standardized units, and sorted to categories based on diameter and transmural location (**Figure 7**). Similarly, existing data on coronary pressure-flow autoregulation in swine (**Table 2**) have been standardized and compiled in an orderly fashion (**Figure 8**). This creates data sets that are simpler to interpret and to use as inputs for models of coronary vascular regulation. Having such data available to analyze may lead to a better understanding of these important physiological phenomena. Our analysis leads us to conclude that coronary myogenic reactivity plays a role in coronary pressure-flow autoregulation in swine. In fact, it can be concluded from our modeling results that coronary myogenic responses are one essential component in producing the phenomenon of coronary pressure-flow autoregulation, as replacing myogenic contractions with pressure-independent vascular tone greatly reduced autoregulatory behavior in the simulations (**Figure 11**). When the composite pressure-diameter relationships of swine coronary arterioles from the literature are used as an input for our model, the predicted coronary pressure-flow autoregulation profile approaches *in vivo* observations (**Figure 12**). We did note some differences between the simulated and composite flow data (e.g., the zero-flow pressure of the simulation was right-shifted and the predicted pressure range of coronary autoregulation was narrower than *in vivo* observation). However, our novel model simulations produce pressure-flow curves that have the same general form and slope as what is observed *in vivo* (**Figure 12A**). Autoregulatory gain in simulations and the composite data show similar trends (**Figure 12B**). More complete and appropriate data are now available to investigate the regulation of coronary blood flow in an animal model that is highly relevant to human cardiovascular health and disease.

Existence of this data set and associated modeling tools for the coronary circulation is important because it has been known for more than 50 years that multiple mechanism (i.e., myogenic, shear stress, and metabolic mechanisms) contribute to the autoregulation of blood flow in skeletal muscle (Stainsby, 1962; Jones and Berne, 1965; Borgstrom and Gestrelius, 1987). In contrast, our understanding of the contribution and interaction of these mechanisms in the coronary circulation has lagged behind, in part, because direct evidence for myogenic contractions in coronary vessels was not available until 1988 (Kuo et al., 1988). As for modeling the interactions of multiple mechanisms in skeletal muscle, Carlson et al. showed that both the myogenic and metabolic responses are needed to overcome shear-dependent effects in skeletal muscle in order to predict autoregulation that is close to experimental observations (Carlson et al., 2008). Their regulatory scheme for skeletal muscle indicates that when arterial pressure is increased, both pressure and flow increase in the arterioles, which produces several interacting effects. First, flow increases oxygen delivery to the tissues, which attenuates the vasodilatory metabolic signal. Second, increased pressure initiates vasoconstriction by the myogenic response. Third, increased flow and pressure exert more shear stress on the vessel wall, causing vasodilation. Thus, myogenic and metabolic responses work together to oppose shear-dependent effects. Moreover, Carlson et al. concluded that the metabolic response contributed more to autoregulation of blood flow than the myogenic response (Carlson et al., 2008). An important question is whether the same conclusions hold true for coronary autoregulation. Namani et al. found that metabolic and myogenic regulation were more important inputs for modeling coronary autoregulation than were shear-dependent effects (Namani et al., 2018). Using the current data set as input for the model produces results which support the previous conclusions of Namani and colleagues for three reasons. First, network flow was highly sensitive to myogenic regulation (evident from the large difference in myogenic and passive curves in **Figure 10**). Second, adding shear stress-dependent effects to the model increases network flow (**Figure 10**). Third, network flow is highly sensitive to metabolic regulation, as full metabolic activation gives a pressure-flow relationship that is very close to the passive curve (**Figure 10**). Thus, in our model of the coronary circulation, while shear has significant effects, metabolism is the major vasodilatory influence. Both shear and metabolism are dilatory and work to oppose myogenic constriction. This finding highlights the need for further study into regulatory mechanisms governing the coronary circulation.

## AUTHOR CONTRIBUTIONS

GD designed the study, analyzed data, and wrote the manuscript. RN, BP, and GK analyzed data and edited the manuscript.

## REFERENCES

Algranati, D., Kassab, G. S., and Lanir, Y. (2010). Mechanisms of myocardium-coronary vessel interaction. *Am. J. Physiol. Heart Circ. Physiol.* 298, H861–H873. doi: 10.1152/ajpheart.00925.2009

Bayliss, W. M. (1902). On the local reactions of the arterial wall to changes of internal pressure. *J. Physiol.* 28, 220–231. doi: 10.1113/jphysiol.1902.sp000911

Berwick, Z. C., Moberly, S. P., Kohr, M. C., Morrical, E. B., Kurian, M. M., Dick, G. M., et al. (2012). Contribution of voltage-dependent K$^+$ and Ca$^{2+}$ channels to coronary pressure-flow autoregulation. *Basic Res. Cardiol.* 107:264. doi: 10.1007/s00395-012-0264-6

Borgstrom, P., and Gestrelius, S. (1987). Integrated myogenic and metabolic control of vascular tone in skeletal muscle during autoregulation of blood flow. *Microvasc. Res.* 33, 353–376. doi: 10.1016/0026-2862(87)90028-8

Burg, M., Grantham, J., Abramow, M., and Orloff, J. (1966). Preparation and study of fragments of single rabbit nephrons. *Am. J. Physiol.* 210, 1293–1298. doi: 10.1152/ajplegacy.1966.210.6.1293

Carlson, B. E., Arciero, J. C., and Secomb, T. W. (2008). Theoretical model of blood flow autoregulation: roles of myogenic, shear-dependent, and metabolic responses. *Am. J. Physiol. Heart Circ. Physiol.* 295, H1572–H1579. doi: 10.1152/ajpheart.00262.2008

Carlson, B. E., and Secomb, T. W. (2005). A theoretical model for the myogenic response based on the length-tension characteristics of vascular smooth muscle. *Microcirculation* 12, 327–338. doi: 10.1080/10739680590934745

Chilian, W. M. (1991). Microvascular pressures and resistances in the left ventricular subepicardium and subendocardium. *Circ. Res.* 69, 561–570. doi: 10.1161/01.RES.69.3.561

Chilian, W. M., and Layne, S. M. (1990). Coronary microvascular responses to reductions in perfusion pressure. Evidence for persistent arteriolar vasomotor tone during coronary hypoperfusion. *Circ. Res.* 66, 1227–1238. doi: 10.1161/01.RES.66.5.1227

Cornelissen, A. J., Dankelman, J., VanBavel, E., and Spaan, J. A. (2002). Balance between myogenic, flow-dependent, and metabolic flow control in coronary arterial tree: a model study. *Am. J. Physiol. Heart Circ. Physiol.* 282, H2224–H2237. doi: 10.1152/ajpheart.00491.2001

Hoffman, J. I., and Spaan, J. A. (1990). Pressure-flow relations in coronary circulation. *Physiol. Rev.* 70, 331–390. doi: 10.1152/physrev.1990.70.2.331

Johnson, P. C. (1980). "The myogenic reponse," in *Handbook of Physiology. The Cardiovascular System. Vascular Smooth Muscle*, eds D. F. Bohr, A. P. Somlyo, and H. V. Sparks (Bethesda, MD: American Physiological. Society), 409–442.

Cornelissen, A. J., Dankelman, J., VanBavel, E., Stassen, H. G., and Spaan, J. A. (2000). Myogenic reactivity and resistance distribution in the coronary arterial tree: a model study. *Am. J. Physiol. Heart Circ. Physiol.* 278, H1490–H1499. doi: 10.1152/ajpheart.2000.278.5.H1490

Davis, M. J. (2012). Perspective: physiological role(s) of the vascular myogenic response. *Microcirculation* 19, 99–114. doi: 10.1111/j.1549-8719.2011.00131.x

DeFily, D. V., and Chilian, W. M. (1995). Coronary microcirculation: autoregulation and metabolic control. *Basic Res. Cardiol.* 90, 112–118. doi: 10.1007/BF00789441

Dole, W. P. (1987). Autoregulation of the coronary circulation. *Prog. Cardiovasc. Dis.* 29, 293–323. doi: 10.1016/S0033-0620(87)80005-1

Duling, B. R., Gore, R. W., Dacey, R. G. Jr., and Damon, D. N. (1981). Methods for isolation, cannulation, and *in vitro* study of single microvessels. *Am. J. Physiol.* 241, H108–H116. doi: 10.1152/ajpheart.1981.241.1.H108

Duncker, D. J., and Bache, R. J. (2008). Regulation of coronary blood flow during exercise. *Physiol. Rev.* 88, 1009–1086. doi: 10.1152/physrev.00045.2006

Duncker, D. J., McFalls, E. O., Krams, R., and Verdouw, P. D. (1992). Pressure-maximal coronary flow relationship in regionally stunned porcine myocardium. *Am. J. Physiol.* 262(6 Pt 2), H1744–H1751. doi: 10.1152/ajpheart.1992.262.6.H1744

Feigl, E. O. (1989). Coronary autoregulation. *J. Hypertens. Suppl.* 7, S55–S58.

Feigl, E. O., Neat, G. W., and Huang, A. H. (1990). Interrelations between coronary artery pressure, myocardial metabolism and coronary blood flow. *J. Mol. Cell. Cardiol.* 22, 375–390. doi: 10.1016/0022-2828(90)91474-L

Goodwill, A. G., Dick, G. M., Kiel, A. M., and Tune, J. D. (2017). Regulation of coronary blood flow. *Compr. Physiol.* 7, 321–382. doi: 10.1002/cphy.c160016

Guth, B. D., Schulz, R., and Heusch, G. (1991). Pressure-flow characteristics in the right and left ventricular perfusion territories of the right coronary artery in swine. *Pflugers Arch.* 419, 622–628. doi: 10.1007/BF00370305

Hamza, L. H., Dang, Q., Lu, X., Mian, A., Molloi, S., and Kassab, G. S. (2003). Effect of passive myocardium on the compliance of porcine coronary arteries. *Am. J. Physiol. Heart Circ. Physiol.* 285, H653–H660. doi: 10.1152/ajpheart.00090.2003

Hill, M. A., and Meininger, G. A. (2012). Arteriolar vascular smooth muscle cells: mechanotransducers in a complex environment. *Int. J. Biochem. Cell Biol.* 44, 1505–1510. doi: 10.1016/j.biocel.2012.05.021

Rajagopalan, S., Dube, S., and Canty, J. M. Jr. (1995). Regulation of coronary diameter by myogenic mechanisms in arterial microvessels greater than 100 microns in diameter. *Am. J. Physiol.* 268(2 Pt 2), H788–H793. doi: 10.1152/ajpheart.1995.268.2.H788

Johnson, P. C. (1986). Autoregulation of blood flow. *Circ. Res.* 59, 483–495. doi: 10.1161/01.RES.59.5.483

Johnson, W. B., Malone, S. A., Pantely, G. A., Anselone, C. G., and Bristow, J. D. (1988). No reflow and extent of infarction during maximal vasodilation in the porcine heart. *Circulation* 78, 462–472. doi: 10.1161/01.CIR.78.2.462

Jones, R. D., and Berne, R. M. (1965). Evidence for a metabolic mechanism in autoregulation of blood flow in skeletal muscle. *Circ. Res.* 17, 540–554. doi: 10.1161/01.RES.17.6.540

Kanatsuka, H., Lamping, K. G., Eastham, C. L., and Marcus, M. L. (1990). Heterogeneous changes in epimyocardial microvascular size during graded coronary stenosis. Evidence of the microvascular site for autoregulation. *Circ. Res.* 66, 389–396. doi: 10.1161/01.RES.66.2.389

Kassab, G. S., Rider, C. A., Tang, N. J., and Fung, Y. C. (1993). Morphometry of pig coronary arterial trees. *Am. J. Physiol.* 265(1 Pt 2), H350–H365. doi: 10.1152/ajpheart.1993.265.1.H350

Kuo, L., Chilian, W. M., and Davis, M. J. (1990a). Coronary arteriolar myogenic response is independent of endothelium. *Circ. Res.* 66, 860–866. doi: 10.1161/01.RES.66.3.860

Kuo, L., Chilian, W. M., and Davis, M. J. (1991). Interaction of pressure- and flow-induced responses in porcine coronary resistance vessels. *Am. J. Physiol.* 261(6 Pt 2), H1706–H1715. doi: 10.1152/ajpheart.1991.261.6.H1706

Kuo, L., Davis, M. J., and Chilian, W. M. (1988). Myogenic activity in isolated subepicardial and subendocardial coronary arterioles. *Am. J. Physiol.* 255(6 Pt 2), H1558–H1562. doi: 10.1152/ajpheart.1988.255.6.H1558

Kuo, L., Davis, M. J., and Chilian, W. M. (1990b). Endothelium-dependent, flow-induced dilation of isolated coronary arterioles. *Am. J. Physiol.* 259(4 Pt 2), H1063–H1070. doi: 10.1152/ajpheart.1990.259.4.H1063

Lelovas, P. P., Kostomitsopoulos, N. G., and Xanthos, T. T. (2014). A comparative anatomic and physiologic overview of the porcine heart. *J. Am. Assoc. Lab. Anim. Sci.* 53, 432–438.

Liao, J. C., and Kuo, L. (1997). Interaction between adenosine and flow-induced dilation in coronary microvascular network. *Am. J. Physiol.* 272(4 Pt 2), H1571–H1581. doi: 10.1152/ajpheart.1997.272.4.H1571

McFalls, E. O., Duncker, D. J., Sassen, L. M., Gho, B. C., and Verdouw, P. D. (1991). Effect of antiischemic therapy on coronary flow reserve and the pressure-maximal coronary flow relationship in anesthetized swine. *J. Cardiovasc. Pharmacol.* 18, 827–836. doi: 10.1097/00005344-199112000-00007

Merkus, D., Vergroesen, I., Hiramatsu, O., Tachibana, H., Nakamoto, H., Toyota, E., et al. (2001). Stenosis differentially affects subendocardial and subepicardial arterioles *in vivo*. *Am. J. Physiol. Heart Circ. Physiol.* 280, H1674–H1682. doi: 10.1152/ajpheart.2001.280.4.H1674

Mosher, P., Ross, J. Jr., McFate, P. A., and Shaw, R. F. (1964). Control of coronary blood flow by an autoregulatory mechanism. *Circ. Res.* 14, 250–259. doi: 10.1161/01.RES.14.3.250

Muller, J. M., Myers, P. R., and Laughlin, M. H. (1993). Exercise training alters myogenic responses in porcine coronary resistance arteries. *J. Appl. Physiol.* 75, 2677–2682. doi: 10.1152/jappl.1993.75.6.2677

Nakayama, K., Osol, G., and Halpern, W. (1988). Reactivity of isolated porcine coronary resistance arteries to cholinergic and adrenergic drugs and transmural pressure changes. *Circ. Res.* 62, 741–748. doi: 10.1161/01.RES.62.4.741

Namani, R., Kassab, G. S., and Lanir, Y. (2018). Integrative model of coronary flow in anatomically based vasculature under myogenic, shear, and metabolic regulation. *J. Gen. Physiol.* 150, 145–168. doi: 10.1085/jgp.201711795

Pantely, G. A., Bristow, J. D., Swenson, L. J., Ladley, H. D., Johnson, W. B., and Anselone, C. G. (1985). Incomplete coronary vasodilation during myocardial ischemia in swine. *Am. J. Physiol.* 249(3 Pt 2), H638–H647. doi: 10.1152/ajpheart.1985.249.3.H638

Schampaert, S., van 't Veer, M., Rutten, M. C., van Tuijl, S., de Hart, J., van de Vosse, F. N., et al. (2013). Autoregulation of coronary blood flow in the isolated beating pig heart. *Artif. Organs* 37, 724–730. doi: 10.1111/aor.12065

Schulz, R., Guth, B. D., and Heusch, G. (1991). No effect of coronary perfusion on regional myocardial function within the autoregulatory range in pigs. Evidence against the Gregg phenomenon. *Circulation* 83, 1390–1403. doi: 10.1161/01.RES.83.4.1390

Shnier, C. B., Cason, B. A., Horton, A. F., and Hickey, R. F. (1994). Coronary blood flow autoregulation and flow heterogeneity in the stunned heart. *Jpn. Heart J.* 35, 654–660. doi: 10.1536/ihj.35.645

Sorop, O., Merkus, D., de Beer, V. J., Houweling, B., Pistea, A., McFalls, E. O., et al. (2008). Functional and structural adaptations of coronary microvessels distal to a chronic coronary artery stenosis. *Circ. Res.* 102, 795–803. doi: 10.1161/CIRCRESAHA.108.172528

Stainsby, W. N. (1962). Autoregulation of blood flow in skeletal muscle during increased metabolic activity. *Am. J. Physiol.* 202, 273–276. doi: 10.1152/ajplegacy.1962.202.2.273

Suzuki, Y., Yeung, A. C., and Ikeno, F. (2011). The representative porcine model for human cardiovascular disease. *J. Biomed. Biotechnol.* 2011:195483. doi: 10.1155/2011/195483

Tofukuji, M., Stamler, A., Li, J., Franklin, A., Wang, S. Y., Hariawala, M. D., et al. (1997a). Effects of magnesium cardioplegia on regulation of the porcine coronary circulation. *J. Surg. Res.* 69, 233–239. doi: 10.1006/jsre.1997.5003

Tofukuji, M., Stamler, A., Li, J., Hariawala, M. D., Franklin, A., and Sellke, F. W. (1997b). Comparative effects of continuous warm blood and intermittent cold blood cardioplegia on coronary reactivity. *Ann. Thorac. Surg.* 64, 1360–1367. doi: 10.1016/S0003-4975(97)00990-9

Tune, J. D. (2014). "Coronary circulation," in *Colloquium Series on Integrated Systems Physiology: From Molecule to Function to Disease*, Vol 6 (Morgan & Claypool Life Sciences), 1–189.

Ueeda, M., Silvia, S. K., and Olsson, R. A. (1992). Nitric oxide modulates coronary autoregulation in the guinea pig. *Circ. Res.* 70, 1296–1303. doi: 10.1161/01.RES.70.6.1296

Wang, S. Y., Friedman, M., Franklin, A., and Sellke, F. W. (1995). Myogenic reactivity of coronary resistance arteries after cardiopulmonary bypass and hyperkalemic cardioplegia. *Circulation* 92, 1590–1596. doi: 10.1161/01.CIR.92.6.1590

Wang, S. Y., Stamler, A., Tofukuji, M., Deuson, T. E., and Sellke, F. W. (1997). Effects of blood and crystalloid cardioplegia on adrenergic and myogenic vascular mechanisms. *Ann. Thorac. Surg.* 63, 41–49. doi: 10.1016/S0003-4975(96)00644-3

Young, J. M., Choy, J. S., Kassab, G. S., and Lanir, Y. (2012). Slackness between vessel and myocardium is necessary for coronary flow reserve. *Am. J. Physiol. Heart Circ. Physiol.* 302, H2230–H2242. doi: 10.1152/ajpheart.01184.2011

3

# Hepatic Hemangiomas Alter Morphometry and Impair Hemodynamics of the Abdominal Aorta and Primary Branches from Computer Simulations

Xiaoping Yin [1†], Xu Huang [2†], Qiao Li [2†], Li Li [2], Pei Niu [2], Minglu Cao [2], Fei Guo [3], Xuechao Li [3], Wenchang Tan [2,4,5] and Yunlong Huo [2,3,4*]

[1] Department of Radiology, Affiliated Hospital of Hebei University, Hebei University, Baoding, China, [2] Department of Mechanics and Engineering Science, College of Engineering, Peking University, Beijing, China, [3] College of Medicine, Hebei University, Baoding, China, [4] PKU-HKUST Shenzhen-Hongkong Institution, Shenzhen, China, [5] Shenzhen Graduate School, Peking University, Shenzhen, China

*Correspondence:
Yunlong Huo
yhuo@pku.edu.cn

[†] These authors have contributed equally to this work.

**Background:** The formation of hepatic hemangiomas (HH) is associated with VEGF and IL-7 that alter conduit arteries and small arterioles. To our knowledge, there are no studies to investigate the effects of HH on the hemodynamics in conduit arteries. The aim of the study is to perform morphometric and hemodynamic analysis in abdominal conduit arteries and bifurcations of HH patients and controls.

**Methods:** Based on morphometry reconstructed from CT images, geometrical models were meshed with prismatic elements for the near wall region and tetrahedral and hexahedral elements for the core region. Simulations were performed for computation of the non-Newtonian blood flow using the Carreau-Yasuda model, based on which multiple hemodynamic parameters were determined.

**Results:** There was an increase of the lumen size, diameter ratio, and curvature in the abdominal arterial tree of HH patients as compared with controls. This significantly increased the surface area ratio of low time-averaged wall shear stress (i.e., $\text{SAR-TAWSS} = \frac{\text{Surface area}_{\text{TAWSS} \leq 4 \text{ dynes·cm}^{-2}}}{\text{Total surface area}} \times 100\%$) ($24.1 \pm 7.9$ vs. $5 \pm 6\%$, $11.6 \pm 12.8$ vs. $< 0.1\%$, and $44.5 \pm 9.2$ vs. $21 \pm 24\%$ at hepatic bifurcations, common hepatic arteries, and abdominal aortas, respectively, between HH and control patients).

**Conclusions:** Morphometric changes caused by HH significantly deteriorated the hemodynamic environment in abdominal conduit arteries and bifurcations, which could be an important risk factor for the incidence and progression of vascular diseases.

Keywords: hepatic hemangioma, computer tomography, abdominal arterial tree, hemodynamics, morphology

## INTRODUCTION

Hemangioma is the most common benign tumor that affects the liver (Gandolfi et al., 1991; John et al., 1994). Hepatic hemangiomas (HH) occur generally in small regions from a few mm to 4 cm despite large HH in the range of 4~40 cm (Sieg et al., 1982; Hoekstra et al., 2013; Toro et al., 2014; Zhao et al., 2015). It was found that HH are associated with microvascular malformations and congenital origin growing slowly from birth (Saegusa et al., 1995; Lehmann et al., 1999). Pregnancy, oral contraceptive use, androgen, or steroid administration were believed to stimulate the incidence and progression of HH (Hoekstra et al., 2013; Toro et al., 2014). The use of specific antibodies against vascular endothelial growth factor (VEGF) and IL-7 was proposed to inhibit the growth of HH (Trastek et al., 1983; Mahajan et al., 2008; Wang et al., 2012). However, the etiology and pathogenesis of HH remain unknown.

Morphometric alteration of large conduit arteries could induce abnormal flow patterns, e.g., stagnation flow, reversal flow, flow vortex, and so on, which were characterized by

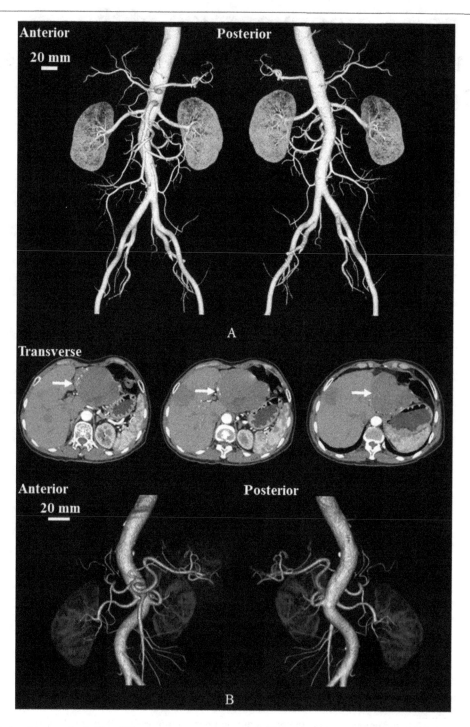

**FIGURE 1 |** Geometrical models reconstructed from CT images of a representative control **(A)** and a representative HH patient **(B)**. **(B)** Also shows CT-axial angiographs, where arrows mark liver hemangiomas.

various hemodynamic risk factors including low time-averaged wall shear stress over a cardiac cycle (low TAWSS), high oscillatory shear index (high OSI), and high TAWSS gradient (high TAWSSG) (Ku, 1997; Kleinstreuer et al., 2001; Huo et al., 2007b, 2008, 2009). Computational fluid dynamics (CFD) has been applied to the hemodynamic analysis in the abdominal arterial tree (Taylor and Draney, 2004). These simulations mainly focused on the flow distribution near stenoses or aneurysms (Boutsianis et al., 2009; Biasetti et al., 2011; Polanczyk et al., 2015; Arzani and Shadden, 2016). To our knowledge, there is lack of studies to show the effects of microvascular malformations on morphometry and hemodynamics in the abdominal aorta and primary branches of HH patients, which could induce hemodynamic impairments to large arteries in the cardiovascular system.

The objective of the study is to demonstrate a comparison of morphometry and hemodynamics in the abdominal aorta and primary branches between HH patients and healthy controls. We hypothesize that HH-induced morphometric changes significantly worsen the hemodynamic environment in abdominal conduit arteries and bifurcations. To test the hypothesis, we reconstructed the large abdominal arterial trees from CT images of 12 HH patients and 9 controls. Flow simulations were performed to solve the Continuity and Navier–Stokes equations with the Carreau-Yasuda model for non-Newtonian blood, similar to a previous study (Yin et al., 2016). The flow velocity waveform was measured at the thoracic aorta of a representative patient and was applied to the inlet of the large abdominal arterial tree with the Womersley velocity profile (Zheng et al., 1985). The fully-developed flow boundary condition was applied to each outlet that considered fractional flow rate (Huo et al., 2013). Based on the computed flow field, multiple hemodynamic parameters, i.e., TAWSS, OSI, and TAWSSG, were determined in the large abdominal arterial trees. Malek et al. showed a threshold $TAWSS \leq 4$ dynes/cm$^2$; Nordgaard et al. indicated a threshold $OSI \geq 0.15$; and Fan et al. proposed a threshold $TAWSSG \geq 500$ dynes/cm$^3$ for the incidence and progression of atherosclerosis (Malek et al., 1999; Nordgaard et al., 2010; Fan et al., 2016). Hence, we used the surface area ratios of low TAWSS (SAR-TAWSS), high OSI (SAR-OSI), and TAWSSG (SAR-TAWSSG) (see the detailed definitions in the Appendix) to characterize the complex hemodynamic environment in abdominal conduit arteries and bifurcations similar to previous studies (Fan et al., 2016, 2017; Yin et al., 2016).

## MATERIALS AND METHODS

### Study Design

We retrospectively analyzed morphometry and hemodynamics of large abdominal arterial trees of HH patients as well as age-matched control subjects, who underwent CT exams at the Affiliated Hospital of Hebei University, China, from January to December 2015. The CT diagnosis of HH in a previous study (Caseiro-Alves et al., 2007) was used, which showed peripheral nodular enhancement at the lesion progressing from the periphery to the center, as shown in **Figure 1**. A total of 12

HH patients (5 males and 7 females from 28 to 69 years) were compared with a total of 9 controls (7 males and 2 females from 31 to 62 years).

The study was approved by the Institutional Review Board (IRB) for the Affiliated Hospital of Hebei University, which conforms the declaration of Helsinki. All patients gave the signed informed consent for all methods of the study performed in accordance with the relevant guidelines and regulations of the IRB for the Affiliated Hospital of Hebei University.

### Imaging Acquisition

CT scans were performed on a Discovery CT750 HD scanner (HDCT, GE Healthcare, Milwaukee, WI, USA). All patients underwent abdomen contrast-enhanced spectral CT from the

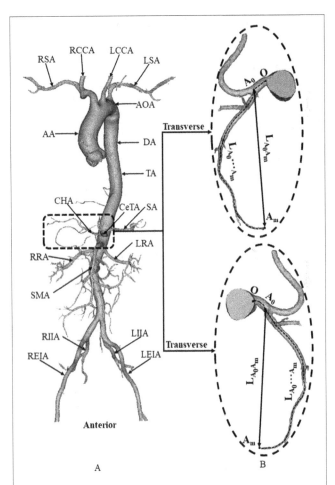

**FIGURE 2 | (A)** Schematic diagram of aorta and primary branches, where AA, ascending aorta; AOA, arch of aorta; DA, descending aorta; TA, thoracic aorta; RSA, right subclavian artery; RCCA, right common carotid artery; LCCA, left common carotid artery; LSA, left subclavian artery; CeTA, celiac trunk artery; CHA, common hepatic artery; SA, splenic artery; RRA, right renal artery; LRA, left renal artery; SMA, superior mesenteric artery; RIIA, right internal iliac artery; REIA, right external iliac artery; LIIA, left internal iliac artery; LEIA, left external iliac artery; and **(B)** zoomed diagram of CeTA and CHA, where the black dotted line represents the centerline, $A_0$ refers to the intersection of centerlines between CeTA and CHA, and $L_{A_0A_m}$ and $L_{A_0\cdots A_m}$ denote the linear and arc lengths from point $A_0$ to $A_m$, respectively.

diaphragm to the edge of the kidney. The spectral CT scan protocol included helical pitch of 0.984:1, rotation speed of 0.5 s, and 50 cm Display Field of View (DFOV). The nonionic contrast media (ioversol, 320 mgl/ml) at the dose of 1.0 ml/kg was injected with a power injector at a rate of 3.0 ml/s through median cubital vein. Arterial phase scanning with an automatic tracking technique with automated scan-triggering software (SmartPrep, GE Healthcare, Milwaukee, WI, USA) started 8 s after the trigger threshold (100 HU) was reached at the level of the celiac trunk (He et al., 2014). The portal venous phase scanning and later delay phase scanning started for 30 and 120 s, respectively, after the beginning of the arterial phase scanning.

## Geometrical Model

Morphometric data of the abdominal aorta and primary branches were extracted from patient CT images using the MIMICS software (Materialise, NV, Belgium), as shown in **Figure 2**. A centerline was formed by a series of center points which were located in the center on the cross–sectional views of the contour of the 3D vessel. Subsequently, the best fit diameter, $D_{fit}$, was calculated as twice the average radius between the point on the centerline and the contour forming the contour of the 3D vessel (Fan et al., 2016; Huang et al., 2016). The CT reconstruction and imaging analysis were performed by researchers (X. Huang, Q. Li and M. Cao) at the College of Engineering, Peking University and (F. Guo and X. Li) at the College of Medicine, Hebei University as well as a Radiologist (X. Yin) at the Affiliated Hospital of Hebei University. The reproducibility of the measurements showed $\kappa$ value equals to 0.87.

## Mesh Generation

Based on morphometric data, geometrical models were meshed with prismatic elements for the near wall region (number of layers = 3, height ratio = 1.2, total height = 1 mm) and tetrahedral and hexahedral elements for the core region (maximal element size = 0.3 mm) using the ANSYS ICEM software (ANSYS Inc., Canonsburg, USA) and then smoothed using the Geomagic Studio software (3D Systems, Rock Hill, USA). Mesh dependency and skewness and orthogonal quality metrics were analyzed to satisfy the quality of the grids such that the relative error in two consecutive mesh refinements was < 1% for the maximum WSS and velocity of steady state flow with inlet flow velocity equal to the time-averaged velocity over a cardiac cycle, similar to previous studies (Chen et al., 2016; Fan et al., 2016; Yin et al., 2016). A total of 3.5–4.5 million hybrid volume elements were necessary to accurately mesh the computational domain. Simulations were demonstrated in a workstation with 3GHz dual Xeon processor and 32-GB of memory, and the computational time for each model ranged from 48 to 72 h.

## Computational Model

Similar to a previous study (Biasetti et al., 2011), the Carreau-Yasuda model for the non-Newtonian blood flow was performed as:

$$\frac{\mu - \mu_\infty}{\mu_0 - \mu_\infty} = \left[1 + (\lambda\dot{\gamma})^a\right]^{(n-1)/a} \tag{1}$$

---

**TABLE 1** | Demographics and morphometry in each patient of control and HH groups.

| Groups | No | Sex | Age | $D_{CHA}$ (mm) | $D_{CeTA}$ (mm) | $D_{TA}$ (mm) | $L_{A_0 A_m}$ (mm) | $L_{A_0 \cdots A_m}$ (mm) | $\frac{D_{CHA}}{D_{CeTA}}$ | $\frac{D_{CHA}}{D_{TA}}$ | $\frac{D_{CeTA}}{D_{TA}}$ | $\frac{L_{A_0 A_m}}{L_{A_0 \cdots A_m}}$ |
|---|---|---|---|---|---|---|---|---|---|---|---|---|
| Control group | 1 | M | 31 | 3.14 | 5.47 | 18.11 | 17.17 | 17.79 | 0.57 | 0.17 | 0.3 | 0.96 |
| | 2 | M | 37 | 3.02 | 7.16 | 20.23 | 58.39 | 84.53 | 0.42 | 0.15 | 0.35 | 0.69 |
| | 3 | M | 40 | 2.62 | 5.08 | 17.83 | 25.96 | 37.91 | 0.52 | 0.15 | 0.28 | 0.68 |
| | 4 | M | 46 | 2.96 | 5.77 | 20.64 | 41.47 | 53.21 | 0.51 | 0.14 | 0.28 | 0.78 |
| | 5 | M | 52 | 3.32 | 7.04 | 18.76 | 50.62 | 53.74 | 0.47 | 0.18 | 0.38 | 0.94 |
| | 6 | M | 52 | 1.99 | 5.93 | 18.14 | 46.43 | 60.47 | 0.34 | 0.11 | 0.33 | 0.77 |
| | 7 | F | 55 | 2.9 | 4.86 | 19.85 | 35.73 | 41.55 | 0.6 | 0.15 | 0.24 | 0.86 |
| | 8 | M | 58 | 3.34 | 4.59 | 20.02 | 33.43 | 33.84 | 0.73 | 0.17 | 0.23 | 0.99 |
| | 9 | F | 62 | 2.91 | 6.35 | 23.78 | 32.78 | 39.03 | 0.46 | 0.12 | 0.27 | 0.84 |
| HH group | 1 | F | 28 | 7.85 | 6.58 | 17.76 | 46.85 | 55.29 | 1.19 | 0.44 | 0.37 | 0.85 |
| | 2 | M | 42 | 4.41 | 7.07 | 21.49 | 46.52 | 75.68 | 0.62 | 0.21 | 0.33 | 0.61 |
| | 3 | M | 43 | 4.88 | 7.54 | 23.76 | 59.23 | 94.12 | 0.65 | 0.21 | 0.32 | 0.63 |
| | 4 | F | 50 | 3.85 | 6.94 | 17.54 | 33.43 | 40.67 | 0.55 | 0.22 | 0.4 | 0.82 |
| | 5 | M | 50 | 4.81 | 7.77 | 21.67 | 52.97 | 66.36 | 0.62 | 0.22 | 0.36 | 0.80 |
| | 6 | F | 50 | 4.21 | 5.94 | 23.3 | 71.82 | 97.12 | 0.71 | 0.18 | 0.25 | 0.74 |
| | 7 | F | 52 | 3.65 | 4.76 | 21.34 | 32.08 | 51.73 | 0.77 | 0.17 | 0.22 | 0.62 |
| | 8 | F | 62 | 5.51 | 5.94 | 19.34 | 36.22 | 44.57 | 0.93 | 0.28 | 0.31 | 0.81 |
| | 9 | M | 63 | 4.92 | 7.24 | 19.97 | 25.07 | 45.48 | 0.68 | 0.25 | 0.36 | 0.55 |
| | 10 | F | 65 | 2.46 | 4.52 | 21.75 | 29.06 | 48.06 | 0.54 | 0.11 | 0.21 | 0.60 |
| | 11 | M | 67 | 5.84 | 7.61 | 25.75 | 37.81 | 54.46 | 0.77 | 0.23 | 0.3 | 0.69 |
| | 12 | F | 69 | 3.76 | 7.08 | 23.69 | 40.95 | 69.94 | 0.53 | 0.16 | 0.3 | 0.59 |

where $\mu_0$ and $\mu_\infty$ equal to 0.16 and 0.0035 Pa·s while $\lambda$ (8.2 s), $n$ (0.02128), and $a$ (0.64) refer to the relaxation time, power-law index and Yasuda exponent, respectively. The viscosity ($\mu$) is associated with the shear rate ($\dot{\gamma}$). The flow velocity waveform was measured at the thoracic aorta of a female patient (**Table 1**. HH Group, No.6) through MRI scans with a one-component cine phase-contrast sequence in a 1.5 T scanner (GE Signa SP, GE Medical Systems, Milwaukee, WI). The velocity waveform was scaled to the Womersley profile (i.e., Equation 3 in Zheng et al., 1985) as the inlet boundary condition. The fully-developed flow boundary condition was set to each outlet, where the diffusion flux for all flow variables in the exit direction are zero. Considering the high number of outflow branches, the flow rate weighting factor (i.e., the sum of flow rate weighting factors is 100%) was set to each outlet. The flow rate weighting factor was set to 24% at the distal abdominal aorta (Xiao et al., 2013) while the weighting factors at other outlets were determined by the flow-diameter scaling law (i.e., $Q \propto D^{7/3}$) (Huo and Kassab, 2012a, 2016; Fan et al., 2016).

The mean Reynolds number (averaged over a cardiac cycle) at the inlet of thoracic aorta has values of $1028 \pm 101$ and $1065 \pm 163$ in control and HH groups, respectively. The commercial software solver FLUENT (ANSYS, Inc., Canonsburg, USA) was used to solve the Navier-Stokes and continuity equations as:

$$\nabla \cdot \vec{u} = 0 \tag{2}$$

$$\rho \frac{\partial \vec{u}}{\partial t} + \rho \vec{u} \cdot \nabla \vec{u} = -\nabla p + \mu \nabla^2 \vec{u} \tag{3}$$

where $p$, $\vec{u}$, and $\rho$ (=1,060 kg/m³) represent the pressure, velocity, and blood density, respectively. An implicit second-order backward Euler method was used with a time step 0.01 s. The convergence of solutions was guaranteed by the globe balance of the conservation equations with a RMS (Root Mean Squared) residual criterion of $10^{-3}$. Four cardiac cycles (0.84 s per cardiac cycle) were conducted to achieve the convergence for the transient analysis similar to previous studies (Fan et al., 2016). Hemodynamic parameters including TAWSS, OSI, and TAWSSG were determined from the computed flow fields in the fourth cardiac cycle, consistent with previous studies (Chen et al., 2016; Fan et al., 2016; Yin et al., 2016). Moreover, we computed SAR-TAWSS, SAR-OSI, and SAR-TAWSSG in abdominal conduit arteries and bifurcations.

## Statistical Analysis

The mean $\pm$ $SD$ (standard deviation) values of various morphometric and hemodynamic parameters were computed by averaging over all subjects in a population. A two-way ANOVA (SigmaStat 3.5) was used to detect the statistical difference of the parameters between control and HH groups. A $p$-value $< 0.05$ was indicative of a significant difference between two populations.

## RESULTS

**Figure 2** shows a schematic representative of aorta and primary branches. **Table 1** lists the morphometry in each patient of

control and HH groups, which have mean $\pm$ SD ages of $48 \pm 10$ and $54 \pm 14$ years, respectively. As shown in **Table 2**, parameters, $D_{CHA}$, $D_{CeTA}$ and $D_{TA}$ refer to the diameters averaged along the entire length of common hepatic artery, celiac trunk artery, and thoracic aorta, respectively. They have mean $\pm$ $SD$ values of $2.9 \pm 0.4$, $5.8 \pm 0.9$, and $19.7 \pm 1.9$ mm in the control group and $4.7 \pm 1.4$, $6.6 \pm 1.1$, and $21.5 \pm 2.5$ in the HH group, which show significant difference of $D_{CHA}$ ($p$-value $< 0.05$). The diameters of CeTA and TA in HH patients are higher than those in controls despite no statistical difference. Moreover, the diameter ratios, $\frac{D_{CHA}}{D_{CeTA}}$ and $\frac{D_{CHA}}{D_{TA}}$, in the HH group are significantly higher than the control group ($p$-value $< 0.05$). On the other hand, there are significantly lower ratios of linear to arc lengths ($\frac{L_{A_0 Am}}{L_{A_0 \cdots Am}}$) in HH CHAs compared with controls ($0.69 \pm 0.11$ vs. $0.84 \pm 0.11$, $p$-value $< 0.05$). This indicates severe curvatures in CHAs of HH patients.

The Reynolds number at the inlet of thoracic aorta with diameters of $21.5 \pm 2.1$ and $22.3 \pm 3.4$ mm has values of 1.028

**TABLE 2** | Statistical analysis of morphometric and hemodynamic parameters in control and HH groups.

| Groups | | Control group | HH group | p-value |
|---|---|---|---|---|
| **MORPHOMETRIC ANALYSIS** | | | | |
| $D_{CHA}$ (mm) | Mean ± SD | 2.9 ± 0.4 | 4.7 ± 1.4 | <0.05 |
| | 95% CI | 2.6–3.2 | 3.8–5.5 | |
| $D_{CeTA}$ (mm) | Mean ± SD | 5.8 ± 0.9 | 6.6 ± 1.1 | 0.099 |
| | 95% CI | 5.1–6.5 | 5.9–7.3 | |
| $D_{TA}$ (mm) | Mean ± SD | 19.7 ± 1.9 | 21.5 ± 2.5 | 0.094 |
| | 95% CI | 18.3–21.1 | 19.9–23.0 | |
| $L_{A_0 Am}$ (mm) | Mean ± SD | 38 ± 12.7 | 42.7 ± 13.6 | 0.432 |
| | 95% CI | 28.2–47.8 | 34.1–51.3 | |
| $L_{A_0 \cdots Am}$ (mm) | Mean ± SD | 46.9 ± 19 | 62.0 ± 19.0 | 0.088 |
| | 95% CI | 32.3–61.5 | 49.9–74.0 | |
| $\frac{D_{CHA}}{D_{CeTA}}$ | Mean ± SD | 0.51 ± 0.11 | 0.71 ± 0.19 | <0.05 |
| | 95% CI | 0.43–0.6 | 0.59–0.83 | |
| $\frac{D_{CHA}}{D_{TA}}$ | Mean ± SD | 0.15 ± 0.02 | 0.22 ± 0.08 | <0.05 |
| | 95% CI | 0.13–0.17 | 0.17–0.27 | |
| $\frac{D_{CeTA}}{D_{TA}}$ | Mean ± SD | 0.3 ± 0.05 | 0.31 ± 0.06 | 0.566 |
| | 95% CI | 0.26–0.33 | 0.27–0.35 | |
| $\frac{L_{A_0 Am}}{L_{A_0 \cdots Am}}$ | Mean ± SD | 0.84 ± 0.11 | 0.69 ± 0.11 | <0.05 |
| | 95% CI | 0.75–0.92 | 0.63–0.76 | |
| **HEMODYNAMIC ANALYSIS** | | | | |
| $D_{Inlet}$ (mm) | | 21.5 ± 2.1 | 22.3 ± 3.4 | 0.704 |
| $Re_{mean}$ | | 1028 ± 101 | 1065 ± 163 | 0.704 |
| **AREA RATIOS AT BIFURCATIONS BETWEEN CeTA AND CHA AND SA** | | | | |
| SAR-TAWSS (%) | | 4 ± 5 | 14.3 ± 4.4 | <0.05 |
| SAR-TAWSSG (%) | | 27 ± 38 | 36.1 ± 28.5 | 0.678 |
| **AREA RATIOS IN CHAs** | | | | |
| SAR-TAWSS (%) | | <0.1 | 6.3 ± 5.1 | <0.05 |
| SAR-TAWSSG (%) | | 68 ± 33 | 55.4 ± 17.1 | 0.445 |
| **AREA RATIOS IN ABDOMINAL AORTAS** | | | | |
| SAR-TAWSS (%) | | 17 ± 22 | 43.6 ± 8.4 | <0.05 |
| SAR-TAWSSG (%) | | 1 ± 1 | 2.1 ± 1.3 | 0.17 |

± 101 and 1.065 ± 163 in control and HH groups, respectively. Hence, the simulation was carried out for computation of flow fields, based on the geometrical models and boundary conditions in **Figure 3**. The highest and lowest flow velocities at the inlet of TA occur at time instances of $t_1$ and $t_2$, as shown in **Figure 3B**. **Figures 4A–C** show the flow streamlines (unit: $s^{-1}$) at time instances of $t_1$ and $t_2$, TAWSS (unit: dynes/cm$^2$) and TAWSSG (unit: dynes/cm$^3$), respectively, in abdominal arterial trees of a representative control as well as a representative HH patient. Accordingly, **Figures 5A,B** show the flow streamlines and vortex cores (unit: $s^{-1}$) at the bifurcation between the celiac trunk artery and common hepatic and splenic arteries. At some time instances in a cardiac cycle, stagnation flow as well as slight reversal flow occurs in three major sites: opposite to flow divider, lateral to junction orifice, and inner curvature, which results in a low TAWSS. Moreover, transient secondary flow leads to complex flow patterns near the bifurcation carina. Hence, we computed SAR-TAWSS and SAR-TAWSSG to analyze the hemodynamics in CHAs and abdominal aortas and at bifurcations between CeTA and CHA and SA in the two groups, as shown in **Table 2**. Since SAR-OSI < 1%, it is neglected here. Hepatic hemangiomas significantly increase SAR-TAWSS (14.3 ± 4.4 vs. 4 ± 5 at bifurcations between CeTA and CHA and SA, 6.3 ± 5.1 vs. < 0.1 in CHAs, and 43.6 ± 8.4 vs. 17 ± 22 in abdominal aortas for HH vs. control groups, $p$-value < 0.05) and impair the hemodynamics in the large abdominal arterial tree. There is no statistical difference of SAR-TAWSSG between control and HH groups.

## DISCUSSION

The study compared morphometry and hemodynamics in the abdominal aorta and primary branches between control and HH patients. The major findings are reported as: (1) HH increase the lumen size in the abdominal arterial tree significantly and show higher $\frac{D_{CHA}}{D_{CeTA}}$ and $\frac{D_{CHA}}{D_{TA}}$ in comparison with controls ($p$-value < 0.05); (2) HH lead to severe curvature in CHAs; and (3) HH result in a significant increase of SAR-TAWSS due to abnormal flow patterns in CHAs and abdominal aortas as well as at bifurcations between CeTA and CHA and SA. The findings are discussed in relation to the potential incidence and progression of cardiovascular diseases.

The prevalence of HH ranges from 0.4 to 7.3% of all space-occupying hepatic lesions (Ishak and Rabin, 1975; John et al., 1994). Since benign HH of small size received little attention (John et al., 1994), previous studies emphasized on the treatment of large HH that cause clinical symptoms (Cui et al., 2003; Zagoria et al., 2004; Tak et al., 2006) and neglected potential impairments of small HH. To our knowledge, the present study

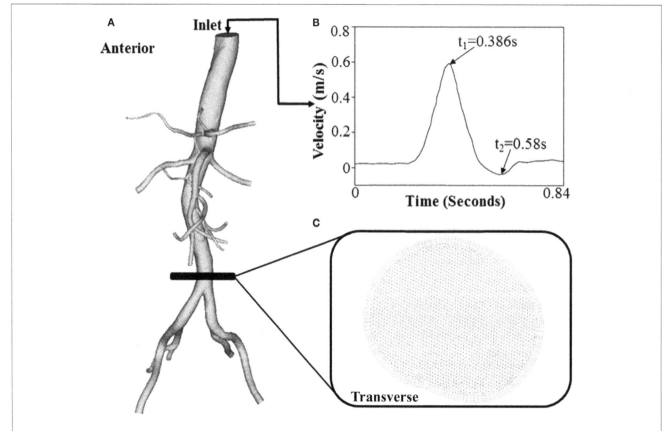

FIGURE 3 | (A) A geometrical model for flow simulations, (B) the inlet flow waveform measured at a patient TA by phase-contrast MRI, and (C) FE meshes at a cross-sectional area.

Hepatic Hemangiomas Alter Morphometry and Impair Hemodynamics of the Abdominal Aorta and Primary...

29

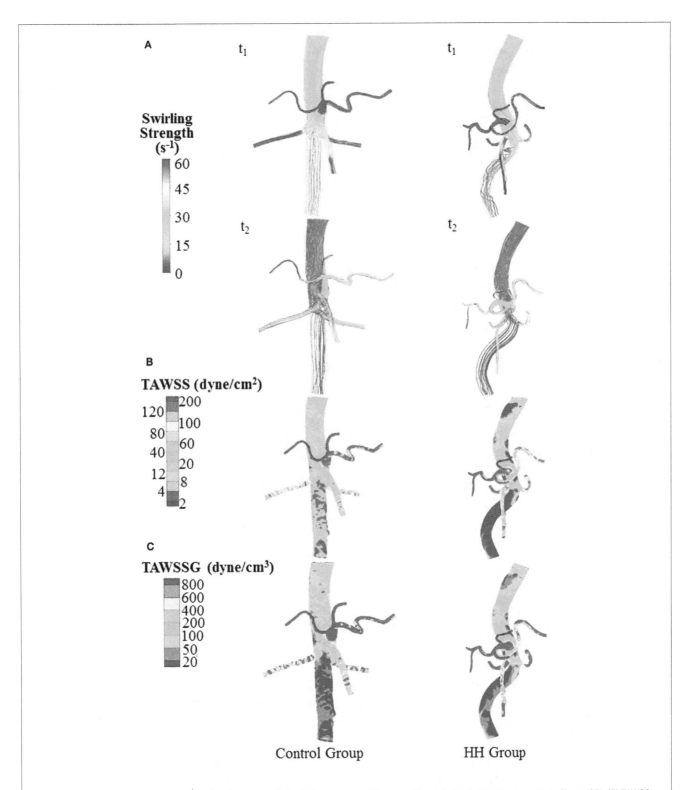

**FIGURE 4 | (A)** Flow streamlines (unit: s$^{-1}$) at time instances with the highest and lowest flow velocities at the inlet of TA (i.e., t$_1$ and t$_2$ in **Figure 3B**), **(B)** TAWSS (unit: dynes/cm$^2$), and **(C)** TAWSSG (unit: dynes/cm$^3$) in a representative control and a representative HH patient.

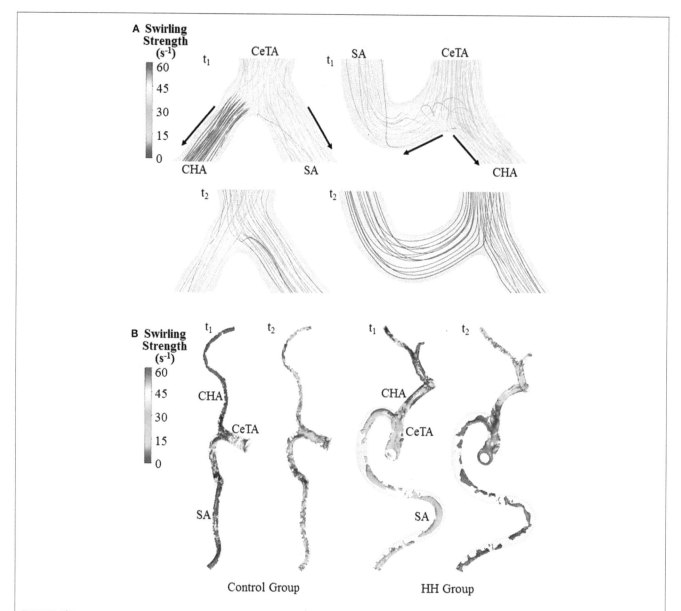

**FIGURE 5 |** Bifurcation flow streamlines **(A)** and vortex cores **(B)** (unit: s$^{-1}$) in a representative control and a representative HH patient at time instances with the highest and lowest flow velocities at the inlet of TA.

first investigates the effects of small HH on morphometry and hemodynamics of the large abdominal arterial tree.

The CT reconstruction showed an increase of lumen size and curvature in the abdominal aorta and primary branches of HH patients. There is higher expression of VEGF and IL-7 in HH patients, which contribute to microvascular malfunctions (Trastek et al., 1983; Mahajan et al., 2008; Wang et al., 2012). The overexpression of VEGF and IL-7 can also be critical risk factors for the morphometric changes of large abdominal arterial trees (Lu and Kassab, 2011; Kim and Byzova, 2014). Moreover, HH are comprised of a chaotic enlargement of distorted micro-vessels such that the flow overload in large conduit arteries occurs to satisfy the balance of supply and demand. The remodeling of

conduit arteries in flow overload should conform to the "uniform normal and shear stress hypothesis" (Kassab et al., 2002; Huo et al., 2007a; Huo and Kassab, 2012b), which results in the increased lumen size and curvature of abdominal conduit arteries (Garcia and Kassab, 1985).

A key finding is the deteriorated hemodynamic environment at bifurcations between CeTA and CHA and SA and in abdominal aortas and CHAs of HH patients. In comparison with controls, the significantly increased $\frac{D_{CHA}}{D_{CeTA}}$ induced more complex flow patterns (e.g., stagnation flow, reversal flow, and second flow) at bifurcations between CeTA and CHA and SA in HH patients, as shown in **Figure 5**. Here, SAR-TAWSS, SAR-OSI, and SAR-TAWSSG were used to characterize the complexity of flow patterns similar to previous studies (Chen et al., 2016; Fan et al., 2016; Yin et al., 2016). The 5-fold increase of SAR-TAWSS and unchanged SAR-OSI and SAR-TAWSSG indicated the deteriorated hemodynamics at bifurcations of HH patients. On the other hand, we have shown low TAWSS on the inner curvature mainly due to the stagnation flow (Huo et al., 2007b, 2008, 2009). The HH-induced curvature significantly increased the values of SAR-TAWSS in both abdominal aortas and CHAs. Therefore, HH impaired the hemodynamics in the large abdominal arterial tree.

## Potential Implications

Low TAWSS, high OSI, and TAWSSG can stimulate the vessel wall to induce abnormal biochemical signals relevant to multiple cardiovascular diseases (Chiu and Chien, 2011). Since most of HH are small and benign, previous studies focused on the microvascular malfunctions and microcirculation, but neglected the possibilities of hemodynamic impairments to abdominal conduit arteries. The present study implies that HH-induced morphometric and hemodynamic changes could lead to the incidence and progression of various vascular diseases (e.g., intimal thickening, atherosclerosis, vascular stiffness, and so on) in abdominal conduit arteries. Moreover, this study implies that the use of antibodies against VEGF and IL-7 could inhibit the development of HH and vascular diseases occurring in large conduit arteries.

## Critique of the Study

The retrospective data were collected from a single center such that the sample size of HH and control patients was relatively small. For further hemodynamic analysis, the large sample size should be collected from multiple centers to ensure the questionnaire sample requirement. Furthermore, prospective studies are required to investigate the effects of HH on various vascular diseases occurring in large conduit arteries. Although the simulation with non-Newtonian model was used to compute the pulsatile blood flow, we neglected the effects of vessel compliance. The FSI (i.e., fluid-structure interaction) simulation should be carried out and validated against the measurements from MRI or 4D flow to investigate hemodynamic changes relevant to the HH-induced abdominal stiffness in the following study.

## CONCLUSIONS

The retrospective study showed the changes of morphometry and hemodynamics in HH patients compared with healthy controls. It was found that HH increased lumen size and curvature of abdominal conduit arteries as well as diameter ratios. The altered morphometry significantly deteriorated the hemodynamics in the large abdominal arterial tree, i.e., an increase of SAR-TAWSS due to abnormal flow patterns in CHAs and abdominal aortas and at bifurcations between CeTA and CHA and SA of HH patients. This implied the possibilities of HH-induced hemodynamic impairments to abdominal conduit arteries. These findings can also improve our understanding of hemodynamic mechanisms relevant to the etiology and pathogenesis of HH.

## AUTHOR CONTRIBUTIONS

The CT reconstruction and imaging analysis were performed by XH, QL, LL, PN, and MC at the College of Engineering, Peking University and FG and XL at the College of Medicine, Hebei University as well as a Radiologist XY at the Affiliated Hospital of Hebei University. Paper was drafted and revised by YH and WT.

## ACKNOWLEDGMENTS

We would like to thank all participants of the study in Peking University and Affiliated Hospital of Hebei University. This research is supported in part by the National Natural Science Foundation of China Grant 11672006 (YH) and 11732001 (WT), the Shenzhen Science and Technology R&D Grant JCYJ20160427170536358 (YH), and the Hebei University Medical Construction Grant 2015A1002 (YH).

## REFERENCES

Arzani, A., and Shadden, S. C. (2016). Characterizations and correlations of wall shear stress in aneurysmal flow. *J. Biomech. Eng.* 138:014503. doi: 10.1115/1.4032056

Biasetti, J., Hussain, F., and Gasser, T. C. (2011). Blood flow and coherent vortices in the normal and aneurysmatic aortas: a fluid dynamical approach to intra-luminal thrombus formation. *J. R. Soc. Interface* 8, 1449–1461. doi: 10.1098/rsif.2011.0041

Boutsianis, E., Guala, M., Olgac, U., Wildermuth, S., Hoyer, K., Ventikos, Y., et al. (2009). CFD and PTV steady flow investigation in an anatomically accurate abdominal aortic aneurysm. *J. Biomech. Eng.* 131:011008. doi: 10.1115/1.3002886

Caseiro-Alves, F., Brito, J., Araujo, A. E., Belo-Soares, P., Rodrigues, H., Cipriano, A., et al. (2007). Liver haemangioma: common and uncommon findings and how to improve the differential diagnosis. *Eur. Radiol.* 17, 1544–1554. doi: 10.1007/s00330-006-0503-z

Chen, X., Gao, Y., Lu, B., Jia, X., Zhong, L., Kassab, G. S., et al. (2016). Hemodynamics in coronary arterial tree of serial stenoses. *PLoS ONE* 11:e0163715. doi: 10.1371/journal.pone.0163715

Chiu, J. J., and Chien, S. (2011). Effects of disturbed flow on vascular endothelium: pathophysiological basis and clinical perspectives. *Physiol. Rev.* 91, 327–387. doi: 10.1152/physrev.00047.2009

Cui, Y., Zhou, L. Y., Dong, M. K., Wang, P., Ji, M., Li, X. O., et al. (2003). Ultrasonography guided percutaneous radiofrequency ablation for hepatic cavernous hemangioma. *World J. Gastroenterol.* 9, 2132–2134. doi: 10.3748/wjg.v9.i9.2132

Fan, T., Feng, Y., Feng, F., Yin, Z., Luo, D., Lu, Y., et al. (2017). A comparison of postoperative morphometric and hemodynamic changes between saphenous vein and left internal mammary artery grafts. *Physiol. Rep.* 5:e13487. doi: 10.14814/phy2.13487

Fan, T., Lu, Y., Gao, Y., Meng, J., Tan, W., Huo, Y., et al. (2016). Hemodynamics of left internal mammary artery bypass graft: effect of anastomotic geometry, coronary artery stenosis, and postoperative time. *J. Biomech.* 49, 645–652. doi: 10.1016/j.jbiomech.2016.01.031

Gandolfi, L., Leo, P., Solmi, L., Vitelli, E., Verros, G., and Colecchia, A. (1991). Natural history of hepatic haemangiomas: clinical and ultrasound study. *Gut* 32, 677–680. doi: 10.1136/gut.32.6.677

Garcia, M., and Kassab, G. S. (1985). Right coronary artery becomes stiffer with increase in elastin and collagen in right ventricular hypertrophy. *J. Appl. Physiol.* 106, 1338–1346. doi: 10.1152/japplphysiol.90592.2008

He, J., Ma, X., Wang, Q., Fan, J., and Sun, Z. (2014). Spectral CT demonstration of the superior mesenteric artery: comparison of monochromatic and polychromatic imaging. *Acad. Radiol.* 21, 364–368. doi: 10.1016/j.acra.2013.11.004

Hoekstra, L. T., Bieze, M., Erdogan, D., Roelofs, J. J., Beuers, U. H., and van Gulik, T. M. (2013). Management of giant liver hemangiomas: an update. *Exp. Rev. Gastroenterol. Hepatol.* 7, 263–268. doi: 10.1586/egh.13.10

Huang, X., Yin, X., Xu, Y., Jia, X., Li, J., Niu, P., et al. (2016). Morphometric and hemodynamic analysis of atherosclerotic progression in human carotid artery bifurcations. *Am. J. Physiol. Heart Circ. Physiol.* 310, H639–H647. doi: 10.1152/ajpheart.00464.2015

Huo, Y., Choy, J. S., Svendsen, M., Sinha, A. K., and Kassab, G. S. (2009). Effects of vessel compliance on flow pattern in porcine epicardial right coronary arterial tree. *J. Biomech.* 42, 594–602. doi: 10.1016/j.jbiomech.2008.12.011

Huo, Y., Guo, X., and Kassab, G. S. (2008). The flow field along the entire length of mouse aorta and primary branches. *Ann. Biomed. Eng.* 36, 685–699. doi: 10.1007/s10439-008-9473-4

Huo, Y., and Kassab, G. S. (2012a). Intraspecific scaling laws of vascular trees. *J. R. Soc. Interface* 9, 190–200. doi: 10.1098/rsif.2011.0270

Huo, Y., and Kassab, G. S. (2012b). Compensatory remodeling of coronary microvasculature maintains shear stress in porcine left-ventricular hypertrophy. *J. Hypertens.* 30, 608–616. doi: 10.1097/HJH.0b013e32834f44dd

Huo, Y., and Kassab, G. S. (2016). Scaling laws of coronary circulation in health and disease. *J. Biomech.* 49, 2531–2539. doi: 10.1016/j.jbiomech.2016.01.044

Huo, Y., Linares, C. O., and Kassab, G. S. (2007a). Capillary perfusion and wall shear stress are restored in the coronary circulation of hypertrophic right ventricle. *Circ. Res.* 100, 273–283. doi: 10.1161/01.RES.0000257777.83431.13

Huo, Y., Luo, T., Guccione, J. M., Teague, S. D., Tan, W., Navia, J. A., et al. (2013). Mild anastomotic stenosis in patient-specific CABG model may enhance graft patency: a new hypothesis. *PLoS ONE* 8:e73769. doi: 10.1371/journal.pone.0073769

Huo, Y., Wischgoll, T., and Kassab, G. S. (2007b). Flow patterns in three-dimensional porcine epicardial coronary arterial tree. *Am. J. Physiol. Heart Circ. Physiol.* 293, H2959–H2970. doi: 10.1152/ajpheart.00586.2007

Ishak, K. G., and Rabin, L. (1975). Benign tumors of the liver. *Med. Clin. North Am.* 59, 995–1013. doi: 10.1016/S0025-7125(16)31998-8

John, T. G., Greig, J. D., Crosbie, J. L., Miles, W. F., and Garden, O. J. (1994). Superior staging of liver tumors with laparoscopy and laparoscopic ultrasound. *Ann. Surg.* 220, 711–719. doi: 10.1097/00000658-199412000-00002

Kassab, G. S., Gregersen, H., Nielsen, S. L., Lu, X., Tanko, L. B., and Falk, E. (2002). Remodelling of the left anterior descending artery in a porcine model of supravalvular aortic stenosis. *J. Hypertens.* 20, 2429–2437. doi: 10.1097/00004872-200212000-00023

Kim, Y. W., and Byzova, T. V. (2014). Oxidative stress in angiogenesis and vascular disease. *Blood* 123, 625–631. doi: 10.1182/blood-2013-09-512749

Kleinstreuer, C., Hyun, S., Buchanan, J. R., Longest, P. W., Archie, J. P., and Truskey, G. A. (2001). Hemodynamic parameters and early intimal thickening in branching blood vessels. *Critic. Rev. Biomed. Eng.* 29, 1–64. doi: 10.1615/CritRevBiomedEng.v29.i1.10

Ku, D. N. (1997). Blood flow in arteries. *Ann. Rev. Fluid Mech.* 29, 399–434. doi: 10.1146/annurev.fluid.29.1.399

Lehmann, F. S., Beglinger, C., Schnabel, K., and Terracciano, L. (1999). Progressive development of diffuse liver hemangiomatosis. *J. Hepatol.* 30, 951–954. doi: 10.1016/S0168-8278(99)80152-4

Lu, D., and Kassab, G. S. (2011). Role of shear stress and stretch in vascular mechanobiology. *J. R. Soc. Interface* 8, 1379–1385. doi: 10.1098/rsif.2011.0177

Mahajan, D., Miller, C., Hirose, K., McCullough, A., and Yerian, L. (2008). Incidental reduction in the size of liver hemangioma following use of VEGF inhibitor bevacizumab. *J. Hepatol.* 49, 867–870. doi: 10.1016/j.jhep.2008.06.028

Malek, A. M., Alper, S. L., and Izumo, S. (1999). Hemodynamic shear stress and its role in atherosclerosis. *JAMA* 282, 2035–2042. doi: 10.1001/jama.282.21.2035

Nordgaard, H., Swillens, A., Nordhaug, D., Kirkeby-Garstad, I., Van Loo, D., Vitale, N., et al. (2010). Impact of competitive flow on wall shear stress in coronary surgery: computational fluid dynamics of a LIMA-LAD model. *Cardiovasc. Res.* 88, 512–519. doi: 10.1093/cvr/cvq210

Polanczyk, A., Podyma, M., Stefanczyk, L., Szubert, W., and Zbicinski, I. (2015). A 3D model of thrombus formation in a stent-graft after implantation in the abdominal aorta. *J. Biomech.* 48, 425–431. doi: 10.1016/j.jbiomech.2014.12.033

Saegusa, T., Ito, K., Oba, N., Matsuda, M., Kojima, K., Tohyama, K., et al. (1995). Enlargement of multiple cavernous hemangioma of the liver in association with pregnancy. *Intern. Med.* 34, 207–211. doi: 10.2169/internalmedicine.34.207

Sieg, A., Stiehl, A., Gotz, R., Konig, R., Schomig, A., and Kommerell, B. (1982). Hepatic hemangioma. *Innere Med.* 9, 365–369.

Tak, W. Y., Park, S. Y., Jeon, S. W., Cho, C. M., Kweon, Y. O., Kim, S. K., et al. (2006). Ultrasonography-guided percutaneous radiofrequency ablation for treatment of a huge symptomatic hepatic cavernous hemangioma. *J. Clin. Gastroenterol.* 40, 167–170. doi: 10.1097/01.mcg.0000196404.07487.1d

Taylor, C. A., and Draney, M. T. (2004). Experimental and computational methods in cardiovascular fluid mechanics. *Ann. Rev. Fluid Mech.* 36, 197–231. doi: 10.1146/annurev.fluid.36.050802.121944

Toro, A., Mahfouz, A. E., Ardiri, A., Malaguarnera, M., Malaguarnera, G., Loria, F., et al. (2014). What is changing in indications and treatment of hepatic hemangiomas. A review. *Ann. Hepatol.* 13, 327–339.

Trastek, V. F., van Heerden, J. A., Sheedy, P. F. II., and Adson, M. A. (1983). Cavernous hemangiomas of the liver, resect or observe? *Am. J. Surg.* 145, 49–53. doi: 10.1016/0002-9610(83)90165-4

Wang, Z., Yuan, Y., Zhuang, H., Jiang, R., Hou, J., Chen, Q., et al. (2012). Hepatic haemangiomas: possible association with IL-17. *J. Clin. Pathol.* 65, 146–151. doi: 10.1136/jclinpath-2011-200365

Xiao, N., Humphrey, J. D., and Figueroa, C. A. (2013). Multi-scale computational model of three-dimensional hemodynamics within a deformable full-body arterial network. *J. Comput. Phys.* 244, 22–40. doi: 10.1016/j.jcp.2012.09.016

Yin, X., Huang, X., Feng, Y., Tan, W., Liu, H., and Huo, Y. (2016). Interplay of proximal flow confluence and distal flow divergence in patient-specific vertebrobasilar system. *PLoS ONE* 11:e0159836. doi: 10.1371/journal.pone.0159836

Zagoria, R. J., Roth, T. J., Levine, E. A., and Kavanagh, P. V. (2004). Radiofrequency ablation of a symptomatic hepatic cavernous hemangioma. *Am. J. Roentgenol.* 182, 210–212. doi: 10.2214/ajr.182.1.1820210

Zhao, W., Guo, X., and Dong, J. (2015). Spontaneous rupture of hepatic hemangioma: a case report and literature review. *Int. J. Clin. Exp. Pathol.* 8, 13426–13428.

Zheng, H., Huo, Y., Svendsen, M., and Kassab, G. S. (1985). Effect of blood pressure on vascular hemodynamics in acute tachycardia. *J. Appl. Physiol.* 109, 1619–1627. doi: 10.1152/japplphysiol.01356.2009

# APPENDIX

1. **SAR-TAWSS at the bifurcation**: surface area ratio of low TAWSS ($= \frac{\text{Surface area}_{\text{TAWSS} \leq 4 \text{ dynes} \cdot \text{cm}^{-2}}}{\text{Bifurcation surface area}} \times 100\%$) at the bifurcation between the celiac trunk artery and common hepatic and splenic arteries. The end-to-side "bifurcation surface area" is defined as the surface area of the proximal graft (5 mm length) to the bifurcation center plus the surface area of the distal arteries (5 mm length) to the bifurcation center. Surface area of TAWSS $\leq 4$ dynes/cm$^2$ refers to the disease-prone site (Malek et al., 1999).

2. **SAR-TAWSS in the artery**: surface area ratio of low TAWSS ($= \frac{\text{Surface area}_{\text{TAWSS} \leq 4 \text{ dynes} \cdot \text{cm}^{-2}}}{\text{Surface area of the artery}} \times 100\%$) in the artery. "Surface area of the artery" refers to the surface area of the celiac trunk artery (or abdominal aorta).

3. **SAR-OSI at the bifurcation**: surface area ratio of high OSI ($= \frac{\text{Surface area}_{\text{OSI} \geq 0.15}}{\text{Bifurcation surface area}} \times 100\%$) at the bifurcation between the celiac trunk artery and common hepatic and splenic arteries. Surface area of OSI $\geq 0.15$ refers to the disease-prone site (Fan et al., 2016).

4. **SAR-OSI in the artery**: surface area ratio of high OSI ($= \frac{\text{Surface area}_{\text{OSI} \geq 0.15}}{\text{Surface area of the artery}} \times 100\%$) in the artery.

5. **SAR-TAWSSG at the bifurcation**: surface area ratio of high TAWSSG ($= \frac{\text{Surface area}_{\text{TAWSSG} \geq 500 \text{ dynes} \cdot \text{cm}^{-3}}}{\text{Bifurcation surface area}} \times 100\%$) at the bifurcation between the celiac trunk artery and common hepatic and splenic arteries. Surface area of TAWSSG $\geq 500$ dynes/cm$^3$ refers to the disease-prone site (Fan et al., 2016).

6. **SAR-TAWSSG in the artery**: surface area ratio of high TAWSSG ($= \frac{\text{Surface area}_{\text{TAWSSG} \geq 500 \text{ dynes} \cdot \text{cm}^{-3}}}{\text{Surface area of the artery}} \times 100\%$) in the artery.

# 4

# Microstructural Infarct Border Zone Remodeling in the Post-Infarct Swine Heart Measured by Diffusion Tensor MRI

Geoffrey L. Kung [1,2], Marmar Vaseghi [3,4], Jin K. Gahm [1,5], Jane Shevtsov [4], Alan Garfinkel [4], Kalyanam Shivkumar [3,4] and Daniel B. Ennis [1,2,6]*

[1] Department of Radiological Sciences, David Geffen School of Medicine, University of California, Los Angeles, Los Angeles, CA, United States, [2] Department of Bioengineering, University of California, Los Angeles, Los Angeles, CA, United States, [3] Cardiac Arrhythmia Center, David Geffen School of Medicine, University of California, Los Angeles, Los Angeles, CA, United States, [4] Department of Medicine (Cardiology), David Geffen School of Medicine, University of California, Los Angeles, Los Angeles, CA, United States, [5] Department of Computer Science, University of California, Los Angeles, Los Angeles, CA, United States, [6] Biomedical Physics Interdepartmental Program, David Geffen School of Medicine, University of California, Los Angeles, Los Angeles, CA, United States

*Correspondence:
Daniel B. Ennis
daniel.ennis@gmail.com

**Introduction:** Computational models of the heart increasingly require detailed microstructural information to capture the impact of tissue remodeling on cardiac electromechanics in, for example, hearts with myocardial infarctions. Myocardial infarctions are surrounded by the infarct border zone (BZ), which is a site of electromechanical property transition. Magnetic resonance imaging (MRI) is an emerging method for characterizing microstructural remodeling and focal myocardial infarcts and the BZ can be identified with late gadolinium enhanced (LGE) MRI. Microstructural remodeling within the BZ, however, remains poorly characterized by MRI due, in part, to the fact that LGE and DT-MRI are not always available for the same heart. Diffusion tensor MRI (DT-MRI) can evaluate microstructural remodeling by quantifying the DT apparent diffusion coefficient (ADC, increased with decreased cellularity), fractional anisotropy (FA, decreased with increased fibrosis), and tissue mode (decreased with increased fiber disarray). The purpose of this work was to use LGE MRI in post-infarct porcine hearts ($N = 7$) to segment remote, BZ, and infarcted myocardium, thereby providing a basis to quantify microstructural remodeling in the BZ and infarcted regions using co-registered DT-MRI.

**Methods:** Chronic porcine infarcts were created by balloon occlusion of the LCx. 6–8 weeks post-infarction, MRI contrast was administered, and the heart was potassium arrested, excised, and imaged with LGE MRI ($0.33 \times 0.33 \times 0.33$ mm) and co-registered DT-MRI ($1 \times 1 \times 3$ mm). Myocardium was segmented as remote, BZ, or infarct by LGE signal intensity thresholds. DT invariants were used to evaluate microstructural remodeling by quantifying ADC, FA, and tissue mode.

**Results:** The BZ significantly remodeled compared to both infarct and remote myocardium. BZ demonstrated a significant decrease in cellularity (increased ADC), significant decrease in tissue organization (decreased FA), and a significant increase in fiber disarray (decreased tissue mode) relative to remote myocardium (all $p < 0.05$). Microstructural remodeling in the infarct was similar, but significantly larger in magnitude (all $p < 0.05$).

**Conclusion:** DT-MRI can identify regions of significant microstructural remodeling in the BZ that are distinct from both remote and infarcted myocardium.

**Keywords: cardiac computational models, diffusion tensor MRI, border zone, cardiac remodeling, cardiac electromechanics**

# INTRODUCTION

Computational modeling of cardiac electromechanics (Krishnamoorthi et al., 2014) can provide mechanistic insight to normal and abnormal cardiac function and electrical wave propagation (Ponnaluri et al., 2016). Chronic myocardial infarction remains a substantial risk factor for both mechanical heart failure and fatal electric rhythm abnormalities. The post-infarct heart is characterized by three distinct regions, including the remote ("normal") myocardium, the dense infarcted scar, and the border zone (BZ) transition region between remote and infarcted myocardium. The infarct BZ is known as a site for electromechanical property transition.

Myocardial fibrosis as a consequence of post-infarct remodeling increases apparent tissue stiffness and decreases anisotropy. Increases in tissue stiffness are implicated in both abnormal diastolic filling and abnormal systolic contraction, ultimately fomenting heart failure. Myocardial fibrosis also disrupts normal electrical wave front propagation, which contributes to the initiation of fatal ventricular arrhythmias (de Bakker et al., 1988, 1993; Morita et al., 2009). In particular, the infarct border zone (BZ) facilitates slow conduction, reentry phenomena, and is implicated in arrhythmogenesis (Anversa et al., 1985; Ursell et al., 1985; de Bakker et al., 1988; Miragoli et al., 2007). Furthermore, anisotropic tissue conduction at epicardial border zones has been shown to influence the occurrence of reentry (Dillon et al., 1988). Methods to identify the BZ for incorporation into computational models of cardiac electromechanics, however, are not currently well established.

Subsequent to administration of a gadolinium-based contrast agent, T1-weighted late gadolinium enhanced (LGE) magnetic resonance imaging (MRI) is recognized as the gold standard for non-invasive myocardial infarct mapping (Kim et al., 2000; Karamitsos et al., 2009; Schelbert et al., 2010). In LGE MRI the slow contrast washout time from the extracellular space gives rise to hyper-enhanced signal intensity (SI) within the infarct (Kim et al., 1996). The adjacent BZ is characterized by a mixture of replacement fibrosis and viable myocytes within the tissue and, as a consequence of partial volume effects, yields an intermediate SI in LGE MRI (Anversa et al., 1985; Schelbert et al., 2010). LGE MRI, however, only indirectly indicates the presence of microstructural remodeling, especially in the infarct and BZ as it only directly reports the presence of the contrast agent. The extent of microstructural remodeling within the LGE identified BZ has not been previously been characterized.

Diffusion tensor MRI (DT-MRI) quantifies the self-diffusion tensor of water undergoing Brownian diffusion within each imaging voxel. This enables the direct quantitative evaluation of microstructural remodeling (e.g., direct and quantitative changes to the tissue microenvironment). Microstructural remodeling is frequently reported using tensor invariants, which saliently characterize important shape attributes of microstructural diffusion and are established as a tool for quantifying differences in regional microstructure (Ennis and Kindlmann, 2006). Complementary information is found in the eigenvectors, which accord with the predominant cardiomyocyte orientation and myolaminar sheetlet orientations (Kung et al., 2011).

A particularly useful set of microstructural remodeling metrics (tensor invariants) consists of the DT's: (1) *apparent diffusion coefficient* (ADC, [$mm^2$/s]), which measures the overall magnitude of isotropic diffusion and increases with decreasing tissue cellularity (Ellingson et al., 2010); (2) *fractional anisotropy* (FA, unitless on [0, 1]), which quantifies the magnitude of anisotropic diffusion and decreases with increasing fibrosis(Wu et al., 2007); and (3) *tissue mode*(Ennis and Kindlmann, 2006) (unitless on [$-1$, 1]), which gauges the kind of tissue anisotropy with mode values near zero indicating orthotropic diffusion indicative of sheet-like structures; mode values near $+1$ indicating rod-like tissue organization; and mode values near $-1$ indicating planar or pancake-like tissue organization.

The objective of this study was to quantify and compare microstructural remodeling in the remote, BZ, and infarcted myocardium of the post-infarct swine using DT-MRI. We hypothesized that microstructural remodeling (changes in ADC, FA, and tissue mode) within the BZ and infarct will constitute a significantly different microstructural environment compared to remote myocardium.

# MATERIALS AND METHODS
## Porcine Heart Preparation

Animal handling and care followed the recommendations of the National Institutes of Health Guide for the Care and Use of Laboratory Animals and the University of California, Los Angeles Institutional Animal Care and Use Committee. Animal protocols were approved by the University of California, Los Angeles Chancellor's Animal Research Committee.

Following a 12-h fasting period, the swine for this study were intramuscularly injected with 1.4 mg/kg Telazol, and then intubated. General anesthesia was maintained with inhaled 2.5% isoflurane. Seven adult female Yorkshire pigs (40–55 kg)

($N = 7$) underwent closed chest myocardial infarction via balloon occlusion and subsequent reperfusion of the left circumflex artery (LCx). An obtuse marginal branch of the LCx was occluded for 150 min with an angioplasty balloon via the retrograde aortic approach using a sheath from the right femoral artery. Evolving infarction was confirmed via ST segment elevation as assessed by continuous electrocardiogram monitoring.

After 6 to 8 weeks, the animals were intubated and placed under general anesthesia as above. Gd-DTPA was injected (0.1 mmol/kg) and allowed to circulate for 15 min before euthanizing with a lethal dose of KCl. Normal adult female Yorkshire pigs (35–50 kg) ($N = 7$) served as the control group undergoing an identical euthanasia procedure without infarct induction.

After sacrifice, each heart was excised by cutting the great cardiac vessels, rinsed with saline and suspended by the root of the aorta in a saline filled container. With the heart suspended, a high viscosity silicone rubber injection compound (Ready-Press Polyvinylsiloxane, Microsonic Inc., Ambridge, PA) was injected first through the pulmonary vein to fill the left ventricle and left atrium then through the superior vena cava to fill the right ventricle and right atrium, in order to maintain an approximate end diastolic cardiac anatomy (Kung et al., 2011). The heart was then removed from saline and placed in a one-liter plastic cylindrical container filled with a magnetic susceptibility matched fluid (Fomblin Y-LVAC 6-06, Solvay Solexis, West Deptford, NJ). The heart was held in place within the container using open-cell foam and oriented to grossly align with the long axis of the container and subsequently the MRI scanner. The combination of the silicone rubber injection compound, magnetic susceptibility matched fluid, and open-cell foam maintains hold the heart rigidly in place during long scan times. These materials also produce very low MRI signals, which significantly facilitates image segmentation.

## *Ex Vivo* Magnetic Resonance Imaging

Imaging was performed using a 3 Tesla (Trio, Siemens AG, Munich, Germany) scanner and a 12-channel head coil. A 3D gradient echo LGE MRI sequence was used with the following pulse sequence parameters: TR/TE = 4.24/9.35 ms, flip angle = 18.5°, bandwidth = 260 Hz/pixel, 9 averages, and scan time = 2:18 (HH:MM). The in-plane imaging resolution was 0.33 mm × 0.33 mm × 0.33 mm (~550 myocytes per voxel) obtained by using a 384 × 384 × 256 encoding matrix and a 128 × 128 × 85.33 mm imaging volume. All MRI exams began within 2 h of sacrifice to ensure Gd-DTPA contrast did not diffuse significantly away from the infarct (Schelbert et al., 2010).

Immediately after LGE imaging, spatially co-registered DT-MRI was performed. A two-dimensional, diffusion weighted, readout-segmented echo-planar pulse sequence (Porter and Heidemann, 2009) was used to acquire DT-MRI data. The following pulse sequence parameters were used for all experiments: TE/TR = 76 ms/6,800 ms, $b$-value = 1,000 s/mm$^2$, 30 non-collinear diffusion gradient encoding directions, one non-diffusion weighted null direction, 15 readout segments, bandwidth = 439 Hz/pixel, and 8–10 averages. The in-plane imaging resolution was 1 mm × 1 mm × 3 mm (~42,000 myocytes per voxel) obtained by using a 150 × 150 encoding

matrix, 43–44 slices and a 150 × 150 × 129–132 mm imaging volume. The total imaging time for each diffusion weighted volume was 3.4 min, for a total DT-MRI acquisition time of 7:00–8:50 (HH:MM) per heart.

Diffusion tensors were reconstructed from the diffusion weighted images using linear regression and custom Matlab (The Mathworks, Natick, MA) code. ADC, FA, and mode (Ennis and Kindlmann, 2006) were calculated for each imaging voxel's diffusion tensor. The diffusion tensors were visualized directly with superquadric glyphs, which are 3D surfaces that depict the tensor's shape and orientation and highlight regional organization and remodeling (Ennis et al., 2005).

## LGE Segmentation and Registration to DT-MRI
### Segmentation

LGE images (**Figure 1A**) were segmented into remote, BZ, and infarcted myocardium and registered to the diffusion tensor images to enable analysis of microstructural remodeling using the validated procedure of Schelbert et al. (2010). First, LGE images were averaged in the slice direction to match the slice thickness of corresponding DT-MRI data. Myocardial voxels were designated as remote, BZ, or infarct based on LGE image signal intensity (SI) thresholds defined for each heart (Ashikaga et al., 2007; Schelbert et al., 2010; Tao et al., 2010). Regions of interest in remote myocardium (myocardial voxels with low SI) and infarct (myocardial voxels with high SI) were drawn in each heart to calculate the SI mean and standard deviation (SD) in each region for each infarcted heart. In accordance with the method used by Schelbert et al. (2010), segmentation of infarct and remote myocardium was defined starting with a threshold halfway between the mean SI of remote myocardium and the mean SI of infarcted myocardium on a per heart basis. The BZ was defined as voxels with SI below the halfway SI level, but greater than two SDs above mean remote myocardium (**Figure 1B**).

### Registration

LGE and DT-MRI studies were performed back-to-back without adjusting the position of the tissue, but small spatial shifts still occurred over the long scan times. Therefore, 3D rigid-body registration was employed between a binary mask created using SI thresholds of the myocardium in the LGE images and binary a mask of the myocardium from the DT-MRI data created using a tensor-based segmentation method (Gahm et al., 2013). The binary LGE masks were down-sampled in the in-plane directions using bicubic interpolation to match the resolution of DT-MRI (**Figure 1C**). LGE and DT-MRI data were registered first in the through-plane direction by aligning the LV apex of both binary mask image sets, then registered via rigid translation in the in-plane direction using two dimensional cross-correlations in Matlab (**Figure 1D**). The registered LGE mask was then applied to the DT-MRI data to label each voxel as remote, BZ or, infarct (**Figure 1E**). The DT-MRI segmentation was further refined by excluding infarct labeled voxels when the connected regions of infarct consisted of three or less voxels (**Figure 1F**), similar to Tao et al. (2010). BZ segmentations were also refined using

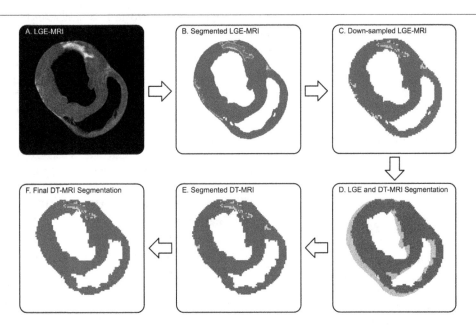

**FIGURE 1 |** Defining remote (blue), borderzone (green), and infarcted (red) myocardium on DT-MRI from co-registered LGE MRI. **(A)** Original high-resolution LGE MRI shows a distinctly bright focal infarct. **(B)** The threshold segmented LGE image is **(C)** down-sampled to match the DT-MRI resolution, then **(D)** co-registered to DT-MRI via 2D cross-correlation. **(E)** The registered LGE segmentation mask is superimposed onto the corresponding myocardial mask of the DT-MRI data. **(F)** Final DT-MRI segmentation refined by excluding islands of high signal intensity consisting of three or less voxels (9 mm$^3$) and removing BZ signal intensities greater than three voxels (3 mm) away from infarct. Note, the LGE to DT-MRI registration required a single pixel-level shift.

morphologic operations to exclude voxels designated as BZ that were greater than three voxels away from infarct labeled regions.

## Statistical Analysis

The central hypothesis of this work is that microstructural remodeling (changes in ADC, FA and mode) within the BZ and infarct constitute a significantly different microstructural environment compared to remote myocardium. Testing this hypothesis required developing the statistically appropriate methods for characterizing significant microstructural remodeling because pixel-based imaging data is spatially correlated and the underlying distribution of the measurement data is non-Gaussian distributed. The key statistical analysis steps include: (1) spatial decorrelation of the data by the auto-correlation length; (2) application of distribution-independent bootstrapped analogs to conventional Gaussian statistical methods; (3) application of boot-strapped analogs of the common $t$-test to enable comparison of medians from non-Gaussian distributions; and (4) use of the boot-strapped analog repeated measures ANOVA to compare groups.

First, the use of inferential statistics requires statistically independent samples. The highly-organized arrangement of myocytes within normal myocardium, however, results in high spatial correlation of the myocardial diffusive properties. For example, adjacent pixels have very similar or spatially correlated tissue properties. This leads to statistically non-independent local diffusion tensors and tensor invariants. To produce statistically independent data points—ADC, FA, and mode were spatially de-correlated in three dimensions within remote, BZ, and infarct

regions via decimation by each region's auto-correlation length (Gahm et al., 2012).

Second, the standard formula-based statistical tests (e.g., $t$-test or ANOVA) require data to be approximately Gaussian in distribution and to have equal variances between comparison groups. The distribution of tensor invariant data, however, is non-Gaussian with unequal variances across different populations (Kung et al., 2011). Therefore, statistical significance tests were performed using bootstrap methods (Gahm et al., 2012).

Third, in order to compare the statistical distributions of tensor invariants between remote, BZ, and infarcted myocardium, we produced bootstrapped histograms by sampling 1,000 times with replacement from the segmented and spatially de-correlated data to define 95% confidence intervals (CIs) within each of 32 histogram bins. When comparing two regions (e.g., remote vs. BZ), if the 95% CIs of the two regions do not overlap within a histogram bin, then the two regions are significantly different within the invariant range of that bin. Similarly, if the 95%-CIs of the bootstrapped medians for two regions within individual hearts do not overlap, then the two regions are significantly different.

Last, to test whether DT invariants significantly remodeled between remote, BZ, and infarct regions for pooled data from all infarcted hearts, we performed a bootstrap analog to repeated measures ANOVA of the de-correlated data (Lazic, 2010). Remote myocardium in infarcted hearts was also compared to myocardium in normal control hearts using a two-group comparison of the medians of de-correlated data. Bootstrapped repeated measures ANOVA and two-group comparisons were performed using the R programming language (http://www.r-project.org), where $p < 0.05$ was regarded as statistically significant. When reporting image quality and auto-correlation lengths, results are reported as mean $\pm$ SD.

## RESULTS

### Infarct Evaluation
Balloon occlusion of the LCx resulted in chronic infarcts that exhibited replacement fibrosis as evidenced by the elevated SI in the LGE images (**Figures 1A**, **2A**). Infarcts regions were predominantly located in the inferior and/or inferoseptal basal to apical LV wall.

### Image Quality and Registration
The mean signal-to-noise ratios (SNR) for the LGE MRI experiments were calculated from each heart by selecting a region of interest (Mewton et al., 2011) in remote/normal myocardium and dividing it by the SD of an ROI of equal area in the background of the same slice for five equally spaced slices within each heart. The mean SNRs from the DT-MRI experiments were calculated from the non-diffusion weighted images for each heart in the same manner as the LGE images. The signal-to-noise ratio of the high resolution LGE images for all hearts was $10 \pm 2$. The SNR of the non-diffusion weighted images of the DT-MRI was $59 \pm 15$. 3D rigid-body registration of LGE and DT-MRI data resulted in shifting of the LGE data by $0.8 \pm 0.9$ and $1.2 \pm 1.5$ mm in the x- and y-directions (in-plane) respectively and $0.2 \pm 0.5$ mm in the z-direction (through-plane), which results in sub pixel-level registration differences.

### Data De-correlation
Auto-correlation lengths were $3.0 \pm 0.6$ voxels ($3.0 \pm 0.6$ mm) in the in-plane x- and y-directions and $1.8 \pm 0.2$ voxels ($5.4 \pm 0.6$ mm) in the through-plane z-direction for normal hearts and remote myocardium in infarcted hearts. Auto-correlation lengths in the BZ were $1.2 \pm 0.1$ voxels ($1.2 \pm 0.1$ mm) in the x- and y-directions and $1.1 \pm 0.2$ voxels ($3.3 \pm 0.6$ mm) in the z-direction. Auto-correlation lengths in the infarct region were $1.7 \pm 0.2$ voxels ($1.7 \pm 0.2$ mm) in the x- and y-directions and $1.2 \pm 0.1$ voxels ($3.6 \pm 0.3$ mm) in the z-direction. The mean values were rounded for data de-correlation.

### Visualization of Microstructural Remodeling
**Figure 2A** depicts a representative short-axis LGE slice from an infarcted heart. Corresponding DT invariant maps are shown in **Figures 2B–D** and show an increase in ADC (**Figure 2B**), a decrease in FA (**Figure 2C**), and little apparent change in tissue mode (**Figure 2D**) within the BZ and infarct regions compared to remote myocardium. **Figure 3A** depicts, in three dimensions, diffusion tensor remodeling within a short-axis slice, a long-axis slice, and the entire infarct highlighted by a transparent isosurface. Each superquadric glyph's long-axis aligns with each voxel's primary eigenvector and is color coded by mapping the primary eigenvector's components to red-green-blue colormap. The brightness of the infarct glyphs is increased for contrast.

**Supplementary Movie 1** is available in the Supplementary Material. **Figure 3B** depicts the same short-axis slice seen in **Figure 3A**. **Figure 3C** depicts the diffusion profile in normal, remote, BZ, and infarcted myocardium by rendering the median microstructural tensors using superquadric glyphs. Superquadric glyphs from the infarct are visibly larger (higher ADC) and more isotropic (lower FA) than the glyphs represented by median invariant values from normal and remote myocardium. Glyphs within the BZ of all infarcted hearts show an intermediate size (intermediate ADC) and intermediate isotropy (intermediate FA) compared to the infarct, normal, and remote myocardium glyphs.

## Quantitative Evaluation of Microstructural Remodeling
LGE based segmentation of the DT-MRI data revealed significant differences in ADC and FA data between all pairwise comparisons of remote, BZ, and infarct regions within each infarcted heart (**Figure 4**, **Table 1**). The BZ within each individual heart is characterized by a significant increase in ADC and significant decreases in both FA and decrease in tissue mode relative to remote myocardium. The infarct region within each heart is characterized by an even larger and significant increase in ADC and significant decreases in both FA and mode.

**Figure 4** depicts pooled histograms with bootstrapped 95%-CIs of the de-correlated DT invariant data for each segmented region. DT invariant medians and their bootstrapped 95% CIs for each pooled region (normal, remote, BZ, and infarct) are listed in **Table 1**. Results from the bootstrapped analog to repeated measures ANOVA revealed significant differences across remote, BZ, and infarct regions for all hearts when comparing ADC ($p < 0.0001$) and FA ($p < 0.0001$), but were not significant for mode ($p = 0.47$). In a comparison of normal myocardium from control swine and remote myocardium from infarcted swine, two-group comparisons of the DT invariants did not reveal significant differences between median values of ADC ($p = 0.18$) and FA ($p = 0.51$), but did show a significant decrease in mode ($p = 0.02$) from normal to remote myocardium.

## DISCUSSION
Replacement fibrosis within an infarct significantly alters the electrophysiological and mechanical properties of the myocardium, leading to electrical abnormalities (e.g., reentrant ventricular arrhythmias) and mechanical dysfunction (e.g., heart failure). The BZ, consisting of a mixture of viable myocytes and fibrotic scar, facilitates slow conduction or reentry and is believed to serve as the substrate for ventricular tachyarrhythmias (Ursell et al., 1985; de Bakker et al., 1988). Furthermore, premature ventricular contractions that can initiate ventricular fibrillation have been shown to elicit from the BZ (Marrouche et al., 2004). Consequently, catheter-based ablation of the BZ is one strategy used to manage ventricular arrhythmias (Marchlinski, 2008) and up to 68% of successful ablation sites reside in the BZ (Verma et al., 2005). Thus, accurate characterization of the BZ is important for developing microstructurally realistic models of cardiac electrophysiology that may aid in identifying

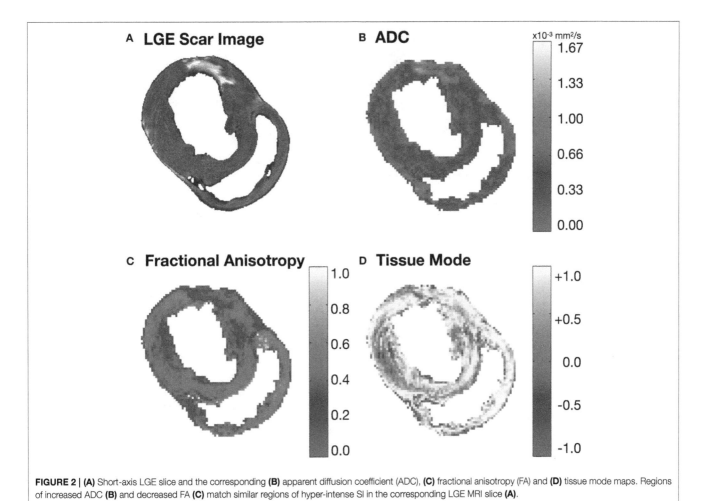

**FIGURE 2 | (A)** Short-axis LGE slice and the corresponding **(B)** apparent diffusion coefficient (ADC), **(C)** fractional anisotropy (FA) and **(D)** tissue mode maps. Regions of increased ADC **(B)** and decreased FA **(C)** match similar regions of hyper-intense SI in the corresponding LGE MRI slice **(A)**.

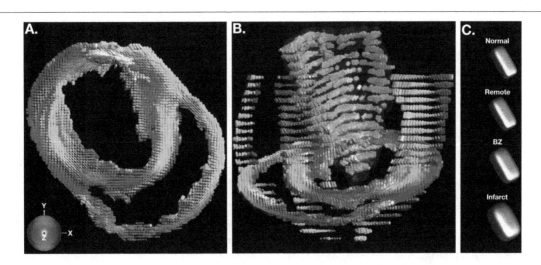

**FIGURE 3 | (A)** Short-axis depiction of diffusion tensor shape and orientation rendered with superquadric glyphs. The long-axis of each glyph is aligned with the primary eigenvector of the diffusion tensor at each voxel. Glyphs are color coded by the primary eigenvector direction with red grossly aligning with the left-right direction, green with the up-down direction, and blue with the through plane direction. The brightness of glyphs in the infarct is enhanced for contrast. **(B)** Short-axis, long-axis and whole-infarct depiction of diffusion tensor shape and orientation rendered with superquadric glyphs. **(C)** Superquadric glyphs of the diffusion tensor shape from normal hearts and remote, borderzone (BZ) and infarcted regions of the heart using the median values of ADC, FA, and tissue mode from **Table 1**. **Supplementary Movie 1** is available in the Supplementary Material.

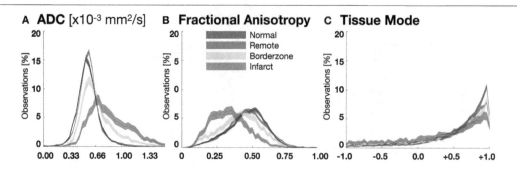

**FIGURE 4 |** Bootstrapped histograms with 95%-CIs (for each bin) for each segmented region (normal myocardium—black, remote—blue, borderzone—green, and infarct—red) using spatially de-correlated data pooled from all hearts for **(A)** apparent diffusion coefficient (ADC), **(B)** fractional anisotropy (FA), and **(C)** tissue mode. Non-overlapping regions between histograms reveal significant differences within a given bin. Significant microstructural remodeling (increase in the median ADC and decrease in median FA) is evident transitioning from normal to remote to borderzone to infarct histograms. Mode changes suggest an increase in fiber disarray (remodeling toward lower tissue mode values) within the borderzone and infarct regions.

**TABLE 1 |** Pooled tensor invariant medians and bootstrapped 95%-CIs of the medians for normal, remote, border zone (BZ), and infarcted myocardium.

| Region | Median ADC [× $10^{-3}$ mm²/s] | 95%-CI of median ADC [× $10^{-3}$ mm²/s] | Median fractional anisotropy | 95%-CI of median FA | Median tissue mode | 95%-CI of median mode |
|---|---|---|---|---|---|---|
| Normal | 0.563 | [0.560, 0.565] | 0.470 | [0.467, 0.473] | 0.743 | [0.736, 0.749] |
| Remote | 0.573[†] | [0.572, 0.577] | 0.464[†] | [0.462, 0.466] | 0.666[‡] | [0.660, 0.672] |
| BZ | 0.647[†] | [0.640, 0.650] | 0.417[†] | [0.412, 0.421] | 0.621 | [0.603, 0.635] |
| Infarct | 0.797[†] | [0.787, 0.807] | 0.330[†] | [0.325, 0.336] | 0.515 | [0.495, 0.538] |

[†]$p < 0.0001$ for bootstrap analog to repeated measures ANOVA.
[‡]$p = 0.02$ for two-group comparison.

of the location of the arrhythmogenic substrate prior to catheter ablation. Previous work by Ashikaga et al. has also suggested that the BZ is characterized by abnormal mechanics (Ashikaga et al., 2005). Therefore, in conjunction with the findings in this study, the BZ exhibits altered mechanics, electrophysiology, and microstructure.

The increase in BZ ADC likely results from the mixture of fibrotic scar and viable myocytes, which increases the extracellular volume and decreases the cellular volume. The larger increase in ADC within the infarct region corresponds to fibrotic scar fully replacing viable myocytes in this region and accords with previous studies observing higher rates of diffusion in infarct regions (Chen et al., 2003; Wu et al., 2007).

The observed decreases in FA within the BZ and infarct regions likely results from two remodeling phenomena: (1) the replacement of myocyte architecture with a more isotropic extracellular collagen network due to replacement fibrosis and; (2) an increase in myofiber disarray, which produces an apparent increase in the isotropy of water diffusion. Such observations of fiber disarray in infarcted myocardium have previously been observed (Chen et al., 2003; Strijkers et al., 2009). Decreased FA within the infarct from this study confirms observations of lower diffusion anisotropy within infarcted myocardium from previous studies (Chen et al., 2003; Wu et al., 2007). The observed decrease in the pairwise comparison of tissue mode within the BZ and infarct may also result from an increase in fiber disarray as local diffusion shifts away from

linear isotropy toward orthotropic or planar diffusion. These changes in ADC, FA, and tissue mode could be used to refine computational models of the heart by proportionally adjusting tissue conductivity (lower in regions of higher ADC) and anisotropy (lower electromechanical anisotropy in regions of lower FA).

Differences in ADC and FA between remote myocardium from infarcted hearts and normal myocardium from control hearts were not statistically significant. Previous studies have shown wall thinning and reduced strain (Weisman et al., 1985, 1988; Bogaert et al., 2000), as well as myocyte lengthening and hypertrophy in remote myocardium when compared to normal controls (Anand et al., 1997). However, collagen volume fraction is not significantly different in remote and control myocardium (Marijianowski et al., 1997), which is consistent with the similar ADC and FA in those regions. The observed tissue mode decrease from normal to remote myocardium indicates an increase in sheet-like structure, which may facilitate the previously observed remote compensatory hyperfunction and increased wall thickening (Sutton and Sharpe, 2000).

Although previous studies have evaluated microstructural remodeling in post-infarct myocardium using DT-MRI (Chen et al., 2003; Wu et al., 2007, 2011; Strijkers et al., 2009), they have used imprecise methods to segment regions into infarct, BZ, and remote regions using short-axis T2-weighted (non-diffusion weighted) images from the DT-MRI experiment. Our study is the first to use LGE MRI to create accurate segmentations of infarct and BZ on a voxel by voxel basis. Previous studies of myocardial remodeling after infarction using DT-MRI have also used *t*-tests to compare DT parameters between regions, however, due to non-Gaussian data sets, spatially correlated data, and unequal variances between data sets standard methods are not appropriate. By de-correlating the data and using bootstrapping methods this is the first study to correctly quantify statistically significant microstructural remodeling of BZ and infarcted myocardium using DT-MRI. These imaging and statistical methods establish that the BZ and infarct are unique microstructural environments.

Methods to evaluate cardiac microstructure with *in vivo* DT-MRI continue to evolve (Aliotta et al., 2017; Nielles-Vallespin et al., 2017). Moving forward studies could be performed that compare the BZ as apparent on *in vivo* LGE MRI to *in vivo* DT-MRI microstructural remodeling. Such studies could lead to important changes to the methods being used to build patient-specific computational models of cardiac disease.

## Limitations

This study used a combination of LGE MRI and DT-MRI to quantify microstructural remodeling in the post-infarct porcine heart, but histological data is not available to confirm the microstructural remodeling results. However, the histological characterization of BZ infarcts has been previously performed in detail. The purpose of this study was to identify MRI-based measures of microstructural remodeling that may aid more

accurate computational model construction. Futhermore, due to resolution constraints, voxels of intermediate SI designating BZ may arise from areas containing an interdigitated mixture of fibrosis and viable myocytes or from adjacent dense infarct and viable myocardium with a single well-defined border (Schelbert et al., 2010). The data from this study was not amenable to distinguishing between these two possible origins of intermediate SI and both were defined as BZ, but may have different electrophysiologic implications. Improvements in DT-MRI resolution and imaging methods may alleviate this ambiguity in BZ segmentation, however, the resolution achieved in this study is similar to those used in previous porcine DT-MRI studies (Wu et al., 2007, 2011).

## CONCLUSION

DT-MRI can identify regions of significant microstructural remodeling in the BZ that are distinct from both remote and infarcted myocardium.

## AUTHOR CONTRIBUTIONS

All authors contributed to the study conception and design. GK, MV, and DE were responsible for acquisition of data. All authors contributed to analysis and/or interpretation of data. drafting/revising the manuscript for intellectual content; and final manuscript approval.

## REFERENCES

Aliotta, E., Wu, H. H., and Ennis, D. B. (2017). Convex optimized diffusion encoding (CODE) gradient waveforms for minimum echo time and bulk motion-compensated diffusion-weighted MRI. *Magn. Reson. Med.* 77, 717–729. doi: 10.1002/mrm.26166

Anand, I. S., Liu, D., Chugh, S. S., Prahash, A. J., Gupta, S., John, R., et al. (1997). Isolated myocyte contractile function is normal in postinfarct remodeled rat heart with systolic dysfunction. *Circulation* 96, 3974–3984. doi: 10.1161/01.CIR.96.11.3974

Anversa, P., Loud, A. V., Levicky, V., and Guideri, G. (1985). Left ventricular failure induced by myocardial infarction. I. Myocyte hypertrophy. *Am. J. Physiol.* 248, H876–H882. doi: 10.1152/ajpheart.1985.248.6.H876

Ashikaga, H., Mickelsen, S. R., Ennis, D. B., Rodriguez, I., Kellman, P., Wen, H., et al. (2005). Electromechanical analysis of infarct border zone in chronic myocardial infarction. *Am. J. Physiol. Heart Circ. Physiol.* 289, H1099–H1105. doi: 10.1152/ajpheart.00423.2005

Ashikaga, H., Sasano, T., Dong, J., Zviman, M. M., Evers, R., Hopenfeld, B., et al. (2007). Magnetic resonance-based anatomical analysis of scar-related ventricular tachycardia: implications for catheter ablation. *Circ. Res.* 101, 939–947. doi: 10.1161/CIRCRESAHA.107.158980

Bogaert, J., Bosmans, H., Maes, A., Suetens, P., Marchal, G., and Rademakers, F. E. (2000). Remote myocardial dysfunction after acute anterior myocardial

Ennis, D. B., Kindlman, G., Rodriguez, I., Helm, P. A., and McVeigh, E. R. (2005). Visualization of tensor fields using superquadric glyphs. *Magn. Reson. Med.* 53, 169–176. doi: 10.1002/mrm.20318

Ennis, D. B., and Kindlmann, G. (2006). Orthogonal tensor invariants and the analysis of diffusion tensor magnetic resonance images. *Magn. Reson. Med.* 55, 136–146. doi: 10.1002/mrm.20741

Gahm, J. G., Kung, G. L., and Ennis, D. B. (2013). "Weighted component-based tensor distance applied to graph-based segmentation of cardiac DT-MRI," in *International Symposium on Biomedical Imaging.*. Available online at: https://ieeexplore.ieee.org/abstract/document/6556522/

infarction: impact of left ventricular shape on regional function: a magnetic resonance myocardial tagging study. *J. Am. Coll. Cardiol.* 35, 1525–1534. doi: 10.1016/S0735-1097(00)00601-X

Chen, J., Song, S. K., Liu, W., McLean, M., Allen, J. S., Tan, J., et al. (2003). Remodeling of cardiac fiber structure after infarction in rats quantified with diffusion tensor MRI. *Am. J. Physiol. Heart Circ. Physiol.* 285, H946–H954. doi: 10.1152/ajpheart.00889.2002

de Bakker, J. M., van Capelle, F. J., Janse, M. J., Tasseron, S., Vermeulen, J. T., de Jonge, N., et al. (1993). Slow conduction in the infarcted human heart. 'Zigzag' course of activation. *Circulation* 88, 915–926. doi: 10.1161/01.CIR.88.3.915

de Bakker, J. M., van Capelle, F. J., Janse, M. J., Wilde, A. A., Coronel, R., Becker, A. E., et al. (1988). Reentry as a cause of ventricular tachycardia in patients with chronic ischemic heart disease: electrophysiologic and anatomic correlation. *Circulation* 77, 589–606. doi: 10.1161/01.CIR.77.3.589

Dillon, S. M., Allessie, M. A., Ursell, P. C., and Wit, A. L. (1988). Influences of anisotropic tissue structure on reentrant circuits in the epicardial border zone of subacute canine infarcts. *Circ Res.* 63, 182–206. doi: 10.1161/01.RES.63.1.182

Ellingson, B. M., Malkin, M. G., Rand, S. D., Connelly, J. M., Quinsey, C., LaViolette, P. S., et al. (2010). Validation of functional diffusion maps (fDMs) as a biomarker for human glioma cellularity. *J. Magn. Reson. Imaging* 31, 538–548. doi: 10.1002/jmri.22068

Ponnaluri, A. V., Perotti, L. E., Liu, M., Qu, Z., Weiss, J. N., Ennis, D. B., et al. (2016). Electrophysiology of heart failure using a rabbit model: from the failing myocyte to ventricular fibrillation. *PLoS Comput. Biol.* 12:e1004968. doi: 10.1371/journal.pcbi.1004968

Porter, D. A., and Heidemann, R. M. (2009). High resolution diffusion-weighted imaging using readout-segmented echo-planar imaging, parallel imaging and a two-dimensional navigator-based reacquisition. *Magn. Reson. Imaging* 62, 468–475. doi: 10.1002/mrm.22024

Schelbert, E. B., Hsu, L. Y., Anderson, S. A., Mohanty, B. D., Karim, S. M., Kellman, P., et al. (2010). Late gadolinium-enhancement cardiac

Gahm, J. K., Wisniewski, N., Kindlmann, G., Kung, G. L., Klug, W. S., Garfinkel, A., et al. (2012). Linear invariant tensor interpolation applied to cardiac diffusion tensor MRI. *Med. Image Comput. Comput. Assist. Interv.* 15, 494–501. doi: 10.1007/978-3-642-33418-4_61

Karamitsos, T. D., Francis, J. M., Myerson, S., Selvanayagam, J. B., and Neubauer, S. (2009). The role of cardiovascular magnetic resonance imaging in heart failure. *J. Am. Coll. Cardiol.* 54, 1407–1424. doi: 10.1016/j.jacc.2009.04.094

Kim, R. J., Chen, E. L., Lima, J. A., and Judd, R. M. (1996). Myocardial Gd-DTPA kinetics determine MRI contrast enhancement and reflect the extent and severity of myocardial injury after acute reperfused infarction. *Circulation* 94, 3318–3326. doi: 10.1161/01.CIR.94.12.3318

Kim, R. J., Wu, E., Rafael, A., Chen, E. L., Parker, M. A., Simonetti, O., et al. (2000). The use of contrast-enhanced magnetic resonance imaging to identify reversible myocardial dysfunction. *N. Engl. J. Med.* 343, 1445–1453. doi: 10.1056/NEJM200011163432003

Krishnamoorthi, S., Perotti, L. E., Borgstrom, N. P., Ajijola, O. A., Frid, A., Ponnaluri, A. V., et al. (2014). Simulation methods and validation criteria for modeling cardiac ventricular electrophysiology. *PLoS ONE* 9:e114494. doi: 10.1371/journal.pone.0114494

Kung, G. L., Nguyen, T. C., Itoh, A., Skare, S., Ingels, N. B. Jr., Miller, D. C., et al. (2011). The presence of two local myocardial sheet populations confirmed by diffusion tensor MRI and histological validation. *J. Magn. Reson. Imaging* 34, 1080–1091. doi: 10.1002/jmri.22725

Lazic, S. E. (2010). The problem of pseudoreplication in neuroscientific studies: is it affecting your analysis? *BMC Neurosci.* 11:5. doi: 10.1186/1471-2202-11-5

Marchlinski, F. E. (2008). Ventricular tachycardia ablation: moving beyond treatment of last resort. *Circ. Arrhythm Electrophysiol.* 1, 147–149. doi: 10.1161/CIRCEP.108.801563

Marijianowski, M. M., Teeling, P., and Becker, A. E. (1997). Remodeling after myocardial infarction in humans is not associated with interstitial fibrosis of noninfarcted myocardium. *J. Am. Coll. Cardiol.* 30, 76–82. doi: 10.1016/S0735-1097(97)00100-9

Marrouche, N. F., Verma, A., Wazni, O., Schweikert, R., Martin, D. O., Saliba, W., et al. (2004). Mode of initiation and ablation of ventricular fibrillation storms in patients with ischemic cardiomyopathy. *J. Am. Coll. Cardiol.* 43, 1715–1720. doi: 10.1016/j.jacc.2004.03.004

Mewton, N., Liu, C. Y., Croisille, P., Bluemke, D., and Lima, J. A. (2011). Assessment of myocardial fibrosis with cardiovascular magnetic resonance. *J. Am. Coll. Cardiol.* 57, 891–903. doi: 10.1016/j.jacc.2010.11.013

Miragoli, M., Salvarani, N., and Rohr, S. (2007). Myofibroblasts induce ectopic activity in cardiac tissue. *Circ Res.* 101, 755–758. doi: 10.1161/CIRCRESAHA.107.160549

Morita, N., Sovari, A. A., Xie, Y., Fishbein, M. C., Mandel, W. J., Garfinkel, A., et al. (2009). Increased susceptibility of aged hearts to ventricular fibrillation during oxidative stress. *Am. J. Physiol. Heart Circ. Physiol.* 297, H1594–H1605. doi: 10.1152/ajpheart.00579.2009

Nielles-Vallespin, S., Khalique, Z., Ferreira, P. F., de Silva, R., Scott, A. D., Kilner, P., et al. (2017). Assessment of myocardial microstructural dynamics by *in vivo* diffusion tensor cardiac magnetic resonance. *J. Am. Coll. Cardiol.* 69, 661–676. doi: 10.1016/j.jacc.2016.11.051

magnetic resonance identifies postinfarction myocardial fibrosis and the border zone at the near cellular level in *ex vivo* rat heart. *Circ. Cardiovasc. Imaging* 3, 743–752. doi: 10.1161/CIRCIMAGING.108.835793

Strijkers, G. J., Bouts, A., Blankesteijn, W. M., Peeters, T. H., Vilanova, A., van Prooijen, M. C., et al. (2009). Diffusion tensor imaging of left ventricular remodeling in response to myocardial infarction in the mouse. *NMR Biomed.* 22, 182–190. doi: 10.1002/nbm.1299

Sutton, M. G., and Sharpe, N. (2000). Left ventricular remodeling after myocardial infarction: pathophysiology and therapy. *Circulation* 101, 2981–2988. doi: 10.1161/01.CIR.101.25.2981

Tao, Q., Milles, J., Zeppenfeld, K., Lamb, H. J., Bax, J. J., Reiber, J. H., et al. (2010). Automated segmentation of myocardial scar in late enhancement MRI using combined intensity and spatial information. *Magn. Reson. Imaging* 64, 586–594. doi: 10.1002/mrm.22422

Ursell, P. C., Gardner, P. I., Albala, A., Fenoglio, J. J. Jr., and Wit, A. L. (1985). Structural and electrophysiological changes in the epicardial border zone of canine myocardial infarcts during infarct healing. *Circ Res.* 56, 436–451. doi: 10.1161/01.RES.56.3.436

Verma, A., Marrouche, N. F., Schweikert, R. A., Saliba, W., Wazni, O., Cummings, J., et al. (2005). Relationship between successful ablation sites and the scar border zone defined by substrate mapping for ventricular tachycardia post-myocardial infarction. *J. Cardiovasc. Electrophysiol.* 16, 465–471. doi: 10.1046/j.1540-8167.2005.40443.x

Weisman, H. F., Bush, D. E., Mannisi, J. A., and Bulkley, B. H. (1985). Global cardiac remodeling after acute myocardial infarction: a study in the rat model. *J. Am. Coll. Cardiol.* 5, 1355–1362. doi: 10.1016/S0735-1097(85)80348-X

Weisman, H. F., Bush, D. E., Mannisi, J. A., Weisfeldt, M. L., and Healy, B. (1988). Cellular mechanisms of myocardial infarct expansion. *Circulation* 78, 186–201. doi: 10.1161/01.CIR.78.1.186

Wu, E. X., Wu, Y., Nicholls, J. M., Wang, J., Liao, S., Zhu, S., et al. (2007). MR diffusion tensor imaging study of postinfarct myocardium structural remodeling in a porcine model. *Magn. Reson. Med.* 58, 687–695. doi: 10.1002/mrm.21350

Wu, Y., Zhang, L. J., Zou, C., Tse, H. F., and Wu, E. X. (2011). Transmural heterogeneity of left ventricular myocardium remodeling in postinfarct porcine model revealed by MR diffusion tensor imaging. *J. Magn. Reson. Imaging* 34, 43–49. doi: 10.1002/jmri.22589

# 5

# Acute Tachycardia Increases Aortic Distensibility, but Reduces Total Arterial Compliance Up to a Moderate Heart Rate

*Yunlong Huo[1,2], Huan Chen[3] and Ghassan S. Kassab[3]\**

[1] PKU-HKUST Shenzhen-Hongkong Institution, Shenzhen, China, [2] Department of Mechanics and Engineering Science, College of Engineering, Peking University, Beijing, China, [3] California Medical Innovations Institute, San Diego, CA, United States

**\*Correspondence:**
Ghassan S. Kassab
gkassab@calmi2.org

**Background:** The differential effects of rapid cardiac pacing on small and large vessels have not been well-established. The objective of this study was to investigate the effect of pacing-induced acute tachycardia on hemodynamics and arterial stiffness.

**Methods:** The pressure and flow waves in ascending aorta and femoral artery of six domestic swine were recorded simultaneously at baseline and heart rates (HR) of 135 and 155 beats per minutes (bpm) and analyzed by the models of Windkessel and Womersley types. Accordingly, the flow waves were simultaneously measured at carotid and femoral arteries to quantify aortic pulse wave velocity (PWV). The arterial distensibility was identified in small branches of coronary, carotid and femoral arteries with diameters of 300–600 $\mu$m by *ex vivo* experiments.

**Results:** The rapid pacing in HR up to 135 bpm reduced the total arterial compliance, stroke volume, systemic pulse pressure, and central systolic pressure by $36 \pm 17$, $38 \pm 26$, $29 \pm 16$, and $23 \pm 12\%$, respectively, despite no statistical difference of mean aortic pressure, cardiac output, peripheral resistance, and vascular flow patterns. The pacing also resulted in a decrease of distensibility of small muscular arteries, but an increase of aortic distensibility. Pacing from 135 to 155 bpm had negligible effects on systemic and local hemodynamics and arterial stiffness.

**Conclusions:** There is an acute mismatch in the response of aorta and small arteries to pacing from basal HR to 135 bpm, which may have important pathological implications under chronic tachycardia conditions.

Keywords: acute tachycardia, total arterial compliance, arterial distensibility, pulse wave velocity, Windkessel model, Womersley model

## INTRODUCTION

Epidemiologic data show that hypertension and atrial fibrillation (AF) often coexist (Dzeshka et al., 2017; Andreadis and Geladari, 2018; Verdecchia et al., 2018). Patients with high blood pressure (BP) show higher risk of developing AF by 50% in men and 40% in women (Benjamin et al., 1994) while >60% of patients with AF have hypertension (Verdecchia et al., 2018). Although multiple clinical studies have shown a direct relationship between BP levels and the risk of AF, the form of the relationship remains unknown (Conen et al., 2009; Grundvold et al., 2012; Verdecchia et al., 2012a,b). Patients with high BP, however, do not benefit from the pharmacological heart rate (HR) lowering (Rimoldi et al., 2016). It is also unclear whether the pharmacological BP control can relieve the incidence and progression of AF (Manolis et al., 2012; Verdecchia et al., 2016; Whelton et al., 2018). Hence, one objective of this study is to quantify the relationship between acute tachycardia and systemic hemodynamics in normotensive swine.

A large number of epidemiological studies have shown that elevated HR increases cardiovascular morbidity and mortality such that high HR is considered as a prognostic factor for the cardiovascular disease independent of other risk factors (e.g., hypertension, hyperlipidemia, diabetes, and so on) (Bergel, 1961; Palatini and Julius, 2004; Diaz et al., 2005; Fox et al., 2007; Lonn et al., 2010; Fox and Ferrari, 2011). The pathophysiology of elevated HR for cardiovascular disease is potentially involved in the decrease of arterial distensibility because a long-term elevated arterial stiffness can be an important determinant of the development and progression of hypertension (Stefanadis et al., 1998; O'Rourke and Hashimoto, 2007; Fox and Ferrari, 2011; Safar, 2018). There is also debate on the mechanical response of large conduit arteries to acute tachycardia (Stefanadis et al., 1998; Liang et al., 1999; Wilkinson et al., 2000; Albaladejo et al., 2001; Lantelme et al., 2002; Haesler et al., 2004) and lack of studies on the mechanical response of small arteries to heart rate changes. Based on the *in vivo* and *ex vivo* measurements, the second objective of this study is to investigate the effects of rapid pacing on arterial distensibility in aorta and small arteries of normotensive swine, which can enhance the understanding of arterial stiffness relevant to elevated HR.

Total arterial compliance and peripheral resistance are two key parameters that have been widely used to characterize systemic hemodynamics (Liu et al., 1986; Stergiopulos et al., 1994, 1995; Westerhof et al., 2009; Nichols and McDonald, 2011). Based on the classical two-element Windkessel model, pulse pressure method has been used to estimate the total arterial compliance accurately (Stergiopulos et al., 1994). To generalize the model, researchers have added more elements (e.g., three-element Windkessel model) (Westerhof et al., 1971; Latson et al., 1988; Laskey et al., 1990) and incorporated non-linearities (Burattini et al., 1987; Li et al., 1990). Moreover, the three-element Windkessel model can be used to quantify aortic characteristic impedance, which is proportional to arterial stiffness (Huo and Kassab, 2006, 2007). On the other hand, pulse wave reflections derived from transmission theory (Westerhof et al., 1972, 2006; Westerhof and Westerhof, 2013) are sensitive to heart rate and peripheral vasculature (Quick et al., 1998). The analytic model of Womersley type features transient flow patterns in aorta and peripheral arteries (Zheng et al., 2010). The third objective of this study is to use the models of Windkessel and Womersley types to perform systemic and local hemodynamic analyses.

We hypothesize that pacing-induced acute tachycardia decreases the acute stiffness of aorta and increases the acute stiffness of small arteries in some pressure range, which results in an acute mismatch. Moreover, pacing-induced acute tachycardia reduces the total arterial compliance, systemic pulse pressure

(PP), central systolic pressure, and stroke volume (SV) in some pressure range despite no statistical difference of mean aortic pressure (MAP), cardiac output (CO), peripheral resistance, and transient flow patterns in aorta and peripheral arteries. To test these hypotheses, the simultaneous measurement of blood pressure, flow, and cross-sectional area (CSA) was performed in ascending aorta and femoral artery of six domestic swine at baseline and during right atrial pacing to HR of 135, 155, and 170 beats per minutes (bpm). Analytic models of Windkessel and Womersley types were used to carry out transient hemodynamic analysis based on these experimental measurements. Aortic pulse wave velocity (PWV) was determined using two simultaneously measured flow waves. In addition to the *in vivo* experiments, the *ex vivo* pulsatile pressure-diameter measurements were demonstrated in small branches of coronary, carotid and femoral arteries when the frequency was varied in the range of 1–3 Hz (mimicking the HR of 60–180 bpm). The physiological implications of initial rapid pacing are discussed along with the limitations and significance of the study.

## MATERIALS AND METHODS
### Animal Preparation
Studies were performed on six domestic swine weighing 71 ± 8 kg for *in vivo* hemodynamic pacing measurements and six controls with similar weights for *ex vivo* measurements of dynamic pressure and diameter waves in small arteries of 300–600 μm in diameter. All animal experiments were performed in accordance with Indiana University, Purdue University, Indianapolis, consistent with the NIH guidelines (Guide for the care and use of laboratory animals) on the protection of animals used for scientific purposes. The experimental protocols were approved by the Institutional Animal Care and Use Committee of Indiana University.

The animal preparation was similar to previous studies (Zheng et al., 2010; Huo and Kassab, 2015). Briefly, surgical anesthesia was induced with TKX (Telaxol 500 mg, Ketamine 250 mg, Xylazine 250 mg) and maintained with 2% isoflurane. The animal was intubated and ventilated with room air and oxygen by a respiratory pump. A side branch from the left jugular vein was dissected and cannulated with 7Fr. sheath for administration of drugs (e.g., heparin, lidocaine, levophed, papaverine, and saline). The right femoral artery was cannulated with a 7Fr. sheath and connected to a pressure transducer (Summit Disposable Pressure Transducer, Baxter Healthcare; error of ±2% at full scale) for monitoring arterial blood pressure.

The right jugular vein was exposed and cannulated with a 9Fr. sheath for the advancement of the pacing lead into the right atrium. The pacing lead (Medtronic 5568) was screwed into the wall of right atrium and connected to a pacemaker (Medtronic Enpulse E2DR01) which was placed into a subcutaneous pocket. The ascending and descending aortas and femoral artery were dissected. Perivascular flow probes (Transonic Systems Inc.; relative error of ±2% at full scale) were mounted on these arteries to measure the volumetric flow rate. Flow and pressure were continuously recorded using a Biopac MP 150 data acquisition system. The cross-sectional area (CSA) of arteries was determined using ultrasound (Philips IE33 ultrasound system).

## *In vivo* Measurements

The heart rate was paced to 135, 155, and 170 bpm as compared with basal HR of about 90 bpm (range of 80–105 bpm). The animals were allowed to recover to basal HR between consecutive pacing sessions. Electrocardiography (ECG) signals were used to monitor HR. The aortic, carotid and femoral flow rates were measured simultaneously. The femoral arterial pressure was measured by the pressure transducer connected to the 7Fr.

sheath. The aortic pressure was determined when the sheath was advanced to aorta under fluoroscopy.

We have shown an abrupt decrease of blood pressure and flow after rapid pacing (initial period) and then recovered close to baseline after about 3–5 min of pacing (recovery period) (Zheng et al., 2010). Since the present study only considered the hemodynamic analysis in the recovery period, the flow and pressure waves as well as ECG signals were continuously recorded for about 10 min under each HR by a data acquisition system (MP 150, Biopac Systems Inc.). Finally, animals were euthanized by an injection of pentobarbital sodium (300 mg/kg).

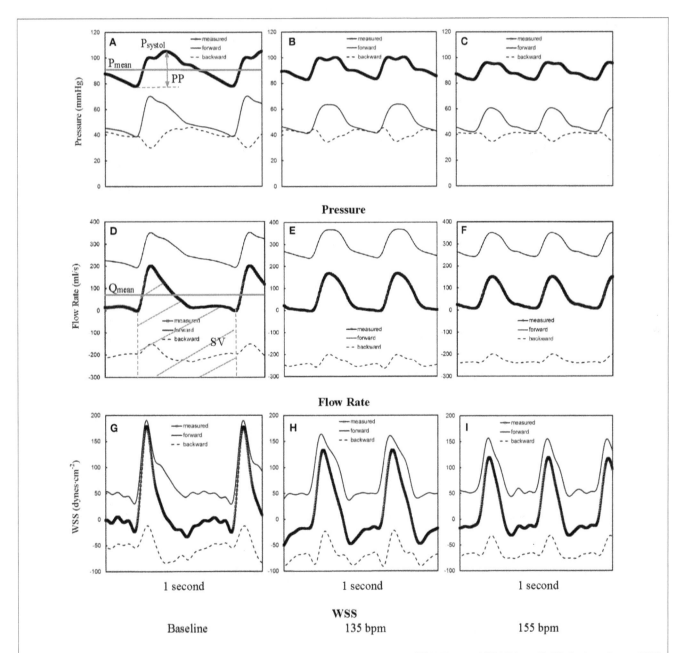

**FIGURE 1** | Pressure waves in ascending aorta **(A)** at baseline and after the heart rate was paced to **(B)** 135 bpm and **(C)** 155 bpm. **(D–F,G–I)** refer to flow and WSS waves, respectively, in ascending aorta corresponding to **A–C**. The marked, solid, and dash lines represent the measured, forward, and backward waves, respectively.

## Ex vivo Measurements in Small Arteries

Similar to previous studies (Huo et al., 2012, 2013; Lu et al., 2017), arteries with diameters of 300–600 μm were dissected free of periarterial tissues. Two black marks were made at the two ends of the artery with waterproof India ink. The image of the vessel was displayed on screen with a CCD camera mounted on the dissection microscope to determine the *in vivo* length (i.e., the length between the two black marks) and then isolated from various positions (i.e., small branches of coronary, carotid, and femoral arteries) and dissected free of fat and connective tissue after euthanasia. The side branches were ligated with suture under dissection microscope in 4°C HEPES PSS (physiological saline solution). An artery specimen was mounted on the two cannulas in an organ bath chamber containing PSS solution. One cannula was connected with a

pressure transducer through a Y tube, while the other was connected with a bottle of PSS solution that induced sawtooth flow wave by a piston pump. The temperature in the bath and bottle was gradually increased to 37°C in 10 min. The vessel was stretched close to the *in vivo* length (axial stretch ratio approximately equals to 1.4). The image of the vessel was displayed on screen with a CCD camera mounted on a stereo microscope and the changes of outer diameter were measured with dimensional analysis software (DIAMTRAK 3+, Australia). The pressure transducer and diameter tracings were interfaced into a computer by a data acquisition system (MP 150, Biopac Systems Inc.), which monitored transient changes of pressure and diameter. The time-averaged pressure over a cardiac cycle equaled to 80 mmHg. We determined the changes of the arterial distensibility as the frequency increases from 1

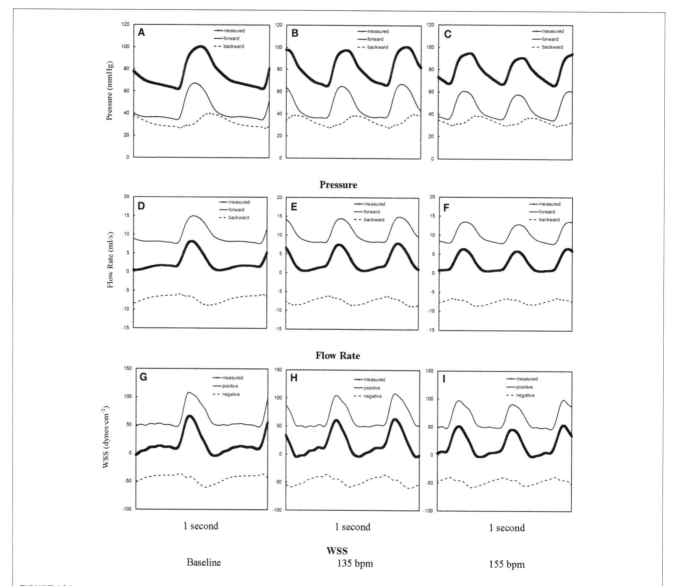

**FIGURE 2 |** Pressure waves in femoral artery **(A)** at baseline and after the heart rate was paced to **(B)** 135 bpm and **(C)** 155 bpm. **(D–F,G–I)** refer to flow and WSS waves, respectively, in femoral artery corresponding to **(A–C)**. The marked, solid, and dash lines represent the measured, forward, and backward waves, respectively.

to 3 Hz (by a step of 0.5 Hz) to mimic HR from 60 to 180 bpm.

## Windkessel Analysis

Based on the *in vivo* measurements of pressure and flow waves in aorta and femoral artery, we determined the time-averaged pressure and flow over a cardiac cycle ($P_{mean}$ and $Q_{mean}$). MAP and PP equal to $P_{mean}$ and the difference of systolic and diastolic pressures, respectively, in ascending aorta. The CO was computed by $Q_{mean} \times 60$ s and the SV was calculated as the ratio of CO to HR. The classical two-element Windkessel model (Stergiopulos et al., 1994) is written as:

$$Z(\omega) = \frac{R}{1 + j\omega RC} \tag{1}$$

where $Z(\omega)$ is the input impedance, $\omega$ the angular frequency after Fourier transformation, C the total arterial compliance [= dV(t)/dP(t), where V(t) is the blood volume of the arterial system and P(t) is the blood pressure of the most proximal artery], and R the peripheral resistance (=$P_{mean}/Q_{mean}$). The peripheral resistance was obtained directly from the measured pressure and flow waves and the total arterial compliance was estimated by the pulse pressure method (Stergiopulos et al., 1994). The

aortic characteristic impedance ($Z_c$) was determined using the three-element Windkessel model (Westerhof et al., 1971) as:

$$Z(\omega) = Z_c + \frac{R - Z_c}{1 + j\omega (R - Z_c) C} \tag{2}$$

where $Z_c$ is the characteristic impedance, i.e., an important parameter to address the relationship between pulsatile pressure and pulsatile flow in an artery when pressure and flow waves are not influenced by wave reflection. Since R and C are determined by experimental measurements and pulse pressure method of Equation (1), $Z_c$ is estimated by minimizing the error between the input impedance by Fourier transformation of the ratio of the measured pressure to flow waves $\left[ \frac{p_{measured}(t)}{q_{measured}(t)} \right]$ and the one predicted by Equation (2), i.e., minimizing $\left[ \frac{|Z_{measured}(\omega) - Z_{estimated}(\omega)|}{|Z_{measured}(\omega)|} \right]$.

## Forward and Backward Waves

The forward [$p_{forward}(t)$, $q_{forward}(t)$] and backward [$p_{backward}(t)$, $q_{backward}(t)$] pressure and flow waves are given as Westerhof et al. (1972):

$$p_{forward}(t) = [p_{measured}(t) + Z_c \cdot q_{measured}(t)]/2;$$
$$q_{forward}(t) = p_{forward}(t)/Z_c \tag{3}$$

TABLE 1 | Hemodynamic parameters in ascending aorta and femoral artery at baseline (80–105 bpm) and HR of 135 and 155 bpm.

| Animals | Ascending aorta | | | | | |
|---|---|---|---|---|---|---|
| | R (mmHg·s/ml) | | | C (ml/mmHg) | | |
| | Baseline | 135 bpm | 155 bpm | Baseline | 135 bpm | 155 bpm |
| 1 | 1.83 | 1.77 | 1.88 | 0.54 | 0.25 | 0.27 |
| 2 | 1.37 | 1.38 | 1.37 | 0.48 | 0.40 | 0.39 |
| 3 | 0.87 | 1.19 | 1.16 | 0.97 | 0.54 | 0.52 |
| 4 | 0.48 | 0.46 | 0.43 | 1.41 | 0.98 | 1.05 |
| 5 | 0.56 | 0.75 | 0.84 | 0.59 | 0.27 | 0.18 |
| 6 | 1.62 | 1.64 | 1.65 | 0.44 | 0.37 | 0.36 |
| Mean ± SD | 1.21 ± 0.57 | 1.20 ± 0.51 | 1.22 ± 0.53 | 0.74 ± 0.38 | 0.47 ± 0.27 | 0.46 ± 0.31 |
| p-value | 0.26 (Baseline-135) | 0.40 (135–155) | | 0.009 (Baseline-135) | 0.77 (135–155) | |

| Animals | Femoral artery | | | | | |
|---|---|---|---|---|---|---|
| | R (mmHg·s/ml) | | | C (ml/mmHg) | | |
| | Baseline | 135 bpm | 155 bpm | Baseline | 135 bpm | 155 bpm |
| 1 | 41.32 | 40.63 | 46.37 | 0.023 | 0.014 | 0.011 |
| 2 | 27.68 | 25.67 | 31.82 | 0.032 | 0.022 | 0.025 |
| 3 | 29.72 | 30.01 | 34.09 | 0.043 | 0.025 | 0.028 |
| 4 | 24.23 | 24.91 | 29.32 | 0.033 | 0.026 | 0.025 |
| 5 | 21.31 | 22.30 | 22.51 | 0.029 | 0.018 | 0.018 |
| 6 | 41.50 | 41.69 | 42.24 | 0.021 | 0.020 | 0.017 |
| Mean ± SD | 30.96 ± 8.59 | 30.87 ± 8.36 | 34.39 ± 8.71 | 0.030 ± 0.008 | 0.021 ± 0.004 | 0.021 ± 0.006 |
| p-value | 0.85 (Baseline-135) | 0.02 (135–155) | | 0.009 (Baseline-135) | 0.89 (135–155) | |

*R and C refer to the peripheral resistance and total arterial compliance, respectively.*

$$p_{backward}(t) = [p_{measured}(t) - Z_c \cdot q_{measured}(t)]/2;$$

$$q_{backward}(t) = -p_{backward}(t)/Z_c \qquad (4)$$

The forward pressure and flow waves have the same shape. The backward pressure and flow waves also have the same shape, but are inverted with respect to another.

## Womersley Analysis

Similar to a previous study (Zheng et al., 2010), the equation for the pulsatile flow velocity profile across the lumen, $u(r, t)$, is given as:

$$u(r,t) = \text{REAL}\left( \frac{2Q(0)\left(R^2 - r^2\right)}{\pi R^4} + \sum_{\omega=1}^{\infty} \frac{\frac{Q(\omega)}{\pi R^2} \cdot \left(1 - \frac{J_0(\Lambda r/R)}{J_0(\Lambda)}\right)}{1 - \frac{2J_1(\Lambda)}{\Lambda J_0(\Lambda)}} e^{i\omega t} \right) \quad (5)$$

where $r$ is the radial coordinate, $R$ is the radius of artery, $\Lambda^2 = i^3\alpha^2$, $q_{measured}(t) = Q(\omega)e^{i\omega t}$, $J_0$ is a Bessel function of zero order and first kind, and $J_1$ is a Bessel function of first order and first kind. Accordingly, wall shear stress (WSS), $\tau(R, t)$, and oscillatory shear index (OSI) for pulsatile blood flow can be written as:

$$\tau(R,t) = \text{REAL}\left( \frac{4\mu}{\pi R^3}Q(0) - \sum_{\omega=1}^{\infty} \frac{\frac{\mu Q(\omega)}{\pi R^3} \cdot \frac{\Lambda J_1(\Lambda)}{J_0(\Lambda)}}{1 - \frac{2J_1(\Lambda)}{\Lambda J_0(\Lambda)}} e^{i\omega t} \right) \quad (6)$$

$$\text{OSI} = \frac{1}{2}\left( 1 - \frac{\left| \frac{1}{T}\int_0^T \tau(R,t) \right|}{\frac{1}{T}\int_0^T |\tau(R,t)|} \right) \quad (7)$$

The viscosity ($\mu$) and density ($\rho$) were assumed to be 4.0 cp and 1.06 g/cm$^3$, respectively. The forward and backward WSS were computed, based on $q_{forward}(t)$ and $q_{backward}(t)$, respectively.

## PWV and Dynamic Elastic Modulus

Aortic PWV is the velocity at which the arterial pulse propagates through the vessel and used clinically as a measure of arterial

**TABLE 2 |** PWV along aorta from carotid to femoral arteries at baseline (80–105 bpm) and HR of 135 and 155 bpm.

| Animals | PWV along aorta from carotid to femoral arteries (m/s) | | |
|---|---|---|---|
| | Baseline | 135 bpm | 155 bpm |
| 1 | 8.45 | 6.14 | 6.31 |
| 2 | 9.33 | 8.81 | 7.97 |
| 3 | 4.95 | 3.75 | 3.50 |
| 4 | 3.61 | 3.30 | 3.25 |
| 5 | 4.50 | 3.72 | 3.63 |
| 6 | 9.34 | 8.35 | 6.99 |
| Mean ± SD | 6.70 ± 2.62 | 5.68 ± 2.47 | 5.28 ± 2.06 |
| p-value | | 0.017 (Baseline-135) | 0.15 (135–155) |

PWV refers to the pulse wave velocity.

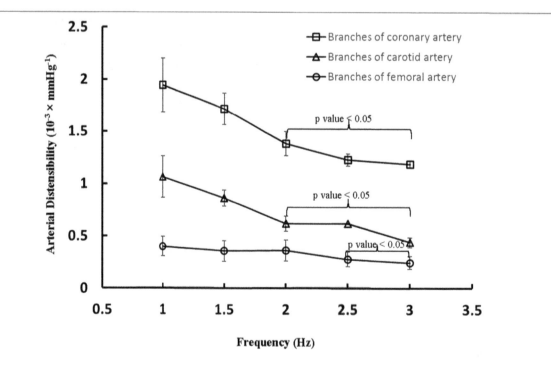

**FIGURE 3 |** Arterial distensibility (Unit: $10^{-3} \times$ mmHg$^{-1}$) as a function of frequency in isolated small branches of coronary, carotid or femoral arteries. There is statistically significant difference ($p < 0.05$) in arterial distensibility between 1.5 Hz (mimicking the HR of 90 bpm) and higher frequencies in parentheses (i.e., $\geq 2$ Hz in branches of coronary and carotid artery and $\geq 2.5$ Hz in branches of femoral artery).

stiffness. Similar to a previous study (Mohiaddin et al., 1993), we determined aortic PWV (PWV = L/ΔT, where L is the distance between carotid and femoral arteries and ΔT is the pulse transit time). The distance, L, was calculated as the distance between the sternal notch and the carotid site subtracted from the distance between the sternal notch and the femoral site using the subtraction method (Butlin et al., 2013) while the pulse transit time, ΔT, was computed using the foot-to-foot method based on the simultaneously measured carotid and femoral flow waves (Mohiaddin et al., 1993).

When tissue is modeled by Kelvin-Voigt model (Bergel, 1961), the vessel dynamic elastic modulus can be written as:

$$E_{dyn} = E' + j\eta\omega = D_{mean} \left| \frac{\Delta p}{\Delta D} \right| \cos\phi + j\eta\omega \quad (8)$$

where $\left| \frac{\Delta p}{\Delta D} \right|$ is the amplitude ratio of sinusoidal pressure and diameter waves and $\phi = \tan^{-1}\left(\frac{\eta\omega}{E}\right)$ is the phase lag of outer diameter behind pressure. Since $\phi$ is small (<0.2 rad), $E_{dyn} \cong E$ such that the dynamic elastic modulus ($\cong D_{mean}\left|\frac{\Delta p}{\Delta D}\right|$) can be determined by Fourier transformation of the *in vitro* measured pulsatile waves. Furthermore, the arterial distensibility ($= \frac{2}{dynamic\ elastic\ modulus}$) was computed in small branches of coronary, carotid and femoral arteries.

## Data Analysis

The measurements were repeated five times and averaged at each HR per animal. The mean and standard deviation (mean ± SD) were computed by averaging over all animals in each HR group. One Way Repeated Measures ANOVA (SigmaStat 3.5) was used to compare the various parameters (e.g., R, C, CO, SV, PWV, $Z_c$, CSA, etc.) between baseline and various HR, where p- < 0.05 represented statistically significant differences.

## RESULTS

**Figures 1A–C** show pressure waves in ascending aorta at baseline and after HR was paced to 135 bpm and 155 bpm, where the marked, solid, and dash lines represent the measured, forward, and backward pressure waves, respectively. Accordingly, **Figures 1D–F** show flow waves and **Figures 1G–I** show WSS waves in ascending aorta at different HR. **Figures 2A–I** show pressure, flow, and WSS waves in femoral artery at baseline, 135 bpm, and 155 bpm in correspondence with **Figures 1A–I**. The ascending aorta and femoral artery of swine had MAP of 91 ± 6 and 86 ± 7 mmHg (averaged over 6 animals), respectively, in the supine position regardless of HR. The CO was 5.9 ± 3.6 and 5.6 ± 3.3 L/min (averaged over 6 animals) at baseline and 135 bpm, respectively. As shown in **Figures 1A,D**, SV, systemic PP, and central systolic pressure were reduced by 38 ± 26%, 29 ± 16%, and 23 ± 12% (averaged over 6 animals, $p < 0.05$), respectively, as HR increased from baseline to 135 bpm. The peripheral resistance was relatively unchanged ($p > 0.25$) as HR increased from baseline to 135 bpm while the total arterial compliance distal to aorta and femoral artery was decreased by 36

± 17 and 29 ± 14% ($p < 0.05$), respectively, as shown in **Table 1**. There was no statistical difference in the total arterial compliance, systemic PP, central systolic pressure, CO, and SV between 135 and 155 bpm.

The aortic (carotid-femoral) PWV was reduced ($p < 0.05$) as HR increased from baseline to 135 bpm, as shown in **Table 2**. There was no statistical difference of PWV ($p = 0.15$) between 135 and 155 bpm. The characteristic impedance in the descending aorta had values of 0.31 ± 0.22, 0.27 ± 0.13, and 0.26 ± 0.13 mmHg·s/ml for baseline, 135, and 155 bpm, respectively. On the other hand, **Figure 3** shows a decrease of arterial distensibility (Unit: $10^{-3} \times mmHg^{-1}$) as the frequency increases in isolated small branches of coronary (square mark), carotid (triangle mark) or femoral (circle mark) arteries. There was statistically significant difference ($p < 0.05$) in arterial distensibility between 1.5 Hz (mimicking the HR of 90 bpm) and higher frequencies (i.e., ≥2 Hz in branches of coronary and carotid artery and ≥2.5 Hz in branches of femoral artery). Moreover, **Figure 4A** shows pressure and flow waves in femoral artery after HR was paced to 170 bpm. There are different amplitudes between consecutive heart beats. **Figure 4B** shows the corresponding waves in femoral artery after I.V. injection of papaverine (100 mg per dose). This restores successive amplitudes of pressure and flow waves.

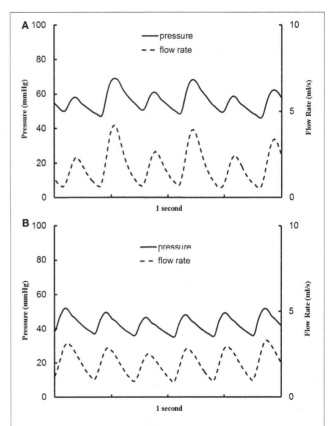

**FIGURE 4 |** Pressure and flow waves in femoral artery **(A)** after the heart rate was paced to 170 bpm and **(B)** after the heart rate was paced to 170 bpm with I.V. injection of papaverine (100 mg per dose).

At baseline, **Figure 5A** shows flow velocity profiles in ascending aorta along the accelerating period of flow waveform and **Figure 5B** shows flow velocity profiles along the decelerating period of flow waveform. **Figures 5C,D** show the corresponding flow velocity profiles at HR of 155 bpm. Peak Reynolds numbers ($Re_{peak}$) are 6,000 and 4,400 for baseline and 155 bpm, respectively, while Womersley numbers (Wo) are 8.9 and 11.7. Moreover, **Figures 6A–D** show flow velocity profiles in femoral artery at baseline and 155 bpm. The femoral artery has peak Reynolds numbers of 690 and 530, and Womersley numbers of 3.2 and 4.2 for baseline and 155 bpm, respectively.

## DISCUSSION

The major finding of the present study was that aortic PWV, determined by the validated techniques in Mohiaddin et al. (1993) and Butlin et al. (2013), and characteristic impedance decreased (i.e., the increase of aortic distensibility) as HR increased from baseline to 135 bpm. We also found that: (1) Total arterial compliance, SV, systemic PP, and central systolic pressure decreased by $36 \pm 17$, $38 \pm 26$, $29 \pm 16$, and $23 \pm 12\%$, respectively, while the MAP, CO and peripheral resistance remained relatively unchanged as HR increased from baseline (HR of 80–105 bpm) to 135 bpm; (2) No statistical difference was found in hemodynamic parameters between 135 and 155 bpm; (3) Arterial distensibility decreased in small arteries as the frequency increased from 1.5 Hz (mimicking 90 bpm) to $\geq 2$ Hz (mimicking HR $\geq$ 120 bpm); and (4) An increase of HR has relatively small effects on flow velocity profiles at HR range of 90–155 bpm, but results in an increase of the turnover of positive and negative WSS.

### Systemic Hemodynamics

It has been documented that pharmacological HR lowering in patients with high BP can result in adverse cardiovascular outcomes (Rimoldi et al., 2016). Here, we showed significantly higher values of SV, systemic PP, and central systolic pressure at baseline as compared to HR of 135 and 155 bpm in swine. A high value of SV due to the prolonged LV (left ventricle) filling time increases LV preload and higher values of systemic PP and central systolic pressure increase LV afterload. This indicates that lowering HR should be considered cautiously in patients, which supports previous conclusion (Rimoldi et al., 2016).

The elevated HR by rapid atrial pacing from baseline to 135 bpm was found to significantly reduce the total arterial compliance (C in Equations 1, 2) distal to the ascending aorta, but remain the peripherical resistance (R in Equations 1, 2) in comparison with the baseline, as shown in **Table 1** and **Figure 1**, which is consistent with a human study (Liang et al., 1999). A decrease of total arterial compliance has been shown to be chronically detrimental for the cardiovascular system (Westerhof et al., 2009). It is known that the total arterial compliance can be estimated by the equation $C = (SV \cdot A_d)/[(A_s + A_d)(P_{ES} - P_d)]$, where $A_s$ and $A_d$ refer to the systolic and diastolic areas under the pressure curve (Liu et al., 1986). $P_d$ refers to the diastolic pressure and $P_{ES}$ refers to the end-systolic aortic pressure (or the pressure at the dicrotic notch). Since the value of $A_d/(A_s +$

$A_d)/(P_{ES} - P_d)$ remains relatively unchanged, the $38 \pm 26\%$ decrease of SV is the major determinant for the $36 \pm 17\%$ decrease of total arterial compliance. In contrast, a decrease of systemic PP ($29 \pm 16\%$) due to the elevated HR may be beneficial for the cardiovascular system because a high value of systemic PP is known to correlate with cardiovascular mortality and morbidity (Benetos et al., 1997). In acute tachycardia, systemic PP is mainly determined by cardiac function while the total arterial compliance distal to the ascending aorta accounts for the entire systemic arteries (Nichols and McDonald, 2011). This suggests different mechanical responses of ventricle and vascular system in response to the rapid atrial pacing from baseline to 135 bpm, which requires further investigations. On the other hand, the relatively unchanged SV, systemic PP, and total arterial compliance as HR increases from 135 to 155 bpm imply a different equilibrium between the ventricle and vascular system from normal range of HR.

### Arterial Distensibility

Acute tachycardia significantly affects the mechanical response of normal conduit arteries given the changes in systemic hemodynamics. We determined the aortic PWV using the foot-to-foot method suggested by expert consensus in European Heart Journal (Laurent et al., 2006). The aortic PWV was found to decrease ($p < 0.05$) with elevated HR from baseline to 135 bpm, which is consistent with the previous studies (Stefanadis et al., 1998; Wilkinson et al., 2000; Albaladejo et al., 2001). There was no statistical difference of PWV between 135 bpm and 155 bpm. The variation of characteristic impedance ($Z_c$ in Equation 2) in descending aorta was consistent with the measured aortic PWV given $Z_c \infty PWV$ (Huo and Kassab, 2006). Clinical studies have investigated the relationship between acute tachycardia and aortic PWV, which have led to contradictory results such as: unchanged PWV (Wilkinson et al., 2000; Albaladejo et al., 2001), decreased PWV (Stefanadis et al., 1998), or increased PWV (Liang et al., 1999; Lantelme et al., 2002; Haesler et al., 2004). Liang et al. found a significant increase of MAP and aortic PWV as patient's HR changed from 56 to 80 bpm, but no significant difference as HR increased from 80 to 100 bpm (Liang et al., 1999). Haesler et al. and Lantelme et al. showed constant MAP and increased PWV in elevated HR (the highest HR was below 100 bpm) in patients with a low degree of atherosclerosis (Haesler et al., 2004) and in subjects with a mean age of 77.8 $\pm$ 8.4 years (Lantelme et al., 2002), respectively. The increase of PWV by rapid pacing is not in agreement with the findings in **Table 2** (normal swine), which may be attributed to aortic diseases such as atherosclerosis (Haesler et al., 2004) and old age (Lantelme et al., 2002) in those patients, or the role of activation of adrenergic system in physiological HR (from 56 to 80 bpm) in young patients not treated with sedative drugs (Liang et al., 1999). Moreover, MAP may be one of the most important factors to affect aortic PWV (Nichols and McDonald, 2011; Townsend et al., 2015). Some recent studies showed that HR dependency of PWV is different at high pressures than at low pressures and HR has a minimal influence on PWV in the lower range of MAP (Safar et al., 2003; Tan et al., 2012). Here, MAP is lower than 100 mmHg such that HR has relatively slight effect on PWV.

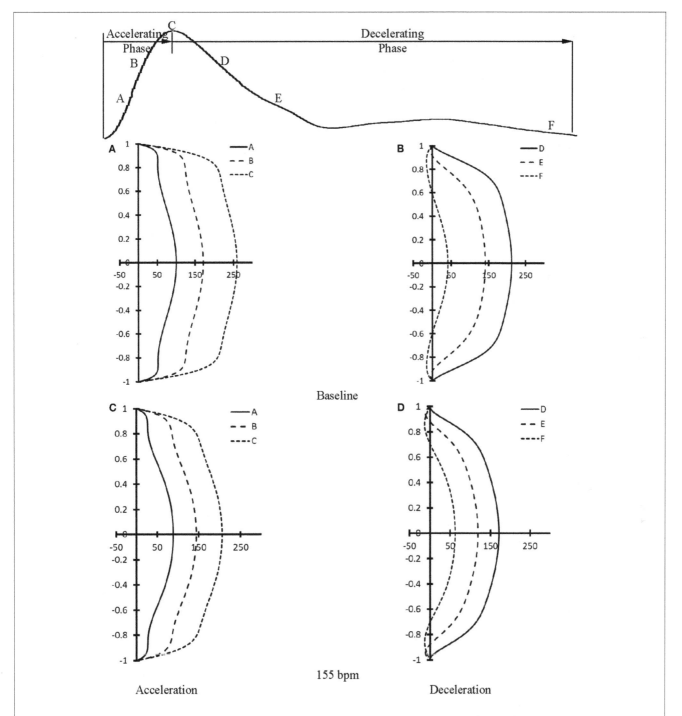

**FIGURE 5 |** Flow velocity profiles in ascending aorta at various time instances during **(A)** accelerating and **(B)** decelerating periods at baseline. **(C,D)** refer to flow velocity profiles in ascending aorta after the heart rate was paced to 155 bpm in correspondence with **(A,B)**. (A–F) in **(A–D)** refer to time instances A–F as shown in the top curve.

A significant decrease of the distensibility of coronary, carotid and femoral arteries (diameters of 300–600 μm) was found as the frequency increased from 1.5 to ≥ 2 Hz. The interaction of incident and reflected pressure and flow waves determines the actual waves, which depends on the mechanical properties of

large elastic arteries, small muscular arteries, and small arterioles (Nichols and McDonald, 2011; Townsend et al., 2015). The peripheral resistance mainly resides in the arteriolar vessels in normal subjects (Chilian, 1991; Huo and Kassab, 2009). The acute tachycardia does not alter the vasoreactivity and mechanical

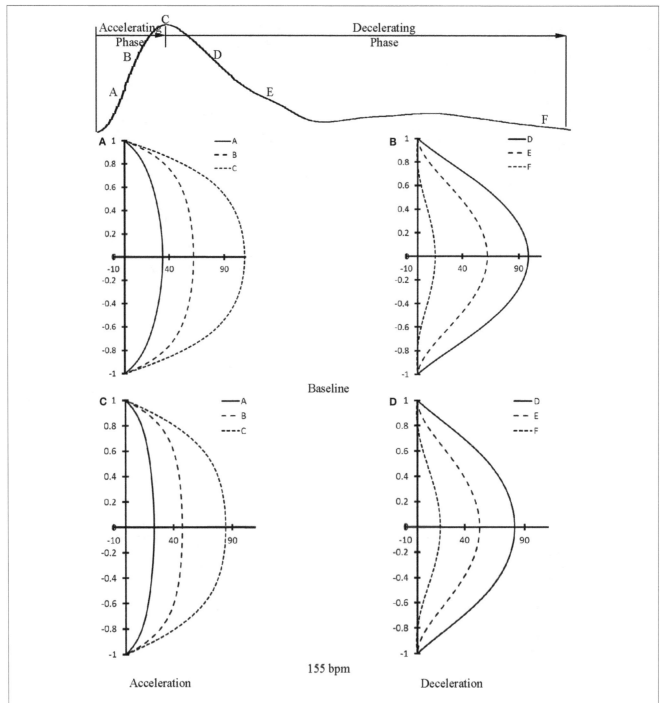

**FIGURE 6 |** Flow velocity profiles in femoral artery at various time instances during **(A)** accelerating and **(B)** decelerating periods at baseline. **(C,D)** refer to flow velocity profiles in femoral artery after the heart rate was paced to 155 bpm in correspondence with **(A,B)**. (A–F) in **(A–D)** refer to time instances A–F as shown in the top curve.

response of the arteriolar bed given the relatively unchanged MAP and peripheral resistance in HR range of 90–155 bpm. In contrast, the irregular pressure and flow waves occurred after the heart was paced to 170 bpm, which disappeared after the injection of papaverine (a smooth muscle relaxant). We have shown that the increased vascular tone significantly increases the arterial stiffness in coronary arteries (Huo et al., 2012, 2013).

These findings imply relatively small effects of vascular tone on the stiffness of small muscular arteries and arterioles in HR range of 90–155 bpm albeit the biology-regulated tone can affect vascular mechanical properties after the heart was paced to 170 bpm. Since the distensibility was determined in isolated small muscular arteries, *in vivo* measurements should be demonstrated to validate the implication. Here, we showed that pacing-induced acute tachycardia affects the elastic response of the arterial wall in small muscular arteries significantly as compared with the aorta, which is consistent with a previous study (Whelton et al., 2013). Moreover, the mismatch between aorta and small muscular arteries in high HR may be a risk factor for adverse cardiovascular events in the long term, which requires further investigations.

## Local Hemodynamics

The accelerating and decelerating phases of pulsatile flow are clearly distinguishable periods in a cardiac cycle, as shown in top curves in **Figures 5, 6**. Since $Re_{peak}$ ($Re_{peak} > 4400$) > $250 \cdot Wo$ ($Wo < 11.7$), the blood flow in aorta should result in turbulence during the decelerating phase of pulsatile flow, but not during the accelerating phase (Nerem and Seed, 1972). Since the present experimental techniques and analytic models did not assess turbulence, we used the Womersley model to simplify the flow velocity profiles. A near-wall flow reversal was found during the decelerating phase, but not during the accelerating phase. Moreover, the ascending aorta has a much larger value of peak Reynolds number than the femoral artery (6,000 vs. 690 at baseline), which leads to the less stable blunt flow velocity profiles as compared with the parabolic profiles in femoral artery. The increased HR, however, seems to have a negligible effect on the flow velocity profiles.

The low time-averaged WSS and high OSI are thought to result in endothelial dysfunction, monocyte deposition, smooth muscle cell proliferation, microemboli formation, and so on (Fan et al., 2016; Huang et al., 2016). In addition, the increased frequency of oscillatory shear stress can cause sustained molecular signaling of pro-inflammatory and proliferative pathways that contribute to endothelial dysfunction and atherosclerosis (Chien, 2008). Elevated HR increases the frequency of oscillatory shear stress while it has very small effects on the time-averaged WSS and OSI. This increased oscillatory shear may be a risk factor for the development of atherosclerosis in arteries, if sustained clinically.

## Critique of Study

The arterial distensibility were measured in isolated small arteries with diameters of 300-600 $\mu$m, which needs to be incorporated into the cardiovascular system for a more systematic analysis. Hence, the hemodynamic analysis in the entire arterial tree including large arteries, small arteries and small arterioles should be implemented to help understand the contribution of both acute and chronic high HR to arterial stiffness and atherosclerosis (Huo and Kassab, 2006, 2007; Huo et al., 2009; Feng et al., 2018). In a review article (Safar et al., 2003), Safar et al. indicated that the aorta and its main branches are highly sensitive to age and changes in MAP while the small muscle arteries are highly sensitive to vasoactive substances (particularly those of endothelial origin). The cellular mechanisms of arterial stiffness in response to chronic high HR (particularly for the regulation of autonomic nervous system and endocrine system) need further investigations in relation to the remodeling of endothelial and smooth muscle cells.

## CONCLUSIONS

This study investigated the role of rapid pacing on systemic and local hemodynamics and arterial stiffness through *in vivo* and *ex vivo* experimental measurements and hemodynamic analysis. The acute increase in HR up to 135 bpm resulted in significant increase/decrease of the distensibility of aorta/small muscular arteries and a mismatch in the response of aorta and small arteries. The mismatch between aorta and small muscular arteries in high HR can be a risk factor for adverse cardiovascular events. The pacing also reduced the total arterial compliance, SV, systemic PP, and central systolic pressure but had no statistical significant effect on MAP, CO, peripheral resistance, and vascular flow patterns. Finally, pacing from 135 to 155 bpm had negligible effect on systemic hemodynamics and arterial stiffness.

## AUTHOR CONTRIBUTIONS

Data analysis were performed by YH at the college of engineering, Peking University and HC at the California Medical Innovations Institute. Paper was drafted and revised by YH and GK at the California Medical Innovations Institute.

## ACKNOWLEDGMENTS

This research is supported in part by the Shenzhen Science and Technology R&D Grant JCYJ20160427170536358 (YH) and National Institute of Health-National Heart, Lung, and Blood Institute Grant HL134841 and HL118738 (GK).

## REFERENCES

Albaladejo, P., Copie, X., Boutouyrie, P., Laloux, B., Déclère, A. D., Smulyan, H., et al. (2001). Heart rate, arterial stiffness, and wave reflections in paced patients. *Hypertension* 38, 949–952. doi: 10.1161/hy1001.096210

Andreadis, E. A., and Geladari, C. V. (2018). Hypertension and atrial fibrillation: a bench to bedside perspective. *Front Biosci.* 10, 276–284. doi: 10.2741/s515

Benetos, A., Safar, M., Rudnichi, A., Smulyan, H., Richard, J. L., Ducimetieère, P., et al. (1997). Pulse pressure: a predictor of long-term cardiovascular mortality in a French male population. *Hypertension* 30, 1410–1415. doi: 10.1161/01.HYP.30.6.1410

Benjamin, E. J., Levy, D., Vaziri, S. M., D'Agostino, R. B., Belanger, A. J., and Wolf, P. A. (1994). Independent risk factors for atrial fibrillation in a population-based cohort. The Framingham Heart Study. *JAMA* 271, 840–844. doi: 10.1001/jama.1994.03510350050036

Bergel, D. H. (1961). The dynamic elastic properties of the arterial wall. *J Physiol.* 156, 458–469. doi: 10.1113/jphysiol.1961.sp006687

Burattini, R., Gnudi, G., Westerhof, N., and Fioretti, S. (1987). Total systemic arterial compliance and aortic characteristic impedance in the dog as a function of pressure - a model based study. *Comput. Biomed. Res.* 20, 154–165. doi: 10.1016/0010-4809(87)90042-5

Butlin, M., Qasem, A., Battista, F., Bozec, E., McEniery, C. M., Millet-Amaury, E., et al. (2013). Carotid-femoral pulse wave velocity assessment using novel cuff-based techniques: comparison with tonometric measurement. *J. Hypertens.* 31, 2237–2243; discussion 2243. doi: 10.1097/HJH.0b013e3283 63c789

Chien, S. (2008). Effects of disturbed flow on endothelial cells. *Ann. Biomed. Eng.* 36, 554–562. doi: 10.1007/s10439-007-9426-3

Chilian, W. M. (1991). Microvascular pressures and resistances in the left ventricular subepicardium and subendocardium. *Circ. Res.* 69, 561–570. doi: 10.1161/01.RES.69.3.561

Conen, D., Tedrow, U. B., Koplan, B. A., Glynn, R. J., Buring, J. E., and Albert, C. M. (2009). Influence of systolic and diastolic blood pressure on the risk of incident atrial fibrillation in women. *Circulation* 119, 2146–2152. doi: 10.1161/CIRCULATIONAHA.108.830042

Diaz, A., Bourassa, M. G., Guertin, M.-C., and Tardif, J.-C. (2005). Long-term prognostic value of resting heart rate in patients with suspected or proven coronary artery disease. *Eur. Heart J.* 26, 967–974. doi: 10.1093/eurheartj/ehi190

Dzeshka, M. S, Shantsila, A., Shantsila, E., and Lip, G. Y. H. (2017). Atrial fibrillation and hypertension. *Hypertension* 70, 854–861. doi: 10.1161/HYPERTENSIONAHA.117.08934

Fan, T., Lu, Y., Gao, Y., Meng, J., Tan, W., Huo, Y., et al. (2016). Hemodynamics of left internal mammary artery bypass graft: effect of anastomotic geometry, coronary artery stenosis, and postoperative time. *J. Biomech.* 49, 645–652. doi: 10.1016/j.jbiomech.2016.01.031

Feng, Y., Wang, X., Fan, T., Li, L., Sun, X., Zhang, W., et al. (2018). Bifurcation asymmetry of small coronary arteries in juvenile and adult mice. *Front. Physiol.* 9:519. doi: 10.3389/fphys.2018.00519

Fox, K., Borer, J. S., Camm, A. J., Danchin, N., Ferrari, R., Lopez Sendon, J. L., et al. (2007). Resting heart rate in cardiovascular disease. *J. Am. Coll. Cardiol.* 50, 823–830. doi: 10.1016/j.jacc.2007.04.079

Fox, K. M., and Ferrari, R. (2011). Heart rate: a forgotten link in coronary artery disease? *Nat. Rev. Cardiol.* 8, 369–79. doi: 10.1038/nrcardio.2011.58

Grundvold, I., Skretteberg, P. T., Liestøl, K., Erikssen, G., Kjeldsen, S. E., Arnesen, H., et al. (2012). Upper normal blood pressures predict incident atrial fibrillation in healthy middle-aged men: a 35-year follow-up study. *Hypertension* 59, 198–204. doi: 10.1161/HYPERTENSIONAHA.111.179713

Haesler, E., Lyon, X., Pruvot, E., Kappenberger, L., and Hayoz, D. (2004). Confounding effects of heart rate on pulse wave velocity in paced patients with a low degree of atherosclerosis. *J. Hypertens.* 22, 1317–1322. doi: 10.1097/01.hjh.0000125447.28861.18

Huang, X., Yin, X., Xu, Y., Jia, X., Li, J., Niu, P., et al. (2016). Morphometric and hemodynamic analysis of atherosclerotic progression in human carotid artery bifurcations. *Am. J. Physiol. Heart Circ. Physiol.* 310, H639–H647. doi: 10.1152/ajpheart.00464.2015

Huo, Y., Cheng, Y., Zhao, X., Lu, X., and Kassab, G. S. (2012). Biaxial vasoactivity of porcine coronary artery. *Am. J. Physiol. Heart Circ. Physiol.* 302, H2058–H2063. doi: 10.1152/ajpheart.00758.2011

Huo, Y., Kaimovitz, B., Lanir, Y., Wischgoll, T., Hoffman, J. I., and Kassab, G. S. (2009). Biophysical model of the spatial heterogeneity of myocardial flow. *Biophys. J.* 96, 4035–4043. doi: 10.1016/j.bpj.2009.02.047

Huo, Y., and Kassab, G. S. (2006). Pulsatile blood flow in the entire coronary arterial tree: theory and experiment. *Am. J. Physiol. Heart Circ. Physiol.* 291, H1074–H1087. doi: 10.1152/ajpheart.00200.2006

Huo, Y., and Kassab, G. S. (2007). A hybrid one-dimensional/Womersley model of pulsatile blood flow in the entire coronary arterial tree. *Am. J. Physiol. Heart Circ. Physiol.* 292, H2623–H2633. doi: 10.1152/ajpheart.00987.2006

Huo, Y., and Kassab, G. S. (2009). Effect of compliance and hematocrit on wall shear stress in a model of the entire coronary arterial tree. *J. Appl. Physiol.* 107, 500–505. doi: 10.1152/japplphysiol.91013.2008

Huo, Y., and Kassab, G. S. (2015). Remodeling of left circumflex coronary arterial tree in pacing-induced heart failure. *J. Appl. Physiol (1985).* 119, 404–411. doi: 10.1152/japplphysiol.00262.2015

Huo, Y., Zhao, X., Cheng, Y., Lu, X., and Kassab, G. S. (2013). Two-layer model of coronary artery vasoactivity. *J. Appl. Physiol (1985).* 114, 1451–1459. doi: 10.1152/japplphysiol.01237.2012

Lantelme, P., Mestre, C., Lievre, M., Gressard, A., and Milon, H. (2002). Heart rate: an important confounder of pulse wave velocity assessment. *Hypertension* 39, 1083–1087. doi: 10.1161/01.HYP.0000019132.41066.95

Laskey, W. K., Parker, H. G., Ferrari, V. A., Kussmaul, W. G., and Noordergraaf, A. (1990). Estimation of total systemic arterial compliance in humans. *J. Appl. Physiol (1985).* 69, 112–119. doi: 10.1152/jappl.1990.69.1.112

Latson, T. W., Hunter, W. C., Katoh, N., and Sagawa, K. (1988). Effect of nitroglycerin on aortic impedance, diameter, and pulse-wave velocity. *Circ. Res.* 62, 884–890. doi: 10.1161/01.RES.62.5.884

Laurent, S., Cockcroft, J., Van Bortel, L., Boutouyrie, P., Giannattasio, C., Hayoz, D., et al. (2006). Expert consensus document on arterial stiffness: methodological issues and clinical applications. *Eur. Heart J.* 27, 2588–2605. doi: 10.1093/eurheartj/ehl254

Li, J. K., Cui, T., and Drzewiecki, G. M. (1990). A nonlinear model of the arterial system incorporating a pressure-dependent compliance. *IEEE Trans. Biomed. Eng.* 37, 673–678. doi: 10.1109/10.55678

Liang, Y. L., Gatzka, C. D., Du, X. J., Cameron, J. D., Kingwell, B. A., and Dart, A. M. (1999). Effects of heart rate on arterial compliance in men. *Clin. Exp. Pharmacol. Physiol.* 26, 342–346. doi: 10.1046/j.1440-1681.1999.03039.x

Liu, Z., Brin, K. P., and Yin, F. C. (1986). Estimation of total arterial compliance: an improved method and evaluation of current methods. *Am. J. Physiol.* 251(3 Pt 2), H588–600.

Lonn, E. M., Rambihar, S., Gao, P., Custodis, F. F., Sliwa, K., Teo, K. K., et al. (2010). Heart rate is associated with increased risk of major cardiovascular events, cardiovascular and all-cause death in patients with stable chronic cardiovascular disease - an analysis of ONTARGET/TRANSCEN. *Clin. Res. Cardiol.* 103, 149–159. doi: 10.1007/s00392-013-0644-4

Lu, Y., Wu, H., Li, J., Gong, Y., Ma, J., Kassab, G. S., et al. (2017). Passive and active triaxial wall mechanics in a two-layer model of porcine coronary artery. *Sci. Rep.* 7:13911. doi: 10.1038/s41598-017-14276-1

Manolis, A. J., Rosei, E. A., Coca, A., Cifkova, R., Erdine, S. E., Kjeldsen, S., et al. (2012). Hypertension and atrial fibrillation: diagnostic approach, prevention and treatment. position paper of the working group 'hypertension arrhythmias and Thrombosis' of the European Society of Hypertension. *J. Hypertens.* 30, 239–252. doi: 10.1097/HJH.0b013e32834f03bf

Mohiaddin, R. H., Firmin, D. N., and Longmore, D. B. (1993). Age-related changes of human aortic flow wave velocity measured noninvasively by magnetic resonance imaging. *J. Appl. Physiol (1985).* 74, 492–497. doi: 10.1152/jappl.1993.74.1.492

Nerem, R. M., and Seed, W. A. (1972). An *in vivo* study of aortic flow disturbances. *Cardiovasc. Res.* 6, 1–14. doi: 10.1093/cvr/6.1.1

Nichols, W. W., and McDonald, D. A. (2011). *McDonald's Blood Flow in Arteries: Theoretic, Experimental, and Clinical Principles*, 6th ed. London: Hodder Arnold. xiv,755 p.

O'Rourke, M. F., and Hashimoto, J. (2007). Mechanical factors in arterial aging: a clinical perspective. *J. Am. Coll. Cardiol.* 50, 1–13. doi: 10.1016/j.jacc.2006.12.050

Palatini, P., and Julius, S. (2004). Elevated heart rate: a major risk factor for cardiovascular disease. *Clin. Exp. Hypertens.* 26, 637–644. doi: 10.1081/CEH-200031959

Quick, C. M., Berger, D. S., and Noordergraaf, A. (1998). Apparent arterial compliance. *Am. J. Physiol.* 274(4 Pt 2), H1393–H1403.

Rimoldi, S. F., Messerli, F. H., Cerny, D., Gloekler, S., Traupe, T., Laurent, S., et al. (2016). Selective heart rate reduction with ivabradine increases central blood pressure in stable coronary artery disease. *Hypertension* 67, 1205–1210. doi: 10.1161/HYPERTENSIONAHA.116.07250

Safar, M. E. (2018). Arterial stiffness as a risk factor for clinical hypertension. *Nat. Rev.Cardiol.* 15, 97–105. doi: 10.1038/nrcardio.2017.155

Safar, M. E., Levy, B. I., and Struijker-Boudier, H. (2003). Current perspectives on arterial stiffness and pulse pressure in hypertension and cardiovascular diseases. *Circulation* 107, 2864–2869. doi: 10.1161/01.CIR.0000096826.36125.B4

Stefanadis, C., Dernellis, J., Vavuranakis, M., Tsiamis, E., Vlachopoulos, C., Toutouzas, K., et al. (1998). Effects of ventricular pacing-induced tachycardia on aortic mechanics in man. *Cardiovasc. Res.* 39, 506–14. doi: 10.1016/S0008-6363(98)00115-1

Stergiopulos, N., Meister, J. J., and Westerhof, N. (1994). Simple and accurate way for estimating total and segmental arterial compliance: the pulse pressure method. *Ann. Biomed. Eng.* 22, 392–7. doi: 10.1007/BF02368245

Stergiopulos, N., Meister, J. J., and Westerhof, N. (1995). Evaluation of methods for estimation of total arterial compliance. *Am. J. Physiol.* 268(4 Pt 2), H1540–H1548.

Tan, I., Butlin, M., Liu, Y. Y., Ng, K., and Avolio, A. P. (2012). Heart rate dependence of aortic pulse wave velocity at different arterial pressures in rats. *Hypertension* 60, 528–533. doi: 10.1161/HYPERTENSIONAHA.112.194225

Townsend, R. R., Wilkinson, I. B., Schiffrin, E. L., Avolio, A. P., Chirinos, J. A., Cockcroft, J. R., et al. (2015). Recommendations for improving and standardizing vascular research on arterial stiffness: a scientific statement from the American Heart Association. *Hypertension* 66, 698–722. doi: 10.1161/HYP.0000000000000033

Verdecchia, P., Angeli, F., Gentile, G., and Reboldi, G. (2016). More versus less intensive blood pressure-lowering strategy: cumulative evidence and trial sequential analysis. *Hypertension* 68, 642–653. doi: 10.1161/HYPERTENSIONAHA.116.07608

Verdecchia, P., Angeli, F., and Reboldi, G. (2018). Hypertension and atrial fibrillation: doubts and certainties from basic and clinical studies. *Circ. Res.* 122, 352–368. doi: 10.1161/CIRCRESAHA.117.311402

Verdecchia, P., Dagenais, G., Healey, J., Gao, P., Dans, A. L., Chazova, I., et al. (2012a). Blood pressure and other determinants of new-onset atrial fibrillation in patients at high cardiovascular risk in the Ongoing Telmisartan Alone and in Combination With Ramipril Global Endpoint Trial/Telmisartan Randomized AssessmeNt Study in ACE iNtolerant subjects with cardiovascular Disease studies. *J. Hypertens.* 30, 1004–1014. doi: 10.1097/HJH.0b013e3283522a51

Verdecchia, P., Mazzotta, G., Angeli, F., and Reboldi, G. (2012b). Above which blood pressure level does the risk of atrial fibrillation increase? *Hypertension* 59, 184–185. doi: 10.1161/HYPERTENSIONAHA.111.187260

Westerhof, B. E., Guelen, I., Westerhof, N., Karemaker, J. M., and Avolio, A. (2006). Quantification of wave reflection in the human aorta from pressure alone: a proof of principle. *Hypertension* 48, 595–601. doi: 10.1161/01.HYP.0000238330.08894.17

Westerhof, N., Elzinga, G., and Sipkema, P. (1971). An artificial arterial system for pumping hearts. *J. Appl. Physiol.* 31, 776–781. doi: 10.1152/jappl.1971.31.5.776

Westerhof, N., Lankhaar, J. W., and Westerhof, B. E. (2009). The arterial Windkessel. *Med. Biol. Eng. Comput.* 47, 131–141. doi: 10.1007/s11517-008-0359-2

Westerhof, N., Sipkema, P., van den Bos, G. C., and Elzinga, G. (1972). Forward and backward waves in the arterial system. *Cardiovasc. Res.* 6, 648–656. doi: 10.1093/cvr/6.6.648

Westerhof, N., and Westerhof, B. E. (2013). Crosstalk proposal: forward and backward pressure waves in the arterial system do represent reality. *J. Physiol.* 591, 1167–9; discussion 1177. doi: 10.1113/jphysiol.2012.249763

Whelton, P. K., Carey, R. M., Aronow, W. S., Casey, D. E. Jr., Collins, K. J., Dennison Himmelfarb, C., et al. (2018). 2017 ACC/AHA/AAPA/ABC/ACPM/AGS/APhA/ASH/ASPC/NMA/PCNA guideline for the prevention, detection, evaluation, and management of high blood pressure in adults: a report of the American College of Cardiology/American Heart Association Task Force on Clinical Practice Guidelines. *J. Am. Coll. Cardiol.* 71, e127–e248. doi: 10.1016/j.jacc.2017.11.006

Whelton, S. P., Blankstein, R., Al-Mallah, M. H., Lima, J. A., Bluemke, D. A., Hundley, W. G., et al. (2013). Association of resting heart rate with carotid and aortic arterial stiffness: multi-ethnic study of atherosclerosis. *Hypertension* 62, 477–484. doi: 10.1161/HYPERTENSIONAHA.113.01605

Wilkinson, I. B., MacCallum, H., Flint, L., Cockcroft, J. R., Newby, D. E., and Webb, D. J. (2000). The influence of heart rate on augmentation index and central arterial pressure in humans. *J. Physiol. (Lond).* 525(Pt 1), 263–270. doi: 10.1111/j.1469-7793.2000.t01-1-00263.x

Zheng, H., Huo, Y., Svendsen, M., and Kassab, G. S. (2010). Effect of blood pressure on vascular hemodynamics in acute tachycardia. *J. Appl. Physiol. (1985)* 109, 1619–1627. doi: 10.1152/japplphysiol.01356.2009

# 6

# High Spatial Resolution Multi-Organ Finite Element Modeling of Ventricular-Arterial Coupling

Sheikh Mohammad Shavik, Zhenxiang Jiang, Seungik Baek and Lik Chuan Lee*

Department of Mechanical Engineering, Michigan State University, East Lansing, MI, United States

*Correspondence:
Lik Chuan Lee
lclee@egr.msu.edu

While it has long been recognized that bi-directional interaction between the heart and the vasculature plays a critical role in the proper functioning of the cardiovascular system, a comprehensive study of this interaction has largely been hampered by a lack of modeling framework capable of simultaneously accommodating high-resolution models of the heart and vasculature. Here, we address this issue and present a computational modeling framework that couples finite element (FE) models of the left ventricle (LV) and aorta to elucidate ventricular—arterial coupling in the systemic circulation. We show in a baseline simulation that the framework predictions of (1) LV pressure—volume loop, (2) aorta pressure—diameter relationship, (3) pressure—waveforms of the aorta, LV, and left atrium (LA) over the cardiac cycle are consistent with the physiological measurements found in healthy human. To develop insights of ventricular-arterial interactions, the framework was then used to simulate how alterations in the geometrical or, material parameter(s) of the aorta affect the LV and vice versa. We show that changing the geometry and microstructure of the aorta model in the framework led to changes in the functional behaviors of both LV and aorta that are consistent with experimental observations. On the other hand, changing contractility and passive stiffness of the LV model in the framework also produced changes in both the LV and aorta functional behaviors that are consistent with physiology principles.

Keywords: left ventricle, finite element modeling, ventricular-arterial coupling, arterial mechanics, cardiac mechanics, systemic circulation

## INTRODUCTION

The heart and vasculature are key components of the cardiovascular system that operate in tandem to deliver oxygen and nutrients to the human body. Physiological adaptation, deterioration, and/or malfunctioning of one component often affects the operation of the other. Indeed, optimal ventricular-arterial interaction (or coupling) is critical to the normal functioning of the cardiovascular system. Any deviations from optimal ventricular-arterial interaction in the cardiovascular system (as indexed by the ratio between arterial stiffness and ventricular elastance) are usually associated with heart diseases (Borlaug and Kass, 2011). In the pulmonary circulatory system, interactions between the right ventricle and the pulmonary vasculature are key determinants of the clinical course of pulmonary hypertension (Naeije and Manes, 2014), specifically, in the transition from compensated to decompensated remodeling. Similarly, in the systemic circulatory system, heart failure with preserved ejection (HFpEF) has been associated with a progressively impaired ventricular-arterial interaction between the left ventricle (LV) and the systemic arteries (Kawaguchi et al., 2003; Borlaug and Kass, 2011). Ventricular-arterial interaction is also reflected at the microstructural level. In particular, remodeling of the vasculature found in these diseases (e.g., smooth muscle hypertrophy/proliferation and deposition of the collagen) (Shimoda and Laurie, 2013; Giamouzis et al., 2016) are often accompanied by similar remodeling in the heart (e.g., myocyte hypertrophy and cardiac fibrosis) (Rain et al., 2013; Hill et al., 2014; Su et al., 2014).

Computational modeling is particularly useful for understanding ventricular-arterial interaction, especially as there are potentially many parameters that can affect this interaction bi-directionally. While ventricular-arterial interactions may be described using electrical analog (or lumped parameter) models of the cardiovascular system (Smith et al., 2004; Arts et al., 2005), the heart and vasculature in such models are represented using highly idealized electrical circuit elements such as resistor, capacitor, and voltage generator. It is difficult, if not impossible, to separate or distinguish between geometrical, material, and microstructural changes from the parameters of these electrical elements. Previous finite element (FE) modeling efforts of the cardiovascular system, however, have focused on either the heart or the vasculature. Specifically, FE models of the heart were developed either in isolation (Wenk et al., 2011; Lee et al., 2013; Gao et al., 2014; Genet et al., 2014), or coupled to an electrical analog of the circulatory system in open (Usyk et al., 2002; Trayanova et al., 2011; Wall et al., 2012; Lee et al., 2016; Xi et al., 2016) or closed loop fashions (Kerckhoffs et al., 2007; Shavik et al., 2017). In an open-loop circulatory modeling framework, the FE ventricular model is generally coupled to a Windkessel model via outlet boundary conditions to simulate the ejection of blood, while the filling and isovolumic phases are, respectively, simulated by increasing and constraining the ventricular cavity volume. Parameters in the modeling framework are then adjusted so that the four distinct cardiac phases form a closed pressure-volume loop. On the other hand, coupling the FE ventricular model to a closed loop circulatory modeling framework is (arguably) more physical since the total blood volume is naturally conserved in the cardiovascular system. Simulation of multiple cardiac cycles is required, however, to obtain a steady state solution. Conversely, FE models of the vasculature were developed either in isolation (Hsu and Bazilevs, 2011; Zeinali-Davarani et al., 2011) or coupled to simplified representation of the heart based on a time-varying elastance function (Kim et al., 2009; Lau and Figueroa, 2015). Although able to describe the heart or vasculature in greater details, these FE modeling frameworks cannot be used to simulate detailed bidirectional ventricular-arterial interactions e.g., how changes in the vasculature mechanical properties affect the deformation and function of the heart and vice versa.

To overcome these limitations, we describe here a novel computational framework that is capable of coupling high spatial resolution FE models of both the vasculature and the heart to describe bidirectional ventricular-arterial coupling in the systemic circulation. Using realistic geometries and microstructure of the LV and aorta, we show that the framework is able to reproduce features that are consistent with measurements made in both compartments. We also performed a parameter study to show how mechanical and geometrical changes in the aorta affect the heart function and vice versa.

## METHODS

### Closed-Loop Systemic Circulatory Model

Finite element models of the aorta and LV were coupled via a closed-loop modeling framework describing the systemic circulatory system. Other components of the circulatory system were modeled using electrical analogs (**Figure 1A**). Mass of blood was conserved by the following equations relating the rate of volume change in each storage compartment of the circulatory system to the inflow and outflow rates

$$\frac{dV_{LA}(t)}{dt} = q_{ven}(t) - q_{mv}(t); \tag{1a}$$

$$\frac{dV_{LV}(t)}{dt} = q_{mv}(t) - q_{ao}(t); \tag{1b}$$

$$\frac{dV_{art}(t)}{dt} = q_{ao}(t) - q_{per}(t); \tag{1c}$$

$$\frac{dV_{ven}(t)}{dt} = q_{per}(t) - q_{ven}(t), \tag{1d}$$

where $V_{LA}$, $V_{LV}$, $V_{art}$, and $V_{ven}$ are volumes of each compartment, and $q_{ven}$, $q_{mv}$, $q_{ao}$, and $q_{per}$ are flow rates at different segments (**Figure 1A**). Flowrate at different segments of the circulatory model depends on their resistance to flow ($R_{ao}$, $R_{per}$, $R_{ven}$, and $R_{mv}$) and the pressure difference between the connecting storage compartments (i.e., pressure gradient). The flow rates are given by

$$q_{ao}(t) = \begin{cases} \frac{P_{LV,cav}(t) - P_{art,cav}(t)}{R_{ao}} & when, P_{LV,cav}(t) \geq P_{art,cav}(t) \\ 0 & when, P_{LV,cav}(t) < P_{art,cav}(t) \end{cases}; \tag{2a}$$

$$q_{per}(t) = \frac{P_{art,cav}(t) - P_{ven}(t)}{R_{per}}; \tag{2b}$$

$$q_{ven}(t) = \frac{P_{ven}(t) - P_{LA}(t)}{R_{ven}}; \tag{2c}$$

$$q_{mv}(t) = \begin{cases} \frac{P_{LA}(t) - P_{LV,cav}(t)}{R_{mv}} & when, P_{LA}(t) \geq P_{LV,cav}(t) \\ 0 & when, P_{LA}(t) < P_{LV,cav}(t) \end{cases}. \tag{2d}$$

Pressure in each storage compartment is a function of its volume. A simplified pressure volume relationship,

$$P_{ven}(t) = \frac{V_{ven}(t) - V_{ven,0}}{C_{ven}}, \tag{3}$$

was prescribed for the veins, where $V_{ven,0}$ is a constant resting volume of the veins and $C_{ven}$ is the total compliance of the venous system. On the other hand, pressure in the left atrium $P_{LA}(t)$ was prescribed to be a function of its volume $V_{LA}(t)$ by the following equations that describe its contraction using a time-varying elastance function $e(t)$:

$$P_{LA}(t) = e(t)P_{es,LA}(V_{LA}(t)) + (1 - e(t))P_{ed,LA}(V_{LA}(t)), \tag{4}$$

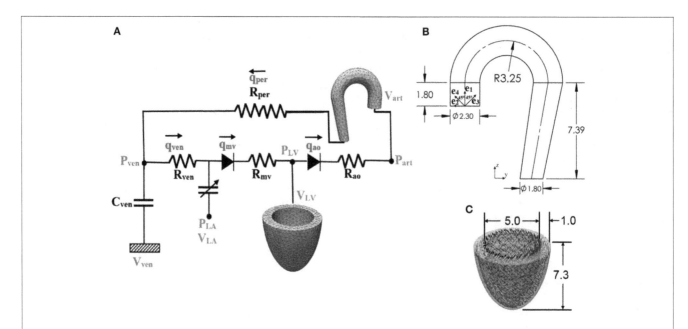

**FIGURE 1 | (A)** Schematic diagram of the ventricular-arterial modeling framework; the LV and aorta were modeled using FE models, rest of the systemic circulation compartments were modeled using their electrical analog. **(B)** unloaded aorta geometry with $e_k$ ($k = 1$–4) showing the directions of the four collagen fiber families, **(C)** unloaded LV geometry with fiber directions varying from 60° at the endocardium to −60° at the epicardium wall (all dimensions are in cm).

where

$$P_{es,LA}(V_{LA}(t)) = E_{es,LA}(V_{LA}(t) - V_{0,LA}), \quad (5a)$$

$$P_{ed,LA}(V_{LA}(t)) = A_{LA}\left(e^{B_{LA}\left(V_{LA}(t) - V_{0,LA}\right)} - 1\right), \quad (5b)$$

and,

$$e(t) = \begin{cases} \frac{1}{2}\left(\sin\left[\left(\frac{\pi}{t_{max}}\right)t - \frac{\pi}{2}\right] + 1\right); & 0 < t \leq 3/2\, t_{max} \\ \frac{1}{2}\,e^{-(t-3/2t_{max})/\tau}; & t > 3/2\, t_{max} \end{cases} \quad (5c)$$

In Equations (5a,b), $E_{es,LA}$ is the end-systolic elastance of the left atrium, $V_{0,LA}$ is the volume axis intercept of the end-systolic pressure volume relationship (ESPVR), and both $A_{LA}$ and $B_{LA}$ are parameters of the end-diastolic pressure volume relationship (EDPVR) of the left atrium. The driving function $e(t)$ is given in Equation (5c) in which $t_{max}$ is the point of maximal chamber elastance and $\tau$ is the time constant of relaxation. The values of $E_{es,LA}$, $V_{0,LA}$, $A_{LA}$, $B_{LA}$, $t_{max}$, and $\tau$ are listed in **Table 1**.

Finally, pressure in the other two storage compartments, namely, LV and aorta, depends on their corresponding volume through non-closed form functions

$$P_{LV,cav}(t) = f^{LV}(V_{LV}(t)), \quad (6)$$

$$P_{art,\,cav}(t) = f^{art}(V_{art}(t)). \quad (7)$$

The functional relationships between pressure and volume in the LV and aorta were obtained using the FE method as described in the next section.

**TABLE 1 |** Parameters of time varying elastance model for the left atrium.

| Parameter | Unit | Values |
|---|---|---|
| End-systolic elastance, $E_{es,LA}$ | Pa/ml | 60 |
| Volume axis intercept, $V_{0,LA}$ | ml | 10 |
| Scaling factor for EDPVR, $A_{LA}$ | Pa | 58.67 |
| Exponent for EDPVR, $B_{LA}$ | ml$^{-1}$ | 0.049 |
| Time to end-systole, $t_{max}$ | ms | 200 |
| Time constant of relaxation, $\tau$ | ms | 35 |

**TABLE 2 |** Parameters of the closed loop lumped parameter circulatory framework.

| Parameter | Unit | Values |
|---|---|---|
| Aortic valve resistance, $R_{ao}$ | Pa ms ml$^{-1}$ | 2,000 |
| Peripheral resistance, $R_{per}$ | Pa ms ml$^{-1}$ | 125,000 |
| Venous resistance, $R_{ven}$ | Pa ms ml$^{-1}$ | 2,000 |
| Mitral valve resistance, $R_{mv}$ | Pa ms ml$^{-1}$ | 2,000 |
| Venous compliance, $C_{ven}$ | ml Pa | 0.3 |
| Resting volume for vein, $V_{ven,0}$ | ml | 3,200 |

## Finite Element Formulation of the Left Ventricle and Aorta

Finite element formulation of the other two storage compartments can be generalized from the minimization of the following Lagrangian functional with the subscript $k = LV$ denoting the LV and $k = art$ denoting the aorta

$$\mathcal{L}_k\left(\boldsymbol{u_k}, p_k, P_{k,cav}, \boldsymbol{c_{1,k}}, \boldsymbol{c_{2,k}}\right) = \int_{\Omega_{0,k}} W_k\left(\boldsymbol{u_k}\right) dV$$

$$- \int_{\Omega_{0,k}} p_k\left(J_k - 1\right) dV - P_{k,cav}\left(V_{k,cav}\left(\boldsymbol{u_k}\right) - V_k\right)$$

$$- \boldsymbol{c_{1,k}} \cdot \int_{\Omega_{0,k}} \boldsymbol{u_k}\, dV - \boldsymbol{c_{2,k}} \cdot \int_{\Omega_{0,k}} \boldsymbol{X_k} \times \boldsymbol{u_k}\, dV. \tag{8}$$

In the above equation, $\boldsymbol{u_k}$ is the displacement field, $P_{k,cav}$ is the Lagrange multiplier to constrain the cavity volume $V_{k,cav}(\boldsymbol{u_k})$ to a prescribed value $V_k$ (Pezzuto and Ambrosi, 2014), $p_k$ is a Lagrange multiplier to enforce incompressibility of the tissue (i.e., Jacobian of the deformation gradient tensor $J_k = 1$), and both $\boldsymbol{c_{1,k}}$ and $\boldsymbol{c_{2,k}}$ are Lagrange multipliers to constrain rigid body translation (i.e., zero mean translation) and rotation (i.e., zero mean rotation) (Pezzuto et al., 2014). The functional relationship between the cavity volumes of the LV and aorta to their respective displacement fields is given by

$$V_{k,cav}\left(\boldsymbol{u_k}\right) = \int_{\Omega_{inner}} dv = -\frac{1}{3}\int_{\Gamma_{inner}} \boldsymbol{x_k} \cdot \boldsymbol{n_k}\, da\,, \tag{9}$$

where $\Omega_{inner}$ is the volume enclosed by the inner surface $\Gamma_{inner}$ and the basal surface at $z = 0$, and $\boldsymbol{n_k}$ is the outward unit normal vector.

Pressure-volume relationships of the LV and aorta required in the lumped parameter circulatory model [i.e., Equations (6, 7)] were defined by the solution obtained from minimizing the functional. Taking the first variation of the functional in Equation (8) leads to the following expression:

$$\delta\mathcal{L}_k\left(\boldsymbol{u_k}, p_k, P_{k,cav}, \boldsymbol{c_{1,k}}, \boldsymbol{c_{2,k}}\right) = \int_{\Omega_{0,k}} \left(\boldsymbol{P_k} - p_k\boldsymbol{F_k}^{-T}\right) : \nabla\delta\boldsymbol{u_k}\, dV$$

$$- \int_{\Omega_{0,k}} \delta p_k\left(J_k - 1\right) dV - P_{k,cav}\int_{\Omega_{0,k}} cof\left(\boldsymbol{F_k}\right) : \nabla\delta\boldsymbol{u_k}\, dV$$

$$- \delta P_{k,cav}\left(V_{k,cav}\left(\boldsymbol{u_k}\right) - V_k\right) - \delta\boldsymbol{c_{1,k}}\cdot\int_{\Omega_{0,k}} \boldsymbol{u_k}\, dV$$

$$- \delta\boldsymbol{c_{2,k}}\cdot\int_{\Omega_{0,k}} \boldsymbol{X_k} \times \boldsymbol{u_k}\, dV - \boldsymbol{c_{1,k}}\cdot\int_{\Omega_{0,k}} \delta\boldsymbol{u_k}\, dV$$

$$- \boldsymbol{c_{2,k}}\cdot\int_{\Omega_{0,k}} \boldsymbol{X_k} \times \delta\boldsymbol{u_k}\, dV. \tag{10}$$

In Equation (10), $\boldsymbol{P_k}$ is the first Piola Kirchhoff stress tensor, $\boldsymbol{F_k}$ is the deformation gradient tensor, $\delta\boldsymbol{u_k}$, $\delta p_k$, $\delta P_{k,cav}$, $\delta\boldsymbol{c_{1,k}}$, $\delta\boldsymbol{c_{2,k}}$ are the variation of the displacement field, Lagrange multipliers for enforcing incompressibility and volume constraint, zero mean translation and rotation, respectively. The Euler-Lagrange problem then becomes finding $\boldsymbol{u_k} \in H^1\left(\Omega_{0,k}\right)$, $p_k \in L^2\left(\Omega_{0,k}\right)$, $P_{k,cav} \in \mathbb{R}$, $\boldsymbol{c_{1,k}} \in \mathbb{R}^3$, $\boldsymbol{c_{2,k}} \in \mathbb{R}^3$ that satisfies

$$\delta\mathcal{L}_k\left(\boldsymbol{u_k}, p_k, P_{k,cav}, \boldsymbol{c_{1,k}}, \boldsymbol{c_{2,k}}\right) = 0 \tag{11}$$

and $\boldsymbol{u_k}\cdot\boldsymbol{n_k}|_{\boldsymbol{base}} = 0$ (for constraining the basal deformation to be in-plane) $\forall\ \delta\boldsymbol{u_k}\ \in H^1\left(\Omega_{0,k}\right)$, $\delta p_k \in L^2\left(\Omega_{0,k}\right)$, $\delta P_{k,cav} \in \mathbb{R}$, $\delta\boldsymbol{c_{1,k}} \in \mathbb{R}^3$, $\delta\boldsymbol{c_{2,k}} \in \mathbb{R}^3$.

An explicit time integration scheme was used to solve the ODEs in Equation (1). Specifically, compartment volumes ($V_{LA}$, $V_{LV}$, $V_{art}$, $V_{ven}$) at each timestep $t_i$ was determined from their respective values and the segmental flow rates ($q_{ven}$, $q_{mv}$, $q_{ao}$, $q_{per}$) at previous timestep $t_{i-1}$ in Equation (1). The computed compartment volumes at $t_i$ were used to update the corresponding pressures ($P_{LA}$, $P_{LV}$, $P_{art}$, $P_{ven}$). Pressures in the left atrium ($P_{LA}$) and veins ($P_{ven}$) were computed from Equations (4) and (3), respectively. On the other hand, pressures in the LV ($P_{LV,cav}$) and aorta ($P_{art,cav}$) were computed from the FE solutions of Equation (11) (for $k = LV$ and $art$) with the volumes ($V_{LV}$, $V_{art}$) at timestep $t_i$ as input. We note here that ($P_{LV,cav}$, $P_{art,cav}$) are scalar Lagrange multipliers in the FE formulation for constraining the cavity volumes to the prescribed values ($V_{LV}$, $V_{art}$). The computed pressures at timestep $t_i$ were then used to update the segmental flow rates in Equation (2) that will be used to compute the compartment volumes at timestep $t_{i+1}$ in the next iteration. Steady-state pressure-volume loop was established by running the simulation over several cardiac cycles, each with a cycle time of 800 ms (equivalent to 75 bpm). All the parameter values used in the circulatory model are listed in **Table 2**.

## Geometry and Microstructure of the LV

The LV geometry was described using a half prolate ellipsoid that was discretized with 1325 quadratic tetrahedral elements. The helix angle associated with the myofiber direction $\boldsymbol{e_{f_0}}$ was varied with a linear transmural variation from $60°$ at the endocardium to $-60°$ at the epicardium in the LV wall based on previous experimental measurements (Streeter et al., 1969) (**Figure 1C**).

## Constitutive Law of the LV

An active stress formulation was used to describe the LV's mechanical behavior in the cardiac cycle. In this formulation, the stress tensor $\boldsymbol{P_{LV}}$ can be decomposed additively into a passive component $\boldsymbol{P_{LV,p}}$ and an active component $\boldsymbol{P_{LV,a}}$ (i.e., $\boldsymbol{P_{LV}} = \boldsymbol{P_{LV,a}} + \boldsymbol{P_{LV,p}}$). The passive stress tensor was defined by $\boldsymbol{P_{LV,p}} = dW_{LV}/d\boldsymbol{F_{LV}}$, where $W_{LV}$ is a strain energy function of a Fung-type transversely-isotropic hyperelastic material (Guccione et al., 1991) given by

$$W_{LV} = \frac{1}{2}C\left(e^Q - 1\right), \tag{12a}$$

where,

$$Q = b_{ff}E_{ff}^2 + b_{xx}\left(E_{ss}^2 + E_{nn}^2 + E_{sn}^2 + E_{ns}^2\right)$$
$$+ b_{fx}\left(E_{fn}^2 + E_{nf}^2 + E_{fs}^2 + E_{sf}^2\right). \tag{12b}$$

In Equation (12), $E_{ij}$ with $(i, j) \in (f, s, n)$ are components of the Green-Lagrange strain tensor $\boldsymbol{E_{LV}}$ with $f$, $s$, $n$ denoting the myocardial fiber, sheet and sheet normal directions, respectively.

Material parameters of the passive constitutive model are denoted by $C$, $b_{ff}$, $b_{xx}$, and $b_{fx}$.

The active stress $\mathbf{P}_{LV,a}$ was calculated along the local fiber direction using a previously developed active contraction model (Guccione et al., 1993; Dang et al., 2005),

$$\mathbf{P}_{LV,a} = T_{max} \frac{Ca_0^2}{Ca_0^2 + ECa_{50}^2} C_t \, \mathbf{e}_f \otimes \mathbf{e}_{f_0}. \tag{13}$$

In the above equation, $\mathbf{e}_f$ and $\mathbf{e}_{f_0}$ are, respectively, the local vectors defining the muscle fiber direction in the current and reference configurations, $T_{max}$ is the isometric tension achieved at the longest sarcomere length and $Ca_0$ denotes the peak intracellular calcium concentration. The length dependent calcium sensitivity $ECa_{50}$ and the variable $C_t$ are given by

$$ECa_{50} = \frac{(Ca_0)_{max}}{\sqrt{\exp\left(B\left(l - l_0\right)\right) - 1}}, \tag{14a}$$

$$C_t = \frac{1}{2}\left(1 - \cos\omega\right). \tag{14b}$$

In Equation (14a), $B$ is a constant, $(Ca_0)_{max}$ is the maximum peak intracellular calcium concentration and $l_0$ is the sarcomere length at which no active tension develops. The variable $\omega$ in Equation (14b) is given by

$$\omega = \begin{cases} \pi \frac{t}{t_0}, & 0 \le t < t_0; \\ \pi \frac{t - t_0 + t_r}{t_r}, & t_0 \le t < t_0 + t_r; \\ 0, & t_0 + t_r \le t. \end{cases} \tag{15}$$

In the above equation, $t_0$ is the time taken to reach peak tension and $t_r$ is the duration of relaxation that depends linearly on the sarcomere length $l$ by

$$t_r = ml + b, \tag{16}$$

where $m$ and $b$ are constants. The sarcomere length $l$ can be calculated from the myofiber stretch $\lambda_{LV}$ by

$$\lambda_{LV} = \sqrt{\mathbf{e}_{f_0} \cdot \mathbf{C}_{LV} \mathbf{e}_{f_0}}, \tag{17a}$$

$$l = \lambda_{LV} l_r. \tag{17b}$$

In Equation (17a), $\mathbf{C}_{LV} = \mathbf{F}_{LV}^T \mathbf{F}_{LV}$ is the right Cauchy-Green deformation tensor and $l_r$ is the relaxed sarcomere length. Parameter values associated with the LV model are tabulated in **Table 3**.

## Geometry and Microstructure of the Aorta

An idealized geometry of the aorta extending from the heart to the thoracic region from a previous study (Vasava et al., 2012) was used here. The geometry was discretized using 1020 quadratic tetrahedral elements. The aorta diameter was assumed to be constant in the first segment starting from the aortic root to the middle of the aortic arch, and then gradually decreased toward the thoracic region. Aortic wall thickness was kept constant (**Figure 1B**).

**TABLE 3 |** Parameters of the LV model.

| Parameter | Description | Value |
|---|---|---|
| $C$ | material parameter, kPa | 0.10 |
| $b_{ff}$ | material parameter | 29.9 |
| $b_{xx}$ | material parameter | 13.3 |
| $b_{fx}$ | material parameter | 26.6 |
| $T_{max}$ | isometric tension under maximal activation, kPa | 200.7 |
| $Ca_0$ | peak intracellular calcium concentration, $\mu$M | 4.35 |
| $(Ca_0)_{max}$ | maximum peak intracellular calcium concentration, $\mu$M | 4.35 |
| $B$ | governs shape of peak isometric tension-sarcomere length relation, $\mu$m$^{-1}$ | 4.75 |
| $l_0$ | sarcomere length at which no active tension develops, $\mu$m | 1.58 |
| $t_0$ | time to peak tension, ms | 171 |
| $m$ | slope of linear relaxation duration-sarcomere length relation, ms $\mu$m$^{-1}$ | 1,049 |
| $b$ | time-intercept of linear relaxation duration-sarcomere length relation, ms | 1,500 |
| $l_r$ | relaxed sarcomere length, $\mu$m | 1.85 |

**TABLE 4 |** Parameters of the aorta model.

| | |
|---|---|
| Elastin | $c_1 = 160$ kPa, $\phi_e = 0.306$ |
| Collagen families | $c_2 = 0.08$ kPa, $c_3 = 2.54$, $\phi_c = 0.544$ ($\phi_1 = 0.1\phi_c$, $\phi_2 = 0.1\phi_c$, $\phi_3 = 0.4\phi_c$, $\phi_4 = 0.4\phi_c$) |
| SMC | $c_4 = 0.01$ kPa, $c_5 = 7.28$, $\phi_m = 0.15$ |
| Others | $\rho = 1050$ kg/m$^3$, $S_m = 54$ kPa, $\lambda_M = 1.4$, $\lambda_0 = 0.8$ |

## Constitutive Law of the Aorta

Stress tensor in the aortic wall was defined by $\mathbf{P}_{art} = dW_{art}/d\mathbf{F}_{art}$, where $W_{art}$ is the sum of the strain energy functions associated with those from the key tissue constituents, namely, elastin-dominated matrix $W_e$, collagen fiber families $W_{c,k}$ and vascular smooth muscle cells (SMC) $W_m$ (Baek et al., 2007; Zeinali-Davarani et al., 2011), i.e.,

$$W_{art} = W_e + \sum_{k=1}^{4} W_{c,k} + W_m. \tag{18}$$

Strain energy function of the elastin-dominated amorphous matrix is given by

$$W_e = M_e \left(\frac{c_1}{2}\right) (tr\,(\mathbf{C}_{art}) - 3), \tag{19}$$

where $M_e$ is the mass per unit volume of the elastin in the tissue, $c_1$ is a material parameter and, $\mathbf{C}_{art} = \mathbf{F}_{art}^T \mathbf{F}_{art}$ is the right Cauchy-Green deformation tensor associated with the aorta.

Four collagen fiber families were considered here. The first and second families of collagen fibers ($k = 1$ and 2) were oriented in the longitudinal and circumferential directions, whereas the third and fourth families of collagen fibers ($k = 3$ and 4) were oriented, respectively, at an angle $\alpha = 45°$ and $-45°$ with respect to the longitudinal axis (**Figure 1B**). We assumed the same strain

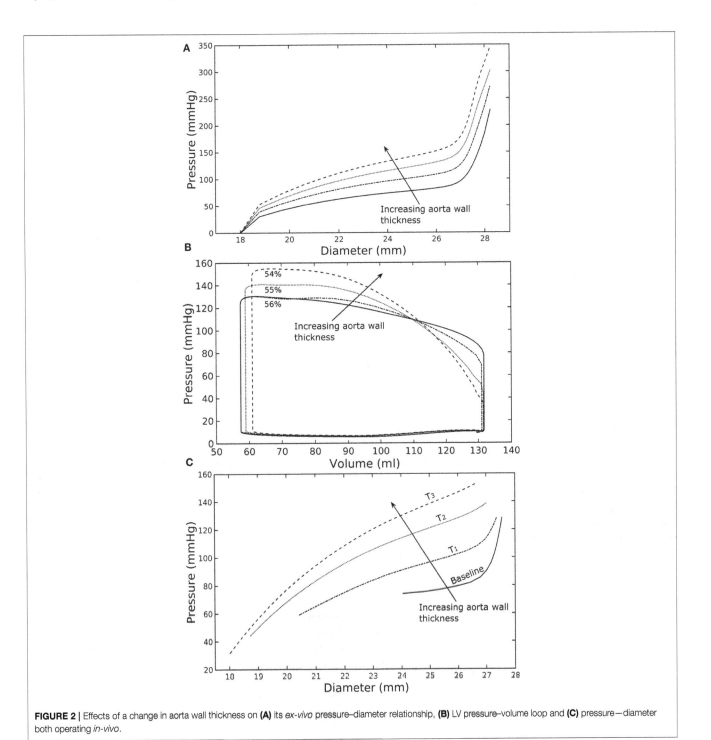

**FIGURE 2 |** Effects of a change in aorta wall thickness on **(A)** its *ex-vivo* pressure–diameter relationship, **(B)** LV pressure–volume loop and **(C)** pressure—diameter both operating *in-vivo*.

energy function for all the families of collagen fibers that is given by

$$W_{c,k} = M_k \frac{c_2}{4c_3} \left\{ \exp\left[ c_3 \left( \lambda_k{}^2 - 1 \right)^2 \right] - 1 \right\}. \qquad (20)$$

In Equation (20), $M_k$ is the mass per unit volume of $k$th family of collagen fibers, $\lambda_k$ is the corresponding stretch of those fibers, and both $c_2$ and $c_3$ are the material parameters. The stretch in the $k$th family of collagen fibers was defined by $\lambda_k = \sqrt{e_{k0} \cdot C_{art} e_{k0}}$,

where $e_{k0}$ is the local unit vector defining the corresponding fibers orientation.

Strain energy function of the smooth muscle cells $W_m$ was additively decomposed into one describing its passive mechanical behavior $W_{m,p}$ and one describing its active behavior $W_{m,a}$ (i.e., $W_m = W_{m,p} + W_{m,a}$). The passive strain energy function is given by

$$W_{m,p} = M_m \frac{c_4}{4c_5} \left\{ exp\left[ c_5 \left( \lambda_m{}^2 - 1 \right)^2 \right] - 1 \right\}. \qquad (21)$$

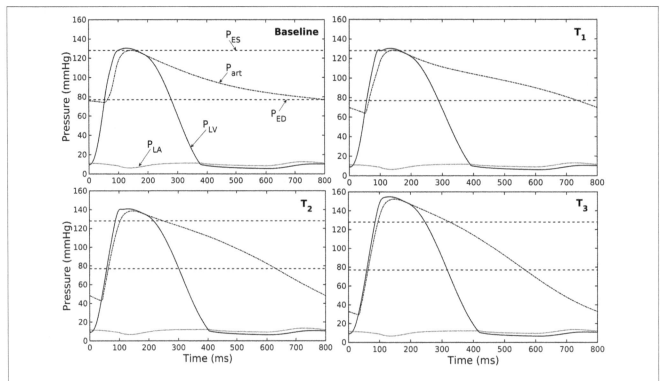

**FIGURE 3 |** Pressure in LV, aorta, and LA during cardiac cycle with increasing aorta wall thickness in ascending order from the Baseline to $T_3$ case ($P_{ES}$ and $P_{ED}$ are respectively, the end-systolic and end-diastolic pressure for the baseline case).

Here, $M_m$ is the mass per unit volume of the smooth muscle in the tissue, $\lambda_m$ is the stretch of the smooth muscle, whereas $c_4$ and $c_5$ are the material parameters. The smooth muscle cells were assumed to be perfectly aligned in the circumferential direction. Its stretch is therefore equivalent to that of the second family of collagen fibers, i.e., $\lambda_m = \lambda_2$. We used the following strain energy function (Zeinali-Davarani et al., 2011) to describe the active tone of vascular smooth muscle,

$$W_{m,a} = M_m \frac{S_m}{\rho} \left[ \lambda_m + \frac{(\lambda_M - \lambda_m)^3}{3 (\lambda_M - \lambda_0)^2} \right]. \qquad (22)$$

In Equation (22), $S_m$ is the stress at maximum contraction, $\rho$ is the density of the tissue, $\lambda_M$ is the prescribed stretch at which the contraction is maximum and $\lambda_0$ is the prescribed stretch at which active force generation ceases. Mass per unit volume for the different constituents were calculated using following relations

$$M_e = \phi_e \rho, \qquad (23a)$$

$$M_m = \phi_m \rho, \qquad (23b)$$

$$M_k = \phi_k (1 - \phi_e - \phi_m) \rho, \qquad (23c)$$

where $\phi_e$, $\phi_m$, and $\phi_k$ denote the mass fraction for elastin, smooth muscle cells and $k$th family of collagen fibers. It was assumed that 20% of the total collagen mass was distributed equally toward the longitudinal and circumferential fiber families and the remaining 80% was distributed equally to the $\alpha = 45°$ and $-45°$ fiber families. Constitutive parameters, mass fraction of each constituents and other parameters of the aorta model are listed in **Table 4**.

The coupled LV-aorta modeling framework, including the solving of FE equations associated with the LV and aorta models, was implemented using the open-source FE library FEniCS (Alnæs et al., 2015).

## RESULTS

A baseline case was established using the LV-aorta coupling framework so that LV pressure-volume loop and aorta pressure-diameter curve were consistent with measurements in the normal human systemic circulation under physiological conditions. Specifically, model prediction of the LV ejection fraction (EF) was 56%, which is within the normal range in humans (**Figure 2B**). Similarly, end-diastolic (ED) and end-systolic (ES) diameters of the aorta in the baseline case (**Figure 2C**) were comparable to *in-vivo* measurements (Greenfield and Patel, 1962; Muraru et al., 2014). We note here that diameter of the aorta mentioned in subsequent text refers to its inner diameter. Pressure waveforms of the LV, aorta, and LA (**Figure 3**) in the baseline case were also within the normal range with an aortic pulse pressure of 50 mmHg (systolic: 128 mmHg, diastolic: 78 mmHg).

## Effects of a Change in Aorta Wall Thickness

Varying the wall thickness in the aorta model led to changes in not only the aorta mechanical behavior but also the LV function (**Figure 2**). The aorta became stiffer (less compliant)

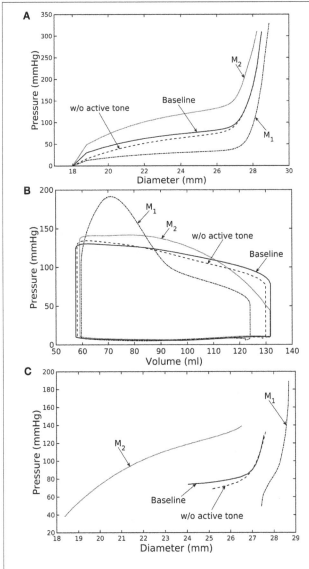

**FIGURE 4 |** Effects of active tone and aorta constituent mass fractions on **(A)** its *ex-vivo* pressure–diameter relationship, **(B)** LV pressure–volume loop and **(C)** pressure—diameter both operating *in-vivo*. (Refer to **Table 5** for cases).

**TABLE 5 |** Mass fractions of the aorta constituents for different cases investigated in the study.

| Case | Mass fractions of the constituents | Comment |
|---|---|---|
| Baseline | Same as **Table 4** | No change |
| Without active | Same as **Table 4** | No active tone in SM, $S_m = 0$ |
| $M_1$ | $\phi_e = 0.122$, $\phi_m = 0.061$, $\phi_c = 0.816$ | Collagen increased by 50%, Elastin and SMC decreased proportionally |
| $M_2$ | $\phi_e = 0.49$, $\phi_m = 0.24$, $\phi_c = 0.272$ | Collagen decreased by 50%, Elastin and SMC increased proportionally |

*For collagen fibers, the distribution of mass in four collagen fiber families was kept the same, i.e., $\phi_1 = 0.1\phi_c$, $\phi_2 = 0.1\phi_c$, $\phi_3 = 0.4\phi_c$, $\phi_4 = 0.4\phi_c$ for all cases.*

## Effect of Changes in Mass Fractions of the Aorta Constituents

Similarly, varying mass fraction of the constituents in the aorta wall (see **Table 5** for the different cases) also led to changes in both the aorta and LV functions. Increasing collagen mass fraction with a corresponding decrease in SMC and elastin mass fractions (case $M_1$) led to a predominantly exponential pressure - diameter response of the aorta that became extremely steep at larger diameter (i.e., >28 mm) (**Figure 4A**). This is because the collagen fibers are stiffer than other constituents at large strain. Under *in vivo* operating condition (as simulated in the LV-aorta coupling framework), an increase in collagen mass fraction resulted in a higher peak systolic pressure and a reduced LV EF (**Figure 4B**). The exponential mechanical response (shown in **Figure 4A**) of the aorta with higher collagen mass fraction was also reflected in the ejection phase of the LV pressure-volume loop, where the pressure-volume curve became steeper toward end-of-systole. With a higher collagen mass fraction, the aorta also operated at a larger diameter than the baseline *in vivo* (**Figure 4C**). Pulse pressure in the aorta with higher collagen mass fraction was much higher and decayed more rapidly when compared to the baseline case (**Figure 5**).

Conversely, reducing collagen mass fraction and increasing elastin and SMC mass fraction proportionally (case $M_2$) led to a dominant neo-Hookean type pressure - diameter behavior, particularly, at smaller diameter (<25 mm). Under *in vivo* operating condition, the peak pressure increased slightly but EF remained nearly unchanged in the LV (**Figure 4B**). The aorta also appeared to be more compliant *in vivo* with a larger change in aortic diameter (~8.1 mm), especially when compared to case $M_1$ that has a higher collagen mass fraction (~1.3 mm) (**Figure 4C**). On the other hand, the aorta also operated at smaller ED and ES diameters than the baseline. Pressure waveforms of the aorta, LV, and LA were not significantly changed compared to the baseline (**Figure 5**).

In the absence of SMC's active tone, the aorta became slightly more compliant than the baseline at diameter smaller than 27 mm (**Figure 4A**). Thus, for a given pressure, the diameter was larger than the baseline. Under *in vivo* operating condition, this change led to a slight increase in the LV and aorta pressure

with increasing wall thickness as reflected by an increase in the slope of the pressure-diameter curves (**Figure 2A**). When operating *in vivo* as simulated in the LV-aorta coupling framework, increasing the aorta wall thickness led to a lower LV EF, a higher peak systolic pressure of the LV (**Figure 2B**) and a leftward shift in the aorta pressure—diameter relationship with smaller diameter at ED and ES (**Figure 2C**). Specifically, an increase in aorta ED wall thickness from 1.8 mm (baseline) to 5.4 mm (T$_3$ case) was accompanied by an increase in pulse pressure from 50 mmHg (in the baseline case) to 120 mmHg. In comparison, the mean aortic pressure changed by only about 10 mmHg (decreased from 102 to 93 mm Hg) for the same increase in wall thickness.

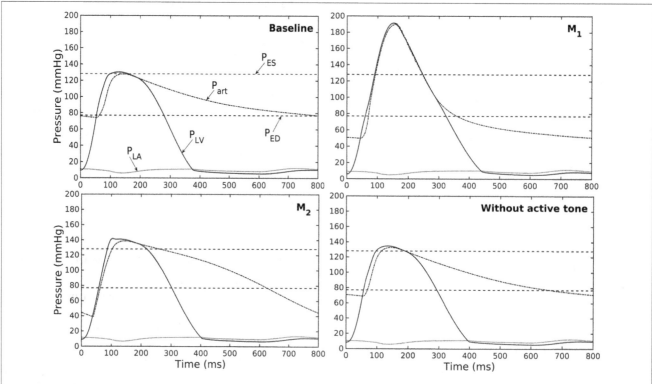

**FIGURE 5 |** Pressure in LV, aorta, and LA during cardiac cycle for different aorta constituent mass fractions and active tone ($P_{ES}$ and $P_{ED}$ are respectively, the end-systolic and end-diastolic pressure for the baseline case).

at ES than the baseline (**Figures 4B,C**). On the other hand, LV and aorta pressure at ED decreased without the active tone (**Figures 4B,C**), resulting in an increase in the aortic pulse pressure compared to baseline (**Figure 5**).

## Effects of a Change in LV contractility

Reducing LV contractility ($T_{max}$) led to a decrease in its peak systolic pressure, end systolic volume and EF (**Figure 6A**). Pressure also dropped accordingly (**Figure 6B**) in the aorta together with the peak stress (**Figure 6C**). With a reduction in LV contractility by 50% (from 200.7 to 100.4 kPa), aorta peak stress was reduced by about 50% compared to the baseline case (from 214 to 110 kPa). The stress was calculated as a root of the sum of the square of all components of the Cauchy stress tensor. Reducing LV contractility also led to changes in the aorta diameter. As a result of lower LV contractility, the aortic pressure decreased that led to less expansion and a decrease in both its ED (from 24.0 mm in baseline to 22.5 mm in case $C_2$) and ES diameter (from 27.5 mm in baseline to 27.0 mm in case $C_2$).

## Effects of a Change in LV Passive Stiffness

Increasing the LV passive stiffness (parameter $C$) in Equation (12a) led to a stiffer end diastolic pressure—volume relationship that was accompanied by a reduction in preload, peak systolic pressure, and EF (as end systolic volume remained nearly unchanged) in the chamber (**Figure 7A**). These changes were translated to a decrease in aortic pressure and peak stress (**Figures 7B,C**) as well as a reduction in its ED (from 24.0 mm in

baseline to 22.4 mm in case $P_2$) and ES (from 27.5 mm in baseline to 27.1 mm in case $P_2$) diameters.

## DISCUSSION

Finite element models of the LV have been widely used in the literature to study its mechanics as well as organ-scale physiological behaviors in the cardiac cycle (Usyk et al., 2002; Kerckhoffs et al., 2007; Lee et al., 2016; Xi et al., 2016; Shavik et al., 2017). In these models, the aorta is usually represented within the lumped parameter circulatory model by its electrical analog, which cannot separate the effects its geometry, microstructure, and constituents' mechanical behavior have on the LV's operating behavior *in vivo* and vice versa. To the best of our knowledge, this is the first computational modeling framework in which FE models of the aorta and LV are coupled in a closed-loop fashion. This framework enables us to take into detailed account of the geometrical, microstructural, and mechanical behavior of the LV and aorta. We have shown here that the coupled LV—aorta FE framework is able to capture physiological behaviors in both the LV and aorta that are consistent with *in vivo* measurements. We also showed that the framework can reasonably predict the effects of changes in geometry and microstructural details the two compartments have on each other over the cardiac cycle.

Using a detailed FE model of the aorta has enabled us to separate the contributions of the key load bearing constituents (elastin, collagen fibers, and SMCs) have on its mechanical

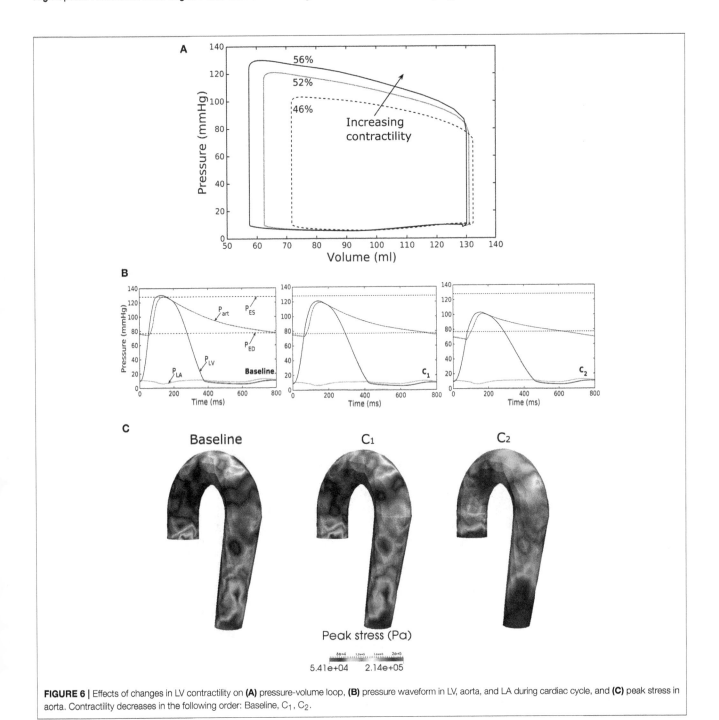

**FIGURE 6 |** Effects of changes in LV contractility on **(A)** pressure-volume loop, **(B)** pressure waveform in LV, aorta, and LA during cardiac cycle, and **(C)** peak stress in aorta. Contractility decreases in the following order: Baseline, $C_1$, $C_2$.

behavior. The aorta FE model predicted a pressure—diameter response in which the mechanical behavior of each constituent is clearly detectable (**Figure 2A**). For instance, mechanical behavior of aorta at lower diameter range (low stretch) is relatively compliant as it is largely endowed by elastin, but exhibits a very stiff behavior at the higher diameter range (high stretch) when more collagen fibers are recruited. The behavior is consistent with previous experimental studies (Roach and Burton, 1957; Schriefl et al., 2012; Kohn et al., 2015). The pressure—diameter relationship predicted by our model (**Figure 2A**) resembled a S-shaped curve with a very stiff response after the inflection point that is a typical feature of large proximal arterial vessels (Bader, 1967; Towfiq et al., 1986).

Our model predicted that an increase in aortic wall thickness led it to become more constricted with smaller ED and ES diameter under *in vivo* operating conditions when coupled to the LV in our modeling framework (**Figure 2C**). Systolic blood pressure and pulse pressure in the aorta increased as a result, and was accompanied by a reduction in stroke volume and an increase in LV peak systolic pressure (**Figure 2B**). Although

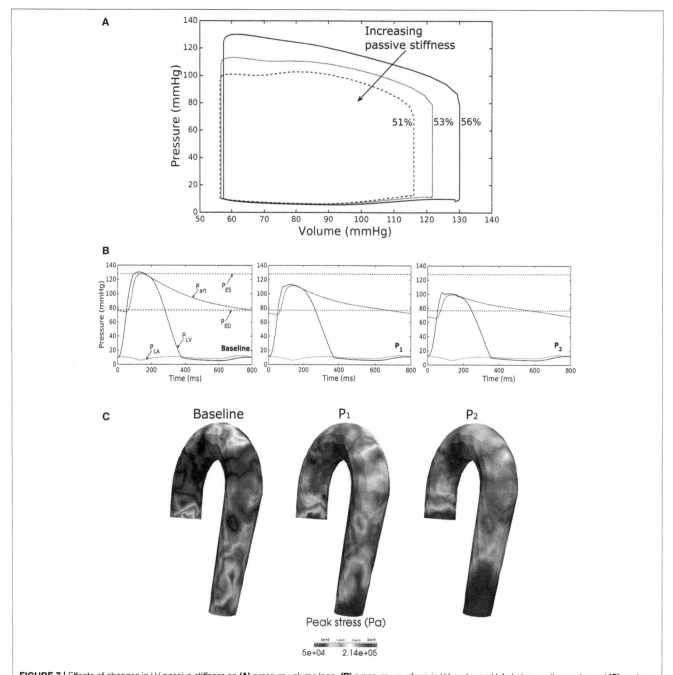

**FIGURE 7** | Effects of changes in LV passive stiffness on **(A)** pressure-volume loop, **(B)** pressure waveform in LV, aorta, and LA during cardiac cycle, and **(C)** peak stress in aorta. Passive stiffness increases in the following order: Baseline, $P_1$, $P_2$.

previous vascular studies suggest that an increase in arterial wall thickness (that may be accompanied by an increase in stiffness) is a result from an increase blood pressure during aging, more recent evidence have suggested that stiffening is a cause for the increase in blood pressure in which a positive feedback loop between them proceeds gradually (Humphrey et al., 2016). These features are consistent with those found in clinical and experimental studies. Specifically, it has been found that the mean aortic wall thickness increases with age (Li et al., 2004; Rosero et al., 2011) in human, which increases the risk of

hypertension and atherosclerosis. Similarly, our model predicted that an increase in aortic wall thickness by 70% elevates the aortic pressure over the hypertensive range (>140 mmHg) (**Figure 3**).

Changes in the aorta microstructure is a feature of pathological remodeling as well as aging. In the systemic vasculature, the proximal aorta has a compliant behavior that helps to keep the systolic blood pressure down. With aging, however, elastin degenerates and is replaced (i.e., compensated) by collagen in the aorta wall (Schlatmann and Becker, 1977; Tsamis et al., 2013; Kohn et al., 2015). Consequently, the collagen fibers bear more of the load that substantially increases the aorta wall stiffness, especially at high stretch. A stiffer aorta leads to many adverse effects including elevated systolic and pulse pressure during ejection, faster decay in the aortic pressure waveform during diastole, and an increase in ventricular afterload that reduces the LV EF (Borlaug and Kass, 2011). These behaviors are all captured in our framework when collagen and elastin mass fractions were increased and decreased, respectively. Specifically, these microstructural changes led to a reduction in EF (**Figure 4B**) and an increase in the aortic systolic and pulse pressure with a faster decay of aortic pressure waveform (**Figure 5**). Our framework also predicted that the aorta underwent more expansion *in vivo* and have a larger operating diameter when collagen mass fraction increases (**Figure 4C**), which is another key characteristic of aging (Bader, 1967; Mao et al., 2008; Craiem et al., 2012). Interestingly, changes in the aorta collagen mass fraction (that lead to it stiffen at high stretch) also affects the shape of the LV pressure volume loop (**Figure 4B**, case $M_1$). Specifically, a rapid steepening of the LV pressure-volume curve near end-of-systole is predicted by our model when collagen mass fraction is increased. This result suggests that the shape of the LV pressure-volume loop may also reflect, to some extent, the accumulation of collagen fibers in the aorta during remodeling.

Our framework also predicted how changes in the contractility and passive stiffness of the LV affects the aorta function. A decrease in LV contractility led to lower LV EF, lower aortic systolic and pulse pressures, as well as a reduction in the aorta peak stress during the cardiac cycle (**Figure 6**). A change in contractility (or inotropic state of the myocardium) produced expected changes (Katz, 1988; Burkhoff, 2005) in the LV pressure—volume loop and aortic pulse pressure. Similarly, the model predicted results from a change in the LV passive stiffness that are consistent with experimental observations (**Figure 7**). With increasing passive stiffness, LV EF decreases and is accompanied by a corresponding decrease in aortic systolic and pulse pressure, as well as peak stress. A change in the passive stiffness of LV (due to such as an alteration in lusitropy), also shows similar changes in the LV pressure—volume loops (Katz, 1988; Burkhoff, 2005) as well as the aortic pressure.

Most clinical studies focus either on the behavior of the LV or aorta. While a number of studies have investigated ventricular—arterial coupling (Kawaguchi et al., 2003; Borlaug and Kass, 2011; Antonini-Canterin et al., 2013; Ky et al., 2013), simplified indices (such as the ratio of end-systolic volume to stroke volume) were used in them to describe this coupling. It is, however, impossible to separate the contribution of microstructure, mechanical behavior, and geometry of the aorta (e.g., diameter or thickness) and LV to any changes in ventricular—arterial coupling. The framework described here helps overcome this limitation and may be useful for developing more insights of the ventricular—arterial interaction. This framework will be extended in future to include the pulmonary vasculature for a more complete understanding of the interactions between the heart and vasculature under different physiological or pathological conditions.

## MODEL LIMITATIONS

We have shown that our coupled LV-aorta FE modeling framework is capable of predicting behaviors that are consistent with measurements. There are, however, some limitations associated with our model. First, idealized geometries were used to represent the aorta and LV models. The idealized half-prolate geometry of the LV used here neglected any asymmetrical geometrical features while the aorta geometry was also simplified and had uniform wall thickness. Because wall thickness decreases slightly along the aorta (Mello et al., 2004), its displacement with the given material parameters may be under-estimated. Second, we have assumed homogeneous material properties in our models. Given that studies have suggested that the mechanical properties may be inhomogeneous in the aorta (Kermani et al., 2017) and LV (Khokhlova and Iribe, 2016), the prescribed material parameters are bulk quantities. While thoracic aortic wall thickness and its stiffness varies, previous experimental studies reported that the aortic structural stiffness (product of intrinsic stiffness and aortic wall thickness) is relatively uniform in the circumferential and longitudinal directions (Kim and Baek, 2011; Kim et al., 2013). Third, the dynamical behavior of fluid and its interaction with the vessel wall were neglected here, and as such, the framework did not take into account the spatial variation of pressure waveform along the aortic tree and shear stress on the luminal surface of the vessel. However, we do not expect this limitation to severely affect our result because wall shear stress in the human aorta ($\sim$50 dyn/cm$^2$ or 0.037 mmHg) (LaDisa et al., 2011) is substantially lower than the pressure (normal stress) (60–120 mm Hg), and the arterial pressure increases by only about 10% from the ascending to the abdominal aorta (Smulyan and Safar, 1997). Fourth, a rule based myofiber orientation in which the helix angle varies linearly across the myocardial wall was used to describe the LV microstructure. Fifth, remodeling of the aorta and LV was simulated by directly manipulating the parameters without consideration of any growth and remodeling mechanisms. Last, we have considered only systemic circulation in this model and ignored the presence of the right ventricle and pulmonary circulatory system that may affect LV and aorta mechanics.

## AUTHOR CONTRIBUTIONS

SMS and LCL developed the theoretical formulation and computational framework of the model. ZJ and SB helped on the development of the theoretical formulation. SMS carried out the simulations for different cases and prepared the results. All authors helped in interpretation of the results and contributed to the final manuscript.

# REFERENCES

Alnæs, M., Blechta, J., Hake, J., Johansson, A., Kehlet, B., Logg, A., et al. (2015). The FEniCS project version 1.5. *Arch. Numer. Softw.* 3, 9–23. doi: 10.11588/ans.2015.100.20553

Antonini-Canterin, F., Poli, S., Vriz, O., Pavan, D., Bello, V. D., and Nicolosi, G. L. (2013). The ventricular-arterial coupling: from basic pathophysiology to clinical application in the echocardiography laboratory. *J. Cardiovasc. Echography* 23:91. doi: 10.4103/2211-4122.127408

Arts, T., Delhaas, T., Bovendeerd, P., Verbeek, X., and Prinzen, F. (2005). Adaptation to mechanical load determines shape and properties of heart and circulation: the circadapt model. *Am. J. Physiol. Heart Circ. Physiol.* 288, 1943–1954. doi: 10.1152/ajpheart.00444.2004

Bader, H. (1967). Dependence of wall stress in the human thoracic aorta on age and pressure. *Circ. Res.* 20, 354–361.

Baek, S., Valentín, A., and Humphrey, J. D. (2007). Biochemomechanics of cerebral vasospasm and its resolution: iconstitutive relations, i., and model simulations. *Ann. Biomed. Eng.* 35, 1498–1509. doi: 10.1007/s10439-007-9322-x

Borlaug, B. A., and Kass, D. A. (2011). Ventricular-vascular interaction in heart failure. *Cardiol. Clin.* 29, 447–459. doi: 10.1016/j.ccl.2011.06.004

Burkhoff, D. (2005). Assessment of systolic and diastolic ventricular properties via pressure-volume analysis: a guide for clinical, translational, and basic researchers. *Am. J .Physiol. Heart Circ. Physiol.* 289, H501–H512. doi: 10.1152/ajpheart.00138.2005

Craiem, D., Casciaro, M. E., Graf, S., Chironi, G., Simon, A., and Armentano, R. L. (2012). Effects of aging on thoracic aorta size and shape: a non-contrast ct study. *Conf. Proc. IEEE. Eng. Med. Biol. Soc.* 2012, 4986–4989. doi: 10.1109/EMBC.2012.6347112

Dang, A. B., Guccione, J. M., Mishell, J. M., Zhang, P. Wallace, A. W., Gorman, R. C., et al. (2005). Akinetic myocardial infarcts must contain contracting myocytes: finite-element model study. *Am. J. Physiol. Heart Circ. Physiol.* 288, H1844–H1850. doi: 10.1152/ajpheart.00961.2003

Gao, H., Wang, H., Berry, C., Luo, X., and Griffith, B. E. (2014). Quasi-Static image-based immersed boundary-finite element model of left ventricle under diastolic loading. *Int. J. Numer. Method. Biomed. Eng.* 30, 1199–1222. doi: 10.1002/cnm.2652

Genet, M., Lee, L. C., Nguyen, R., Haraldsson, H., Acevedo-Bolton, G., Zhang, Z., et al. (2014). Distribution of normal human left ventricular myofiber stress at end diastole and end systole: a target for *in silico* design of heart failure treatments. *J. Appl. Physiol.* 117, 142–152. doi: 10.1152/japplphysiol.00255.2014

Giamouzis, G., Schelbert, E. B., and Butler, J. (2016). Growing evidence linking microvascular dysfunction with heart failure with preserved ejection fraction. *J. Am. Heart Assoc.* 5:e003259. doi: 10.1161/JAHA.116.003259

Greenfield, J. C., and Patel, D. J. (1962). Relation between pressure and diameter in the ascending aorta of man. *Circ. Res.* 10, 778–781. doi: 10.1161/01.RES.10.5.778

Guccione, J. M., McCulloch, A. D., and Waldman, L. K. (1991). Passive material properties of intact ventricular myocardium determined from a cylindrical model. *J. Biomech. Eng.* 113, 42–55. doi: 10.1115/1.2894084

Guccione, J. M., Waldman, L. K., and McCulloch, A. D. (1993). Mechanics of active contraction in cardiac muscle: part ii–cylindrical models of the systolic left ventricle. *J. Biomech. Eng.* 115, 82–90. doi: 10.1115/1.2895474

Hill, M. R., Simon, M. A., Valdez-Jasso, D., Zhang, W., Champion, H. C., and Sacks. M. S. (2014). Structural and mechanical adaptations of right ventricle free wall myocardium to pressure overload. *Ann. Biomed. Eng.* 42, 2451–2465. doi: 10.1007/s10439-014-1096-3

Hsu, M. C., and Bazilevs, Y. (2011). Blood vessel tissue prestress modeling for vascular fluidstructure interaction simulation. *Finite Elem. Anal. Design* 47, 593–599. doi: 10.1016/j.finel.2010.12.015

Humphrey, J. D., Harrioson, D. G., Figueroa, C. A., Lacolley, P., and Laurent, S. (2016). Central artery stiffness in hypertension and aging: a problem with cause and consequence. *Circ. Res.* 118, 379–381. doi: 10.1161/CIRCRESAHA.115.307722

Katz, A. M. (1988). Influence of altered inotropy and lusitropy on ventricular pressure-volume loops. *J. Am. Coll. Cardiol.* 11, 438–445. doi: 10.1016/0735-1097(88)90113-1

Kawaguchi, M., Hay, I., Fetics, B., and Kass, D. A. (2003). Combined ventricular systolic and arterial stiffening in patients with heart failure and preserved

ejection fraction: implications for systolic and diastolic reserve limitations. *Circulation* 107, 714–720. doi: 10.1161/01.CIR.0000048123.22359.A0

Kerckhoffs, R. C. P., Neal, M. L., Gu, Q., Bassingthwaighte, J. B., Omens, J. H., and McCulloch, A. D. (2007). Coupling of a 3D finite element model of cardiac ventricular mechanics to lumped systems models of the systemic and pulmonic circulation. *Ann. Biomed. Eng.* 35, 1–18. doi: 10.1007/s10439-006-9212-7

Kermani, G., Hemmasizadeh, A., Assari, S., Autieri, M., and Darvish, K. (2017). Investigation of inhomogeneous and anisotropic material behavior of porcine thoracic aorta using nano-indentation tests. *J. Mech. Behav. Biomed. Mater.* 69, 50–56. doi: 10.1016/j.jmbbm.2016.12.022

Khokhlova, A. D., and Iribe, G. (2016). Transmural differences in mechanical properties of isolated subendocardial and subepicardial cardiomyocytes. *Bull. Exp. Biol. Med.* 162, 48–50. doi: 10.1007/s10517-016-3542-8

Kim, H. J., Vignon-Clementel, I. E., Figueroa, C. A., Ladisa, J. F., Jansen, K. E., Feinstein, J. A., et al. (2009). On coupling a lumped parameter heart model and a three-dimensional finite element aorta model. *Ann. Biomed. Eng.* 37, 2153–2169. doi: 10.1007/s10439-009-9760-8

Kim, J., Hong, J. W., and Baek, S. (2013). Longitudinal differences in the mechanical properties of the thoracic aorta depend on circumferential regions. *J. Biomed. Mater. Res. A* 101, 1525–1529. doi: 10.1002/jbm.a.34445

Kim, J., and Baek, S. (2011). Circumferential variations of mechanical behavior of the porcine thoracic aorta during the inflation test. *J. Biomech.* 44, 1941–1947. doi: 10.1016/j.jbiomech.2011.04.022

Kohn, J. C., Lampi, M. C., and Reinhart-King, C. A. (2015). Age-related vascular stiffening: causes and consequences. *Front. Genet.* 6:112. doi: 10.3389/fgene.2015.00112

Ky, B., French, B., Khan, A. M., Plappert, T., Wang, A., Chirinos, J. A., et al. (2013). ventricular-arterial coupling, remodeling, and prognosis in chronic heart failure. *J. Am. Coll. Cardiol.* 62, 1165–1172. doi: 10.1016/j.jacc.2013.03.085

LaDisa, J. F., Dholakia, R. J., Figueroa, C. A., Vignon-Clementel, I. E., Chan, F. P., Samyn, M. M., et al. (2011). Computational simulations demonstrate altered wall shear stress in aortic coarctation patients treated by resection with end-to-end anastomosis. *Congenit. Heart Dis.* 6, 432–443. doi: 10.1111/j.1747-0803.2011.00553.x

Lau, K. D., and Figueroa, C. A. (2015). simulation of short-term pressure regulation during the tilt test in a coupled 3D–0D closed-loop model of the circulation. *Biomech. Model. Mechanobiol.* 14, 915–929. doi: 10.1007/s10237-014-0645-x

Lee, L. C., Wenk, J. F., Zhong, L., Klepach, D., Zhang, Z., Ge, L., et al. (2013). analysis of patient-specific surgical ventricular restoration: importance of an ellipsoidal left ventricular geometry for diastolic and systolic function. *J. Appl. Physiol.* 115, 136–144. doi: 10.1152/japplphysiol.00662.2012

Lee, L. C., Sundnes, J., Genet, M., Wenk, J. F., and Wall, S. T. (2016).An integrated electromechanical-growth heart model for simulating cardiac therapies. *Biomech. Model. Mechanobiol.* 15, 791–803. doi: 10.1007/s10237-015-0723-8

Li, A. E., Kamel, I., Rando, F., Anderson, M., Kumbasar, B., Lima, J. A. C. et al. (2004). Using MRI to assess aortic wall thickness in the multiethnic study of atherosclerosis: distribution by race, sex, and age. *Am. J. Roentgenol.* 182, 593–597. doi: 10.2214/ajr.183.3.1820593

Mao, S. S., Ahmadi, N., Shah, B., Beckmann, D., Chen, A., Ngo, L., et al. (2008). Normal thoracic aorta diameter on cardiac computed tomography in healthy asymptomatic adults. *Acad. Radiol.* 15, 827–834. doi: 10.1016/j.acra.2008.02.001

Mello, J. M., de Orsi, A. M., and Padovani, C. R. (2004). Structure of the aortic wall in the guinea pig and rat. *Braz. J. Morphol.* 21, 35–38.

Muraru, D., Maffessanti, F., Kocabay, G., Peluso, D., Dal Bianco, L., Piasentini, E., et al. (2014). Ascending aorta diameters measured by echocardiography using both leading edge-to-leading edge and inner edge-to-inner edge conventions in healthy volunteers. *Eur. Heart J. Cardiovasc. Imaging* 15, 415–422. doi: 10.1093/ehjci/jet173

Naeije, R., and Manes, A. (2014). The right ventricle in pulmonary arterial hypertension. *Eur. Respir. Rev.* 23, 476–487. doi: 10.1183/09059180.00007414

Pezzuto, S., and Ambrosi, D. (2014). Active contraction of the cardiac ventricle and distortion of the microstructural architecture. *Int. J. Numer. Method. Biomed. Eng.* 30, 1578–1596. doi: 10.1002/cnm.2690

Pezzuto, S., Ambrosi, D., and Quarteroni, A. (2014). An orthotropic active-strain model for the myocardium mechanics and its numerical approximation. *Eur. J. Mech. A Solids* 48, 83–96. doi: 10.1016/j.euromechsol.2014.03.006

Rain, S., Handoko, M. L., Trip, P., Gan, C. T., Westerhof, N., Stienen, G. J., et al. (2013). Right ventricular diastolic impairment in patients with pulmonary arterial hypertension. *Circulation* 128, 2016–2025, 1–10. doi: 10.1161/CIRCULATIONAHA.113.001873

Roach, M. R., and Burton, A. C. (1957). The reason for the shape of the distensibility curves of arteries. *Can. J. Biochem. Physiol.* 3568, 1–90. doi: 10.1139/o57-080

Rosero, E. B., Peshock, R. M., Khera, A., Clagett, P., Lo, H., and Timaran, C. H. (2011). Sex, race, and age distributions of mean aortic wall thickness in a multiethnic population-based sample. *J. Vasc. Surg.* 53, 950–957. doi: 10.1016/j.jvs.2010.10.073

Schlatmann, T. J.M., and Becker, A. E. (1977). Histologic changes in the normal aging aorta: implications for dissecting aortic aneurysm. *Am. J. Cardiol.* 39, 13–20. doi: 10.1016/S0002-9149(77)80004-0

Schriefl, A. J., Zeindlinger, G., Pierce, D. M., Regitnig, P., and Holzapfel, G. A. (2012). Determination of the layer-specific distributed collagen fibre orientations in human thoracic and abdominal aortas and common iliac arteries. *J. R. Soc. Interface* 9, 1275–1286. doi: 10.1098/rsif.2011.0727

Shavik, S. M., Wall, S. T., Sundnes, J., Burkhoff, D., and Lee, L. C. (2017). Organ-level validation of a cross-bridge cycling descriptor in a left ventricular finite element model: effects of ventricular loading on myocardial strains. *Physiol. Rep.* 5:e13392. doi: 10.14814/phy2.13392

Shimoda, L. A., and Laurie, S. S. (2013). Vascular remodeling in pulmonary hypertension. *J. Mol. Med.* 91, 297–309. doi: 10.1007/s00109-013-0998-0

Smith, B. W., Chase, J. G., Nokes, R. I., Shaw, G. M., and Wake., G. (2004). Minimal haemodynamic system model including ventricular interaction and valve dynamics. *Med. Eng. Phys.* 26, 131–139. doi: 10.1016/j.medengphy.2003.10.001

Smulyan, H., and Safar, M. E. (1997). Systolic blood pressure revisited. *J. Am. Col. Cardiol.* 29, 1407–1413. doi: 10.1016/S0735-1097(97)00081-8

Streeter, D. D., Spotnitz, H. M., Patel, D. P., Ross, J., and Sonnenblick., E. H. (1969). Fiber orientation in the canine left ventricle during diastole and systole. *Circ. Res.* 24, 339–347. doi: 10.1161/01.RES.24.3.339

Su, M. Y., Lin, L. Y., Tseng, Y. H., Chang, C. C., Wu, C. K., Lin, J. L., et al. (2014). CMR-verified diffuse myocardial fibrosis is associated with diastolic dysfunction in HFpEF. *JACC Cardiovasc. Imaging* 7, 991–997. doi: 10.1016/j.jcmg.2014.04.022

Towfiq, B. A., Weir, J., and Rawles., J. M. (1986). Effect of age and blood pressure on aortic size and stroke distance. *Br. Heart J.* 55, 560–568. doi: 10.1136/hrt.55.6.560

Trayanova, N. A., Constantino, J., and Gurev., V. (2011). Electromechanical models of the ventricles. *Am. J. Physiol. Heart Circ. Physiol.* 301, H279–H286. doi: 10.1152/ajpheart.00324.2011

Tsamis, A., Krawiec, J. T., and Vorp., D. A. (2013). Elastin and collagen fibre microstructure of the human aorta in ageing and disease: a review. *J. R. Soc. Interface* 10:20121004 doi: 10.1098/rsif.2012.1004

Usyk, T. P., LeGrice, I. J., and McCulloch., A. D. (2002). Computational model of three-dimensional cardiac electromechanics. *Comput. Vis. Sci.* 4, 249–257. doi: 10.1007/s00791-002-0081-9

Vasava, P., Jalali, P., Dabagh, M., and Kolari., P. J. (2012). Finite element modelling of pulsatile blood flow in idealized model of human aortic arch: study of hypotension and hypertension. *Comput. Math. Methods Med.* 2012:861837. doi: 10.1155/2012/861837

Wall, S. T., Guccione, J. M., Ratcliffe, M. B., and Sundnes., J. S. (2012). Electromechanical feedback with reduced cellular connectivity alters electrical activity in an infarct injured left ventricle: a finite element model study. *Am. J. Physiol. Heart. Circ. Physiol.* 302, H206–H214. doi: 10.1152/ajpheart.00272.2011

Wenk, J. F., Sun, K., Zhang, Z., Soleimani, M., Ge, L., Saloner, D., et al. (2011). Regional left ventricular myocardial contractility and stress in a finite element model of posterobasal myocardial infarction. *J. Biomech. Eng.* 133:44501. doi: 10.1115/1.4003438

Xi, C., Latnie, C., Zhao, X., Tan, J. L., Wall, S. T., Genet, M., et al. (2016). Patient-specific computational analysis of ventricular mechanics in pulmonary arterial hypertension. *J. Biomech. Eng.* 138:111001. doi: 10.1115/1.4034559

Zeinali-Davarani, S., Sheidaei, A., and Baek, S. (2011). A finite element model of stress-mediated vascular adaptation: application to abdominal aortic aneurysms. *Comput. Methods Biomech. Biomed. Eng.* 14, 803–817. doi: 10.1080/10255842.2010.495344

# Bifurcation Asymmetry of Small Coronary Arteries in Juvenile and Adult Mice

Yundi Feng[1], Xuan Wang[1], Tingting Fan[1], Li Li[1], Xiaotong Sun[1], Wenxi Zhang[1], Minglu Cao[1], Jian Liu[2*], Jianping Li[3*] and Yunlong Huo[1*]

[1] Department of Mechanics and Engineering Science, College of Engineering, Peking University, Beijing, China, [2] Department of Cardiology, Peking University People's Hospital, Beijing, China, [3] Department of Cardiology, Peking University First Hospital, Beijing, China

*Correspondence:
Jian Liu
drjianliu@163.com
Jianping Li
lijianping@medmail.com.cn
Yunlong Huo
yhuo@pku.edu.cn

**Background:** Microvascular bifurcation asymmetry is of significance for regulation of coronary flow heterogeneity during juvenile and adult growth. The aim of the study is to investigate the morphometric and hemodynamic variation of coronary arterial bifurcations in mice of different ages.

**Methods:** Pulsatile blood flows were computed from a Womersley-type model in the reconstructed left coronary arterial (LCA) trees from Micro-CT images in normal mice at ages of 3 weeks, 6 weeks, 12 weeks, 5-6 months, and >8 months. Diameter and flow ratios and bifurcation angles were determined in each bifurcation of the LCA trees.

**Results:** The blood volume and inlet flow rate of LCA trees increase and decrease during juvenile and adult growth, respectively. As vessel diameters decrease, the increased ratios of small to large daughter vessel diameters ($D_s/D_l$) result in more uniform flows and lower velocities. There are significant structure-functional changes of LCA trees in mice of >8 months compared with mice of <8 months. As $D_s/D_l$ increases, the variation trend of bifurcation angle during juvenile growth is different from that during adult growth.

**Conclusions:** Although inlet flows are different in adult vs. juvenile mice, the adult still have uniform flow and low velocity. This is accomplished through a decrease in diameter. The design ensures ordered dispersion of red cells through asymmetric branching patterns into the capillaries.

Keywords: coronary arterial tree, bifurcation asymmetry, bifurcation angle, advancing age, mouse model

## INTRODUCTION

The structure and function of coronary arterial trees undergo changes during normal growth and aging (Wei, 1992; LeBlanc and Hoying, 2016). For example, an increase of vessel density was found in the adult primarily owing to angiogenesis in which new daughter vessel segments grow (sprouting) or split (intussusception) from existing mother segments (Carmeliet and Jain, 2011; LeBlanc and Hoying, 2016). We have recently shown an age-independent exponent in the length-volume scaling law of an entire coronary arterial tree in juvenile and adult mice (Chen et al., 2015) because of fractal-like tree features (Huo and Kassab, 2016). In comparison with the unchanged "global" hierarchy of a vascular tree structure, the "local" branching patterns characterize the age-dependent anatomy of coronary arterial trees and affect flow patterns at junctions

(Huo et al., 2009a; Huo Y. L. et al., 2012). The change of flow patterns can lead to low wall shear stress, high oscillatory shear index, high spacial gradient of wall shear stress, and so on (Huo et al., 2007a, 2008, 2009b). These hemodynamic parameters are related to stagnation, reversal and vortical flows (Asakura and Karino, 1990; Kleinstreuer et al., 2001; Huo et al., 2007a), which result in abnormal biological responses such as dysfunction of endothelial cells, monocyte deposition, elevated wall permeability to macromolecules, particle migration into the vessel wall, smooth muscle cell proliferation, microemboli formation, and so on (Malek et al., 1999; Chiu and Chien, 2011). The current studies of advancing age in the coronary vasculature are generally confined to large epicardial arteries (LeBlanc and Hoying, 2016). To our knowledge, there is, however, lack of studies to show the effects of normal growth and development on the "local" branching patterns in coronary resistance vasculature (vessel diameter <200 $\mu$m).

Coronary blood flows in arterioles and small arteries play a fundamental role for regulation of total vascular resistance under physiological and pathological conditions (Chilian et al., 1989; Chilian, 1991; Pries and Secomb, 2005; Reglin et al., 2017). The flows are affected by multiple factors, e.g., Fahraeus-Lindqvist effects, bifurcation laws, and so on (Pries et al., 1995; Gompper and Fedosov, 2016; Secomb, 2017). Based on the constructal law, Bejan and Lorente indicated that an efficient transport system requires more symmetric bifurcations to keep fractional flows as uniform as possible (Bejan and Lorente, 2010). According to the morphometric measurements, normal arteriolar bifurcations are more symmetric than ischemia-regenerated or tumor-induced branching patterns to ensure ordered dispersion of red cells though the capillary network (Baish and Jain, 2000; Arpino et al., 2017).

The objective of the study is to investigate the changes of bifurcation asymmetry in coronary arterial trees of mice during juvenile and adult growth. We hypothesize that the bifurcation changes of small coronary arteries (i.e., diameter ratio and bifurcation angle) result in more uniform flows and lower velocities as vessel diameters decrease in mice of different ages. The inlet flow rate and blood volume of coronary arterial trees are also assumed to have different variation trends between juvenile and adult growth. To test the hypothesis, we analyzed diameter ratios and bifurcation angles in each bifurcation of coronary arterial trees reconstructed from Micro-CT ($\mu$CT) images of mice at ages of 3, 6, 12 weeks, 5-6 months and >8 months. Pulsatile blood flows in each tree were computed from a Womersley-type model (Huo and Kassab, 2006), based on which the flow and velocity ratios were determined in each bifurcation. The significance and limitation of the morphometric and hemodynamic analysis were discussed relevant to the microcirculation.

## MATERIALS AND METHODS

### Morphometric Data

We have reconstructed coronary arterial trees of ICR (Institute of Cancer Research) mice from $\mu$CT images. All animal experiments were performed in accordance with Chinese National and Hebei University ethical guidelines regarding the use of animals in research, consistent with the NIH guidelines (Guide for the care and use of laboratory animals) on the protection of animals used for scientific purposes. The experimental protocols were approved by the Animal Care and Use Committee of Hebei University, China.

The reconstructed left coronary arterial (LCA) trees (including 9 LCA trees in 3 weeks group, 9 LCA trees in 6 weeks group, 7 LCA trees in 12 weeks group, 8 LCA trees in 5-6 months group and 9 LCA trees in > 8 months group) were used to analyze the changes in bifurcations of normal mice at different ages (from 3 weeks to >8 months), as shown in **Figures 1A-E**. Similar to a previous study (Chen et al., 2015), animals were anesthetized with pentobarbital sodium (60 mg/Kg) and heparinized with undiluted heparin (1 ml, 1,000 USPU/ml). After midline incision for laparotomy, animals were terminated by injecting an overdose of pentobarbital sodium through the inferior vena cava. The thoracic aorta was perfused with MICROFIL (Flow Tech, Carver, MA) at a constant pressure of 100 mmHg after the termination. The flow of cast solution was zero during the 90 min prior to hardening of cast at a constant pressure of 100 mmHg. The animal was stored in 10% formalin in the refrigerator for 24 h. The hearts were dissected and stored in 10% formalin in refrigerator until $\mu$CT scans. Morphometric data of LCA trees (including the diameter and rectangular coordinates of center points which were located in the center on the cross–sectional views of the contour of the 3D vessel) were extracted from $\mu$CT images using a gray-scale threshold method (with a low CT-threshold of 100) in the MIMICS software (Materialize, NV, Belgium).

A centerline was formed by a series of center points. Subsequently, the best fit diameter, $D_{fit}$, was calculated as twice the average radius between the center point and the contour forming the 3D vessel. The blurring of small vessel edges was corrected to yield $D_{correct}$ by fitting a Gaussian distribution function to the line profiles followed by computation of the input square wave. Since a vessel (a segment between two nodes of bifurcation) included 10-80 center points, the length and volume of a vessel were defined as:

$$L = \sum_{i=0}^{N-1} \sqrt{(x_{i+1} - x_i)^2 + (y_{i+1} - y_i)^2 + (z_{i+1} - z_i)^2} \text{ and } V = \sum_{i=0}^{N-1} \left( \frac{\pi D_{correct}^2}{4} \cdot \sqrt{(x_{i+1} - x_i)^2 + (y_{i+1} - y_i)^2 + (z_{i+1} - z_i)^2} \right),$$

where $(x, y, z)$ refers to rectangular coordinates of center points from inlet ($i = 0$) to outlet ($i = N$) of the vessel. The cross-section area (CSA) of a vessel equaled to the intravascular volume divided by the length. A linear least-squares fit of all center points was used to determine the spatial direction of a vessel. The mother, large daughter, and small daughter diameters and lengths, $(D_m, L_m)$, $(D_l, L_l)$, and $(D_s, L_s)$, as well as bifurcation angles were determined at all bifurcations of coronary arterial trees, as shown in **Figure 1F**. The LCA trees with vessel diameter $\geq 40 \mu$m (twice the voxel size) were used to reduce the sampling error of the finite discrete grid. Unless otherwise stated, the terminal vessels of $\mu$CT-determined LCA trees have diameter $\geq 40 \mu$m.

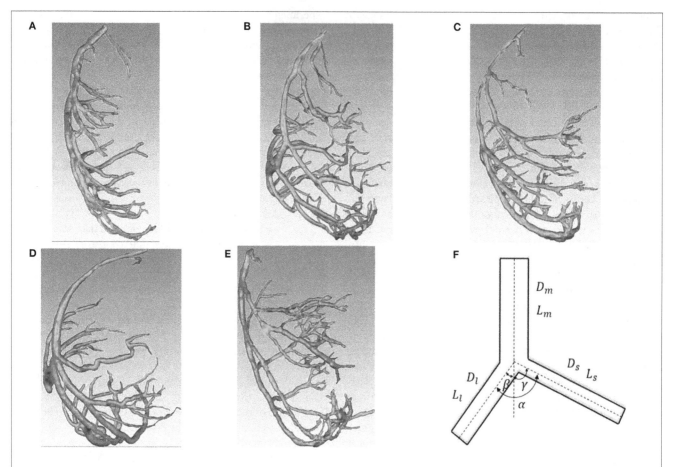

**FIGURE 1 | (A-E)** LCA trees of mice at ages of 3 weeks **(A)**, 6 weeks **(B)**, 12 weeks **(C)**, 5-6 months **(D)** and >8 months **(E)** reconstructed from μCT images; **(F)** Schematic representation of a coronary bifurcation.

## Womersley-Type Model

Similar to a previous study (Huo and Kassab, 2006), a mathematical model is used to analyze pulsatile blood flow of coronary arteries in diastole in the absence of vessel tone. The governing equations for flow and pressure in a vessel (x = 0 and x = L refer to the inlet and outlet, respectively) can be written as:

$$Q(x, \omega) = a \cdot \cos\left(\frac{\omega x}{c}\right) + b \cdot \sin(\frac{\omega x}{c}) \quad (1)$$

$$P(x, \omega) = iZ_1 \left[ -a \cdot \sin\left(\frac{\omega x}{c}\right) + b \cdot \cos\left(\frac{\omega x}{c}\right) \right] \quad (2)$$

where $a$ and $b$ are arbitrary constants of integration, $\omega$ the angular frequency, $c = \sqrt{1 - F_{10}(\acute{\alpha})} \cdot c_0$ ($c_0 = \sqrt{\frac{Eh}{\rho R}}$ and $\acute{\alpha}$ is the Womersley number) the wave velocity, $Y_0 = \frac{A(n)}{\rho c_0}$ the characteristic admittance, $Z_0 = \frac{1}{Y_0}$ the characteristic impedance, and $Z_1 = Z_0 / \sqrt{1 - F_{10}(\acute{\alpha})}$. Moreover, we define the impedance and admittance as:

$$Z(x, \omega) = \frac{P(x, \omega)}{Q(x, \omega)} \text{ and } Y(x, \omega) = \frac{Q(x, \omega)}{P(x, \omega)} \quad (3)$$

In a given vessel segment, at x = 0 and x = L, we have the respective inlet and outlet impedances:

$$Z(0, \omega) = \frac{iZ_1 \cdot b}{a} \text{ and}$$

$$Z(L, \omega) = \frac{iZ_1 \left[ -a \cdot \sin\left(\frac{\omega L}{c}\right) + b \cdot \cos\left(\frac{\omega L}{c}\right) \right]}{a \cdot \cos\left(\frac{\omega L}{c}\right) + b \cdot \sin\left(\frac{\omega L}{c}\right)} \quad (4)$$

From Equation (4), we obtain:

$$Z(0, \omega) = \frac{iZ_1 \cdot \sin\left(\frac{\omega L}{c}\right) + Z(L, \omega) \cdot \cos\left(\frac{\omega L}{c}\right)}{\cos\left(\frac{\omega L}{c}\right) + iY_1 \cdot Z(L, \omega) \cdot \sin\left(\frac{\omega L}{c}\right)} \quad (5)$$

Equation (5) was used to calculate the impedance/admittance in a tree from inlet to the terminal vessels.

## Method of Solution

The characteristic impedance, characteristic admittance and velocity (including the viscous effect) were first calculated for every vessel segment. We assume that mass is conserved and pressure is continuous at each bifurcation, which may be written as:

$$Q_m(\omega) = Q_l(\omega) + Q_s(\omega) \text{ and } P_m(\omega) = P_l(\omega) = P_s(\omega) \quad (6)$$

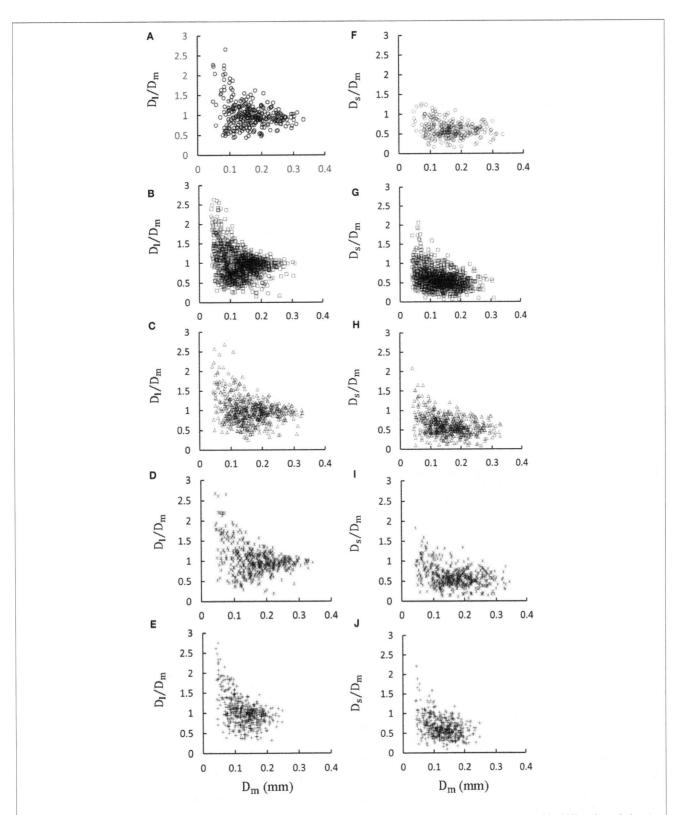

**FIGURE 2 | (A–E)** Relationship between $D_l/D_m$ (diameter ratio of large daughter to mother vessels) and $D_m$ (diameter of mother vessel) in all bifurcations of mice at ages of 3 weeks **(A)**, 6 weeks **(B)**, 12 weeks **(C)**, 5-6 months **(D)** and >8 months **(E)**; **(F-J)** Relationship between $D_s/D_m$ (diameter ratio of small daughter to mother vessels) and $D_m$ in all bifurcations of mice at ages of 3 weeks **(F)**, 6 weeks **(G)**, 12 weeks **(H)**, 5-6 months **(I),** and >8 months **(J)**. There is significant difference of $D_l/D_m$ and $D_s/D_m$ between mice of >8 months and 3 weeks, between mice of >8 months and 6 weeks, between mice of >8 months and 12 weeks, and between mice of >8 months and 5-6 months while there is no statistical difference between mice of other ages.

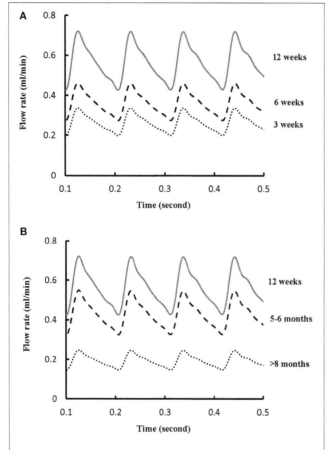

**FIGURE 3 | (A)** Pulsatile blood flows at the inlet of LCA trees of mice during juvenile growth (from 3 to 12 weeks) and **(B)** Pulsatile blood flows at the inlet of LCA trees of mice during adult growth (≥12 weeks). The mean ± SD values of time-averaged flow rates over a cardiac cycle equal to 0.26 ± 0.17, 0.36 ± 0.23, 0.51 ± 0.18, 0.43 ± 0.22, and 0.21 ± 0.15 ml/min for mice at ages of 3, 6, 12 weeks, 5-6 months and >8 months, respectively.

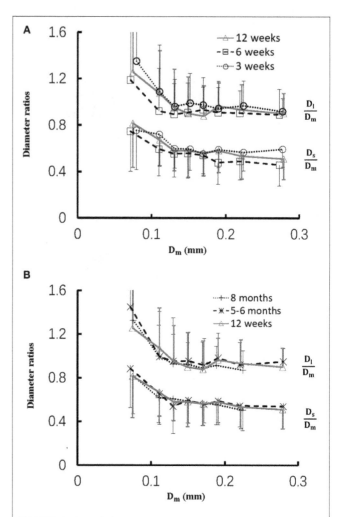

**FIGURE 4 | (A)** Relationship between $D_l/D_m$, $D_s/D_m$, and $D_m$ in 8 diameter ranges of coronary arterial trees of mice during juvenile growth (from 3 to 12 weeks) and **(B)** Relationship between $D_l/D_m$, $D_s/D_m$, and $D_m$ in 8 diameter ranges of coronary arterial trees of mice during adult growth (≥12 weeks). Error bars refer to the SDs of those parameters in each diameter ranges. There is no statistical difference of $D_l/D_m$ and $D_s/D_m$ between mice of various ages in each single diameter range. For mice of all ages, there is significant difference of $D_l/D_m$ and $D_s/D_m$ between range 1 and other ranges and between range 2 and other ranges.

From Equation (6), we obtain:

$$Y_m(L, \omega) = Y_l(0, \omega) + Y_s(0, \omega) \tag{7}$$

Once the terminal impedance/admittance is computed, we proceed backwards to iteratively calculate the impedance/admittance in the entire coronary tree by using Equations (5) and (7) similar to a previous study (Huo and Kassab, 2006). The aortic pressure was obtained from a previous study (Huo et al., 2008) and discretized by a Fourier transformation to determine the constants $a$ and $b$ in Equations (1) and (2). The flow and pressure were then calculated by using Equations (1) and (2).

The blood flow density ($\rho$) in coronary arteries was assumed to be 1.06 g/cm$^3$ (Chen et al., 2016; Fan et al., 2016; Yin et al., 2016). The variation of viscosity ($\mu$) with vessel diameter and hematocrit was based on Pries' viscosity model (Pries et al., 1992). The coronary wall thickness was assumed to be one-tenth of the vessel diameter. The static Young's modulus was ~8.0 × 10$^6$ (dynes/cm$^2$) and the dynamic Young's modulus was also

considered consistent with the previous study (Huo and Kassab, 2006). Symmetric arteriolar subtrees were pasted to all terminal vessels. A symmetric arteriolar subtree was constructed from the terminal vessel down to the first capillaries, based on two scaling relationships, $DR = 2^{\frac{-1}{1.07+2}}$ and $LR = 2^{\frac{-1}{3-0.42}}$ (DR and LR refer to the diameter and length ratio) (see Table 2 in Huo and Kassab, 2012a). The outlet impedances at the first capillaries were computed by the steady value; i.e., $\frac{128\mu_{capillary}L_{capillary}}{\pi D_{capillary}^4}$ (g · sec/cm$^4$).

## Statistical Analysis

The fraction of volumetric blood flow is mainly determined by diameter ratios ($\frac{D_l}{D_m}$, $\frac{D_s}{D_m}$, and $\frac{D_s}{D_l}$) while the change of flow velocities from mother to daughter vessels is characterized by

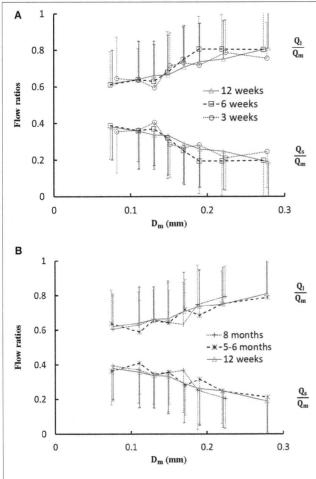

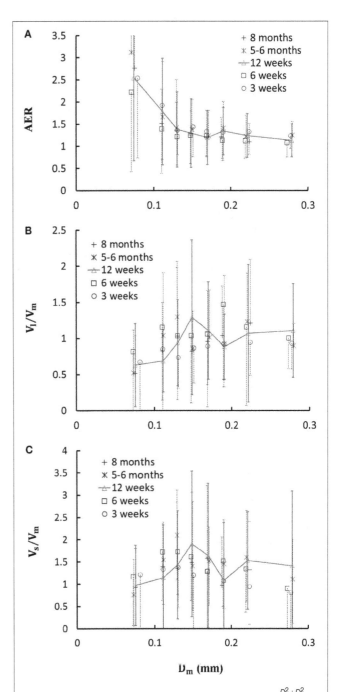

**FIGURE 5 | (A)** Relationship between $Q_l/Q_m$, $Q_s/Q_m$, and $D_m$ in 8 diameter ranges of coronary arterial trees of mice during juvenile growth (from 3 to 12 weeks) and **(B)** Relationship between $Q_l/Q_m$, $Q_s/Q_m$, and $D_m$ in 8 diameter ranges of coronary arterial trees of mice during adult growth ($\geq$12 weeks). Error bars refer to the SDs of those parameters in each diameter ranges. There is no statistical difference of $Q_l/Q_m$ and $Q_s/Q_m$ between mice of various ages in each single diameter range. For mice of all ages, there is no statistical difference between different ranges.

**FIGURE 6 | (A)** Relationship between area expansion ratio ($AER = \frac{D_l^2 + D_s^2}{D_m^2}$) and $D_m$; **(B)** Relationship between $V_l/V_m$ and $D_m$; and **(C)** Relationship between $V_s/V_m$ and $D_m$ in 8 diameter ranges of coronary arterial trees of mice during juvenile and adult growth. Error bars refer to the SDs of those parameters in each diameter ranges. For mice of all ages, there is significant difference of AER, $V_l/V_m$ and $V_s/V_m$ between range 1 and other ranges and between range 2 and other ranges.

the area expansion ratio ($AER = \frac{D_l^2 + D_s^2}{D_m^2}$) (VanBavel and Spaan, 1992; Kaimovitz et al., 2008). Bifurcation angle in small arteries regulates the spacial heterogeneity of coronary blood flow albeit it is a critical risk factor for atherosclerotic plaques and stenting restenosis in large epicardial coronary arteries (Huo et al., 2012b; Huo Y. et al., 2012a). Hence, similar to previous studies (Huo et al., 2007b; Huo and Kassab, 2012b), diameter ratios ($\frac{D_l}{D_m}$, $\frac{D_s}{D_m}$, and $\frac{D_s}{D_l}$), area expansion ratios ($AER = \frac{D_l^2 + D_s^2}{D_m^2}$), flow ratios ($\frac{Q_l}{Q_m}$, $\frac{Q_s}{Q_m}$, and $\frac{Q_s}{Q_l}$), and velocity ratios ($\frac{V_l}{V_m}$, $\frac{V_s}{V_m}$, and $\frac{V_s}{V_l}$) in a LCA tree were analyzed in eight mother diameter (i.e., $D_m$) ranges as: Range 1 (<100 $\mu$m), Range 2 (100-120 $\mu$m), Range 3 (120-140 $\mu$m), Range 4 (140-160 $\mu$m), Range 5 (160-180 $\mu$m), Range 6 (180-200 $\mu$m), Range 7 (200-250 $\mu$m) and Range 8 ($\geq$250 $\mu$m). Moreover, bifurcation angles in a LCA

tree were summarized in four $\frac{D_s}{D_l}$ ranges as: Range 1 (<0.4), Range 2 (0.4-0.6), Range 3 (0.6-0.8) and Range 4 ($\geq$0.8). The mean and standard deviation (mean$\pm$SD) were computed by averaging over all bifurcations in each group. Two Way Repeated

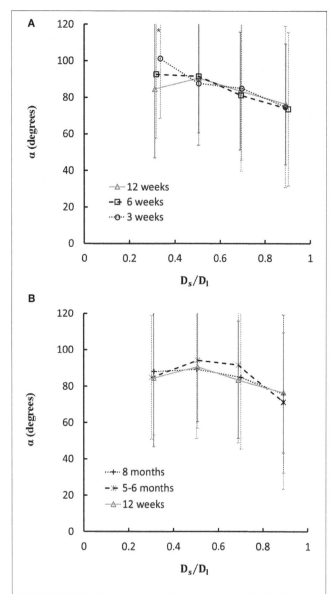

**FIGURE 7 | (A)** Relationship between bifurcation angles and $D_s/D_l$ (diameter ratio of small to large daughter vessels) in mice during juvenile growth and **(B)** Relationship between bifurcation angles and $D_s/D_l$ in mice during adult growth. Error bars refer to the SDs of bifurcation angles in each $D_s/D_l$ ranges. Symbol "*" refers to the statistical difference in mice of 3 weeks vs. 6 weeks, 3 weeks vs. 12 weeks, 3 weeks vs. 5-6 months, and 3 weeks vs. >8 months.

Measures ANOVA (SigmaStat 3.5) was used to compare those morphometric and hemodynamic parameters in bifurcations between different ages and between different diameter ranges, where $p < 0.05$ represented a statistically significant difference.

## RESULTS

**Figures 1A-E** show LCA trees of mice at ages of 3, 6, 12 weeks, 5-6 months, and >8 months reconstructed from μCT images. Accordingly, the LCA trees have blood volumes of 7.1 ± 4.1, 9.9 ± 3.7, 16.1 ± 4.7, 13.8 ± 4.0, and 5.5 ± 3.4 (×$10^{-4}$) cm³

(averaged over all LCA trees in each group) and the animals have body weights (BW) of 11.0 ± 0.8, 17.4 ± 1.5, 37.6 ± 3.9, 36.1 ± 4.1, and 38.1 ± 4.8 g (averaged over all animals in each group). **Figures 2A-E** show the changes of $D_l/D_m$ (diameter ratio of large daughter to mother vessels) as a function of $D_m$ (diameter of mother vessel) in all bifurcations of mice at different age groups. **Figures 2F-J** show the corresponding changes of $D_s/D_m$ (diameter ratio of small daughter to mother vessels) with $D_m$. A comparison in all bifurcations shows that mice of >8 months have significant difference of $D_l/D_m$ and $D_s/D_m$ from mice of <8 months ($p < 0.05$ between mice of >8 months and 3 weeks, between mice of >8 months and 6 weeks, between mice of >8 months and 12 weeks, and between mice of >8 months and 5-6 months) despite no statistical difference between mice of other ages. **Figures 3A,B** show pulsatile blood flows (waves averaged over all mice at the same age) at the inlet of LCA trees of mice during juvenile and adult growth, respectively. The time-averaged flow rate over a cardiac cycle has mean ± SD values of 0.26 ± 0.17, 0.36 ± 0.23, 0.51 ± 0.18, 0.43 ± 0.22, and 0.21 ± 0.15 ml/min for mice at ages of 3, 6, 12 weeks, 5-6 months and >8 months, which are proportional to the blood volumes of LCA trees. Similar to the changes of $D_l/D_m$ and $D_s/D_m$, a comparison in all bifurcations shows mice of >8 months have significant difference of $Q_l/Q_m$ and $Q_s/Q_m$ from mice of <8 months despite no statistical difference between mice of other ages. Moreover, there is significant difference of $V_l/V_m$ and $V_s/V_m$ between mice of 3 and 6 weeks, between mice of 3 and 12 weeks, and between mice of 3 weeks and 5-6 months as well as between mice of >8 months and 6 weeks, between mice of >8 months and 12 weeks, and between mice of >8 months and 5-6 months.

**Figure 4** shows the changes of diameter ratios as a function of mother diameter during juvenile and adult growth while **Figure 5** shows the changes of flow ratios. **Figures 6A-C** show the relationships between AER and $D_m$, between $V_l/V_m$ and $D_m$, and between $V_s/V_m$ and $D_m$ in coronary arterial trees of mice during juvenile and adult growth. A comparison of those parameters in each single diameter range shows no statistical difference between mice of different ages. As mother vessel diameter increases in mice of 3, 6, 12 weeks, 5-6 months and >8 months, AER and diameter ratios ($D_l/D_m$ and $D_s/D_m$) decrease abruptly when $D_m < 140$ μm and remain relatively unchanged when $D_m \geq 140$ μm ($p < 0.05$ between range 1 and other ranges and between range 2 and other ranges). Moreover, $D_s/D_l$ values when $D_m < 140$ μm are slightly higher than those when $D_m > 200$ μm. There are gradual increase and decrease of $Q_l/Q_m$ and $Q_s/Q_m$, respectively, with the increase of mother vessel diameter. There is an abrupt decrease of $V_l/V_m$, and $V_s/V_m$ as mother vessel diameter decreases from 140 to 40 μm ($p < 0.05$ between range 1 and other ranges and between range 2 and other ranges).

On the other hand, **Figures 7A,B** show the relationships between the measured bifurcation angles ($\alpha_{measured}$) and $D_s/D_l$ during juvenile and adult growth, respectively. There is a monotonical decrease of $\alpha_{measured}$ with the increase of $D_s/D_l$ at ages of 3 and 6 weeks, but a parabolic curve with peak values (~90°) when $D_s/D_l = 0.5$ at ages of 12 weeks, 5-6 months, and >8 months ($p < 0.05$ for 3 weeks vs. 6 weeks, 3 weeks vs. 12

weeks, 3 weeks vs. 5-6 months, and 3 weeks vs. >8 months when $D_s/D_l < 0.4$).

## DISCUSSION

The present study used a Womersley-type mathematical model to compute pulsatile blood flows in LCA trees of mice. The computed flow rates at the inlet of LCA trees vary in the range of 0.2-0.5 ml/min in agreement with the Doppler measurements (Teng et al., 2016). The inlet flow rate and blood volume of LCA trees increase in mice from 3 to 12 weeks and decrease during adult growth. Myocardial flows were estimated to be 9.45, 8.28, 5.43, 4.76, and 2.21 ml/min/g, respectively, in mice of 3, 6, 12 weeks, 5-6 months and >8 months. Myocardial flows in mice of <8 months are significantly higher than those in porcine ($\sim$2.25 mL/min/g in Huo et al., 2009a). On the other hand, the waveform is preserved at the inlet of LCA trees in diastole in the absence of vessel tone during juvenile and adult growth, as shown in **Figure 3**. Furthermore, **Figure 5** showed the development of relatively uniform flows as vessel diameters decrease from the inlet to 40 μm in LCA trees of mice, which agrees with previous findings (Bejan and Lorente, 2010). This is mainly attributed to the design of branching patterns as shown in **Figures 1, 4**.

A key finding of the study is that diameter ratios ($D_l/D_m$ and $D_s/D_m$) and AER when 40 μm $\leq D_m <$ 140 μm in mice are significantly higher than those in porcine (Kaimovitz et al., 2008) despite their similarity at 140 μm $\leq D_m <$ 350 μm, which leads to an abrupt decrease of velocity ratios ($V_l/V_m$ and $V_s/V_m$) as vessel diameters decrease from 140 to 40 μm in **Figure 6** (Kassab, 2005). Mice at the age of <8 months have significantly higher myocardial flows (>two-fold) than large animals. Owing to the proportional relation between myocardial flow and metabolic rate, a significant increase of diameter ratios and AER reduces the flow velocity in vessels of 40 μm $\leq D_m <$ 140 μm to satisfy the metabolism in the mouse heart compared with large animals in that microvascular blood flow per unit of time is to ensure the needed exchange of substances between tissue and blood compartments (Jacob et al., 2016). We also demonstrated a comparison of diameter and flow ratios to show the effects of normal growth and development on morphometry and hemodynamics of LCA trees of mice. The statistical analysis at all bifurcations showed significant difference of diameter and flow ratios between mice of >8 months and others as well as no statistical difference between mice of <8 months. Myocardial flows in mice of >8 months were also significantly lower than others. Diameter ranges 1-7 showed no statistical difference between mice of different ages while mice of >8 months have no arteries in diameter range 8 ($\geq$250 μm). Hence, the structure-functional change of LCA trees in mice of >8 months is mainly attributed to the regression of blood vessels (blood volumes of 7.1 $\pm$ 4.1, 9.9 $\pm$ 3.7, 16.1 $\pm$ 4.7, and 13.8 $\pm$ 4.0 vs. 5.5 $\pm$ 3.4 ($\times 10^{-4}$) cm$^3$).

On the other hand, we showed the linear relationship between bifurcation angles and $D_s/D_l$ in LCA trees of mice at ages of 3 and 6 weeks, but the parabolic curve with the peak bifurcation angles ($\sim$90°) at $D_s/D_l = 0.5$ in mice at ages of 12 weeks, 5-6 months and > 8 months. The linear relationship may be caused by the progression of mouse heart during juvenile growth while the parabolic curve is associated with the mature and stable heart size during adult growth, which requires further investigations with considering how the spatial heterogeneity of myocardial flows is altered by the age-dependent bifurcation angles.

### Critique of the Study

The present study carried out the pulsatile blood flow analysis in coronary arterial trees of mice during normal juvenile and adult growth, which brings in some complexities. For example, although coronary arterial trees with diameter > 40 μm were reconstructed from μCT images, symmetric arteriolar subtrees with diameters from 40 μm down to the first capillaries were generated from two scaling relationships. The simple Womersley-type model was derived for Newtonian fluids in straight pipes. Here, the non-Newtonian effect was partly captured in small arteries by using a diameter-dependent viscosity. Based on a more realistic model with considering non-Newtonian fluids, the hemodynamic analysis should be performed to accurately validate morphometric predictions when arteriolar trees with diameter <40 μm are available. Moreover, the following studies should relate vessel tone and metabolic signals to the 3D spatial bifurcation asymmetry for understanding the microcirculation and myocardial heterogeneity deeply.

## CONCLUSIONS

This study analyzed the morphometric and hemodynamic variation of microvascular bifurcations in LCA trees of normal mice at ages of 3, 6, 12 weeks, 5-6 months and >8 months. The inlet flow rate and blood volume of LCA trees increase during juvenile growth and decrease during adult growth while the flow waveform is preserved in diastole in the absence of vessel tone. The blood flow becomes more uniform as vessel diameters decrease from the inlet to 40 μm owing to the changes of diameter ratios ($D_l/D_m$ and $D_s/D_m$). The changes of diameter ratios and AER also lead to an abrupt decrease of velocity ratios with the decrease of vessel diameter from 140 to 40 μm. Mice of >8 months show structure-functional difference from others.

## AUTHOR CONTRIBUTIONS

The data analysis was done by YF, XW, TF, and XS. Micro-CT images were collected by LL, WZ, and MC. The manuscript was drafted and revised by YH, JLiu and JLi.

## ACKNOWLEDGMENTS

We would like to thank all participants in Peking University. The study is supported in part by the National Natural Science Foundation of China Grant 11672006, China MOST Grant 2014DFG32740 (YH), and Shenzhen Science and Technology R&D Grant JCYJ20160427170536358 (YH), and Capital's Funds for Health Improvement and Research 2016-2-4073 (JLi).

# REFERENCES

Arpino, J. M., Nong, Z. X., Li, F. Y., Yin, H., Ghonaim, N., Milkovich, S., et al. (2017). Four-Dimensional microvascular analysis reveals that regenerative angiogenesis in ischemic muscle produces a flawed microcirculation. *Circ. Res.* 120, 1453-1465. doi: 10.1161/CIRCRESAHA.116.310535

Asakura, T., and Karino, T. (1990). Flow patterns and spatial distribution of atherosclerotic lesions in human coronary arteries. *Circ. Res.* 66, 1045-1066

Baish, J. W., and Jain, R. K. (2000). Fractals and cancer. *Cancer Res.* 60, 3683-3688.

Bejan, A., and Lorente, S. (2010). The constructal law of design and evolution in nature. *Philos. Trans. R. Soc. Lond. B Biol. Sci.* 365, 1335-1347. doi: 10.1098/rstb.2009.0302

Carmeliet, P., and Jain, R. K. (2011). Molecular mechanisms and clinical applications of angiogenesis. *Nature* 473, 298-307. doi: 10.1038/nature10144

Chen, X., Gao, Y., Lu, B., Jia, X., Zhong, L., Kassab, G. S., et al. (2016). Hemodynamics in coronary arterial tree of serial stenoses. *PLoS ONE* 11:e0163715. doi: 10.1371/journal.pone.0163715

Chen, X., Niu, P., Niu, X., Shen, W., Duan, F., Ding, L., et al. (2015). Growth, ageing and scaling laws of coronary arterial trees. *J. R. Soc. Interface* 12:20150830. doi: 10.1098/rsif.2015.0830

Chilian, W. M. (1991). Microvascular pressures and resistances in the left ventricular subepicardium and subendocardium. *Circ. Res.* 69, 561-570

Chilian, W. M., Layne, S. M., Klausner, E. C., Eastham, C. L., and Marcus, M. L. (1989). Redistribution of coronary microvascular resistance produced by dipyridamole. *Am. J. Physiol.* 256(2 Pt 2), H383-H390. doi: 10.1152/ajpheart.1989.256.2.H383

Chiu, J. J., and Chien, S. (2011). Effects of disturbed flow on vascular endothelium: pathophysiological basis and clinical perspectives. *Physiol. Rev.* 91, 327-387. doi: 10.1152/physrev.00047.2009

Fan, T., Lu, Y., Gao, Y., Meng, J., Tan, W., Huo, Y., et al. (2016). Hemodynamics of left internal mammary artery bypass graft: effect of anastomotic geometry, coronary artery stenosis, and postoperative time. *J. Biomech.* 49, 645-652. doi: 10.1016/j.jbiomech.2016.01.031

Gompper, G., and Fedosov, D. A. (2016). Modeling microcirculatory blood flow: current state and future perspectives. *Wiley Interdiscip. Rev. Syst. Biol. Med.* 8, 157-168. doi: 10.1002/wsbm.1326

Huo, Y., Cheng, Y., Zhao, X., Lu, X., and Kassab, G. S. (2012b). Biaxial vasoactivity of porcine coronary artery. *Am. J. Physiol. Heart Circ. Physiol.* 302, H2058-H2063. doi: 10.1152/ajpheart.00758.2011

Huo, Y., Choy, J. S., Svendsen, M., Sinha, A. K., and Kassab, G. S. (2009b). Effects of vessel compliance on flow pattern in porcine epicardial right coronary arterial tree. *J. Biomech.* 42, 594-602. doi: 10.1016/j.jbiomech.2008.12.011

Huo, Y., Finet, G., Lefevre, T., Louvard, Y., Moussa, I., and Kassab, G. S. (2012a). Which diameter and angle rule provides optimal flow patterns in a coronary bifurcation? *J. Biomech.* 45, 1273-1279. doi: 10.1016/j.jbiomech.2012.01.033

Huo, Y., Guo, X., and Kassab, G. S. (2008). The flow field along the entire length of mouse aorta and primary branches. *Ann. Biomed. Eng.* 36, 685-699. doi: 10.1007/s10439-008-9473-4

Huo, Y., Kaimovitz, B., Lanir, Y., Wischgoll, T., Hoffman, J. I., and Kassab, G. S. (2009a). Biophysical model of the spatial heterogeneity of myocardial flow. *Biophys. J.* 96, 4035-4043. doi: 10.1016/j.bpj.2009.02.047

Huo, Y., and Kassab, G. S. (2006). Pulsatile blood flow in the entire coronary arterial tree: theory and experiment. *Am. J. Physiol. Heart Circ. Physiol.* 291, H1074-H1087. doi: 10.1152/ajpheart.00200.2006

Huo, Y., and Kassab, G. S. (2012a). Intraspecific scaling laws of vascular trees. *J. R. Soc. Interface* 9, 190-200. doi: 10.1098/rsif.2011.0270

Huo, Y., and Kassab, G. S. (2012b). Compensatory remodeling of coronary microvasculature maintains shear stress in porcine left-ventricular hypertrophy. *J. Hypertens.* 30, 608-616. doi: 10.1097/HJH.0b013e32834f44dd

Huo, Y., and Kassab, G. S. (2016). Scaling laws of coronary circulation in health and disease. *J. Biomech.* 49, 2531-2539. doi: 10.1016/j.jbiomech.2016.01.044

Huo, Y. L., Finet, G., Lefevre, T., Louvard, Y., Moussa, I., and Kassab, G. S. (2012). Optimal diameter of diseased bifurcation segment: a practical rule for percutaneous coronary intervention. *EuroIntervention* 7, 1310-1316. doi: 10.4244/EIJV7I11A206

Huo, Y., Linares, C. O., and Kassab, G. S. (2007b). Capillary perfusion and wall shear stress are restored in the coronary circulation of hypertrophic right ventricle. *Circ. Res.* 100, 273-283 doi: 10.1161/01.RES.0000257777.83431.13

Huo, Y., Wischgoll, T., and Kassab, G. S. (2007a). Flow patterns in three-dimensional porcine epicardial coronary arterial tree. *Am. J. Physiol. Heart Circ. Physiol.* 293, H2959-H2970. doi: 10.1152/ajpheart.00586.2007

Jacob, M., Chappell, D., and Becker, B. F. (2016). Regulation of blood flow and volume exchange across the microcirculation. *Crit. Care* 20:319. doi: 10.1186/s13054-016-1485-0

Kaimovitz, B., Huo, Y., Lanir, Y., and Kassab, G. S. (2008). Diameter asymmetry of porcine coronary arterial trees: structural and functional implications. *Am. J. Physiol. Heart Circ. Physiol.* 294, H714-H723. doi: 10.1152/ajpheart.00818.2007

Kassab, G. S. (2005). Functional hierarchy of coronary circulation: direct evidence of a structure-function relation. *Am. J. Physiol. Heart Circ. Physiol.* 289, H2559-H2565. doi: 10.1152/ajpheart.00561.2005

Kleinstreuer, C., Hyun, S., Buchanan, J. R., Longest, P. W., Archie, J. P., and Truskey, G. A. (2001). Hemodynamic parameters and early intimal thickening in branching blood vessels. *Crit. Rev. Biomed. Eng.* 29, 1-64. doi: 10.1615/CritRevBiomedEng.v29.i1.10

LeBlanc, A. J., and Hoying, J. B. (2016). Adaptation of the coronary microcirculation in aging. *Microcirculation* 23, 157-167. doi: 10.1111/micc.12264

Malek, A. M., Alper, S. L., and Izumo, S. (1999). Hemodynamic shear stress and its role in atherosclerosis. *JAMA* 282, 2035-2042.

Pries, A. R., Neuhaus, D., and Gaehtgens, P. (1992). Blood viscosity in tube flow: dependence on diameter and hematocrit. *Am. J. Physiol.* 263(6 Pt 2), H1770-H1778. doi: 10.1152/ajpheart.1992.263.6.H1770

Pries, A. R., and Secomb, T. W. (2005). Microvascular blood viscosity *in vivo* and the endothelial surface layer. *Am. J. Physiol. Heart Circ. Physiol.* 289, H2657-H2664. doi: 10.1152/ajpheart.00297.2005

Pries, A. R., Secomb, T. W., and Gaehtgens, P. (1995). Design Principles Of Vascular Beds. *Circ. Res.* 77, 1017-1023

Reglin, B., Secomb, T. W., and Pries, A. R. (2017). Structural control of microvessel diameters: origins of metabolic signals. *Front. Physiol.* 8:813. doi: 10.3389/fphys.2017.00813

Secomb, T. W. (2017). Blood flow in the microcirculation. *Annu. Rev. Fluid Mech.* 49, 443-461. doi: 10.1146/annurev-fluid-010816-060302

Teng, B., Tilley, S. L., Ledent, C., and Mustafa, S. J. (2016). *In vivo* assessment of coronary flow and cardiac function after bolus adenosine injection in adenosine receptor knockout mice. *Physiol. Rep.* 4:e12818. doi: 10.14814/phy2.12818

VanBavel, E., and Spaan, J. A. (1992). Branching patterns in the porcine coronary arterial tree. Estimation of flow heterogeneity. *Circ. Res.* 71, 1200-1212

Wei, J. Y. (1992). Age and the cardiovascular system. *N. Engl. J. Med.* 327, 1735-1739

Yin, X., Huang, X., Feng, Y., Tan, W., Liu, H., and Huo, Y. (2016). Interplay of proximal flow confluence and distal flow divergence in patient-specific vertebrobasilar system. *PLoS ONE* 11:e0159836. doi: 10.1371/journal.pone.0159836

# 8

# Application of Patient-Specific Computational Fluid Dynamics in Coronary and Intra-Cardiac Flow Simulations: Challenges and Opportunities

Liang Zhong [1,2*†], Jun-Mei Zhang [1,2†], Boyang Su [1], Ru San Tan [1,2*], John C. Allen [2] and Ghassan S. Kassab [3]

[1] National Heart Centre Singapore, National Heart Research Institute of Singapore, Singapore, Singapore, [2] Duke-NUS Medical School, Singapore, Singapore, [3] California Medical Innovations Institute, San Diego, CA, United States

*Correspondence:
Liang Zhong
zhong.liang@nhcs.com.sg
Ru San Tan
tan.ru.san@singhealth.com.sg

[†] These authors have contributed equally to this work and are joint first author.

The emergence of new cardiac diagnostics and therapeutics of the heart has given rise to the challenging field of virtual design and testing of technologies in a patient-specific environment. Given the recent advances in medical imaging, computational power and mathematical algorithms, patient-specific cardiac models can be produced from cardiac images faster, and more efficiently than ever before. The emergence of patient-specific computational fluid dynamics (CFD) has paved the way for the new field of computer-aided diagnostics. This article provides a review of CFD methods, challenges and opportunities in coronary and intra-cardiac flow simulations. It includes a review of market products and clinical trials. Key components of patient-specific CFD are covered briefly which include image segmentation, geometry reconstruction, mesh generation, fluid-structure interaction, and solver techniques.

Keywords: blood flow, computational fluid dynamics (CFD), patient-specific, cardiovascular, coronary, intra-cardiac flow simulation

## INTRODUCTION—CORONARY ARTERY DISEASE, CARDIAC DYSFUNCTION, AND DIAGNOSIS

In coronary artery disease (CAD) atherosclerotic build-up can narrow the arterial lumen, resulting in myocardial ischemia. Prevalence of CAD is 6% in the general population and up to 20% in those aged over 65 years. About 13% of deaths are due to CAD. By 2030, it is projected that 15% of male deaths will be attributable to CAD (World Health Organization, 2011).

CAD can be diagnosed by means of either an anatomic parameter, such as diameter stenosis or a functional parameter linked to coronary territory myocardial ischemia. Stenosis does not invariably impair distal coronary flow, and this is particularly true with regard to the intermediate coronary artery lesions (i.e., diameter stenosis between 30 and 70%). Non-invasive tests of myocardial ischemia (e.g., nuclear myocardial perfusion imaging, stress echocardiography) identify areas of the most severely reduced relative coronary flow reserve. They are fairly accurate for myocardial ischemia detection on a per-patient basis, but these perform less well in quantifying severity of individual coronary territory ischemia. The latter is relevant in multi-vessel percutaneous coronary intervention (PCI), where coronary physiological information, overlaid on detailed maps of patient-specific coronary artery anatomy, dictates management decisions. Fractional flow reserve (FFR) measured during invasive coronary angiography (ICA) under adenosine-induced hyperemia has emerged as the gold standard for assessment of coronary flow physiology and coronary territory ischemia (Johnson et al., 2012).

Diagnosis of heart contractile dysfunction requires demonstration of either diastolic or systolic function abnormalities. The gold standard for determining diastolic dysfunction is an increase in invasively measured ventricular end-diastolic pressure–>15 mmHg in the case of the left ventricle (LV) (Nishimura and Tajik, 1997). Systolic dysfunction is assessed by the change in maximal ventricular pressure (P) during isovolumic contraction, $dP/dt_{max}$ (Yamada et al., 1998). Multiple ventricular pressure-volume loops assayed using a conductance catheter under varying loading conditions can yield end-diastolic ($E_{ed}$) and end-systolic elastances ($E_{es}$) that characterize ventricular diastolic and systolic dysfunction, respectively (Burkhoff et al., 2005). Emerging noninvasive echocardiographic and cardiac magnetic resonance (MRI) imaging techniques enable corroborative assessment of regional and global cardiac chamber dysfunction involving strain and strain rate (Zhong et al., 2012), curvedness (a descriptor of three-dimensional ventricular shape) and curvedness rate (Zhong et al., 2009), ventricular contractility $d\sigma^*/dt_{max}$, where $\sigma^*$ is pressure-normalized wall stress (Zhong et al., 2014), and atrio-ventricular velocities (Leng et al., 2016).

Patient-specific computational fluid dynamics (CFD) modeling is a recent development. Non-invasive FFR ($FFR_{CT}$) is derived from CFD modeling of images acquired using computed tomography coronary angiography (CTCA). With invasive FFR as the gold standard, $FFR_{CT} \leq 0.80$ is superior to both CTCA and ICA determined diameter stenosis for ascertaining ischemia on a coronary artery territory basis (Min et al., 2012). $FFR_{CT}$ analysis is solely available via a centralized commercial web-based service of the HeartFlow® company. Time-consuming computational demands and high costs—6 h and $2000 USD to process a case (Kimura et al., 2015)—hamper widespread clinical adoption. The requisite offsite handling of sensitive confidential patient information and associated medical conditions is a highly delicate issue involving IT-security, potential for data abuse, etc.

Unlike coronary blood flow simulation, CFD studies on intra-cardiac flows are primarily confined to research purposes owing to the complexity of modeling intra-cardiac flows. In truth, coronary and intra-cardiac flows are closely connected. Coronary artery dysfunction leads to myocardium ischemia, and intra-cardiac flows provide blood for circulation throughout the body, including the coronary circulation. Prolonged and untreated myocardial ischemia could increase the risk for death or myocardial infarction (Iskander and Iskandrian, 1998). Future integration of both coronary and intra-cardiac flow simulations is desirable to enable a comprehensive assessment of cardiac circulatory pathophysiology. This paper aims to pave the way for integrated simulations and focuses on a progress review of CFD applications in modeling coronary and intra-cardiac flow. Other applications of CFD in cardiovascular disease can be found in Morris et al. (2015).

## CORONARY FLOW SIMULATION

## Challenges and Opportunities in Patient-Specific Simulation Techniques for Studying Blood Flow in Coronary Arteries

In general, the tasks involved in performing CFD simulation for a patient-specific coronary artery tree are as follows: (1) Image acquisition and segmentation to reconstruct a 3D patient-specific coronary model; (2) CFD preprocessing to discretize the domain with meshes and define the boundary conditions; and (3) Solving the fluid governing equations using a fluid solver and post-processing to visualize the flow field (**Figure 1**). If fluid structure interaction (FSI) is considered, an additional solid solver is used, and coupling between fluid and solid solvers is implemented. **Table 1** summarizes the challenges involved.

Coronary anatomy can be imaged using ICA, intravascular ultrasound (IVUS), optical coherence tomography (OCT), CTCA, and MRI (Zhang et al., 2014). Invasive IVUS and OCT yields high-resolution cross-sectional views of the coronary arteries, and can be used in conjunction with biplane ICA to reconstruct the 3D vessel model. Since non-invasive CTCA possesses higher spatial resolution than MRI and echocardiography, it is widely used for 3D patient-specific coronary model reconstruction. However present CTCA has a spatial resolution of about 0.3 mm, which limits its use to coronary arteries of 1 mm or greater in diameter. Although CAD is not generally characterized nor is FFR measured in such small vessels, the latter is essential for characterizing coronary microcirculation.

Sophisticated segmentation approaches such as level-set segmentation (Bekkers and Taylor, 2008) have been applied to reconstruct 2D and 3D patient-specific coronary models, either by fusion of biplane ICA with IVUS images (Papafaklis et al., 2007) or directly from CTCA images (Torii et al., 2009). Commercial (e.g., 3D Doctor, Mimics, SliceOmatic, Amira) and open-source general image processing tools [e.g., VTK, ITK, ITK-SNAP, VTK, Analyze, and ImageJ (or Fiji)], make reconstruction of patient-specific models from medical images possible. Furthermore, their plug-in capability allows easy customization of segmentation tools. Artifacts such as calcification, motion and mis-registration are not easily overcome by segmentation techniques, and remain challenging.

In terms of simulation tools, commercial software such as ANSYS (including ICEM, FLUENT, CFX), STAR-CCM, and open-source tools (e.g., OpenFOAM) is applicable to general CFD simulations, including simulating the blood flow in coronary arteries. SimVascular (Schmidt et al., 2008) is a special tool designed for simulating the blood flow in vessels. These tools allow users specifications on mesh generation, boundary conditions settings and etc. As regards meshes, mesh generation schemes can be classified as structured or unstructured meshes. Structured grid generators, including "block-structured" techniques (used in ICEM CFD, TrueGrid, and IA-FEMesh)

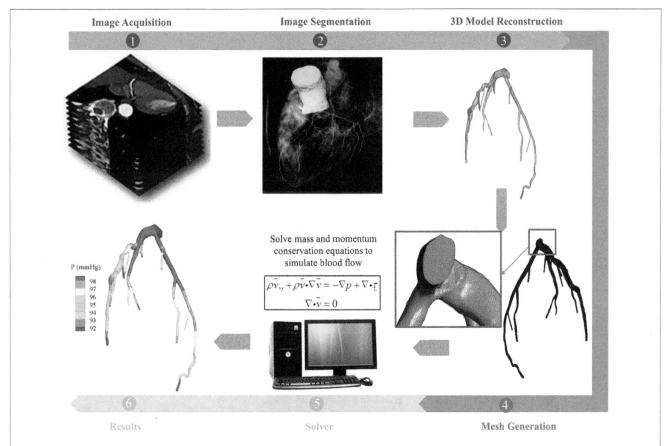

**FIGURE 1 |** Schematic drawings for the procedures of patient-specific simulations for blood flow in coronary arteries, including (1) acquisition of CTA or ICA images (2) segmentation of acquired images (3) reconstruction of 3D model (4) mesh generation to discretize the 3D model (5) solving the mass and momentum conservation equations to simulate the blood flow in coronary arteries, if FSI is taken into consideration, solid solver will also be activated, and (6) presentation of simulations.

generally require complex iterative smoothing procedures to align elements with boundaries or physical domain. For the complex 3D coronary artery models reconstructed from medical images, unstructured meshes are commonly needed, which are built based on node coordinates and the connections between nodes to form elements. Commercial packages (e.g., ANSYS, TGrid) and open-source (e.g., TetGen, gmesh) allow automatic discretization of complex geometry with tetrahedral meshes. However quality control of tetrahedral meshes can be challenging and varies according to the mesh generation method employed (Wittek et al., 2016). The advancing front method, such as the Delaunay triangulation method, can provide better control of the mesh quality, but at the expense of prolonged computational time. In addition, 4-noded tetrahedral elements are involved with artificial stiffening, which presents challenges in modeling soft tissue, such as the coronary artery wall (Wittek et al., 2010). Higher-order and mixed-formulation tetrahedral elements can assist in overcoming these challenges. Nevertheless their computational cost is about four times higher than the 4-noded tetrahedral elements (Bourdin et al., 2007). To overcome the difficulty of generating good quality meshes for complex geometry with limited time and the convergence difficulties in modeling structures with large deformations, meshless

methods have been recognized as one possible solution (Doblare et al., 2005). Meshless methods discretize the computational domain into a cloud of nodal points (Belinha, 2016). This discretization flexibility may allow direct model generation from CTCA or MRI images. However, meshless methods also have substantial shortcomings: (i) limited strict mathematical proof, (ii) incomplete theory, and (iii) lower computation efficiency compared to traditional computational methods using meshes (Zhang et al., 2012).

To achieve an acceptable simulation of blood flow in the coronary arteries, proper boundary conditions are paramount. Although flow and pressure waveforms can be obtained from the literature, *in-vitro* and *in-vivo* measurements are necessary for accurate simulations. For many CFD applications, it is virtually impossible to know flow and/or pressure waveforms a *priori* due to the difficulty of obtaining simultaneous measurements in coronary arteries. To solve this problem, multi-scale simulations have been developed that couple 3D simulation with reduced-order (1 or 0-dimensional) models at the boundaries. These models characterize pressure and flow rate in upstream and downstream vasculatures (Kim et al., 2010) as resistance, compliance, and impedance. How to determine the values of these patient-specific parameters remains a dilemma. Although

**TABLE 1 |** Current challenges and opportunities in numerical simulation of coronary arteries.

| Simulation procedures | | Current challenges and opportunities |
|---|---|---|
| Image acquisition | | • Current spatial resolution for CTCA and ICA was around 0.3 mm (Kantor et al., 2007; Lewis et al., 2016; Galassi et al., 2018). This limits their use to coronary arteries of 1 mm or greater in diameter. The ideal spatial resolution is 0.1 mm (Lewis et al., 2016).<br>Severe motion artifacts, stair-step artifacts, image noise, or calcium blooming may lead to non-diagnostic CTCA images (Alkadhi et al., 2008).<br>Image resolution and quality can be mitigated to an extent by extracting images in different cardiac phases and using multiple imaging modalities for reconstruction (Sankaran et al., 2016). |
| Segmentation and 3D model reconstruction | | • It is challenging to segment images with severe motion and stair-step artifacts, image noise, calcification, or misregistration.<br>• Segmentation of coronary artery tree may take a few hours. |
| Fluid dynamics simulation | Fluid mesh generation | • Quality control of tetrahedral meshes can be challenging (Wittek et al., 2016).<br>Meshless methods discretize the computational domain into a cloud of nodal points (Belinha, 2016), which may allow direct model generation from CTCA or MRI images. |
| | Boundary conditions | • Both prescribed and lumped parameter (0 or 1-order) models can be used as boundary conditions. The lumped parameters (e.g., resistance, compliance, etc.) may be tuned via numerical optimization (Spilker et al., 2007). |
| | Fluid solver | • Both robust implicit approaches and explicit methods can be used to solve the flow-governing equations.<br>• Explicit methods are generally less robust compared to the implicit fully coupled methods (Kim et al., 2010; Sankaran et al., 2012). |
| FSI coupling | | • Traditional FSI techniques based on ALE method requires expensive computational cost due to re-meshing (Hecht and Pironneau, 2017).<br>Immersed boundary (Peskin, 2003) and coupled momentum methods (Figueroa et al., 2006) are alternatives to treat coronary vessels as compliant. |

morphologic information (e.g., scaling law) is widely used, numerical optimization may be necessary to tune these patient-specific parameters (Spilker et al., 2007).

Another obstacle in multi-scale simulation is how to solve the flow-governing equations using reduced-order models as boundary conditions. Both robust implicit approaches and explicit methods have been used. Explicit methods do not require changing the numerical algorithms to solve the governing equations (Sankaran et al., 2012), although they are generally less robust compared to the implicit fully coupled methods (Kim et al., 2010).

Recent progress in FSI techniques has allowed treating the coronary vessels as compliant. In the traditional Arbitrary Lagrangian-Eulerian (ALE) method (Malvè et al., 2012), boundaries and interfaces of both fluid and structural computational domains are precisely tracked during the iterations. When taking heart movement into consideration, re-meshing computational domains is often necessary to maintain mesh quality, which substantially increases computational cost. Over the years, stability of the ALE method has been improved (Hecht and Pironneau, 2017).

Alternative FSI techniques used to simulate flow in the presence of a moving boundary include immersed boundary and coupled momentum methods. These use fixed fluid meshes with boundaries defined by a set of moving Lagrangian points (Peskin, 2003) or linear membrane (Figueroa et al., 2006). Although prescribed heart motion has been used for simulating the blood flow in left (Prosi et al., 2004) and right (Torii et al., 2010)

coronary arteries, more efficient, and robust FSI techniques are necessary to model large deformations of coronary arteries when taking heart motion during a cardiac cycle into account.

Recent development of fluid-solid-growth modeling incorporates vascular wall geometry, structure and properties governed by stress-mediated growth and remodeling (G&R) into FSI simulation (Figueroa et al., 2009). In this way, biofluid mechanics, biosolid mechanics, and biotransport phenomena, such as arterial growth, remodeling, and adaptation (Valentín et al., 2013) can be better understood. Recently, machine learning has been adopted into the CFD simulation to reduce the computational time incorporating features trained by a database generated from a set of offline CFD simulations (Sankaran et al., 2015; Itu et al., 2016). Sankaran and Marsden (2011) developed an adaptive collocation algorithm to quantify the effect of input uncertainties on cardiovascular simulation. Using a data-driven framework, Sankaran et al. (2016) studied the impact of anatomic and physiologic uncertainty (e.g., various boundary conditions and blood viscosity) on blood flow simulation. These data-driven modeling approaches wherein CFD data is used to enrich and refine the models may become popular in the future.

In addition, the assumption of blood as a Newtonian fluid is only valid for shear rate higher than $100$ s$^{-1}$, which may not be true when a flow recirculation region is formed near a coronary stenosis. The influence of non-Newtonian properties of blood on the velocity distribution and shear-thinning has been studied via various single and multi-phase non-Newtonian hemodynamic models (Jung et al., 2006). An effect of non-Newtonian properties on overall pressure drop across the arterial stenosis was exhibited at a flow with the Reynolds number of 100 or less (Cho and Kensey, 1991).

## Challenges and Opportunities in Applying Patient-Specific CFD Technologies for Diagnosing the Severity of Coronary Artery Disease

Recent patient-specific CFD simulations provide detailed hemodynamic parameter (HP) information, such as pressure (P), wall pressure gradient (WPG) (Liu et al., 2012), wall shear stress (WSS) (Papafaklis et al., 2007; Stone et al., 2012), oscillatory shear index (OSI), relative residence time (RRT), and stress phase angle (SPA) (Knight et al., 2010), enabling characterization of HP distributions on coronary vessel walls. Definitions of these HPs (**Table 2**) and illustrations of their distributions in a left coronary artery tree (**Figure 2**) are presented. In the simulations, pressure and resistance boundary conditions were assigned to the inlet and outlets, respectively. A non-slip condition was imposed on the wall (Zhang et al., 2015).

Among the HPs, pressure was closely related to FFR (Johnson et al., 2012), where FFR is the ratio of pressure distal to stenosis and aortic pressure at hyperemia, obtained during ICA. Alternative approaches for calculating FFR non-invasively have been attempted by several groups.

The Heart Flow company is a pioneer to combine CTCA images with CFD for calculating non-invasive FFR$_{CT}$ in CAD diagnosis. Kim et al (Kim et al., 2010) pioneered non-invasive FFR$_{CT}$ by reconstructing 3D patient-specific coronary artery model from CTCA images and coupling lumped parameter models to an implicit solver of fluid-governing equations (**Figure 3A**). Multicenter clinical trials DISCOVER-FLOW, DeFACTO, and NXT (Koo et al., 2011; Min et al., 2012; Nørgaard et al., 2014) demonstrated superior diagnostic accuracy for FFR$_{CT}$ vs. CTCA alone. PLATFORM trial (Douglas et al., 2015) (Lu et al., 2017) demonstrated the feasibility and safety of FFR$_{CT}$ as a diagnostic strategy in triage of patients with suspected CAD compared to standard of care. REAL-FFR$_{CT}$ (Kawaji et al., 2017) demonstrated good diagnostic performance of FFR$_{CT}$ even in patients with severely calcified vessels. Recently HeartFlow's FFR$_{CT}$ software has been approved by FDA for measuring coronary blockages non-invasively. However it used cloud technology for uploading CTCA images and downloading FFR$_{CT}$ report. This could involve data security issues that would hinder the on-site computation.

To facilitate on-site FFR computation supported by Siemens Company, Coenen et al. modeled coronary vessel as 1D segment and employed a reduced-order model for simulating the coronary circulation. In this way, the computational time was reduced to 5–10 min per patient (Coenen et al., 2015). Calculated pressure information, viz. computational FFR (cFFR), was mapped onto a 3D model reconstructed from CTCA images (**Figure 3B**). The correlation between cFFR and FFR, however, was poor ($r = 0.59$). To further reduce the computational time, Itu and colleagues from Siemens applied machine-learning approach for computing cFFR$_{ML}$ with features extracted from training database (Itu et al., 2016). The database

consisted of synthetically generated coronary artery models and corresponding FFR values computed from the CFD algorithm (**Figure 3C**).

Another attempt to reduce the computation time to be <30 min was conducted by Ko and colleagues from Toshiba Medical Systems Corp. core laboratory (Ko et al., 2017). Differing from the above studies, 4 CTCA images were acquired and reconstructed at phases of 70, 80, 90, and 99% of the R-R interval. The arterial luminal deformation was taken into consideration and a reduced-order fluid model was used to simulate a 1-dimensional pressure and flow distribution in coronary tree (**Figure 3D**). In this approach, the interaction between fluid and structure is taken into account to some extent, although it is not a fully-coupled FSI simulation.

With the exception of CTCA images, attempts have been made to derive FFR$_{QCA}$ using CFD simulation in patient-specific coronary artery models reconstructed from ICA In a study involving 77 coronary vessels (Tu et al., 2014), FFR$_{QCA}$ correlated well with the gold standard FFR ($r = 0.81$, $p < 0.001$). Invasive FFR$_{QCA}$ obviates the need for pressure wire/catheter and adenosine. QFR was further derived from 3 flow models using fixed empiric flow velocity; modeled hyperemic flow velocity derived from measured angiography without administration of adenosine, and measured hyperemic flow velocity, respectively (Tu et al., 2016). Diagnostic accuracy of QFR was tested in the FAVOR II China (Xu et al., 2017) and WIFI II (Westra et al., 2018) studies. Based on this method, Medis QAngio 3D XA software was developed to calculate QFR.

Combining coronary angiogram images with CFD simulation was also studied by Morris et al. (2013) to estimate virtual fractional flow reserve (vFFR) with generic boundary conditions. VIRTUheart software was therefore developed to facilitate the calculation of vFFR. CathWorks is another tool available for FFR simulation-based service through the combination of coronary angiograms and CFD simulation.

Infusion OCT with a coronary angiogram was used by Poon et al. (2015, 2017) in an attempt to reconstruct the vessel and calculate virtually derived FFR.

Other HPs (**Table 2**) have been considered in relation to CAD based on biomechanical forces involved in regulation of blood vessel structure (Langille and O'Donnell, 1986). Among them, WSS has been the most studied. WSS is the frictional force of blood exerted tangentially to the luminal surface of the blood vessel per unit area. WSS is typically within the range of 15–20 dynes/cm$^2$ (Kassab and Navia, 2006) for normal arteries; abnormal WSS outside this range promotes atherogenesis. There are two competing theories. In *in-vitro* experiments on canine thoracic aorta endothelial cells (ECs), ECs became abnormal for WSS >379 dynes/cm$^2$ (Fry, 1968). This implied that high WSS might injure and denudate the ECs resulting in atherogenesis. Conversely, Caro et al. found intimal thickening and atherosclerosis with WSS <6 dynes/cm$^2$ (Caro et al., 1969). They conjectured that low WSS was associated with prolonged particle retention time, and increased intimal accumulation of lipids, leading to atherogenesis. Indeed, Rutsch et al. proposed several signaling pathways relating disturbed WSS with EC mechanico-chemical transductions (Rutsch et al., 2011).

**TABLE 2 |** Hemodynamic parameters (HPs) predicted by CFD (Computational Fluid Dynamics) to link with CAD (Coronary Artery Disease).

| HPs | Units | Definition and Formula | Related hypothesis | Related studies | Remark |
|---|---|---|---|---|---|
| P | Pa | Force acting perpendicularly on the vessel wall per unit area | Elevated blood pressure is associated with atherosclerotic formation (Glagov et al., 1989) | Aueron and Gruentzig, 1984 | FFR is the pressure based indicator for CAD diagnosis (Johnson et al., 2012). Recent coupling between CFD and medical images leads to new indictors, such as $FFR_{CT}$, $FFR_{QCA}$, $_CFFR$ and $FFR_B$ (Nørgaard et al., 2014; Tu et al., 2014; Coenen et al., 2015; Zhang et al., 2016, 2018) |
| WPG | Pa/m | Spatial gradient of the wall pressure $$WPG = \sqrt{\left(\frac{\partial P}{\partial x}\right)^2 + \left(\frac{\partial P}{\partial y}\right)^2 + \left(\frac{\partial P}{\partial z}\right)^2}$$ Note: $P$ is pressure exerted on the wall; $x$, $y$ and $z$ are coordinates in different directions | WPG may represent important local modulators of endothelial gene expression in atherogenesis and may result in the redistribution of the initially accumulated atheromatic material within the sub-endothelial layer | Liu et al., 2012 | |
| WSS | Pa | Frictional force of blood exerted tangential to the luminal surface of the blood vessel per unit area $$wss = \tau_w = \mu\left(\frac{\partial \vec{u}}{\partial \vec{n}}\right)\bigg|_{wall}$$ Note: $\vec{u}$ and $\vec{n}$ are the velocity vector and the direction vector normal to the wall, respectively | WSS over normal coronary artery was found to within the range of 15–20 dynes/cm$^2$ a. High WSS is conjectured to injure and denude the vessel wall of endothelial cells, resulting in atherosclerotic plaque (Fry, 1968) b. Low WSS is suspected to prolong particle retention time and increase intimal accumulation of lipids, leading to atherosclerosis formation (Caro et al., 1969) | Combing CFD with IVUS images and biplane coronary angiography helps to predict WSS, which is correlated with baseline luminal narrowing or plaque thickness (Stone et al., 2003; Papafaklis et al., 2007; Gijsen et al., 2008); Habib (Eshtehardi et al., 2012; Stone et al., 2012) | Among them, PREDICTION study (Stone et al., 2012) is impressive. Study recruited 506 patients. Results revealed that low local WSS and large plaque burden could identify plaques that develop progressively and lead to lumen narrowing |
| OSI | | A measure to quantify the change in direction and magnitude of the WSS (Ku et al., 1985) $$OSI = \frac{1}{2}\left(1 - \left|\int_0^T \tau_w dt\right| / \int_0^T |\tau_w|\, dt\right)$$ Note: $T$ is the duration of one cardiac cycle | Marked oscillations in the direction of WSS could be captured by high OSI values, which may lead to atherogenesis (Knight et al., 2010) | Knight et al. (2010) obtained CT images of 30 patients with 120 plaques. By virtually removing the plaques, CFD predicted OSI was correlated with plaque location | It was found that OSI has higher positive prediction value (PPV) than WSS |
| RRT | Pa$^{-1}$ | The residence time of a particle in the vicinity of vascular endothelium (Himburg et al., 2004) $$RRT = \frac{1}{(1-2\times OSI)\times TAWSS}$$ Note: TAWSS is the time-averaged WSS | Prolonged residence time of blood, viz. higher RRT, may increase the likelihood of adhesion of platelets and leukocytes to the endothelium and lead to the smooth muscle cell proliferation | Kleinstreuer et al., 2001; Knight et al., 2010 | It was found that RRT had higher PPV than WSS |
| SPA | | Time-averaged temporal phase angle between circumferential stress (CS) and WSS on the arterial wall to quantify the time lag arises between the pulsatile WSS and CS (Qiu and Tarbell, 1996) $$SPA = \varphi(D - \tau_w)$$ Note: $\varphi(D - \tau_w)$ is the time-averaged phase difference between lumen diameter circumferential direction and WSS | SPA measures the degree of asynchrony between pressure and flow waveforms | Torii et al., 2009; Zhang et al., 2015 | SPA is proposed to be a useful indicator in predicting sites prone to atherosclerosis |

CFD has been applied in the study of HP distributions, particularly WSS, in both idealized and patient-specific coronary artery models (Papafaklis et al., 2007). The PREDICTION study (Stone et al., 2012) enrolled 506 PCI patients and studied the natural history of plaque development in a subset of 374 (74%) over a 6- to 10-month period post-PCI. WSS was calculated for 3D coronary artery models reconstructed by combining intracoronary IVUS and biplane ICA images. Large plaque burden and low local WSS were found to be independent and additive predictors of plaque

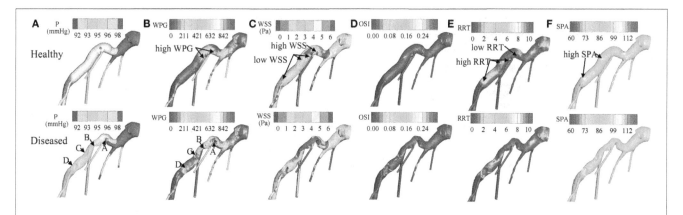

**FIGURE 2 |** Distributions of **(A)** P (Pressure), **(B)** WPG (wall pressure gradient), **(C)** WSS (wall shear stress), **(D)** OSI (oscillatory shear index), **(E)** RRT (relative residence time), and **(F)** SPA (stress phase angle) on the virtually healthy and diseased left coronary artery trees respectively. Labels of **(A–D)** indicate the stenosis locations. In the virtually healthy artery model, low WSS, and high RRT was exhibited in three of the four locations, where the stenoses were formed, and high WSS with low RRT was exhibited in the fourth. These findings suggest that coronary plaque is more likely to form in locations with low- WSS- and- high- RRT or high- WSS- and- low- RRT. From Zhang et al. (2015).

progression and luminal narrowing. Other clinical trials are currently underway investigating potential links between HPs and coronary atherogenesis (Antoniadis et al., 2015). These presage exciting possibilities for identifying indicators that may be useful for CAD diagnosis and patient management.

## INTRA-CARDIAC FLOW SIMULATION

## Challenges and Opportunities in Patient-Specific Simulations for Studying Intra-Cardiac Flow

**Figure 4** illustrates the general process of CFD simulation of blood flow in the LV based on cardiac MRI images (Su et al., 2015). Images comprise the long-axis and a stack of 12–14 short-axis images covering the LV from apex to base. Typical slice thickness is 8 mm; and typical frame rate 20–40 per cardiac cycle. Short-axis images are segmented either manually or automatically wherein blood pool is distinguished from heart muscle, and papillary muscles are included in blood pool. Long-axis images are used to track the mitral annulus at the intersection of the LV and the left atrium, which cannot be segmented easily on short-axis images due to through-plane displacement. A similar method is applied to construct the aortic annulus at the LV outflow tract. A patient-specific model based on segmentations is thereby generated (steps are highlighted by red rectangle in 1.1 of **Figure 4**).

Next, the complex 3D models are discretized into tetrahedral, hexahedral or polyhedral grids using either in-house or commercial mesh generators such as ANSYS ICEM CFD, STAR-CCM+. A tetrahedral mesh is frequently adopted, which requires re-meshing when spring-based smoothing fails to cope with large deformations. Polyhedral meshes confer superior convergence speed (Spiegel et al., 2011) and can be easily implemented for FSI simulation. To factor in wall motion during numerical simulation, surface mesh numbers and their connectivity must match at each time step. By exploiting consistent topology within

the patient-specific model, surface meshes at other time frames are generated based on the corresponding LV geometry, and the correlation between the 3D model and the surface mesh at the first time step. Cubic-spline interpolation is commonly applied, as the frame rate of MRI is inadequate for numerical simulation.

In simulations that use the immersed boundary method (Peskin, 2003), a Cartesian mesh is typically applied to the blood domain, where the LV surface consists of triangular facets. In other words, the discretization step can be skipped by using the patient-specific model directly.

Boundary conditions at inlet and outlet are initialized with appropriate blood properties prior to solving the Navier-Stokes equations. Cardiac flow profiles measured from velocity-encoded imaging modalities such as phase-contrast MRI scans can be used to specify inlet and outlet boundary conditions (Wong et al., 2017). Aortic/pulmonary pressure can only be measured invasively, which might not always be possible.

In addition, the heart is a complex multi-scale system involving the interaction of cardiac electrophysiology with muscle tissue, rapid valve opening and closure, and large wall deformation during the cardiac cycle (Quarteroni et al., 2017). To consider the coupling between electrophysiology and heart mechanics, fiber orientation/ architecture information is necessary for modeling electrical conduction and associated force generation (Crozier et al., 2016). As *in-vivo* acquisition of the fiber architecture is difficult (Toussaint et al., 2013), "Rule-based" methods was used to assign fiber orientation to ventricular cardiac models, which did not include the fiber structure within endocardial and intramural structures (Bayer et al., 2012). "Atlas-based" approaches used a mesh warping process to map the meshes associated with diffusion tensor MRI fiber data on an idealized template mesh. In this way, the fiber architecture information can be automatically incorporated into new patient-specific model (Vadakkumpadan et al., 2012).

The appropriate choice of constitutive models and material parameters to represent valves in computational studies is another topic related to the heart valve mechanics. In the

| | Diagrams | Characteristics |
|---|---|---|
| (a) Heart Flow (FFR$_{CT}$) (Gaur et al., 2013) | | i. 3D model reconstructed from CTCA + transient CFD with lumped parameter models<br>ii. Accuracy: 84% (Discover-Flow:159 vessels), 86% (NXT: 484 vessels)<br>iii. Cloud service<br>iv. Service Charge: about US $1,500/case<br>v. Computational Time: about 8-12 hours<br>vi. Data security issue<br>vii. FDA clearance |
| (b) Siemens (1$^{st}$ generation, cFFR) (Coenen et al., 2015) | | i. 1D model reconstructed from CTCA + transient CFD<br>ii. Onsite computation<br>iii. Computational Time: 5-10 minutes/case<br>iv. Accuracy: 74% (189 vessels) |
| (c) Siemens (2$^{nd}$ generation, cFFR$_{ML}$) (Itu et al., 2016) | | i. Machine learning from CFD simulation on 12,000 synthetic coronary artery trees<br>ii. Computational Time for new case: 1-4 minutes/case<br>iii. Accuracy: 83.2% (125 vessels) |
| (d) Toshiba (CT-FFR) (Ko et al., 2017) | | i. Bundled with Toshiba scanner<br>ii. Four diastolic phase images acquisition between 70% and 100% (typically 70%, 80%, 90%, 99% of R-R interval), higher radiation involved in contract to normal one phase image acquisition<br>iii. Reduced order (1D) fluid model<br>iv. Accuracy: 83.9% (56 vessels) |

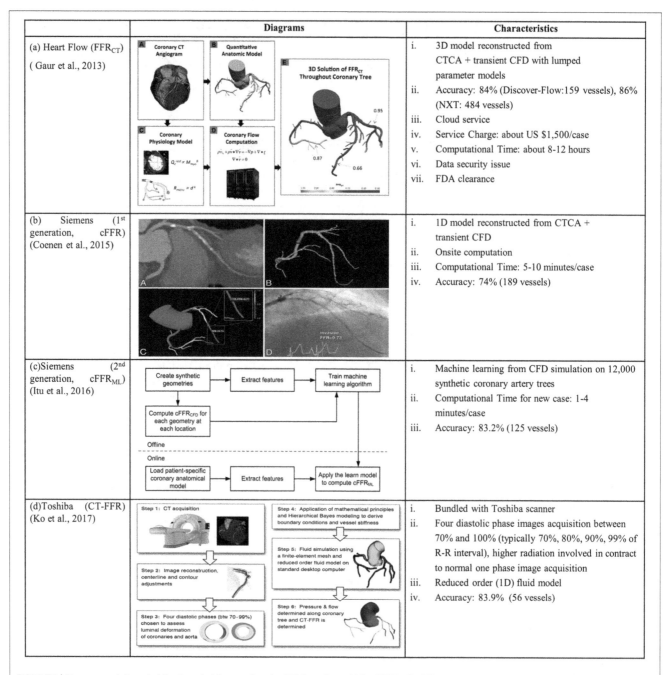

**FIGURE 3 |** Diagrams and characteristics for calculating non-invasive FFR through combining CTCA with CFD by the companies of **(A)** Heart Flow: FFR$_{CT}$ (Gaur et al., 2013); **(B)** Siemens (1st generation: cFFR) (Coenen et al., 2015); **(C)** Siemens (2nd generation: cFFR$_{ML}$) (Itu et al., 2016); and **(D)** Toshiba: CT-FFR (Ko et al., 2017).

study of Rausch et al. (2013), mitral valves were modeled as follows: (i) the Neo-Hooken isotropic nonlinear hyperplastic model (neglecting the anisotropic microstructure of mitral leaflet tissue; (ii) the coupled May-Newman model to characterize the heterogeneous response of the entire mitral valve complex; (iii) the decoupled Holzapfel model to represent the anisotropic properties of arterial tissue. The last two models resulted in smaller local displacement errors relative to the first model.

Cardiac tissue properties are the other important parameters for modeling the cardiac multi-scale interaction. However *in-vitro* measurement of tissue properties using a cardiac tissue mechanics testing system (Golob et al., 2014) is not applicable to the circumference in most cases. Estimating the material stiffness from pressure-volume loop analysis might be a practical way (Pironet et al., 2013). Modeling flow-mediated thrombus generation becomes feasible by coupling the hemodynamic equations to the biochemical convection–diffusion–reaction

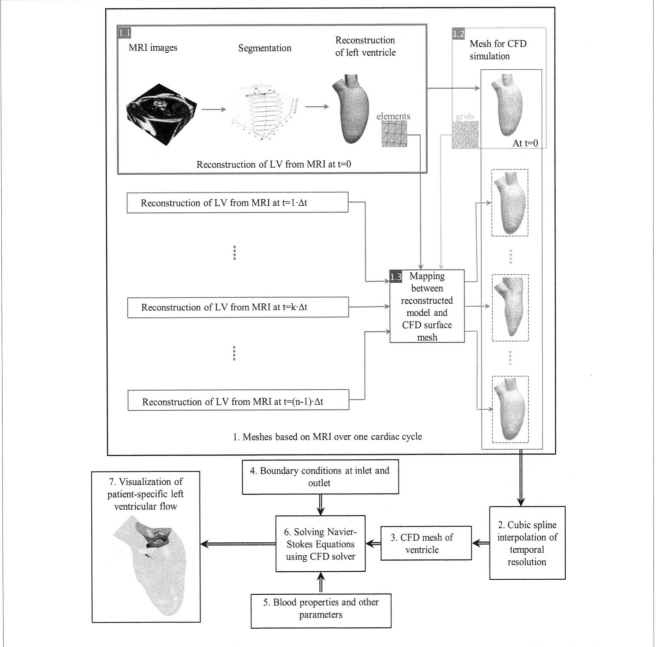

**FIGURE 4 |** Flow chart of CFD simulation of patient-specific intra-cardiac flow. Black box: each step of numerical simulation (Su et al., 2016). Red box: left ventricle reconstruction from MRI images. Green box: CFD mesh generation. Violet box: Mapping between reconstructed model and CFD surface mesh. Dotted blue box: CFD mesh resulted from mapping. Blue box: A series of CFD meshes at each frame. Elements (blue) and grids (green) are for reconstructed geometry and CFD mesh, respectively.

(CDR) equations (Mittal et al., 2016). Challenges of patient-specific intra-cardiac flow simulation are summarized in **Table 3**.

**Figure 5** summarizes various post-processing analyses of intra-cardiac flow. The flow mapping facilitates visualization of flow patterns throughout the cardiac cycle. Characteristic of diastolic flow is the clockwise anterior vortex, which is believed to preserve momentum and direct the flow toward the outflow tract

(Chnafa et al., 2014). The flow mapping depicts one 2D slice of the complex 3D LV flow at a time. Therefore, 3D vortex structure is superior, and has been widely applied in the literature.

In a normal subject, a vortex ring is observed during the rapid filling phase, which results from flow separation at the mitral valve tip (Seo et al., 2014). The vortex ring interacts with endocardium and dissipates (i.e., breaking into smaller eddies during diastasis). Another vortex ring is again generated

**TABLE 3** | Current challenges and opportunities in numerical simulation of intra-cardiac flow.

| Simulation procedures | | Current challenges and opportunities |
|---|---|---|
| Image acquisition | | • Current spatial and time resolution for cardiac MRI was around 1–1.5 mm/40–50 ms respectively (Saeed et al., 2015), which are inadequate for assessing the rapid opening and closing of thin heart valves. |
| Segmentation and 3D model reconstruction | | • Segmentation and 3D model reconstruction of the valves and right ventricle is challenging due to the limited spatial resolution of current MRI technology. |
| Fluid dynamics simulation | Fluid mesh generation | • To factor in wall motion during numerical simulation with dynamic meshes, the number of surface meshes and their connectivity must match at various time frames. Cubic-spline interpolation is usually needed to achieve adequate number of meshes for transient numerical simulation. This might be challenging for a complex heart chamber with valves, especially for the patients with heart disease.<br>• Cartesian meshes can be used when the blood flow is simulated using the immersed boundary method (Peskin, 2003). |
| | Boundary conditions | • Realistic pressure and flow information could be provided through phase-contrast MRI, cardiac catheterization and etc. |
| | Fluid solver | • Improvement of computational speed to solve complex flow phenomena for heart chamber and valves are essential for the multi-physics coupling. |
| Multi-physics coupling and others | | • Besides FSI, coupling electrophysiology with mechanics is also important in understanding heart function (Quarteroni et al., 2017)<br>The definitions of fiber orientation (Crozier et al., 2016) and tissue properties (Golob et al., 2014) are important for modeling the cardiac multiscale interaction. |

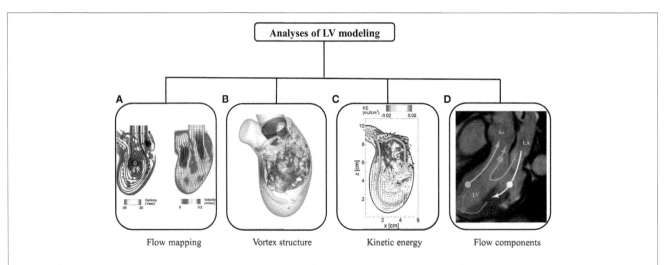

**FIGURE 5** | Post-processing of intra-cardiac flow showing **(A)** flow mapping (Seo et al., 2014); **(B)** vortex structure (Seo et al., 2014); **(C)** kinetic energy (Seo and Mittal, 2013); and **(D)** flow component (Svalbring et al., 2016).

during atrial contraction, albeit weaker in terms of penetration distance. Both 2D flow mapping and 3D vortex structure provide quantitative analyses of LV flow.

A number of parameters have been proposed to quantify kinetic energy and energy loss during cardiac motion. Pumping efficiency during systole is defined as the ratio of total flux of mechanical energy through the aorta and power expended on blood flow by heart muscle (Seo et al., 2014). In contrast, myocardial efficiency based on the pressure-volume loop is defined as the ratio of systole work and energy consumption of heart muscle. Kinetic energy dissipation is closely related to flow field, and is the energy dissipated into heat. Relatively higher energy dissipation is expected in regions with complex flow fields

due to vortex formation. Since energy dissipation is sensitive to flow field, it has been used to diagnose ventricular dysfunction (Mangual et al., 2013).

To quantify blood transit across the LV, numerous trajectories of massless particles are obtained over a few cardiac cycles (Pedrizzetti and Domenichini, 2014). According to flow trajectories, end-diastolic volume is categorized into volumes of four subgroups: (i) direct flow, blood that passes through ventricle during one heartbeat; (ii) retained flow, blood that enters during diastole but does not exit at end of systole in one heartbeat; (iii) delayed ejection flow, blood that enters ventricle in earlier cardiac cycles but exits in current cycle; and (iv) residual volume, blood that resides in ventricle over a number of

**TABLE 4** | Published patient-specific CFD simulations of heart ventricles.

| First author and year | Chamber | Imaging | Normal | PAH | DCM | SVR | SV | HCM | MI | MS | Valve | Dimensions | Method |
|---|---|---|---|---|---|---|---|---|---|---|---|---|---|
| Doost et al., 2017 | LV | MRI | 1 | – | – | – | – | – | – | – | N | 2D | DM |
| Imanparast et al., 2016 | LV | MRI | 1 | – | – | – | – | – | – | – | N | 3D | DM |
| Su et al., 2016 | LV | MRI | 1 | 1 | – | – | – | – | – | – | Y | 3D | DM |
| Doost et al., 2016 | LV | MRI | 1 | – | – | – | – | – | – | – | N | 3D | DM |
| Chnafa et al., 2016 | LV | CT | 1 | – | – | – | – | – | – | – | Y | 3D | DM |
| Bavo et al., 2016 | LV | Echo | 2 | – | 1 | – | – | – | – | – | Y | 3D | DM |
| Vedula et al., 2015 | LV | CT | 1 | – | – | – | – | – | – | – | Y | 3D | DM |
| Su et al., 2014a | LV | MRI | 1 | – | – | – | – | 1 | – | – | N | 3D | DM |
| Su et al., 2014b | LV | MRI | 1 | – | – | – | – | – | – | – | N | 2D | DM |
| Khalafvand et al., 2014 | LV | MRI | – | – | – | 1 | – | – | – | – | N | 3D | DM |
| Moosavi et al., 2014 | LV | MRI | 1 | – | – | – | – | – | – | – | N | 3D | DM |
| Seo et al., 2014# | LV | CT | 1 | – | – | – | – | – | – | – | Y | 3D | IBM |
| Chnafa et al., 2014* | LV | CT | – | – | – | – | – | – | – | – | Y | 3D | DM |
| Corsini et al., 2014 | RV | MRI | – | – | – | – | 1 | – | – | – | N | 3D | DM |
| De Vecchi et al., 2014 | LV/RV | Echo | – | – | – | – | 1 | – | – | 1 | N | 3D | DM |
| Seo and Mittal, 2013# | LV | CT | 1 | – | – | – | – | – | – | – | N | 3D | IBM |
| Mangual et al., 2013 | LV | Echo | 20 | – | 8 | – | – | – | – | – | N | 3D | IBM |
| Nguyen et al., 2013 | LV | MRI | 1 | – | – | – | – | – | – | – | N | 3D | DM |
| Le and Sotiropoulos, 2012 | LV | MRI | 1 | – | – | – | – | – | – | – | N | 3D | IBM |
| Mangual et al., 2012 | RV | Echo | 1 | – | – | – | – | – | – | – | N | 3D | IBM |
| Dahl and Vierendeels, 2012 | LV | Echo | 1 | – | – | – | – | – | – | – | Y | 2D | DM |
| Khalafvand et al., 2012 | LV | MRI | 3 | – | – | – | – | – | 3 | – | N | 2D | DM |
| Tay et al., 2011 | LV | MRI | 1 | – | – | – | – | – | – | – | N | 3D | IBM |
| Mihalef et al., 2011 | LV/RV | CT | – | – | – | – | – | – | – | 1 | Y | 3D | DM |
| Krittian et al., 2010 | LV | MRI | 1 | – | – | – | – | – | – | – | N | 3D | DM |
| Doenst et al., 2009 | LV | MRI | 1 | – | – | 1 | – | – | – | – | N | 3D | IBM |
| Schenkel et al., 2009 | LV | MRI | 1 | – | – | – | – | – | – | – | N | 3D | DM |
| Long et al., 2008 | LV | MRI | 6 | – | – | – | – | – | – | – | N | 3D | DM |
| Saber et al., 2003 | LV | MRI | 1 | – | – | – | – | – | – | – | N | 3D | DM |
| Saber et al., 2001 | LV | MRI | 1 | – | – | – | – | – | – | – | N | 3D | DM |

*PAH, Pulmonary Arterial Hypertension; DCM, Dilated Cardiomyopathy; SVR, Surgical Ventricular Restoration; SV, Single Ventricle; HCM, Hypertrophic Cardiomyopathy; MI, Myocardial Infarction; MS, Mitral Stenosis; DM, Dynamic Mesh; IBM, Immersed Boundary Method; \*, The type of heart disease was not specified in the manuscript; #, Only the initial shape is based on patient-specific data.*

cardiac cycles. *In-vivo* studies demonstrate direct and residual flow ($\geq 2$ cycles) constitute about 37 and 30%, respectively, of end-diastolic volume, respectively (Eriksson et al., 2011). Although it is believed that larger residual volume may promote thrombogenesis, clinical significance of the relative distribution of the four volumes of subgroups has not been elucidated. The considerable differences among numerical studies (Mangual et al., 2013; Seo and Mittal, 2013) could be due to uncertainties, differing assumptions and the methodologies adopted.

## Challenges and Opportunities in Use of Patient-Specific CFD Technologies for Diagnosing Heart Dysfunction

A promising application of numerical models is found in surgical and interventional planning for predicting procedural outcomes.

Corsini and coworkers compared two surgical options for a patient with single ventricle malformation (Corsini et al., 2014). A secondary application is to advance the understanding of the effects of myocardial disease and surgery on ventricular flow. Su and colleagues deduced that HCM retarded the formation of vortex ring during diastole because the narrowed LV chamber delayed flow separation and escalated energy dissipation (Su et al., 2014a). Although various effects of myocardial disease on ventricular flow have been investigated, sample sizes in these numerical studies were too small to provide meaningful insights.

Since the 1990s, numerical studies have been conducted to study heart function (Hunter et al., 2003; Sugiura et al., 2012) including intraventricular flows. The early studies were focused on ideal models due to limitations of imaging techniques, particularly for segmenting images from noisy data. More contemporary published patient-specific numerical studies are

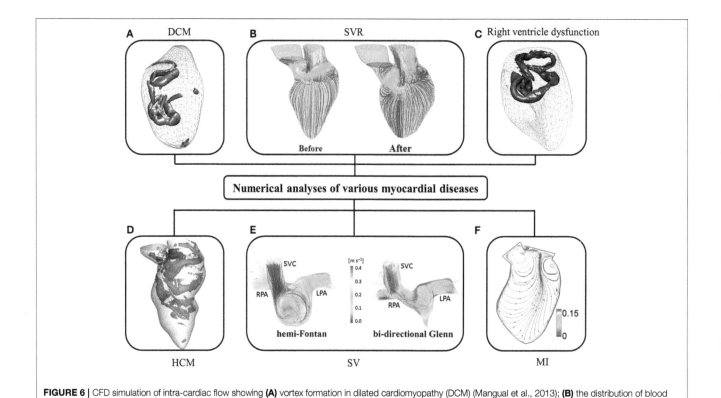

**FIGURE 6 |** CFD simulation of intra-cardiac flow showing **(A)** vortex formation in dilated cardiomyopathy (DCM) (Mangual et al., 2013); **(B)** the distribution of blood velocity before and after surgical ventricular restoration (SVR) (Khalafvand et al., 2014); **(C)** vortex formation in right ventricle (Mangual et al., 2012); **(D)** vortex formation in hypertrophic cardiomyopathy (HCM); **(E)** distribution of blood velocity in a single ventricle (SV) (SVC, superior vena cava; RPA, right pulmonary artery; LPA, left pulmonary artery); **(F)** the distribution of blood velocity in the LV with myocardial infarction (MI) (Khalafvand et al., 2012).

summarized in **Table 4**, in which the majority of studies focus on the LV rather than the RV (where the geometry is more complex than LV). As shown in **Table 4**, very few studies employed reconstructed 3D models from echocardiographic images (Mangual et al., 2013). Among imaging modalities, MRI is the most widely used owing to superior soft tissue contrast, and absence of ionizing radiation. In our experience, the accuracy of current commercial (e.g., 3D Doctor, Mimics, SliceOmatic, Amira) and open (e.g., ITK, ITK-SNAP, VTK, Analyze) segmentation software packages depends on the experience of the user who processes the MRI images. This is a hurdle to wider adoption of numerical studies. Most studies focus on normal subjects, with relatively few myocardial disease cases, for example, right ventricle (RV) dysfunction (Mangual et al., 2012), dilated cardiomyopathy (Mangual et al., 2013), hypertrophic cardiomyopathy (HCM) (Su et al., 2014a), single ventricle (Corsini et al., 2014), and myocardial infarction (Khalafvand et al., 2012) (**Figure 6**).

Although valve leaflet dynamics influence intraventricular flow development relative to vortex formation mechanisms and penetration depth, they are not taken into consideration in most studies as current spatiotemporal resolution of MRI and CT images are inadequate for assessing the rapid opening and closing of thin heart valves. Although the mitral valve was incorporated by Seo et al. (2014), the model was not a full patient-specific model. Only the initial geometry was based on patient-specific CT data, while the remaining geometries were simply dilated

according to an ideal model. In addition, the mitral valve motion was pre-defined rather than based on patient-specific data. Mihalef et al. (2011) studied a patient with severe mitral stenosis and regurgitation. The expected strong forward jet toward the apex during diastole and the reversal toward the atrium during systole balanced out, preempting a mismatch between the leaflet dynamics and LV volumetric changes in this selected case.

One feasible solution to model valvular motion is the FSI (Khalafvand et al., 2011; Domenichini and Pedrizzetti, 2014; Doost et al., 2016), which to date has been applied only in 2D studies (**Table 4**). Basically, there are two methods for modeling myocardium deformation during a cardiac cycle: dynamic mesh and immersed boundary method. Volumetric mesh deforms to cope with the motion of the boundary (e.g., the ventricle) in the dynamic mesh method; while in the immersed boundary method, modeling is accomplished using stationary grids and adding force near the boundary in the Navier-Stokes equations to take ventricular wall effects into account. Although the immersed boundary method avoids the issues of potential meshing failure during mesh generation and deformation, additional functions must be added to obtain the solution, which results in extra computational cost.

## CONCLUSIONS

Regulatory authorities such as US Food and Drug Administration have recognized the value of computer modeling and simulation in the regulatory approval process (Malinauskas et al., 2017). Authorities encourage use of the simulation to complement bench, animal and human testing. There are an increasing number of FDA applications that include simulations. The Heart Flow's $FFR_{CT}$ software has been approved by the US FDA for measuring coronary blockages non-invasively. Because most healthcare practitioners and organizations are unfamiliar to the technical, computational and simulation methodologies of patient-specific CFD, and the methodology is not yet fully developed, there is an understandable hesitancy to embrace the approach. This is in addition to the presently unrealized ability of researchers and practitioners advocates to effectively communicate the potential benefits of patient-specific CFD. One possible reason for the lack of interest by clinicians could be the lack of a validation protocol in general. A general validation protocol would stipulate procedures and methods for measuring a specified clinical quantity using a standard technique and comparing it to a CFD computation.

However, the virtual absence of specific clinical quantities with recognized links to the vast majority of pathologies—with the exception of FFR for PCI—upon which decisions could be predicted, creates a particularly challenging obstacle in the validation of patient-specific models. In addition, development of patient-specific models is a time-consuming task that requires patient-specific geometries, material properties, and realistic boundary conditions. These represent formidable challenges, but at the same time significant opportunities to interject precision medicine into clinical practice for improved clinical outcomes.

## AUTHOR CONTRIBUTIONS

LZ, J-MZ and BS: conception or design of the work; LZ, J-MZ, BS, RT, JA, and GK: draft the work or revise it critically for important intellectual content. All authors have seen and approved the final version of manuscript.

## REFERENCES

Alkadhi, H., Stolzmann, P., Scheffel, H., Desbiolles, L., Baumüller, S., Plass, A., et al. (2008). Radiation dose of cardiac dual-source CT: the effect of tailoring the protocol to patient-specific parameters. *Eur. J. Radiol.* 68, 385–391. doi: 10.1016/j.ejrad.2008.08.015

Antoniadis, A., Mortier, P., Kassab, G., Dubini, G., Foin, N., Murasato, Y., et al. (2015). Biomechanical modeling to improve coronary artery bifurcation stenting: expert review document on techniques and clinical implementation. *JACC Cardiovasc. Interv.* 8, 1281–1296. doi: 10.1016/j.jcin.2015.06.015

Aueron, F. M., and Gruentzig, A. R. (1984). Percutaneous transluminal coronary angioplasty: indication and current status. *Prim Cardiol.* 10, 97–107.

Bavo, A. M., Pouch, A. M., Degroote, J., Vierendeels, J., Gorman, J. H., Gorman, R. C., et al. (2016). Patient-specific CFD models for intraventricular flow analysis from 3D ultrasound imaing: comparison of three clinical cases. *J. Biomech.* 50, 144–150. doi: 10.1016/j.jbiomech.2016.11.039

Bayer, J. D., Blake, R. C., Plank, G., and Trayanova, N. (2012). A novel rule-based algorithm for assigning myocardial fiber orientation to computational heart models. *Ann. Biomed. Eng.* 40, 2243–2254. doi: 10.1007/s10439-012-0593-5

Bekkers, E. J., and Taylor, C. A. (2008). Multiscale vascular surface model generation from medical imaging data using hierarchical features. *IEEE Trans. Med. Imaging* 27, 331–341. doi: 10.1109/TMI.2007.905081

Belinha, J. (2016). Meshless methods: the future of computational biomechanical simulation. *J. Biom. Biostat.* 7:325. doi: 10.4172/2155-6180.1000325

Bourdin, X. X., Torsseille, X., Petit, P., and Beillas, P. (2007). "Comparison of tetrahedral and hexahedral meshes for organ finite element modeling: an application kidney impact," in *20th International Technical Conference on the Enhanced Safety of Vehicles* (Lyon: NHTSA).

Burkhoff, D., Mirsky, I., and Suga, H. (2005). Assessment of systolic and diastolic ventricular properties via pressure-volume analysis: a guide for clinical, translational, and basic researchers. *Am. J. Physiol. Heart Circ. Physiol.* 289, H501–H512. doi: 10.1152/ajpheart.00138.2005

Caro, C. G., Fitz-Geraldm, J. M., and Schroter, R. C. (1969). Arterial wall shear and distribution of early atheroma in man. *Nature* 223, 1159–1160. doi: 10.1038/2231159a0

Chnafa, C., Mendez, S., and Nicoud, F. (2014). Image-based large-eddy simulation in a realistic left heart. *Comput. Fluids* 94, 173–187. doi: 10.1016/j.compfluid.2014.01.030

Doost, S. N., Ghista, D., Su, B., Zhong, L., and Morsi, Y. S. (2016). Heart blood flow simulation: a perspective review. *BioMed. Engin. Online* 15:101. doi: 10.1186/s12938-016-0224-8

Doost, S. N., Zhong, L., Su, B., and Morsi, Y. S. (2017). Two-dimensional intraventricular flow pattern visualization using the image-based computational fluid dynamics. *Comput. Methods Biomechanics Biomed. Engin.* 20, 492–507. doi: 10.1080/10255842.2016.12 50891

Chnafa, C., Mendez, S., and Nicoud, F. (2016). Image-based simulations show important flow fluctuations in a normal left ventricle: what could be the implications? *Ann. Biomed. Eng.* 44, 3346–3358. doi: 10.1007/s10439-016-1614-6

Cho, Y. I., and Kensey, K. R. (1991). Effects of the non-Newtonian viscosity of blood on flows in a diseased arterial vessel. Part 1: steady flows. *Biorheology* 28, 241–262. doi: 10.3233/BIR-1991-283-415

Coenen, A., Lubbers, M., Kurata, A., Kono, A., Dedic, A., Chelu, R. G., et al. (2015). Fractional flow reserve computed from noninvasive CT angiography data: diagnostic performance of an on-site clinician-operated computational fluid dynamics algorithm. *Radiology* 274, 674–683. doi: 10.1148/radiol.141 40992

Corsini, C., Baker, C., Kung, E., Schievano, S., Arbia, G., Baretta, A., et al. (2014). An integrated approach to patient-specific predictive modeling for single ventricle heart palliation. *Comput. Methods Biomech. Biomed. Engin.* 17, 1572–1589. doi: 10.1080/10255842.2012.758254

Crozier, A., Augustin, C. M., Neic, A., Prassl, A. J., Holler, M., Fastl, T. E., et al. (2016). Image-based personalization of cardiac anatomy for coupled electromechanical modeling. *Ann. Biomed. Eng.* 44, 58–70. doi: 10.1007/s10439-015-1474-5

Dahl, S., and Vierendeels, J. (2012). FSI simulation of asymmetric mitral valve dynamics during diastolic filling. *Comput. Methods Biomech. Biomed. Engin.* 15, 121–130. doi: 10.1080/10255842.2010.517200

De Vecchi, C., Caudron, J., Dubourg, B., Pirot, N., Lefebvre, V., Bauer, F., et al. (2014). Effect of the ellipsoid shape of the left ventricular outflow tract on the echocardiographic assessment of aortic valve area in aortic stenosis. *J. Cardiovasc. Comput. Tomogr.* 8, 52–57. doi: 10.1016/j.jcct.2013.12.006

Doblare, M., Cueto, E., Calvo, B., Martinez, M. A., Garcia, J. M., and Cegonino, J. (2005). On the employ of meshless methods in biomechanics. *Comput. Methods Appl. Mech.* 194, 801–821. doi: 10.1016/j.cma.2004. 06.031

Doenst, T., Spiegel, K., Reik, M., Markl, M., Hennig, J., Nitzsche, S., et al. (2009). Fluid-dynamic modeling of the human left ventricle: methodology and application to surgical ventricular reconstruction. *Ann. Thorac. Surg.* 87, 1187–1195. doi: 10.1016/j.athoracsur.2009.01.036

Domenichini, F., and Pedrizzetti, G. (2014). Asymptotic model of fluid–tissue interaction for mitral valve dynamics. *Cardiovasc. Engin. Technol.* 6, 95–104. doi: 10.1007/s13239-014-0201-y

Iskander, S., and Iskandrian, A. E. (1998). Risk assessment using single-photon emission computed tomographic technetium-99m sestamibi imaging. *J. Am. Coll. Cardiol.* 32, 57–62. doi: 10.1016/S0735-1097(98)00177-6

Itu, L., Rapaka, S., Passerini, T., Georgescu, B., Schwemmer, C., Schoebinger, M., et al. (2016). A machine-learning approach for computation of fractional flow reserve from coronary computed tomography. *J. Appl. Physiol.* 121, 42–52. doi: 10.1152/japplphysiol.00752.2015

Douglas, P. S., Pontone, G., Hlatky, M. A., Patel, M. R., Norgaard, B. L., Byrne, R. A., et al. (2015). Clinical outcomes of fractional flow reserve by computed tomographic angiography-guided diagnostic strategies vs. usual care in patients with suspected coronary artery disease: the prospective longitudinal trial of FFRct: outcome and resource impacts stud. *Eur. Heart J.* 36, 3359–3367. doi: 10.1093/eurheartj/ehv444

Eriksson, J., Dyverfeldt, P., Engvall, J., Bolger, A. F., Ebbers, T., and Carlhäll, C. J. (2011). Quantification of presystolic blood flow organization and energetics in the human left ventricle. *Am. J. Physiol. Heart Circ. Physiol.* 300, H2135–H2141. doi: 10.1152/ajpheart.00993.2010

Eshtehardi, P., McDaniel, M. C., Suo, J., Dhawan, S. S., Timmins, L. H., Binongo, J. N. G., et al. (2012). Association of coronary wall shear stress with atherosclerotic plaque burden, composition, and distribution in patients with coronary artery disease. *J. Am. Heart Assoc.* 1:e002543. doi: 10.1161/JAHA.112.002543

Figueroa, C. A., Baek, S., Taylor, C. A., and Humphrey, J. D. (2009). A computational framework for fluid-solid-growth modeling in cardiovascular simulations. *Comput. Methods Appl. Mech. Eng.* 198, 3583–3602. doi: 10.1016/j.cma.2008.09.013

Figueroa, C. A., Vignon-clementel, I. E., Jansen, K. E., Hughes, T. J. R., and Taylor, C. A. (2006). A coupled momentum method for modeling blood flow in three-dimensional deformable arteries. *Comput. Methods Appl. Mech. Engin.* 195, 5685–5706. doi: 10.1016/j.cma.2005.11.011

Fry, D. L. (1968). Acute vascular endothelial changes associated with increased blood velocity gradients. *Circ. Res.* 22, 165–197. doi: 10.1161/01.RES.22.2.165

Galassi, F., Alkhalil, M., Lee, R., Martindale, P., Kharbanda, R. K., Channon, K. M., et al. (2018). 3D reconstruction of coronary arteries from 2D angiographic projections using nonuniform rational basis splines (NURBS) for accurate modelling of coronary stenoses. *PLoS ONE* 13:e0190650. doi: 10.1371/journal.pone.0190650

Gaur, S., Achenbach, S., Leipsic, J., Mauri, L., Bezerra, H. G., Jensen, J. M., et al. (2013). Rationale and design of the HeartFlowNXT (HeartFlow analysis of coronary blood flow using CT angiography: NeXt sTeps) study. *J. Cardiovasc. Comput. Tomogr.* 7, 279–288. doi: 10.1016/j.jcct.2013.09.003

Gijsen, F. J., Wentzel, J. J., Thury, A., Mastik, F., Schaar, J. A., Schuurbiers, J. C. H., et al. (2008). Strain distribution over plaques in human coronary arteries relates to shear stress. *Am. J. Physiol. Heart Circ. Physiol.* 295, H1608–H1614. doi: 10.1152/ajpheart.01081.2007

Glagov, S., Zarins, C. K., Giddens, D. P., and Ku, D. N. (1989). "Mechanical factors in the pathogenesis, localization and evolution of atherosclerotic plaques," in *Diseases of the Arterial Wall*, eds B. Camilleri and B. Fiessinger (Berlin: Springer-Verlag), 217–239.

Golob, M., Moss, R. L., and Chesler, N. C. (2014). Cardiac tissue structure, properties, and performance: a materials science perspective. *Ann. Biomed. Eng.* 42, 2003–2013. doi: 10.1007/s10439-014-1071-z

Hecht, F., and Pironneau, O. (2017). An energy stable monolithic Eulerian fluid-structure finite element method. *Int. J. Numer. Methods Fluids* 85, 430–446. doi: 10.1002/fld.4388

Himburg, H. A., Grzybowski, D. M., Hazel, A. L., LaMack, J. A., and Friedman, M. H. (2004). Spatial comparison between wall shear stress measures and porcine arterial endothelial permeability. *Am. J. Physiol. Heart. Circ. Physiol.* 286, 1916–1922. doi: 10.1152/ajpheart.00897.2003

Hunter, P. J., Pullan, A. J., and Smaill, B. H. (2003). Modeling total heart function. *Annu. Rev. Biomed. Eng.* 5, 147–177. doi: 10.1146/annurev.bioeng.5.040202.121537

Imanparast, A., Fatouraee, N., and Sharif, F. (2016). The impact of valve simplifications on left ventricular hemodynamics in a three dimensional simulation based on *in vivo* MRI data. *J. Biomech.* 49, 1482–1489. doi: 10.1016/j.jbiomech.2016.03.021

Johnson, N. P., Kirkeeide, R. L. L., and Gould, K. L. L. (2012). Is discordance of coronary flow reserve and fractional flow reserve due to methodology or clinically relevant coronary pathophysiology? *JACC Cardiovasc. Imaging* 5, 193–202. doi: 10.1016/j.jcmg.2011.09.020

Langille, B. L., and O'Donnell, F. (1986). Reductions in arterial diameter produced by chronic decreases in blood flow are endothelium-dependent. *Science* 23, 405–407.

Le, T., and Sotiropoulos, F. (2012). On the three-dimensional vortical structure of early distolic flow in a patient-specific left ventricle. *Eur. J. Mech. B Fluids* 35, 20–24. doi: 10.1016/j.euromechflu.2012.01.013

Jung, J., Lyczkowski, R. W., Panchal, C. B., and Hassanein, A. (2006). Multiphase hemodynamic simulation of pulsatile flow in a coronary artery. *J. Biomech.* 39, 2064–2073. doi: 10.1016/j.jbiomech.2005.06.023

Kantor, B., Kuzo, R. S., and Gerber, T. C. (2007). Coronary computed tomographic angiography: current and future uses. *Heart Metab.* 34, 5–9.

Kassab, G. S., and Navia, J. A. (2006). Biomechanical considerations in the design of graft: the homeostasis hypothesis. *Annu. Rev. Biomed. Eng.* 8, 499–535. doi: 10.1146/annurev.bioeng.8.010506.105023

Kawaji, T., Shiomi, H., Morishita, H., Morimoto, T., Taylor, C. A., Kanao, S., et al. (2017). Feasibility and diagnostic performance of fractional flow reserve measurement derived from coronary computed tomography angiography in real clinical practice. *Int. J. Cardiovasc. Imaging* 33, 271–281. doi: 10.1007/s10554-016-0995-9

Khalafvand, S. S., Ng, E. Y. K., and Zhong, L. (2011). CFD simulation of flow through heart: a perspective review. *Comput. Methods Biomech. Biomed. Engin.* 14, 113–132. doi: 10.1080/10255842.2010.493515

Khalafvand, S. S., Ng, E. Y. K., Zhong, L., and Hung, T. K. (2012). Fluid-dynamics modelling of the human left ventricle with dynamic mesh for normal and myocardial infarction: preliminary study. *Comput. Biol. Med.* 42, 863–870. doi: 10.1016/j.compbiomed.2012.06.010

Khalafvand, S. S., Zhong, L., and Ng, E. Y. K. (2014). Three-dimensional CFD/MRI modeling reveals that ventricular surgical restoration improves ventricular function by modifying intraventricular blood flow. *Int. J. Numer. Method. Biomed. Eng.* 30, 1044–1056. doi: 10.1002/cnm.2643

Kim, H. J., Vignon-Clementel, I. E., Coogan, J. S., Figueroa, C. A., Jansen, K. E., and Taylor, C. A. (2010). Patient-specific modeling of blood flow and pressure in human coronary arteries. *Ann. Biomed. Eng.* 38, 3195–3209. doi: 10.1007/s10439-010-0083-6

Kimura, T., Shiomi, H., Kuribayashi, S., Isshiki, T., Kanazawa, S., Ito, H., et al. (2015). Cost analysis of non-invasive fractional flow reserve derived from coronary computed tomographic angiography in Japan. *Cardiovasc. Interv. Ther.* 30, 38–44. doi: 10.1007/s12928-014-0285-1

Kleinstreuer, C., Hyun, S., Buchanan, J. R., Longest, P. W., Archie, J. P., and Truskey, G. A. (2001). Hemodynamic parameters and early intimal thickening in branching blood vessels. *Crit. Rev. Biomed. Eng.* 29, 1–64. doi: 10.1615/CritRevBiomedEng.v29.i1.10

Knight, J., Olgac, U., Saur, S. C., Poulikakos, D., Marshall, W. Jr., Cattin, P. C., et al. (2010). Choosing the optimal wall shear parameter for the prediction of plaque location-A patient-specific computational study in human right coronary arteries. *Atherosclerosis* 211, 445–450. doi: 10.1016/j.atherosclerosis.2010.03.001

Ko, B. S., Cameron, J. D., Munnur, R. K., Wong, D. T. L., Fujisawa, Y., Sakaguchi, T., et al. (2017). Noninvasive CT-derived FFR based on structural and fluid analysis: a comparison with invasive FFR for detection of functionally significant stenosis. *JACC Cardiovasc. Imaging* 10, 663–673. doi: 10.1016/j.jcmg.2016.07.005

Koo, B. K., Erglis, A., Doh, J.-H., Daniels, D. V., Jegere, S., Kim, H. S., et al. (2011). Diagnosis of ischemia-causing coronary stenoses by noninvasive fractional flow reserve computed from coronary computed tomographic angiograms. Results from the prospective multicenter DISCOVER-FLOW (Diagnosis of Ischemia-Causing Stenoses Obtained via Noninvasive Fractional Flow Reserve) study. *J. Am. Coll. Cardiol.* 58, 1989–1997. doi: 10.1016/j.jacc.2011.06.066

Krittian, S., Janoske, U., Oertel, H., and Böhlke, T. (2010). Partitioned fluid-solid coupling for cardiovascular blood flow: left-ventricular fluid mechanics. *Ann. Biomed. Eng.* 38, 1426–1441. doi: 10.1007/s10439-009-9895-7

Ku, D. N., Giddens, D. P., Zarins, C. K., and Glagov, S. (1985). Pulsatile flow and atherosclerosis in the human carotid bifurcation. Positive correlation between plaque location and low oscillating shear stress. *Arteriosclerosis* 5, 293–302. doi: 10.1161/01.ATV.5.3.293

Nishimura, R. A., and Tajik, A. J. (1997). Evaluation of diastolic filling of left ventricle in health and disease: doppler echocardiography is the clinician's Rosetta Stone. *J. Am. Coll. Cardiol.* 30, 8–18.

Nørgaard, B., Leipsic, J., Gaur, S., Seneviratne, S., Ko, B. S., Ito, H., et al. (2014). Diagnostic performance of non-invasive fractional flow reserve derived from coronary CT angiography in suspected coronary artery disease: the NXT trial. *J. Am. Coll. Cardiol.* 63, 1145–1155. doi: 10.1016/j.jacc.2013.11.043

Leng, S., Jiang, M., Zhao, X. D., Allen, J. C., Kassab, G. S., Ouyang, R. Z., et al. (2016). Three-dimensional tricuspid annular motion analysis from cardiac magnetic resonance feature-tracking. *Ann. Biomed. Eng.* 44, 3522–3538. doi: 10.1007/s10439-016-1695-2

Lewis, M. A., Pascoal, A., Keevil, S. F., and Lewis, C. A. (2016). Selecting a CT scanner for cardiac imaging: the heart of the matter. *Br. J. Radiol.* 89, 569–590. doi: 10.1259/bjr.20160376

Liu, B., Zheng, J., Bach, R., and Tang, D. (2012). Correlations of coronary plaque wall thickness with wall pressure and wall pressure gradient: a representative case study. *Biomed. Eng. Online* 11:43. doi: 10.1186/1475-925X-11-43

Long, Q., Merrifield, R., Xu, X. Y., Kilner, P., Firmin, D. N., and G-Z, Y. (2008). Subject-specific computational simulation of left ventricular flow based on magnetic resonance imaging. *Proc. Inst. Mech. Eng. H.* 222, 475–485. doi: 10.1243/09544119JEIM310

Lu, M. T., Ferencik, M., Roberts, R. S., Lee, K. L., Ivanov, A., Adami, E., et al. (2017). Noninvasive FFR derived from coronary CT angiography: management and outcomes in the PROMISE trial. *JACC Cardiovasc. Imaging* 10, 1350–1358. doi: 10.1016/j.jcmg.2016.11.024

Malinauskas, R. A., Hariharan, P., Day, S. W., Herbertson, L. H., Buesen, M., Steinseifer, U., et al. (2017). FDA benchmark medical device flow models for CFD validation. *ASAIO J.* 63, 150–160. doi: 10.1097/MAT.0000000000000499

Malvè, M., García, A., Ohayon, J., and Martínez, M. A. (2012). Unsteady blood flow and mass transfer of a human left coronary artery bifurcation: FSI vs. CFD. *Int. Commun. Heat Mass Transf.* 39, 745–751. doi: 10.1016/j.icheatmasstransfer.2012.04.009

Mangual, J. O., Domenichini, F., and Pedrizzetti, G. (2012). Three dimensional numerical assessment of the right ventricular flow using 4D echocardiography boundary data. *Eur. J. Mech. B Fluids* 35, 25–30. doi: 10.1016/j.euromechflu.2012.01.022

Mangual, J. O., Kraigher-Krainer, E., De Luca, A., Toncelli, L., Shah, A., Solomon, S., et al. (2013). Comparative numerical study on left ventricular fluid dynamics after dilated cardiomyopathy. *J. Biomech.* 46, 1611–1617. doi: 10.1016/j.jbiomech.2013.04.012

Mihalef, V., Ionasec, R. I., Sharma, P., Georgescu, B., Voigt, I., Suehling, M., et al. (2011). Patient-specific modelling of whole heart anatomy, dynamics and haemodynamics from four-dimensional cardiac CT images. *Interface Focus.* 1, 286–296. doi: 10.1098/rsfs.2010.0036

Min, J. K., Leipsic, J., Pencina, M. J., Berman, D. S., Koo, B. K., van Mieghem, C., et al. (2012). Diagnostic accuracy of fractional flow reserve from anatomic CT angiography. *JAMA.* 308, 1237–1245. doi: 10.1001/2012.jama.11274

Mittal, R., Seo, J. H., Vedula, V., Choi, Y. J., Liu, H., Huang, H. H., et al. (2016). Computational modeling of cardiac hemodynamics: current status and future outlook. *J. Comput. Phys.* 305, 1065–1082. doi: 10.1016/j.jcp.2015.11.022

Moosavi, M. H., Fatouraee, N., Katoozian, H., Pashaei, A., Camara, O., and Frangi, A. E. (2014). Numerical simulation of blood flow in the left ventricle and aortic sinus using magnetic resonance imaging and computational fluid dyanmics. *Comput. Methods Biomech. Biomed. Engin.* 17, 740–749. doi: 10.1080/10255842.2012.715638

Morris, P. D., Narracott, A., von Tengg-Kobligk, H., Soto, D. A. S., Hsiao, S., Lungu, A., et al. (2015). Computational fluid dynamics modelling in cardiovascular medicine. *Heart* 102, 18–28. doi: 10.1136/heartjnl-2015-308044

Morris, P. D., Ryan, D., Morton, A. C., Lycett, R., Lawford, P. V., Hose, D. R., et al. (2013). Virtual fractional flow reserve from coronary angiography: modeling the significance of coronary lesions. Results from the VIRTU-1 (VIRTUal fractional flow reserve from coronary angiography) study. *JACC Cardiovasc. Interv.* 6, 149–157. doi: 10.1016/j.jcin.2012.08.024

Nguyen, V. T., Loon, C. J., Nguyen, H. H., Liang, Z., and Leo, H. L. (2013). A semi-automated method for patient-specific computational flow modelling of left ventricles. *Comput. Methods Biomech. Biomed. Engin.* 18, 401–413. doi: 10.1080/10255842.2013.803534

Sankaran, S., Moghadam, M. E., Kahn, A. M., Tseng, E. E., Guccione, J. M., and Marsden, A. L. (2012). Patient-specific multiscale modeling of blood flow for coronary artery bypass graft surgery. *Ann. Biomed. Eng.* 40, 2228–2242. doi: 10.1007/s10439-012-0579-3

Schenkel, T., Malve, M., Reik, M., Markl, M., Jung, B., and Oertel, H. (2009). MRI-based CFD analysis of flow in a human left ventricle: methodology and application to a healthy heart. *Ann. Biomed. Eng.* 37, 503–515. doi: 10.1007/s10439-008-9627-4

Papafaklis, M. I., Bourantas, C. V., Theodorakis, P. E., Katsouras, C. S., Fotiadis, D. I., and Michalis, L. K. (2007). Association of endothelial shear stress with plaque thickness in a real three-dimensional left main coronary artery bifurcation model. *Int. J. Cardiol.* 115, 276–278. doi: 10.1016/j.ijcard.2006.04.030

Pedrizzetti, G., and Domenichini, F. (2014). Left ventricular fluid mechanics: the long way from theoretical models to clinical applications. *Ann. Biomed. Eng.* 43, 26–40. doi: 10.1007/s10439-014-1101-x

Peskin, C. S. (2003). The immersed boundary method. *Acta. Numer.* 11, 479–517. doi: 10.1017/S0962492902000077

Pironet, A., Desaive, T., Kosta, S., Lucas, A., Paeme, S., Collet, A., et al. (2013). A multi-scale cardiovascular system model can account for the load-dependence of the end-systolic pressure-volume relationship. *Biomed. Eng. Online* 12:8. doi: 10.1186/1475-925X-12-8

Poon, E. K. W., Hayat, U., Thondapu, V., Ooi, A. S. H., Haq, M. A. U., Moore, S., et al. (2015). Advances in three-dimensional coronary imaging and computational fluid dynamics: Is virtual fractional flow reserve more than just a pretty picture? *Coron. Artery Dis.* 26, e43–e54. doi: 10.1097/MCA.0000000000000219

Poon, E. K. W., Thondapu, B., Revalor, E., Ooi, A., and Barlis, P. (2017). Coronary optical coherence tomography-derived virtual fractional flow reserve (FFR): anatomy and physiology all-in-one. *Eur. Heart J.* 38, 3604–3605. doi: 10.1093/eurheartj/ehx594

Prosi, M., Perktold, K., Ding, Z., and Friedman, M. H. (2004). Influence of curvature dynamics on pulsatile coronary artery flow in a realistic bifurcation model. *J. Biomech.* 37, 1767–1775. doi: 10.1016/j.jbiomech.2004.01.021

Qiu, Y., and Tarbell, J. M. (1996). Computational simulation of flow in the end-to-end anastomosis of a rigid graft and a compliant artery. *ASAIO J.* 42, M702–M709. doi: 10.1097/00002480-199609000-00078

Quarteroni, A., Lassila, T., Rossi, S., and Ruiz-Baier, R. (2017). Integrated heart—coupling multiscale and multiphysics models for the simulation of the cardiac function. *Comput. Methods Appl. Mech. Eng.* 314, 345–407. doi: 10.1016/j.cma.2016.05.031

Rausch, M. K., Famaey, N., Shultz, T. O. B., Bothe, W., Miller, D. C., and Kuhl, E. (2013). Mechanics of the mitral valve: a critical review, an *in vivo* parameter identification, and the effect of prestrain. *Biomech. Model. Mechanobiol.* 12, 1053–1071. doi: 10.1007/s10237-012-0462-z

Rutsch, F., Nitschke, Y., and Terkeltaub, R. (2011). Genetics in arterial calcification: pieces of a puzzle and cogs in a wheel. *Circ. Res.* 109, 578–592. doi: 10.1161/CIRCRESAHA.111.247965

Saber, N. R., Gosman, A. D., Wood, N. B., Kilner, P. J., Charrier, C. L., and Firmin, D. N. (2001). Computational flow modeling of the left ventricle based on *in vivo* MRI data: initial experience. *Ann. Biomed. Eng.* 29, 275–283. doi: 10.1114/1.1359452

Saber, N. R., Wood, N. B., Gosman, A. D., Merrifield, R. D., Yang, G. Z., Charrier, C. L., et al. (2003). Progress towards patient-specific computational flow modeling of the left heart via combination of magnetic resonance imaging with computational fluid dynamics. *Ann. Biomed. Eng.* 31, 42–52. doi: 10.1114/1.1533073

Saeed, M., Van, T. A., Krug, R., Hetts, S. W., and Wilson, M. W. (2015). Cardiac MR imaging: current status and future direction. *Cardiovasc. Diagn. Ther.* 5, 290–310. doi: 10.3978/j.issn.2223-3652.2015.06.07

Sankaran, S., and Marsden, A. L. (2011). A stochastic collocation method for uncertainty quantification and propagation in cardiovascular simulations. *J. Biomech. Eng.* 133:031001. doi: 10.1115/1.4003259

Sankaran, S., Grady, L., and Taylor, C. A. (2015). Impact of geometric uncertainty on hemodynamic simulations using machine learning. *Comput. Methods Appl. Mech. Eng.* 297, 167–190. doi: 10.1016/j.cma.2015.08.014

Sankaran, S., Kim, H. J., Choi, G., and Taylor, C. A. (2016). Uncertainty quantification in coronary blood flow simulations: impact of geometry, boundary conditions and blood viscosity. *J. Biomech.* 49, 2540–2547. doi: 10.1016/j.jbiomech.2016.01.002

Toussaint, N., Stoeck, C. T., Schaeffter, T., Kozerke, S., Sermesant, M., and Batchelor, P. G. (2013). *In vivo* human cardiac fibre architecture estimation using shape-based diffusion tensor processing. *Med. Image Anal.* 17, 1243–1255. doi: 10.1016/j.media.2013.02.008

Tu, S., Barbato, E., Köszegi, Z., Yang, J., Sun, Z., Holm, N. R., et al. (2014). Fractional flow reserve calculation from 3-dimensional quantitative coronary angiography and TIMI frame count: a fast computer model to quantify the functional significance of moderately obstructed coronary arteries. *JACC Cardiovasc. Interv.* 7, 768–777. doi: 10.1016/j.jcin.2014.03.004

Schmidt, J. P., Delp, S. L., Sherman, M. A., Taylor, C. A., Pande, V. S., and Altman, R. B. (2008). The simbios national center: systems biology in motion. *Proc. IEEE.* 96, 1266–1280. doi: 10.1109/JPROC.2008.925454

Seo, J. H., and Mittal, R. (2013). Effect of diastolic flow patterns on the function of the left ventricle. *Phys. Fluids* 25:110801. doi: 10.1063/1.4819067

Seo, J. H., Vedula, V., Abraham, T., Lardo, A. C., Dawoud, F., Luo, H., et al. (2014). Effect of the mitral valve on diastolic flow patterns. *Phys. Fluids* 26:121901. doi: 10.1063/1.4904094

Spiegel, M., Redel, T., Zhang, Y. J., Struffert, T., Hornegger, J., Grossman, R. G., et al. (2011). Tetrahedral vs. polyhedral mesh size evaluation on flow velocity and wall shear stress for cerebral hemodynamic simulation. *Comput. Methods Biomech. Biomed. Engin.* 14, 9–22. doi: 10.1080/10255842.2010.518565

Spilker, R. L., Feinstein, J. A., Parker, D. W., Reddy, V. M., and Taylor, C. A. (2007). Morphometry-based impedance boundary conditions for patient-specific modeling of blood flow in pulmonary arteries. *Ann. Biomed. Eng.* 35, 546–559. doi: 10.1007/s10439-006-9240-3

Stone, P. H., Coskun, A. U., Kinlay, S., Clark, M. E., Sonka, M., Wahle, A., et al. (2003). Effect of endothelial shear stress on the progression of coronary artery disease, vascular remodeling, and in-stent restenosis in humans: *in vivo* 6-month follow-up study. *Circulation* 108, 438–444. doi: 10.1161/01.CIR.0000080882.35274.AD

Stone, P. H., Saito, S., Takahashi, S., Makita, Y., Nakamura, S., Kawasaki, T., et al. (2012). Prediction of progression of coronary artery disease and clinical outcomes using vascular profiling of endothelial shear stress and arterial plaque characteristics: the PREDICTION study. *Circulation* 126, 172–181. doi: 10.1161/CIRCULATIONAHA.112.096438

Su, B., Kabinejadian, F., Phang, H. Q., Kumar, G. P., Cui, F., Kim, S., et al. (2015). Numerical modeling of intraventricular flow during diastole after implantation of BMHV. *PLoS ONE* 10:e0126315. doi: 10.1371/journal.pone.0126315

Su, B., Tan, R. S., Tan, J. L., Guo, K. W. Q., Zhang, J. M., Leng, S., et al. (2016). Cardiac MRI based numerical modeling of left ventricular fluid dynamics with mitral valve incorporated. *J. Biomech.* 49, 1199–1205. doi: 10.1016/j.jbiomech.2016.03.008

Su, B., Zhang, J. M., Tang, H. C., Wan, M. Lim, C. C. W., Su, Y., et al. (2014a). "Patient-specific blood flows and vortex formations in patients with hypertrophic cardiomyopathy using computational fluid dynamics," in *Biomedical Engineering and Sciences (IECBES), Conference on IEEE*, (Sarawak) 276–280.

Su, B., Zhong, L., Wang, X. K., Zhang, J. M., Tan, R. S., Allen, J. C., et al. (2014b). Numerical simulation of patient-specific left ventricular model with both mitral and aortic valves by FSI approach. *Comput. Methods Programs Biomed.* 113, 474–482. doi: 10.1016/j.cmpb.2013.11.009

Sugiura, S., Washio, T., Hatano, A., Okada, J., Watanabe, H., and Hisada, T. (2012). Multi-scale simulations of cardiac electrophysiology and mechanics using the University of Tokyo heart simulator. *Prog. Biophys. Mol. Biol.* 110, 380–389. doi: 10.1016/j.pbiomolbio.2012.07.001

Svalbring, E., Fredriksson, A., Eriksson, J., Dyverfeldt, P., Ebbers, T., Bolger, A. F., et al. (2016). Altered diastolic flow patterns and kinetic energy in subtle left ventricular remodeling and dysfunction detected by 4D flow MRI. *PLoS ONE* 11:e0161391. doi: 10.1371/journal.pone.0161391.

Tay, W. B., Tseng, Y. H., Lin, L. Y., and Tseng, W. Y. (2011). Towards patient-specific cardiovascular modeling system using the immersed boundary technique. *Biomed. Eng. Online* 10:52. doi: 10.1186/1475-925X-10-52

Torii, R., Keegan, J., Wood, N. B., Dowsey, A. W., Hughes, A. D., Yang, G. Z., et al. (2010). MR image-based geometric and hemodynamic investigation of the right coronary artery with dynamic vessel motion. *Ann. Biomed. Eng.* 38, 2606–2620. doi: 10.1007/s10439-010-0008-4

Torii, R., Wood, N. B., Hadjiloizou, N., Dowsey, A. W., Wright, A. R., Hughes, A. D., et al. (2009). Stress phase angle depicts differences in coronary artery hemodynamics due to changes in flow and geometry after percutaneous coronary intervention. *Am. J. Physiol. Heart Circ. Physiol.* 296, H765–H776. doi: 10.1152/ajpheart.01166.2007

Tu, S., Westra, J., Yang, J., von Birgelen, C., Ferrara, A., Pellicano, M., et al. (2016). Diagnostic accuracy of fast computational approaches to derive fractional flow reserve from diagnostic coronary angiography: the international multicenter FAVOR pilot study. *JACC Cardiovasc. Interv.* 9, 2024–2035. doi: 10.1016/j.jcin.2016.07.013

Vadakkumpadan, F., Arevalo, H., Ceritoglu, C., Miller, M., and Trayanova, N. (2012).Image-based estimation of ventricular fiber orientations for personalized modeling of cardiac electrophysiology. *IEEE Trans. Med. Imaging* 31, 1051–1060. doi: 10.1109/TMI.2012.2184799

Valentín, A., Humphrey, J. D., and Holzapfel, G. A. (2013). A finite element-based constrained mixture implementation for arterial growth, remodeling, and adaptation: theory and numerical verification. *Int. J. Numer. Method. Biomed. Eng.* 29, 822–849. doi: 10.1002/cnm.2555

Vedula, V., George, R., Younes, L., and Mittal, R. (2015). Hemodynamics in the left atrium and its effect on ventricular flow patterns. *J. Biomech. Eng.* 137:111003. doi: 10.1115/1.4031487

Westra, J., Tu, S., Winther, S., Nissen, L., Vestergaard, M.-B., Andersen, B. K., et al. (2018). Evaluation of coronary artery stenosis by quantitative flow ratio during invasive coronary angiography. *Circ. Cardiovasc. Imaging* 11:e007107. doi: 10.1161/CIRCIMAGING.117.007107

Wittek, A., Grosland, N. M., Joldes, G. R., Magnotta, V., and Miller, K. (2016). From finite element meshes to clouds of points: a review of methods for generation of computational biomechanics models for patient-specific applications. *Ann. Biomed. Eng.* 44, 3–15. doi: 10.1007/s10439-015-1469-2

Wittek, A., Joldes, G., Couton, M., Warfield, S. K., and Miller, K. (2010). Patient-specific non-linear finite element modelling for predicting soft organ deformation in real-time; application to non-rigid neuroimage registration. *Prog. Biophys. Mol. Biol.* 103, 292–303. doi: 10.1016/j.pbiomolbio.2010.09.001

Wong, K. K., Wang, D., Ko, J. K. L., Mazumdar, J., Le, T. T., and Ghista, D. (2017). Computational medical imaging and hemodynamics framework for functional analysis and assessment of cardiovascular structures. *Biomed. Eng. Online* 16:35. doi: 10.1186/s12938-017-0326-y

World Health Organization (2011). *Burden: Mortality, Morbidity and Risk Factors*. Global Status Report on Noncommunicable Diseases 2010, 9–31.

Xu, B., Tu, S., Qiao, S., Qu, X., Chen, Y., Yang, J., et al. (2017). Diagnostic accuracy of angiography-Based quantitative flow ratio measurements for online assessment of coronary stenosis. *J. Am. Coll. Cardiol.* 70, 3077–3087. doi: 10.1016/j.jacc.2017.10.035

Yamada, H., Oki, T., Tabata, T., Iuchi, A., and Ito, S. (1998). Assessment of left ventricular systolic wall motion velocity with pulsed tissue Doppler imaging: comparison with peak dP/dt of the left ventricular pressure curve. *J. Am. Soc. Echocardiogr.* 11, 442–449. doi: 10.1016/S0894-7317(98)70024-0

Zhang, J. M., Luo, T., Tan, S. Y., Lomarda, A. M., Wong, A. S., Keng, F. Y., et al. (2015). Hemodynamic analysis of patient-specific coronary artery tree. *Int. J. Numer. Methods Biomed. Eng.* 31:e02708. doi: 10.1002/cnm.2708

Zhang, J. M., Shuang, D., Baskaran, L., Wu, W., Teo, S. K., Huang, W., et al. (2018). Advanced analyses of computed tomography coronary angiography can help discriminate ischemic lesions. *Int. J. Cardiol.* doi: 10.1016/j.ijcard.2018.04.020 . [Epub ahead print].

Zhang, J. M., Zhong, L., Luo, T., Lomarda, A. M., Huo, Y., Yap, J., et al. (2016). Simplified models of non-invasive fractional flow reserve based on CT images. *PLoS ONE* 11:e0153070. doi: 10.1371/journal.pone.0153070

Zhang, J. M., Zhong, L., Su, B., Wan, M., Yap, J. S., Tham, J. P., et al. (2014). Perspective on CFD studies of coronary artery disease lesions and hemodynamics: a review. *Int. J. Numer. Methods Biomed. Eng.* 30, 659–680. doi: 10.1002/cnm.2625

Zhang, X., Zhang, P., and Zhang, L. (2012). A simple technique to improve computational efficiency of meshless methods. *Proc. Engin.* 31, 1102–1107. doi: 10.1016/j.proeng.2012.01.1149

Zhong, L., Gobeawan, L., Su, Y., Tan, J. L., Ghista, D., Chua, T., et al. (2012). Right ventricular regional wall curvedness and area strain in patients with repaired tetralogy of fallot. *Am. J. Physiol. Heart Circ. Physiol.* 302, H1306–H1316. doi: 10.1152/ajpheart.00679.2011

Zhong, L., Huang, F. Q., Tan, L. K., Allen, J. C., Ding, Z. P., Kassab, G., et al. (2014). Age and gender-specific changes in left ventricular systolic function in human volunteers. *Int. J. Cardiol.* 172, e102–e105. doi: 10.1016/j.ijcard.2013.12.128

Zhong, L., Su, Y., Yeo, S. Y., Tan, R. S., Ghista, D. N., and Kassab, G. (2009). Left ventricular regional wall curvedness and wall stress in patients with ischemic dilated cardiomyopathy. *Am. J. Physiol. Heart Circ. Physiol.* 296, H573–H584. doi: 10.1152/ajpheart.00525.2008

# 9

# Quantification of Biventricular Strains in Heart Failure with Preserved Ejection Fraction Patient Using Hyperelastic Warping Method

Hua Zou[1], Ce Xi[2], Xiaodan Zhao[1], Angela S. Koh[1,3], Fei Gao[1], Yi Su[4], Ru-San Tan[1,3], John Allen[3], Lik Chuan Lee[2], Martin Genet[5,6] and Liang Zhong[1,3]*

[1] National Heart Centre Singapore, Singapore, Singapore, [2] Department of Mechanical Engineering, Michigan State University, East Lansing, MI, United States, [3] Duke-NUS Medical School, National University of Singapore, Singapore, Singapore, [4] Institute of High Performance Computing, A*STAR, Singapore, Singapore, [5] Mechanics Department and Solid Mechanics Laboratory, École Polytechnique, C.N.R.S., Université Paris-Saclay, Palaiseau, France, [6] M3DISIM Team, I.N.R.I.A, Université Paris-Saclay, Palaiseau, France

*Correspondence:
Liang Zhong
zhong.liang@nhcs.com.sg;
zhong.liang@duke-nus.edu.sg

Heart failure (HF) imposes a major global health care burden on society and suffering on the individual. About 50% of HF patients have preserved ejection fraction (HFpEF). More intricate and comprehensive measurement-focused imaging of multiple strain components may aid in the diagnosis and elucidation of this disease. Here, we describe the development of a semi-automated hyperelastic warping method for rapid comprehensive assessment of biventricular circumferential, longitudinal, and radial strains that is physiological meaningful and reproducible. We recruited and performed cardiac magnetic resonance (CMR) imaging on 30 subjects [10 HFpEF, 10 HF with reduced ejection fraction patients (HFrEF) and 10 healthy controls]. In each subject, a three-dimensional heart model including left ventricle (LV), right ventricle (RV), and septum was reconstructed from CMR images. The hyperelastic warping method was used to reference the segmented model with the target images and biventricular circumferential, longitudinal, and radial strain–time curves were obtained. The peak systolic strains are then measured and analyzed in this study. Intra- and inter-observer reproducibility of the biventricular peak systolic strains was excellent with all ICCs > 0.92. LV peak systolic circumferential, longitudinal, and radial strain, respectively, exhibited a progressive decrease in magnitude from healthy control→HFpEF→HFrEF: control (−15.5 ± 1.90, −15.6 ± 2.06, 41.4 ± 12.2%); HFpEF (−9.37 ± 3.23, −11.3 ± 1.76, 22.8 ± 13.1%); HFrEF (−4.75 ± 2.74, −7.55 ± 1.75, 10.8 ± 4.61%). A similar progressive decrease in magnitude was observed for RV peak systolic circumferential, longitudinal and radial strain: control (−9.91 ± 2.25, −14.5 ± 2.63, 26.8 ± 7.16%); HFpEF (−7.38 ± 3.17, −12.0 ± 2.45, 21.5 ± 10.0%); HFrEF (−5.92 ± 3.13, −8.63 ± 2.79, 15.2 ± 6.33%). Furthermore, septum peak systolic circumferential, longitudinal, and radial strain magnitude decreased gradually from healthy control to HFrEF: control (−7.11 ± 1.81, 16.3 ± 3.23, 18.5 ± 8.64%); HFpEF

$(-6.11 \pm 3.98, -13.4 \pm 3.02, 12.5 \pm 6.38\%)$; HFrEF $(-1.42 \pm 1.36, -8.99 \pm 2.96, 3.35 \pm 2.95\%)$. The ROC analysis indicated LV peak systolic circumferential strain to be the most sensitive marker for differentiating HFpEF from healthy controls. Our results suggest that the hyperelastic warping method with the CMR-derived strains may reveal subtle impairment in HF biventricular mechanics, in particular despite a "normal" ventricular ejection fraction in HFpEF.

**Keywords: heart failure with preserved ejection fraction, left ventricle, right ventricle, strain, hyperelastic warping**

## INTRODUCTION

Heart failure (HF) with preserved ejection fraction is a clinical syndrome in which patients have symptoms and signs of HF but normal or near-normal left ventricle ejection fraction (LVEF). Nearly 30–50% of patients worldwide with HF have HFpEF (Hogg et al., 2004), including Singapore (Zhong et al., 2013), and the prevalence appears to be rising. Based on large community and admission cohorts, some studies have suggested recently that the prognosis may not differ significantly between HFrEF and HFpEF patients, making HFpEF a substantially challenging public health issue with an increasing burden on the elderly population (Lo et al., 2013). Characterized by diastolic dysfunctions with increased LV stiffness, slow LV filling, and elevated LV end-diastolic pressure, HFpEF is most frequently associated with myocardial fibrosis or hypertrophy. Despite normal or nearly normal LVEF, ventricular contractility indexes used in both Western and Asian population indicate that systolic dysfunction is common in HFpEF patients (Borlaug et al., 2009; Zhong et al., 2011, 2013). Impaired LV systolic function may be revealed by measuring ventricular strain (Lo et al., 2013; Choudhary et al., 2016; Genet et al., 2016a).

In most studies, ventricular strain is measured using tissue doppler or 2-D speckle-tracking echocardiography (Flachskampf et al., 2015). However, tissue doppler-based assessment of LV longitudinal function is angle dependent and typically assesses only mitral annular motion (Koyama et al., 2003). Speckle-tracking is the most widely available imaging modality for quantitative assessment of the LV and RV structure and functions (Kraigher-Krainer et al., 2014); image quality of the RV is, however, often poor and somewhat subjective with quantitation accuracy limited by the complex chamber geometry (Haddad et al., 2008; De Siqueira et al., 2016). Cardiac magnetic resonance (CMR) imaging has emerged as the gold standard for quantitative assessment of LV and RV volumes and functions (Marcelo et al., 2016). It is superior to echocardiography for evaluating segmental wall motion abnormalities and extra cardiac

findings due to its higher spatial resolution (Hussein et al., 2013). In addition, CMR was demonstrated to have superior reproducibility over two-dimensional (2D) echocardiography (Kleijn et al., 2012; Leng et al., 2015).

Interest in the RV function in HF arises from community-based studies showing that 83% of HFpEF patients have associated pulmonary hypertension and one-third of them have right ventricular dysfunction (Kanwar et al., 2016). These findings have generated interest to study RV function in HFpEF. However, very few studies have been undertaken to quantify motion in the RV myocardium and ventricular septum for the assessment of RV function and interaction between LV and RV. Here, we utilized a hyperelastic warping approach to quantify ventricular motion and function by estimating bi-ventricular strains from CMR images. The hyperelastic warping is a deformable image registration technique integrating finite deformation continuum mechanics with image-based data to obtain strain measurements from medical images such as MRI, positron emission tomography (PET), and computed tomography (CT; Rabbitt et al., 1995; Veress et al., 2002, 2013). In the hyperelastic warping method, a finite element (FE) model of the region of interest is deformed by a body force that depends on the difference in image intensities between the template and target images. Hyperelastic strain energy based on continuum mechanics is applied to constrain and regularize the deformation (Veress et al., 2005; Genet et al., 2015, 2016b). Note that other regularizers have also been proposed, such as incompressibility (Mansi et al., 2011), or equilibrium gap (Claire et al., 2004; Genet et al., 2018). Application of the hyperelastic warping approach in cardiac motion and function has focused primarily on quantifying LV strains (Veress et al., 2008, 2013; Genet et al., 2016b) that has been verified by tagged MRI (Phatak et al., 2009) and 3D CSPAMM MR images (Genet et al., 2015). This method has also been applied to quantify circumferential strain in individual patient with HFpEF (Zou et al., 2016) and pulmonary hypertension (Xi et al., 2016).

In this work, we performed further bi-ventricular strain measurement using the hyperelastic warping method to extract circumferential, longitudinal, and radial strains in three regions of the bi-ventricular unit, namely, LV, RV, and septum. The goals of this study are threefold: (i) develop a framework to simultaneously quantify circumferential, longitudinal, and radial strains in the bi-ventricle model, (ii) detect abnormalities in these three types of strains in HFpEF patients compared to HFrEF and normal controls, and (iii) study the inter- and intra-observer reproducibility of the hyperelastic warping approach in its application in HF patients.

---

**Abbreviations:** EF, ejection fraction; HFpEF, heart failure with preserved ejection fraction; HFrEF, heart failure with reduced ejection fraction; LV, left ventricle; $\varepsilon_{CC}^{LV}$, left ventricular peak systolic circumferential strain; $\varepsilon_{LL}^{LV}$, left ventricular peak systolic longitudinal strain; $\varepsilon_{RR}^{LV}$, left ventricular peak systolic radial strain; MRI, magnetic resonance imaging; RV, right ventricle; $\varepsilon_{CC}^{RV}$ right ventricular peak systolic circumferential strain; $\varepsilon_{LL}^{RV}$, right ventricular peak systolic longitudinal strain; $\varepsilon_{RR}^{RV}$, right ventricular peak systolic radial strain; $\varepsilon_{CC}^{Sep}$, septum peak systolic circumferential strain; $\varepsilon_{LL}^{Sep}$, septum peak systolic longitudinal strain; $\varepsilon_{RR}^{Sep}$, septum peak systolic radial strain.

## MATERIALS AND METHODS

### Study Population

The HF patients were recruited from the Curvedness-based Imaging Study (CBIS), a prospective study initiated in 2012. The normal control subjects were recruited from the Cardiac Aging Study (CAS) (Koh et al., 2018), a prospective study initiated in 2014. Ten paired sub-groups of subjects were enrolled and underwent CMR scans. One control, one HFrEF patient, and one HFpEF patient were recruited for each sub-group. They were age-comparable and gender-matched. Normal controls had no known cardiovascular disease or other co-morbidities. Patients with a clinical history of HF were recruited as HF patients. Using 40% as an LVEF cut-off value, HF patients with LVEF > 40% were treated as HFpEF while those with LVEF < 40% as HFrEF. The studies were approved by the local Institutional Review Board,

and all enrolled participants gave written informed consent. The demographics of the study groups are summarized in **Table 1**.

### CMR Image Acquisition

As part of the routine clinical protocol, HFpEF and HFrEF patients underwent CMR evaluation on a 3T system (Ingenia, Philips Healthcare, Netherlands) with a dStream Torso coil (maximal number of channels 32). The same imaging protocol was applied to the control subjects. Balanced turbo field echo (BTFE) end-expiratory breath hold cine images were acquired in multi-planner short-axis and long-axis views. The short-axis view included the images from the apex to basal. The long-axis images included the two-chamber, three-chamber, and four-chamber views. The following typical sequence parameters were used: TR/TE 3/1 ms, flip angle 45°, slice thickness 8 mm for short-axis, pixel bandwidth 1797 Hz, field of view 280–450 mm,

**TABLE 1 |** Demographics of study populations.

| Characteristics | Normal (n = 10) | HFpEF (n = 10) | HFrEF (n = 10) | HFpEF *versus* HFrEF§ |
|---|---|---|---|---|
| Age (year) | 52.1 ± 12.7 | 52.4 ± 12.5 | 52.7 ± 11.6 | NS |
| Gender (F/M) | 2/8 | 2/8 | 2/8 | NS |
| Height (cm) | 167.9 ± 8.6 | 164.1 ± 7.4 | 167.3 ± 10.8 | NS |
| Weight (kg) | 69.7 ± 11.4 | 76.5 ± 16.7 | 86.2 ± 22.2* | NS |
| BSA (m²) | 1.79 ± 0.18 | 1.85 ± 0.23 | 1.97 ± 0.30 | NS |
| SBP (mmHg) | 133.7 ± 11.6 | 136.1 ± 34.1 | 124.2 ± 19.6 | NS |
| DBP(mmHg) | 81 ± 9.37 | 75.7 ± 25.8 | 71.9 ± 13.1 | NS |
| LVEF (%) | 65 ± 6 | 53 ± 7* | 25 ± 9* | <0.05 |
| LVEDV index (ml/m²) | 71.0 ± 12.8 | 89.7 ± 17.0* | 148.3 ± 53.1* | <0.05 |
| LVESV index (ml/m²) | 25.0 ± 6.6 | 43.1 ± 13.2* | 114.0 ± 50.0* | <0.05 |
| LVSV index (ml/m²) | 46.1 ± 8.7 | 46.7 ± 7.4 | 34.3 ± 13.1 | 0.053 |
| LV mass index (g/m²) | 47.8 ± 6.6 | 69.1 ± 19.5* | 79.3 ± 27.2* | NS |
| RVEF (%) | 56 ± 6 | 57 ± 7 | 40 ± 12* | <0.05 |
| RVEDV index (ml/m²) | 79.5 ± 15.2 | 76.1 ± 16.7 | 89.6 ± 29.9 | NS |
| RVESV index (ml/m²) | 35.7 ± 9.4 | 33.1 ± 9.6 | 54.8 ± 26.3* | <0.05 |
| RVSV index (g/m²) | 43.7 ± 7.2 | 43.3 ± 9.7 | 34.7 ± 13.3 | NS |
| Pulse (BPM) | 72 ± 10 | 58 ± 10 | 83 ± 24 | <0.05 |
| NYHA (I), n (%) | N.A | 3 (30) | 4 (30) | NS |
| NYHA (II), n (%) | N.A | 5 (50) | 4 (30) | NS |
| NYHA (III), n (%) | N.A | 1 (10) | 2 (20) | NS |
| NYHA (IV), n (%) | N.A | 1 (10) | 0 (0) | NS |
| Atrial flutter/fibrillation, n (%) | N.A | 2 (20) | 1 (10) | NS |
| Cancer within last five years, n (%) | N.A | 0 (0) | 0 (0) | NS |
| Chronic renal insufficiency, n (%) | N.A | 2 (20) | 0 (0) | NS |
| Current smoker, n (%) | N.A | 4 (40) | 1 (10) | NS |
| Depression, n (%) | N.A | 0 (0) | 0 (0) | NS |
| Diabetes, n (%) | N.A | 3 (30) | 6 (60) | NS |
| Hyperlipidemia, n (%) | N.A | 7 (70) | 5 (50) | NS |
| Hypertension, n (%) | N.A | 8 (80) | 5 (50) | NS |
| Peripheral vascular disease, n (%) | N.A | 1 (10) | 0 (0) | NS |
| Myocardial infarction, n (%) | N.A | 1 (10) | 0 (0) | NS |
| Stroke, n (%) | N.A | 0 (0) | 1 (10) | NS |
| NTproBNP | N.A | 2667.2 ± 2519.6 | 921.6 ± 837.7 | <0.05 |

*Data are mean ± SD. BSA, body surface area; SBP, systolic blood pressure; DBP, diastolic blood pressure; LV, left ventricular; EF, ejection fraction; EDV, end-diastolic volume; ESV, end-systolic volume; SV, stroke volume; RV, right ventricular; HFrEF, heart failure with reduced EF; HFpEF, heart failure with preserved EF; NYHA, New York Heart Association; NTproBNP: N-terminal pro b-type natriuretic peptide. § Wilcoxon rank-sum test. *Statistically significant difference between HFpEF vs normal controls, HFrEF vs normal controls, Wilcoxon rank-sum test (p < 0.05).*

temporal resolution ≈ 28 ms, in plane spatial resolution 0.6 mm × 0.6mm–1.1 mm × 1.1 mm, and frame rate was selected as 30 or 40 frames per cardiac cycle. Among these 30 subjects, 30 frames are used for all the short-axis view. For long-axis view, 26 subjects had 30 frames, and the other four had 40 frames.

## Framework to Obtain the Circumferential, Longitudinal, and Radial Strains

The strain acquisition framework was implemented using a combination of open-source software: MeVisLab (MeVis Medical Solution AG, Bremen, Germany), Gmsh (Geuzaine and Remacle, 2009), Fenics (Alnaes et al., 2015), and in-house code (Genet et al., 2014, 2015). The overall workflow is shown in **Figure 1**.

### CMR Images

**Figure 2** shows an example of the short-axis and long-axis CMR images covering the LV and RV. They were used in contour segmentation and surface reconstruction, including short-axis images from basal to apex, and the four-chamber long-axis images.

### Contours Segmentation and Model Reconstruction

**Figures 3A,B** show the contour segmentation from the short-axis and long-axis images for LV endocardium, RV endocardium, and

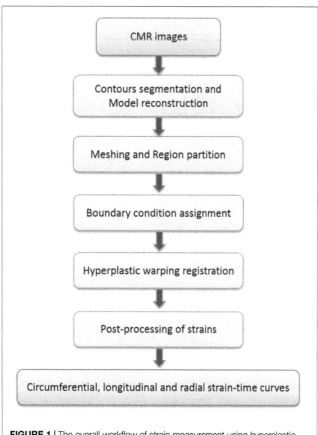

**FIGURE 1 |** The overall workflow of strain measurement using hyperelastic warping method.

bi-ventricular epicardium (from top to bottom, respectively). End of systole (ES) was chosen to be the time point to manually delineate the contours for model reconstruction – this is the cardiac phase when the aorta valve in three-chamber view starts to close. Depending on the size of the heart and the quality of the image, around 3–10 short-axis images and the four-chamber long-axis image were utilized. **Figures 3C,D** show, respectively, the contours used for surface reconstruction and the generated surfaces for the LV, RV, and bi-ventricular epicardium. Papillary muscles and trabeculated structures were not included as myocardium. After reconstruction, the model is corrected using a "WEMReducePolygons" module in Mevislab if there were mis-registration of the images.

### FE Mesh Discretization and Region Partition

Following reconstruction of the three surfaces, they were assembled together to form the bi-ventricle model. **Figure 4A** shows the three-dimensional bi-ventricle model, and **Figure 4B** shows the FEmesh model generated by GMSH (Geuzaine and Remacle, 2009). Considering the computational time as well as the accuracy, we employed 0.3 as the mesh size. For these 30 cases, the number of FE nodes (points) ranged from 2286 to 3288 and the number of cells ranged from 7013 to 11,985. As previously mentioned, the model was partitioned into three regions (i.e., LV, RV, and septum) for strain study as shown in **Figure 4C**.

### Boundary Conditions Assignment

The short-axis images were used in the hyperelastic warping method. However, with the heart in motion, there was an excursion in the long-axis direction, thus a displacement was applied in the long-axis direction as a boundary condition in the hyperelastic warping method. The magnitude of the displacement was estimated by the mitral annular plane systolic excursion (MAPSE) at the septum measured in the four-chamber view in MeVisLab, as shown in **Figure 5**. During the dynamic deformation, the prescribed longitudinal displacement was controlled by a sine function.

### Hyperelastic Warping Theory

Hyperelastic warping is a deformable image registration technique that can be used to measure cardiac strain derived from analysis of medical images such as MRI, ultrasound, and microPET imaging (Veress et al., 2013). In the hyperelastic warping method, a FE mesh (**Figure 4B**) was deformed along with a set of short-axis images during a cardiac cycle. The deformation of the FE mesh was defined as the mapping $\phi(X) = X + u(X)$, where $u$ is the displacement field and $X$ is the position. The deformation gradient was defined as

$$F(X) = \frac{\partial \phi}{\partial X} \qquad (1)$$

The forces responsible for driving the registration deformation were derived from the difference in image intensity field between

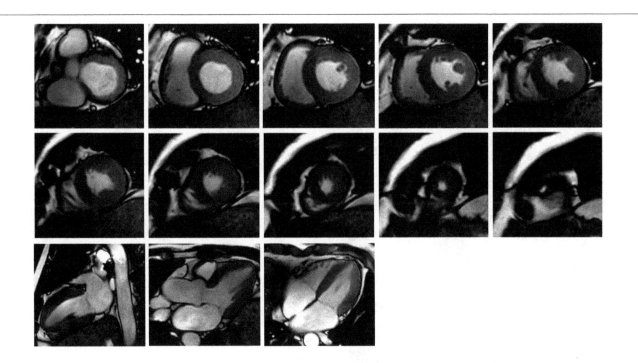

**FIGURE 2** | Cardiac MR images corresponding to 10 short-axis slices (the upper two rows) and three long-axis slices (the third row).

two volumetric image data sets by minimizing the following energy expression

$$E(\varphi) = \int W(X, C)\frac{dv}{J} - \int U(R(X) - T(\phi))\frac{dv}{J} \quad (2)$$

Here, $W$ is the hyperelastic strain density energy function related to the material model of myocardium and $C = F^T F$ is the Cauchy–Green deformation tensor. A Neo–Hookean strain energy density function was used to define $W$, which is given as

$$W(X, C) = C_1\,(I_1\text{-}3) \quad (3)$$

where $C_1$ is a material constant and $I_1$ is the first invariant of the right Cauchy–Green deformation tensor. The energy term $U$ produced an image force field responsible for the local registration of the discretized reference image $R$ to the target image $T$ and is expressed as

$$U(X, \phi) = \frac{\gamma}{2}(R(X) - T(\phi))^2 \quad (4)$$

where $\gamma$ is the penalty factor enforcing the alignment of the reference image to the target image. In summary, the FE mesh model was deformed to align with the target images via a computed image-based local body force term that depends on (1) the difference in image intensity between the template and target images, (2) the target image intensity gradient, and (3) a prescribed penalty factor.

The hyperelastic warping approach was implemented using FEniCS (Logg et al., 2012; Alnaes et al., 2015). The penalty parameter $\gamma$ in Eq. 3 was set as 0.005 for all the cases. The method to optimize $\gamma$ is referred to (Genet et al., 2017).

**Figure 6** shows an example of the resultant deformation in the biventricular model from a normal subject computed from the hyperelastic warping method. As shown in the figure, the deformed biventricular model matched closely with the myocardium in CMR short-axis images at different cardiac time points.

## Post-processing of Strains

The ES biventricular geometry was used as the initial configuration for tracking because we found that the image registration worked better when the myocardial wall at all subsequent time points is thinner than the initial one, which always revealed an image intensity gradient within the initial wall volume. Since the deformation gradient $F$ was defined with ES as the initial configuration, the local Green-Lagrange strain tensor with end-diastole (ED) as the reference configuration – a more commonly used metric – was defined as

$$E = \frac{1}{2}\left(F^T F_{ED}^{-T} F F_{ED}^{-1} - I\right) \quad (5)$$

In Eq. 5, $I$ is the identity tensor and $F_{ED}$ is the deformation gradient tensor at ED. Normal strains in the circumferential $\varepsilon_{CC}$, longitudinal $\varepsilon_{LL}$, and radial $\varepsilon_{RR}$ directions were computed by projecting $E$ onto these directions using $\varepsilon_{ii} = e_i \bullet E e_i$ with $i \in (C, L, R)$. The circumferential $e_C$, longitudinal $e_L$, and radial $e_R$ were prescribed using a Laplace–Dirichlet rule-based (LDRB) algorithm (Bayer et al., 2012) with myofiber angle prescribed to be zero.

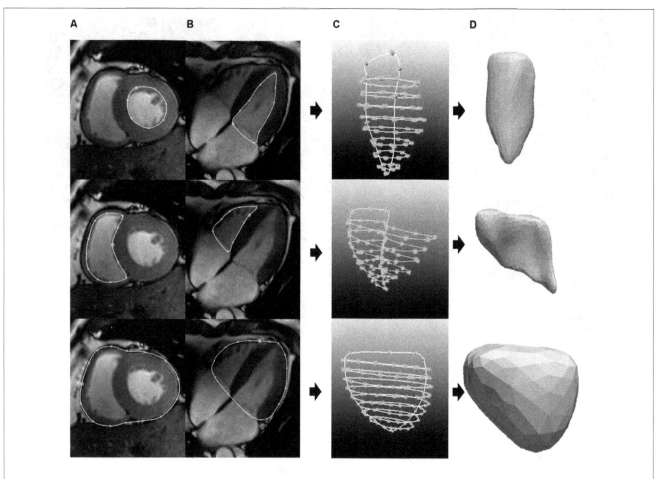

**FIGURE 3 |** Generating the surface for LV endo (top), RV endo (middle), and bi-ventricular epicardia (bottom). **(A)** Short-axis contours segmentation. **(B)** Long-axis contours segmentation. **(C)** All the contours for surface generation. **(D)** LV endo, RV endo, and bi-ventricular epicardia surfaces.

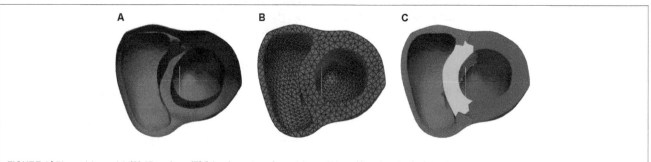

**FIGURE 4 |** Bi-ventricle model: **(A)** 3D surface, **(B)** finite element mesh model, and **(C)** partition of region (red: RV free wall; green: septum; blue: LV free wall).

## Strain–Time Curves

**Figure 7A** shows the circumferential direction assigned on the model and the circumferential strain-time curve, **Figure 7B** the longitudinal direction and longitudinal strain–time curve, and **Figure 7C** shows the radial direction and radial strain–time curve. These strain components were computed at each cardiac time point to construct the strain–time curves. The strain curves were computed by averaging the strains over all the elements with respect to the three regions: RV free wall, septum, and LV free wall as shown in **Figure 4C**. The effects of atrial contraction at late filling (i.e., "atrial kick") are visible in the strain–time curves, particularly, in those associated with the LV.

## Reproducibility

Assessment of inter- and intra-observer variability of the hyperelastic warping method was performed on a random selection of nine cases: three controls, three HFpEF, and three HFrEF patients. Inter-observer variability was assessed by comparing measurements made by two independent observers from two different centers. Intra-observation variability was

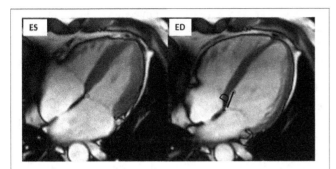

**FIGURE 5 |** Measurement of septal displacement of septal in four-chamber view.

obtained from repeated measurements on these nine cases, 1 month apart, by the same observer.

## Statistical Analysis

Data were analyzed using SPSS (version 17.0, Chicago, IL, United States) and SAS (version 9.3, Cary, NC, United States). Comparisons of demographics, patient characteristics, and CMR measurements between patients and control subjects were performed using independent $t$-tests for normally distributed data, Mann–Whitney $U$-tests for non-normally distributed data, and Fisher's exact tests for categorical data. Intra- and Inter-observer variability in peak circumferential, longitudinal, and radial strains were assessed by mean bias $\pm$ SD, limits of agreement, coefficient of variation (CV), and intra-class correlation coefficient (ICC) using data from nine randomly chosen subjects. ICC between 0.4 and 0.59 was considered fair, good between 0.60 and 0.74, and excellent when ≥0.75 (Aarsæther et al., 2012).

## RESULTS

### Patient Demographics

Study subjects in each group consist of eight males and two females with a mean $\pm$ SD age of 52.1 $\pm$ 12.7, 52.4 $\pm$ 12.5, and 52.7 $\pm$ 11.6 years for controls, HFpEF, and HFrEF patients, respectively. Demographic and clinical characteristic of study subjects are given in **Table 1**. Compared with normal controls, LVEF was lower in both HF groups. Between the HF groups, LVEF was larger in HFpEF patients (53 $\pm$ 7%) than the HFrEF

group (25 $\pm$ 9%). Both HF groups were comparable to controls with respect to height, BSA, SBP, DBP, LVSV index, RVEDV index, and RVSV index, but exhibited higher LVEDV index, LVESV index, and LV mass index than the controls ($p < 0.05$). The HFpEF patients had comparable RVEF and RVESV index to controls, while the HFrEF patients had lower RVEF and higher RVESV index than both controls and HFpEF patients ($p < 0.05$). HF groups were comparable relative to disease history, including NYHA class, atrial flutter/fibrillation, cancer within 5 years, chronic renal insufficiency, current smoker, depression, diabetes, hyperlipidemia, hypertension, peripheral vascular disease, myocardial infarction, and stroke. NTproBNP was much higher in HFpEF patients than in HFrEF patients ($p < 0.05$).

## Peak Systolic Circumferential, Longitudinal, and Radial Strains

**Table 2** shows the average values of the peak circumferential, longitudinal, and radial strains in different regions (LV, RV, and septum) for control, HFpEF, and HFrEF patients. All the peak circumferential, longitudinal, and radial strains in the LV were, respectively, found to gradually decrease in magnitude ($p < 0.05$) from control → HFpEF→ HFrEF groups (circumferential: $-15.5 \pm 1.90$, $-9.37 \pm 3.23$, $-4.75 \pm 2.74$; longitudinal: $-15.6 \pm 2.06$, $-11.3 \pm 1.76$, $-7.55 \pm 1.75$; radial: $41.4 \pm 12.2$, $22.8 \pm 13.1$, $10.8 \pm 4.61$; **Table 2**). This may reveal impaired systolic LV function in both HF groups. **Figure 8** shows scatter plots for the three strains in the LV. Excellent separation of controls from both the HFpEF and HFrEF patients was observed in the peak circumferential strain (**Figure 8A**). Almost no overlap was found between the controls and the two HF groups of patients. Similar to the peak circumferential strain, peak longitudinal strain exhibited negligible overlap of controls with HFpEF and HFrEF (**Figure 8B**). Significant differences were found between the peak radial strain of normal controls and patients. However, there was some overlap between the normal controls and the patients (**Figure 8C**).

Circumferential and radial strains in RV were smaller in HFpEF patients compared with the Controls but no significant difference was observed ($-9.91 \pm 2.25$ vs. $-7.38 \pm 3.17$ for circumferential strain and $26.8 \pm 7.16$ vs. $21.5 \pm 10.0$ for radial strain). However, longitudinal strain in RV was significantly decreased in the HFpEF group when compared to the controls ($-14.5 \pm 2.63$ vs. $-12.0 \pm 2.45$; $p < 0.05$,

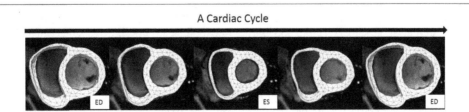

**FIGURE 6 |** Registration of the bi-ventricular model with the CMR images during a cardiac cycle. Note: biventricular model was reconstructed only from the CMR images at ES.

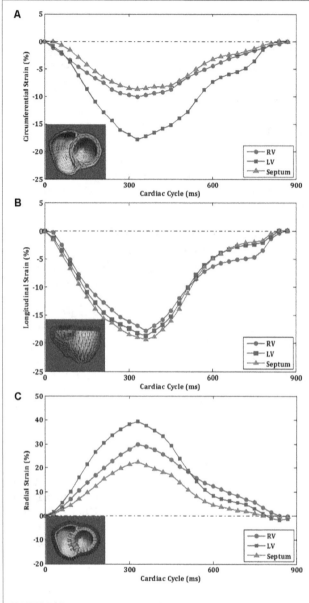

**FIGURE 7** | Strain orientation and strain–time curves of LV, RV, and septum for one cardiac cycle. **(A)** Circumferential strain. **(B)** Longitudinal strain. **(C)** Radial strain.

$(12.5 \pm 6.38$ vs. $18.5 \pm 8.64)$. Circumferential, longitudinal, and radial strains in the septum were all depressed in the HFrEF group compared with Controls ($p < 0.05$, **Table 2**). The scatter plot of strains for septum is shown in **Figure 10**.

## ROC Analysis and Cut-Off Values

Receiver operating characteristic (ROC) curve analysis showed that LV circumferential and longitudinal strains were superior to the septal strain for differentiating normal controls from HFpEF patients (**Figure 11**). Area under the ROC curve (AUC) for LV circumferential strain was 1.00 with corresponding sensitivity and specificity of 1.00. AUC for LV longitudinal strain was 0.95 with sensitivity 0.90 and specificity 0.90 (**Table 3**).

## Reproducibility

**Table 4** shows both intra- and inter-observer variability for nine randomly chosen cases (three normal controls, three HFpEF, and three HFrEF). In the Bland–Altman analysis, peak circumferential strain for LV had the best intra-observer agreement (bias, $0.08 \pm 0.63$; 95% CI, $-1.16$ to $1.32$) and inter-observer agreement (bias, $0.67 \pm 0.90$; 95% CI, $-1.10$ to $2.45$). Peak radial strain RV exhibited the largest intra-observer variability (bias, $1.28 \pm 4.23$; 95% CI, $-7.01$ to $9.57$) and peak radial strain for LV had the largest inter-observer variability (bias, $5.6 \pm 8.30$; 95% CI, $-10.63$ to $21.9$). All parameters had an excellent intra- and inter-observer agreement (ICC $\geq 0.92$).

## DISCUSSION

In this study, we compared myocardial strains estimated using a hyperelastic warping approach in the control, HFpEF, and HFrEF patients that are comparable in age and gender. To the best of our knowledge, this research work is the first to study biventricular three-dimensional strain (longitudinal, circumferential, and radial) based on CMR images in HF patients using the hyperelastic warping method. The major contributions of our study are as follows: (1) development of a novel framework for assessment of the biventricular mechanics of HF from CMR and (2) implementation of a viable and reproducible hyperelastic warping method for simultaneous evaluation of 3D circumferential, longitudinal, and radial strains for HF patients. The key findings from our study are as follows: (1) strains estimated in cine CMR images of HF patients using the hyperelastic are feasible and reproducible, (2) peak (absolute) circumferential, longitudinal, and radial strains in the RV, LV, and septum are highest in the normal controls followed by HFpEF to HFrEF patients, and (3) peak LV circumferential and longitudinal strain can better differentiate HFpEF patients from healthy subjects. These findings may provide a new method for simultaneous assessment of 3D biventricular strains in HF patients.

## LV Strain

We have found that all the three strain components (circumferential, longitudinal, and radial strains) in HFpEF and HFrEF patients were decreased compared to the normal

**Table 2**). Significant differences were found for all the three strain components between HFrEF and normal controls ($-5.92 \pm 3.13$ vs. $-9.91 \pm 2.25$ for circumferential strain; $-8.63 \pm 2.79$ vs. $-14.5 \pm 2.63$ for longitudinal strain; and $15.2 \pm 6.33$ vs. $26.8 \pm 7.16$ for radial strain; all $p < 0.05$, **Table 2**). Only longitudinal strain was observed to differ significantly between HFrEF and HFpEF ($-8.63 \pm 2.79$ vs. $-12.04 \pm 2.45$; $p < 0.05$, **Table 2**). Scatter plots of RV strains are shown in **Figure 9**.

Circumferential and longitudinal strains in the septum were depressed in HFpEF patients compared to the controls ($-6.11 \pm 3.98$ vs. $-7.11 \pm 1.81$ for circumferential strain; $-13.4 \pm 3.02$ vs. $-16.3 \pm 3.23$ for longitudinal strain; all $p < 0.05$, **Table 2**). Radial strain was smaller but not significantly different

**TABLE 2** | Average circumferential, longitudinal, and radial strains for RV, LV, and septum.

| Strain parameters | Normal | HFpEF | HFrEF | HFpEF vs. HFrEF§ |
|---|---|---|---|---|
| $\varepsilon_{CC}^{RV}$ (%) | −9.91 ± 2.25 | −7.38 ± 3.17 | −5.92 ± 3.13* | NS |
| $\varepsilon_{CC}^{LV}$ (%) | −15.49 ± 1.90 | −9.37 ± 3.23* | −4.75 ± 2.74* | <0.05 |
| $\varepsilon_{CC}^{Sep}$ (%) | −7.11 ± 1.81 | −6.11 ± 3.98* | −1.42 ± 1.36* | <0.05 |
| $\varepsilon_{LL}^{RV}$ (%) | −14.49 ± 2.63 | −12.04 ± 2.45* | −8.63 ± 2.79* | <0.05 |
| $\varepsilon_{LL}^{LV}$ (%) | −15.58 ± 2.06 | −11.30 ± 1.76* | −7.55 ± 1.75* | <0.05 |
| $\varepsilon_{LL}^{Sep}$ (%) | −16.26 ± 3.23 | −13.38 ± 3.02* | −8.89 ± 2.96* | <0.05 |
| $\varepsilon_{RR}^{RV}$ (%) | 26.79 ± 7.16 | 21.49 ± 10.01 | 15.15 ± 6.33* | NS |
| $\varepsilon_{RR}^{LV}$ (%) | 41.41 ± 12.20 | 22.81 ± 13.05* | 10.84 ± 4.61* | <0.05 |
| $\varepsilon_{RR}^{Sep}$ (%) | 18.51 ± 8.64 | 12.45 ± 6.38 | 3.35 ± 2.95* | <0.05 |

*Values are mean ± SD. $\varepsilon_{CC}^{RV}$, right ventricular peak circumferential strain; $\varepsilon_{CC}^{LV}$, left ventricular peak circumferential strain; $\varepsilon_{CC}^{Sep}$, septum peak circumferential strain; $\varepsilon_{LL}^{RV}$, right ventricular peak longitudinal strain; $\varepsilon_{LL}^{LV}$, left ventricular peak longitudinal strain; $\varepsilon_{LL}^{Sep}$, septum peak longitudinal strain; $\varepsilon_{RR}^{RV}$, right ventricular peak radial strain; $\varepsilon_{RR}^{LV}$, left ventricular peak radial strain; $\varepsilon_{RR}^{Sep}$, septum peak radial strain; HFrEF, heart failure with reduced ejection fraction; HFpEF, heart failure with preserved ejection fraction. § Wilcoxon rank-sum test. *Statistically significant difference between HFPEF vs. normal, HFREF vs. normal controls, Wilcoxon rank-sum test (p < 0.05).*

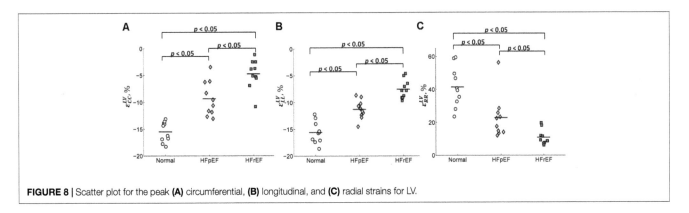

**FIGURE 8** | Scatter plot for the peak **(A)** circumferential, **(B)** longitudinal, and **(C)** radial strains for LV.

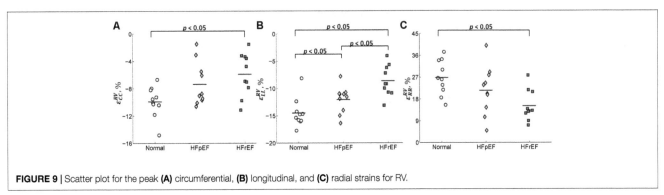

**FIGURE 9** | Scatter plot for the peak **(A)** circumferential, **(B)** longitudinal, and **(C)** radial strains for RV.

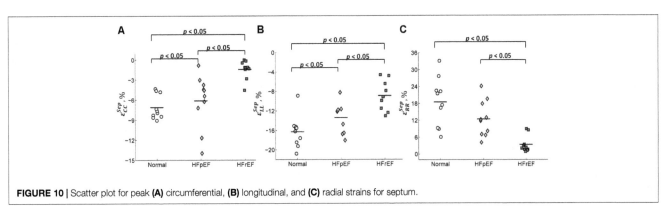

**FIGURE 10** | Scatter plot for peak **(A)** circumferential, **(B)** longitudinal, and **(C)** radial strains for septum.

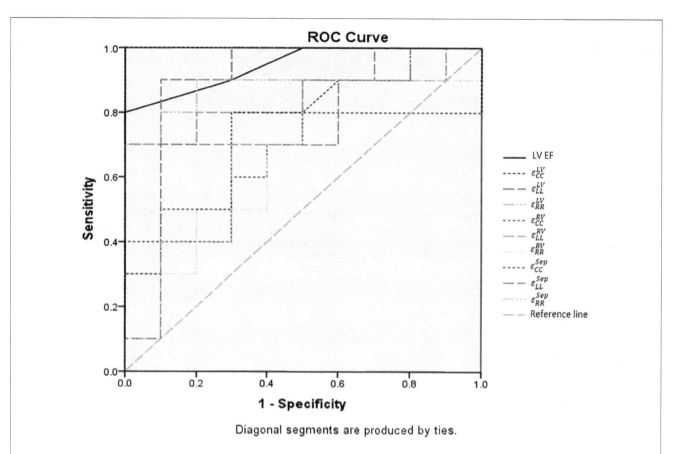

**FIGURE 11 |** ROC curves of all strain parameters and LVEF for differentiating normal controls with HFpEF patients. LVEF, left ventricular ejection fraction; $\varepsilon_{CC}^{RV}$, right ventricular peak circumferential strain; $\varepsilon_{CC}^{LV}$, left ventricular peak circumferential strain; $\varepsilon_{CC}^{Sep}$, septum peak circumferential strain; $\varepsilon_{LL}^{RV}$, right ventricular peak longitudinal strain; $\varepsilon_{LL}^{LV}$, left ventricular peak longitudinal strain; $\varepsilon_{LL}^{Sep}$: septum peak longitudinal strain; $\varepsilon_{RR}^{RV}$, right ventricular peak radial strain; $\varepsilon_{RR}^{LV}$, left ventricular peak radial strain; $\varepsilon_{RR}^{Sep}$, septum peak radial strain.

subjects. Similar conclusions are also found in Yip et al. (2011), where they found a similar trend in global 2D circumferential, radial, and longitudinal strain (as well as torsion) using standard 2D Doppler and speckle-tracking echocardiography.

Several studies (MacIver and Townsend, 2007; MacIver, 2008, 2011; Maciver et al., 2015) have used mathematical modeling to explain the apparent paradox of a reduction in longitudinal, circumferential, and radial strain but with a preserved LVEF.

**TABLE 3 |** Sensitivity, specificity and AUC of the strains and LVEF for differentiating normal controls and HFpEF.

| Parameters | Patient type | Cut-off value | Sensitivity | Specificity | AUC |
|---|---|---|---|---|---|
| $\varepsilon_{CC}^{RV}$ (%) | HFpEF | 6.39 | 0.400 | 1.000 | 0.715 |
| $\varepsilon_{CC}^{LV}$ (%) | HFpEF | 13.10 | 1.000 | 1.000 | 1.000 |
| $\varepsilon_{CC}^{Sep}$ (%) | HFpEF | 7.26 | 0.800 | 0.700 | 0.690 |
| $\varepsilon_{LL}^{RV}$ (%) | HFpEF | 14.12 | 0.800 | 0.800 | 0.780 |
| $\varepsilon_{LL}^{LV}$ (%) | HFpEF | 12.85 | 0.900 | 0.900 | 0.950 |
| $\varepsilon_{LL}^{Sep}$ (%) | HFpEF | 14.90 | 0.700 | 0.900 | 0.750 |
| $\varepsilon_{RR}^{RV}$ (%) | HFpEF | 25.26 | 0.700 | 0.600 | 0.660 |
| $\varepsilon_{RR}^{LV}$ (%) | HFpEF | 30.53 | 0.900 | 0.800 | 0.890 |
| $\varepsilon_{RR}^{Sep}$ (%) | HFpEF | 20.51 | 0.900 | 0.500 | 0.700 |
| LVEF | HFpEF | 59 | 0.800 | 1.000 | 0.945 |

$\varepsilon_{CC}^{RV}$, right ventricular peak circumferential strain; $\varepsilon_{CC}^{LV}$, left ventricular peak circumferential strain; $\varepsilon_{CC}^{Sep}$, septum peak circumferential strain; $\varepsilon_{LL}^{RV}$, right ventricular peak longitudinal strain; $\varepsilon_{LL}^{LV}$, left ventricular peak longitudinal strain; $\varepsilon_{LL}^{Sep}$, septum peak longitudinal strain; $\varepsilon_{RR}^{RV}$, right ventricular peak radial strain; $\varepsilon_{RR}^{LV}$, left ventricular peak radial strain; $\varepsilon_{RR}^{Sep}$, septum peak radial strain; LVEF, left ventricular ejection fraction.

**TABLE 4 |** Inter- and intra-observer agreement for nine randomly chosen cases (three control, three HFpEF, and three HFrEF).

| Variable | Variability | Mean bias ± SD | Limits of agreement | Coefficient of variation (%) | ICC (95% CI) |
|---|---|---|---|---|---|
| $\varepsilon_{CC}^{RV}$ | Intra-observer | 0.20 ± 1.31 | −2.38 to 2.78 | 10.40 | 0.954 (0.799, 0.990) |
| | Inter-observer | 1.00 ± 1.24 | −1.43 to 3.43 | 11.89 | 0.964 (0.839, 0.992) |
| $\varepsilon_{CC}^{LV}$ | Intra-observer | 0.08 ± 0.63 | −1.16 to 1.32 | 4.18 | 0.997 (0.988, 0.999) |
| | Inter-observer | 0.67 ± 0.90 | −1.10 to 2.45 | 7.27 | 0.994 (0.973, 0.999) |
| $\varepsilon_{CC}^{Sep}$ | Intra-observer | 0.56 ± 0.51 | −0.45 to 1.58 | 11.27 | 0.989 (0.843, 0.998) |
| | Inter-observer | 0.55 ± 1.73 | −2.85 to 3.95 | 23.35 | 0.952 (0.787, 0.989) |
| $\varepsilon_{LL}^{RV}$ | Intra-observer | −0.91 ± 1.56 | −3.97 to 2.15 | 9.30 | 0.940 (0.728, 0.987) |
| | Inter-observer | −0.27 ± 1.57 | −3.35 to 2.81 | 8.48 | 0.945 (0.758, 0.988) |
| $\varepsilon_{LL}^{LV}$ | Intra-observer | −0.54 ± 0.86 | −2.23 to 1.14 | 5.77 | 0.989 (0.944, 0.998) |
| | Inter-observer | −0.56 ± 1.42 | −3.35 to 2.23 | 8.98 | 0.974 (0.883, 0.994) |
| $\varepsilon_{LL}^{Sep}$ | Intra-observer | −1.23 ± 1.35 | −3.89 to 1.42 | 9.11 | 0.963 (0.692, 0.993) |
| | Inter-observer | −1.32 ± 2.38 | −6.00 to 3.35 | 14.78 | 0.921 (0.649, 0.982) |
| $\varepsilon_{RR}^{RV}$ | Intra-observer | 1.28 ± 4.23 | −7.01 to 9.57 | 12.41 | 0.953 (0.805, 0.989) |
| | Inter-observer | 4.97 ± 3.52 | −1.94 to 11.88 | 20.39 | 0.953 (0.794, 0.990) |
| $\varepsilon_{RR}^{LV}$ | Intra-observer | 0.47 ± 2.47 | −4.36 to 5.31 | 6.15 | 0.997 (0.987, 0.999) |
| | Inter-observer | 5.63 ± 8.30 | −10.63 to 21.90 | 28.09 | 0.948 (0.769, 0.988) |
| $\varepsilon_{RR}^{Sep}$ | Intra-observer | −0.87 ± 1.12 | −3.06 to 1.31 | 8.74 | 0.995 (0.965, 0.999) |
| | Inter-observer | 1.00 ± 2.29 | −3.49 to 5.50 | 15.33 | 0.986 (0.939, 0.977) |

$\varepsilon_{CC}^{RV}$, right ventricular peak circumferential strain; $\varepsilon_{CC}^{LV}$, left ventricular peak circumferential strain; $\varepsilon_{CC}^{Sep}$, septum peak circumferential strain; $\varepsilon_{LL}^{RV}$, right ventricular peak longitudinal strain; $\varepsilon_{LL}^{LV}$, left ventricular peak longitudinal strain; $\varepsilon_{LL}^{Sep}$, septum peak longitudinal strain; $\varepsilon_{RR}^{RV}$, right ventricular peak radial strain; $\varepsilon_{RR}^{LV}$, left ventricular peak radial strain; $\varepsilon_{RR}^{Sep}$, septum peak radial strain.

These studies suggest that the normal ejection fraction in patients with HF can be explained by the presence of left ventricular hypertrophy, which is found in the HFpEF patients of this study (LV mass index: 47.8 ± 6.6 g/m$^2$ for normal controls vs. 69.1 ± 19.5 g/m$^2$ for HFpEF, $p < 0.05$, **Table 1**).

In the literature, decreasing longitudinal strain was found in HFpEF patients (Borlaug, 2014). Specifically, a high prevalence of patients hospitalized with acute HFpEF with abnormal LV longitudinal strain suggests the presence of some previously unrecognized myocardial systolic dysfunction associated with this disease (Buggey et al., 2017). Consistent with our findings, a clinical trial including 219 HFpEF patients also demonstrated that LV longitudinal and circumferential strains are significantly lower in HFpEF patients when compared with normal controls (Kraigher-Krainer et al., 2014). Peak global longitudinal strain and strain rate in HFpEF patients are also found to be higher than those found in HFrEF patients (Carluccio et al., 2011). However, reports are conflicted with respect to the peak LV circumferential and radial strains in HFpEF patients. Some investigators suggest that reduced peak longitudinal strain in the presence of normal LVEF in HFpEF patients is due to a compensatory increase in circumferential and/or radial function (Fang et al., 2004; Paulus et al., 2007; Edvardsen and Haugaa, 2011; Vitarelli et al., 2015). Others suggest that peak radial strain in LV is increased in asymptomatic mildly hypertensive patients but decreases as LV hypertrophy (LVH) progresses and the severity of HF increases. Longitudinal and radial strains in the LV were reduced, but circumferential deformation and twist were normal in HFpEF patients in a study by Wang et al. (2008). To the contrary, longitudinal, radial, and circumferential deformation and twist are consistently reduced in patients with HFrEF.

## RV Strain

Right ventricular systolic dysfunction is a common feature in HFrEF that is associated with impaired functional capacity and portended a poor prognosis (Mohammed et al., 2014). The prevalence as well as the functional and prognostic implications of RV dysfunction in HFpEF are, however, less clear. Here, although there are no significant differences in all RV functional parameters (e.g., RVEF, RVEDV index, RVESV index, and RVSV index) between HFpEF patients and normal controls – see **Table 1**, we found that the peak RV longitudinal strain is significantly decreased in HFpEF patients compared with normal controls. This finding suggests that RV function may be impaired in HFpEF patients, and peak RV longitudinal strain may be a useful in detecting this change. Consistent with previous findings, all the three RV strain components are significantly reduced in HFrEF patients. This is also consistent with the significant difference in RVEF and RVESV index between HFrEF patients and normal subjects.

Systematic assessment of RV function is a widely recognized challenge owing to: (1) its complex geometry, (2) the limited definition of the RV endocardial surface occasioned by trabeculated myocardium, and (3) the retrosternal position of the RV that limits echocardiographic imaging windows (Cameli et al., 2014). It is, however, also becoming increasingly clear that assessing RV strain is important in analyzing HF. Meris et al. (2010) found that RV strain accurately identified reduced global RV function. Moreover, there is also mounting evidence that pulmonary hypertension with RV dysfunction is associated with a reduced regional longitudinal strain. A large body of data showing that pulmonary hypertension and RV dysfunction are also common in HFpEF (Gorter et al., 2016). However, the focus is on tricuspid annular plane systolic excursion (TAPSE), fractional area change (FAC), and tricuspid annular systolic velocity (RV S; Melenovsky et al., 2014; Leng et al., 2016). Studies reporting on RV strain, in particular those using CMR, are scarce. Our study on the evaluation of the longitudinal, circumferential, and radial strains in the RV suggests that hyperelastic warping method may be helpful.

## Septum Strain
Septum shape and deformation (i.e., area strain) has been studied in repaired tetralogy of Fallot patients with volume overloading (Zhong et al., 2012). However, septum strains by using warping method were investigated for the first time in HFpEF. The results revealed that circumferential and longitudinal strains decreased gradually from controls→HFpEF→HFrEF. The observed decrease in radial strain was approximately 50% for HFpEF compared to controls. However, due to the wide band of radial strain exhibited in the normal controls, the difference was not statistically significant. We emphasize that longitudinal strain was reduced in the septal region, as well as in the LV and RV.

## Reproducibility
Overall, LV strains have better reproducibility than the septum and RV, which is expected due to its thicker wall. Circumferential and longitudinal strains have excellent intra- and inter-observer agreement, although this is less so for radial strains that still possesses acceptable reproducibility. Peak LV circumferential strain has the best reproducibility, followed by peak LV longitudinal strain. On the other hand, peak radial strain has the worst reproducibility.

## Comparability of Strain Values to Other Published Results
Absolute peak strains obtained here appear to be smaller compared with previous studies. In normal subjects, peak LV circumferential, longitudinal and radial strains were $-18.4 \pm 2.9\%$, $-19.1 \pm 4.1\%$, and $39.8 \pm 8.3\%$ for Western population (Taylor et al., 2015); and $-24.3 \pm 3.1\%$, $-22.4 \pm 2.9\%$, and $79.0 \pm 19.4\%$ for Chinese population (Peng et al., 2018), respectively using CMR feature tracking. Comparing the peak values, those found here are relative smaller in the circumferential ($-15.5 \pm 1.90\%$) and longitudinal directions ($-15.6 \pm 2.06\%$), but slightly different in the radial direction ($41.4 \pm 12.2\%$). This disparity may be explained by a difference in strain definition used in that and our studies. Specifically, we have used Green–Lagrange strain that expressed as $\frac{\Delta L}{L} + \frac{1}{2}\left(\frac{\Delta L}{L}\right)^2$ in the one-dimensional case whereas Biot strain, reduced to $\frac{\Delta L}{L}$

in one-dimension was used in previous study. The additional term $\frac{1}{2}\left(\frac{\Delta L}{L}\right)^2$ leads to the Green–Lagrange strain having a lower peak value in the shortening (circumferential and longitudinal) directions and a larger peak value in the lengthening (radial) direction during systole. The disparity in strain estimated from feature tracking technique and deformable registration method was also discussed previously (Mangion et al., 2016).

## Limitations
First, to address the poor out-of-plane tracking at the ventricular base that arises because of the large out-of-plane resolution in the short-axis clinical CMR images, we have imposed a basal longitudinal displacement that varies sinusoidally with time. Despite able to obtain reasonable results even with this assumption, having a higher out-of-plane resolution (smaller slice thickness) may obviate the need to impose such an assumption.

Second, sample size in this study is relatively small. A larger sample size will be used in future studies to the increase statistical power.

## CONCLUSION

An advanced image registration method based on continuum mechanics was used to estimate three-dimensional peak circumferential, longitudinal, and radial strain in the bi-ventricular model. By dividing the biventricular unit into LV, RV, and septum, a new perspective was introduced for investigating strain in HFpEF and HFrEF and for studying the physiology of HFpEF disease. Diminishing magnitude in strain components from controls, HFpEF to HFrEF demonstrated subtle functional impairment in the LV and RV in HFpEF patients.

## AUTHOR CONTRIBUTIONS

HZ and LZ contributed to the conception of the hypothesis of the study, implementation of all the analysis, and were involved in the evaluation of the results and preparation of the manuscript. CX contributed to the development of the code and inter-observer variability. XZ contributed to data preparation and analysis. AK and R-ST contributed to patient recruitment and image acquisition. FG and JA contributed to data analysis and statistics. LCL contributed to development of the code and critically revising of the work. MG contributed to development of the code. YS contributed to the evaluation of the results and preparation of the manuscript.

## REFERENCES

Aarsæther, E., Rösner, A., Straumbotn, E., and Busund, R. (2012). Peak longitudinal strain most accurately reflects myocardial segmental viability following acute myocardial infarction - an experimental study in open-chest pigs. *Cardiovasc. Ultrasound* 10:23. doi: 10.1186/1476-7120-10-23

Alnaes, M. S., Blechta, J., Hake, J., Johansson, A., Kehlet, B., Logg, A., et al. (2015). The FEniCS Project Version 1.5. *Arch. Numer. Softw.* 3, 9–23. doi: 10.11588/ans.2015.100.20553

Bayer, J. D., Blake, R. C., Plank, G., and Trayanova, N. A. (2012). A novel rule-based algorithm for assigning myocardial fiber orientation to computational heart models. *Ann. Biomed. Eng.* 40, 2243–2254. doi: 10.1007/s10439-012-0593-5

Borlaug, B. A. (2014). The pathophysiology of heart failure with preserved ejection fraction. *Nat. Rev. Cardiol.* 11, 507–515. doi: 10.1038/nrcardio.2014.83

Borlaug, B. A., Lam, C. S., Roger, V. L., Rodeheffer, R. J., and Redfiled, M. M. (2009). Contractiltiy and ventricular systolic stiffening in hypertensive heart disease: insights into the pathogenesis of heart failure with preserved ejection fraction. *J. Am. Coll. Cardiol.* 54, 410–418. doi: 10.1016/j.jacc.2009.05.013

Buggey, J., Alenezi, F., Yoon, H. J., Phelan, M., DeVore, A. D., Khouri, M. G., et al. (2017). Left ventricular global longitudinal strain in patients with heart failure with preserved ejection fraction: outcomes following an acute heart failure hospitalization. *ESC Heart Fail* 4, 432–439. doi: 10.1002/ehf2.12159

Cameli, M., Righini, F. M., Lisi, M., and Mondillo, S. (2014). Right ventricular strain as a novel approach to analyze right ventricular performance in patients with heart failure. *Heart Fail. Rev.* 19, 603–610. doi: 10.1007/s10741-013-9414-7

Carluccio, E., Biagioli, P., Alunni, G., Murrone, A., Leonelli, V., Pantano, P., et al. (2011). Advantages of deformation indices over systolic velocities in assessment of longitudinal systolic function in patients with heart failure and normal ejection fraction. *Eur. J. Heart Fail.* 13, 292–302. doi: 10.1093/eurjhf/hfq203

Choudhary, N., Duncanson, L., Butler, J., Reichek, N., Vittorio, T., Young, A., et al. (2016). MRI feature trccking strain profiles distinguish patients with left ventricular systolic and diastolic dysfunction with and without clinical heart failure. *J. Cardiovsc. Magn. Reson.* 18:O79. doi: 10.1186/1532-429X-18-S1-O79

Claire, D., Hild, F., and Roux, S. (2004). A finite element formulation to identify damage fields: the equilibrium gap method. *Int. J. Numer. Methods Eng.* 61, 189–208. doi: 10.1002/nme.1057

De Siqueira, M. E. M., Pozo, E., Fernandes, V. R., Sengupta, P. P., Modesto, K., Gupta, S. S., et al. (2016). Characterization and clinical significance of right ventricular mechanics in pulmonary hypertension evaluated with cardiovascular magnetic resonance feature tracking. *J. Cardiovasc. Magn. Reson.* 18, 39. doi: 10.1186/s12968-016-0258-x

Edvardsen, T., and Haugaa, K. H. (2011). Imaging assessment of ventricular mechanics. *Heart* 97, 1349–1356. doi: 10.1136/pgmj.2009.184390rep

Fang, Z. Y., Leano, R., and Marwick, T. H. (2004). Relationship between longitudinal and radial contractility in subclinical diabetic heart disease. *Clin. Sci.* 106, 53–60. doi: 10.1042/CS20030153

Flachskampf, F. A., Biering-Sørensen, T., Solomon, S. D., Duvernoy, O., Bjerner, T., and Smiseth, O. A. (2015). cardiac imaging to evaluate left ventricular diastolic function. *JACC Cardiovasc. Imaging* 8, 1071–1093. doi: 10.1016/j.jcmg.2015.07.004

Genet, M., Chuan Lee, L., Ge, L., Acevedo-Bolton, G., Jeung, N., Martin, A. J., et al. (2015). A novel method for quantifying smooth regional variations in myocardial contractility within an infarcted human left ventricle based on delay-enhanced magnetic resonance imaging. *J. Biomech. Eng.* 137:P081009. doi: 10.1115/1.4030667

Genet, M., Lee, L. C., Baillargeon, B., Guccione, J. M., and Kuhl, E. (2016a). Modeling pathologies of diastolic and systolic heart failure. *Ann. Biomed. Eng.* 44, 112–127. doi: 10.1007/s10439-015-1351-2

Genet, M., Lee, L. C., and Kozerke, S. (2017). "A continuum finite strain formulation of the equilibrium gap regularizer for finite element image correlation," in *Proceedings of 13ème Colloque National en Calcul des Structures (CSMA2017)*, France. Available at: https://hal.archives-ouvertes.fr/hal-01661810

Genet, M., Stoeck, C. T., Deuster, C. V., Lee, L. C., Guccione, J. M., and Kozerke, S. (2016b). "Finite element digital image correlation for cardiac strain analysis from 3D whole-heart tagging," in *Proceedings of the 24rd Annual Meeting of the International Society for Magnetic Resonance in Medicine (ISMRM2016)*, Singapore.

Genet, M., Lee, L. C., Nguyen, R., Haraldsson, H., Acevedo-bolton, G., Zhang, Z., et al. (2014). Distribution of normal human left ventricular myofiber stress at end diastole and end systole: a target for in silico design of heart failure treatments. *J. Appl. Physiol.* 117, 142–152. doi: 10.1152/japplphysiol.00255.2014

Genet, M., Stoeck, C. T., von Deuster, C., Lee, L. C., and Kozerke, S. (2018). Equilibrated warping: finite element image registration with finite strain equilibrium gap regularization. *Med. Image Anal.* 50, 1–22. doi: 10.1016/j.media.2018.07.007

Geuzaine, C., and Remacle, J. F. (2009). Gmsh: a 3-D finite element mesh generator with built-in pre- and post-processing facilities. *Int. J. Numer. Methods Eng.* 79, 1309–1331. doi: 10.1002/nme.2579

Gorter, T. M., Hoendermis, E. S., van Veldhuisen, D. J., Voors, A. A., Lam, C. S. P., Geelhoed, B., et al. (2016). Right ventricular dysfunction in heart failure with preserved ejection fraction: a systematic review and meta-analysis. *Eur. J. Heart Fail.* 18, 1472–1487. doi: 10.1002/ejhf.630

Haddad, F., Hunt, S. A., Rosenthal, D. N., and Murphy, D. J. (2008). Right ventricular function in cardiovascular disease, part I: anatomy, physiology, aging, and functional assessment of the right ventricle. *Circulation* 117, 1436–1448. doi: 10.1161/CIRCULATIONAHA.107.653576

Hogg, K., Swedberg, K., and McMurray, J. (2004). Heart failure with preserved left ventricular systolic function: epidemiology, clinical characteristics, and prognosis. *J. Am. Coll. Cardiol.* 43, 317–327.

Hussein, R. S., Ibrahim, A. S., Abd El-Hameed, A. M., El-Fiky, A. A., and Tantawy, W. H. (2013). Does CMR have an additive role over echo in evaluating ischemic LV dysfunction? *Egypt. J. Radiol. Nucl. Med.* 44, 475–482. doi: 10.1016/j.ejrnm.2013.06.004

Kanwar, M., Walter, C., Clarke, M., and Patarroyo-Aponte, M. (2016). Targeting heart failure with preserved ejection fraction: current status and future prospects. *Vasc. Health Risk Manag.* 12, 129–141. doi: 10.2147/VHRM.S83662

Kleijn, S. A., Brouwer, W. P., Aly, M. F. A., Rüssel, I. K., De Roest, G. J., Beek, A. M., et al. (2012). Comparison between three-dimensional speckle-tracking echocardiography and cardiac magnetic resonance imaging for quantification of left ventricular volumes and function. *Eur. Heart J. Cardiovasc. Imaging* 13, 834–839. doi: 10.1093/ehjci/jes030

Koh, A. S., Gao, F., Leng, S., Kovalik, J.-P., Zhao, X., Tan, R. S., et al. (2018). Dissecting clinical and metabolomics associations of left atrial phasic function by cardiac magnetic resonance feature tracking. *Sci. Rep.* 8:8138. doi: 10.1038/s41598-018-26456-8

Koyama, J., Ray-Sequin, P. A., and Falk, R. H. (2003). Longitudinal myocardial function assessed by tissue velocity, strain, and strain rate tissue doppler echocardiography in patients with AL (primary) cardiac amyloidosis. *Circulation* 107, 2446–2452. doi: 10.1161/01.CIR.0000068313.67758.4F

Kraigher-Krainer, E., Shah, A. M., Gupta, D. K., Santos, A., Claggett, B., Pieske, B., et al. (2014). Impaired systolic function by strain imaging in heart failure with preserved ejection fraction. *J. Am. Coll. Cardiol.* 63, 447–456. doi: 10.1016/j.jacc.2013.09.052

Leng, S., Jiang, M., Zhao, X.-D., Allen, J. C., Kassab, G. S., Ouyang, R.-Z., et al. (2016). Three-dimensional tricuspid annular motion analysis from cardiac magnetic resonance feature-tracking. *Ann. Biomed. Eng.* 44, 3522–3538. doi: 10.1007/s10439-016-1695-2

Leng, S., Zhao, X.-D., Huang, F.-Q., Wong, J.-J., Su, B.-Y., Allen, J. C., et al. (2015). Automated quantitative assessment of cardiovascular magnetic resonance-derived atrioventricular junction velocities. *Am. J. Physiol. Heart Circ. Physiol.* 309, H1923–H1935. doi: 10.1152/ajpheart.00284.2015

Lo, C., Lai, Y., Wu, J., Yun, C., Hung, C., Bulwer, B. E., et al. (2013). Cardiac systolic mechanics in heart failure with preserved ejection fraction: new insights and controversies. *Acta Cardiol. Sin.* 29, 515–523.

Logg, A., Mardal, K., and Wells, G. (2012). *Fenics: Automated Solution of Differential Equations by the Finite Element Method*. Heidelberg: Springer. doi: 10.1007/978-3-642-23099-8

MacIver, D. H. (2008). A mathematical model of left ventricular contraction and its application in heart disease. *WIT Trans. State Art Sci. Eng.* 35, 65–86. doi: 10.2495/978-1-84564-096-5/04

MacIver, D. H. (2011). A new method for quantification of left ventricular systolic function using a corrected ejection fraction. *Eur. J. Echocardiogr.* 12, 228–234. doi: 10.1093/ejechocard/jeq185

Maciver, D. H., Adeniran, I., and Zhang, H. (2015). Left ventricular ejection fraction is determined by both global myocardial strain and wall thickness. *Ijcha* 7, 113–118. doi: 10.1016/j.ijcha.2015.03.007

MacIver, D. H., and Townsend, M. (2007). A novel mechanism of heart failure with normal ejection fraction. *Heart* 94, 446–449. doi: 10.1136/hrt.2006.114082

Mangion, K., Gao, H., McComb, C., Carrick, D., Clerfond, G., Zhong, X., et al. (2016). A novel method for estimating myocardial strain: assessment of deformation tracking against reference magnetic resonance methods in healthy volunteers. *Sci. Rep.* 6:38774. doi: 10.1038/srep38774

Mansi, T., Pennec, X., Sermesant, M., Delingette, H., and Ayache, N. (2011). ILogDemons: a demons-based registration algorithm for tracking incompressible elastic biological tissues. *Int. J. Comput. Vis.* 92, 92–111. doi: 10.1007/s11263-010-0405-z

Marcelo, F. D. C., Tal, G., and Ravin, D. (2016). The future of cardiovascular imaging. *Circulation* 133, 2640–2661. doi: 10.116/circulationaha.116.023511

Melenovsky, V., Hwang, S.-J., Lin, G., Redfield, M. M., and Borlaug, B. A. (2014). Right heart dysfunction in heart failure with preserved ejection fraction. *Eur. Heart J.* 35, 3452–3462. doi: 10.1093/eurheartj/ehu193

Meris, A., Faletra, F., Conca, C., Klersy, C., Regoli, F., Klimusina, J., et al. (2010). Timing and magnitude of regional right ventricular function: a speckle tracking-derived strain study of normal subjects and patients with right ventricular dysfunction. *J. Am. Soc. Echocardiogr.* 23, 823–831. doi: 10.1016/j.echo.2010.05.009

Mohammed, S. F., Hussain, I., AbouEzzeddine, O. F., Abou Ezzeddine, O. F., Takahama, H., Kwon, S. H., et al. (2014). Right ventricular function in heart failure with preserved ejection fraction: a community-based study. *Circulation* 130, 2310–2320. doi: 10.1161/CIRCULATIONAHA.113.008461

Paulus, W. J., Tschöpe, C., Sanderson, J. E., Rusconi, C., Flachskampf, F. A., Rademakers, F. E., et al. (2007). How to diagnose diastolic heart failure: A consensus statement on the diagnosis of heart failure with normal left ventricular ejection fraction by the heart failure and echocardiography associations of the european society of cardiology. *Eur. Heart J.* 28, 2539–2550. doi: 10.1093/eurheartj/ehm037

Peng, J., Zhao, X., Zhao, L., Fan, Z., Wang, Z., Chen, H., et al. (2018). Normal values of myocardial deformation assessed by cardiovascular magnetic resonance feature tracking in a healthy chinese population: a multicenter study. *Front. Physiol.* 9:1181. doi: 10.3389/fphys.2018.01181

Phatak, N. S., Maas, S. A., Veress, A. I., Pack, N. A., Di, E. V. R., and Weiss, J. A. (2009). Strain measurement in the left ventricle during systole with deformable image registration q. *Med. Image Anal.* 13, 354–361. doi: 10.1016/j.media.2008.07.004

Rabbitt, R. D., Weiss, J. A., Christensen, G. E., Inst, M., Louis, S., and Miller, M. I. (1995). Mapping of hyperelastic deformable templates using the finite element method. *Proc. SPIE* 2573, 252–265.

Taylor, R. J., Moody, W. E., Umar, F., Edwards, N. C., Taylor, T. J., Stegemann, B., et al. (2015). Myocardial strain measurement with feature-tracking cardiovascular magnetic resonance: normal values. *Eur. Heart J. Cardiovasc. Imaging* 16, 871–881. doi: 10.1093/ehjci/jev006

Veress, A. I., Gullberg, G. T., and Weiss, J. A. (2005). Measurement of strain in the left ventricle with cine-MRI and deformable image registration. *J. Biomech. Eng.* 127, 1195–1207. doi: 10.1115/1.2073677

Veress, A. I., Klein, G., and Gullberg, G. T. (2013). A comparison of hyperelastic warping of pet images with tagged MRI for the analysis of cardiac deformation. *Int. J. Biomed. Imaging* 2013:728624. doi: 10.1155/2013/728624

Veress, A. I., Weiss, J. A., Huesman, R. H., Reutter, B. W., Scott, E., Sitek, A., et al. (2008). Measuring Regional Changes in the Diastolic Deformation of the Left Ventricle of SHR Rats Using microPET Technology and Hyperelastic Warping. *Ann. Biomed. Eng.* 36, 1104–1117.

Veress, A. I., Weiss, J. A., Klein, G. J., Gullberg, G. T., and Berkeley, L. (2002). "Quantification' of 3D left ventricular deformation using hyperelastic warping: comparisons between MRI and PET imaging," in *Proceedings of the Computers in Cardiology* (Memphis, TN: IEEE), 709–712. doi: 10.1109/CIC.2002.1166871

Vitarelli, A., Mangieri, E., Terzano, C., Gaudio, C., Salsano, F., Rosato, E., et al. (2015). Three-dimensional echocardiography and 2D-3D speckle-tracking imaging in chronic pulmonary hypertension: Diagnostic accuracy in detecting hemodynamic signs of right ventricular (RV) failure. *J. Am. Heart Assoc.* 4, 1–14. doi: 10.1161/JAHA.114.001584

Wang, J., Khoury, D. S., Yue, Y., Torre-Amione, G., and Nagueh, S. F. (2008). Preserved left ventricular twist and circumferential deformation, but depressed longitudinal and radial deformation in patients with diastolic heart failure. *Eur. Heart J.* 29, 1283–1289. doi: 10.1093/eurheartj/ehn141

Xi, C., Latnie, C., Zhao, X., Tan, J., Le Wall, S. T., Genet, M., et al. (2016). Patient-specific computational analysis of ventricular mechanics in pulmonary arterial hypertension. *J. Biomech. Eng.* 138, 1–9. doi: 10.1115/1.4034559

Yip, G. W.-K., Zhang, Q., Xie, J.-M., Liang, Y.-J., Liu, Y.-M., Yan, B., et al. (2011). Resting global and regional left ventricular contractility in patients with heart failure and normal ejection fraction: insights from speckle-tracking echocardiography. *Heart* 97, 287–294. doi: 10.1136/hrt.2010.205815

Zhong, L., Gobeawan, L., Su, Y., Tan, J.-L., Ghista, D., Chua, T., et al. (2012). Right ventricular regional wall curvedness and area strain in patients with repaired tetralogy of Fallot. *Am. J. Physiol. Heart Circ. Physiol.* 302, H1306–H1316. doi: 10.1152/ajpheart.00679.2011

Zhong, L., Ng, K. K., Sim, L. L., Allen, J. C., Lau, Y. H., Sim, D. K., et al. (2013). Myocardial contractile dysfunction associated with increased 3-month and 1-year mortality in hospitalized patients with heart failure and preserved ejection fraction. *Int. J. Cardiol.* 168, 1975–1983. doi: 10.1016/j.ijcard.2012.12.084

Zhong, L., Poh, K. K., Lee, L. C., Le, T. T., and Tan, R. S. (2011). Attenuation of stress-based ventricular contractility in patients with heart failure and normal ejection fraction. *Ann. Acad. Med. Singapore* 40, 179–185.

Zou, H., Zhao, X., Ce, X., Lee, L. C., Genet, M., Su, Y., et al. (2016). "Characterization of patient - specific biventricular mechanics in heart failure with preserved ejection fraction: hyperelastic warping," in *Proceedings of the 38th Annual International Conference of the IEEE Engineering in Medicine and Biology Society (EMBC)*, Orlando, FL, 4149–4152.

# 10

# Electrical Conductance Device for Stent Sizing

*Ghassan S. Kassab\**

*California Medical Innovations Institute, San Diego, CA, United States*

*\*Correspondence:*
*Ghassan S. Kassab*
*gkassab@calmi2.org*

The minimum stent area (MSA) has been clinically established as a significant predictor of restenosis, thrombosis, and ischemia using intra-vascular ultrasound (IVUS). Unfortunately, IVUS measurements are far from routine because of significant cost of IVUS, the training required, the subjectivity of image interpretation and the time added to the procedure. The objective of this study is to verify the accuracy of a conductance catheter for stent sizing. Here, we introduce an easy and entirely objective device and method for real time determination of MSA. A 10 kHz, 35 μA rms current is passed through the external electrodes of an intravascular catheter while the conductance is measured across a separate set of electrodes. Both phantom and *ex vivo* validations of metal stent sizing in five porcine carotid arteries were confirmed. The accuracy of the measurements were found to be excellent in phantoms (root mean square, rms, of 3.4% of actual value) and in *ex-vivo* vessels (rms = 3.2% of measured value). An offset of conductance occurs when a conductive metal stent (e.g., bare metal stent) is deployed in the vessel, while the slope remains the same. This offset is absent in the case of drug eluting stent where the metal is coated (i.e., insulated) or non-metal bioresorbable stent. The present device makes easy, accurate and reproducible measurements of the size of stented blood vessels within 3.2% rms error. This device provides an alternative method to sizing of stent (i.e., MSA) in real-time without subjective interpretation and with less cost than IVUS.

Keywords: minimum stent area, lumen sizing, diameter, conductance catheter, drug eluting stents

## INTRODUCTION

Many studies have shown that the minimum stent area (MSA) is an important predictor of prognosis and later events such as restenosis, thrombosis, myocardial ischemia, and so on (Kasaoka et al., 1998; Wu et al., 2003; Fujii et al., 2004, 2005). This observation has led to the notion of "bigger is better" (Di Mario and Karvouni, 2000). The limit to such larger size is, of course, vessel injury, dissection and edge stenosis when the vessel is overly distended. Hence, it is clinically important to determine the MSA accurately.

Angiography, intra-vascular ultrasound (IVUS) and optical coherence tomography (OCT) are techniques than can be currently used to determine the size of a vessel after stenting. A difficulty with angiography is the poor resolution with the two-dimensional view, typically obtained from a single x-ray projection. Furthermore, trapping of contrast agent near the stent lattice often creates hazing or fuzziness in the angiogram, which further reduces the accuracy of measurement (Ziada et al., 1997; Grewal et al., 2001). IVUS, on the other hand, is more accurate and reliable. Other factors, however, limit its routine clinical use. The cost of IVUS (device and console), the significant training required, and the subjectivity of image interpretation have significantly limited its usage to less than 20% of routine procedures despite being on the market for over 20 years. Finally, OCT is primarily used as a research tool for high spatial resolution images to assess the interaction of struts with vessel wall but has limited penetration and is even more expensive than IVUS. Hence, it is desirable to introduce easier, more cost effective and entirely objective tools for MSA measurements to improve clinical outcome.

Kassab (Kassab et al., 2005, 2009; Hermiller et al., 2011; Nair et al., 2018) introduced an impedance catheter and guidewires that allows real time vessel lumen sizing based on an electric impedance principle. These devices were validated in silico, *in vitro* and *in vivo* in swine (Kassab et al., 2005, 2009) and patients (Hermiller et al., 2011; Nair et al., 2018). As a proof of concept, we modify the catheter and technique of determining vessel size in the presence of a stent (typically a metal; either bare metal or drug coated). It is noted that contact of the impedance electrodes with bare metal stent (BMS) can cause electrical shorting of signal and significant resulting noise, which prohibits accurate measurements. Furthermore, the presence of a bare metal in the measurement field also affects the conductance and introduces an offset. The present study proposes solutions to overcome these issues. The major conclusion is that, with a small modification of the catheter, accurate measurements of MSA can be made with the current device. Since most stents used clinical are drug eluting (coated and hence electrically insulated), no modification of the device is needed as described below.

## MATERIALS AND METHODS

### Design Modification of Impedance Catheter for Stent Sizing

The impedance catheters were similar to those used in previous studies (Kassab et al., 2005). Four holes were made in the catheter 5 mm, 9 mm, 10 mm, and 14 mm from the tip (i.e., 4-1-4 mm spacings). One insulated wire was threaded through each hole. The portion of the wire exposed through each hole was then stripped of its insulation and wrapped around the catheter. Previously, the four electrodes were exposed at the surface of the catheter where direct contact with stent was possible. In the present study, a design was proposed where grooves are made into the catheter such that the wires were made sub-surface as shown in **Figure 1**. This design decreases surface contact of wires or electrodes with the stent while allowing the necessary exposure for the conducting electrode in the measurement field.

The exteriorized portions of the four wires through the lumen were connected to an electronic conductance module constructed in our laboratory. This module drives a 10 kHz, 35 μA (root mean squared, rms) constant current between the two outermost electrodes and measures the resultant voltage between the two inner electrodes. The voltage detected, moderated in amplitude by the impedance change through the NaCl solution, has a frequency of approximately 10 kHz. The data acquisition rate has a frequency of 10 kHz, with current injected and detected voltage channels.

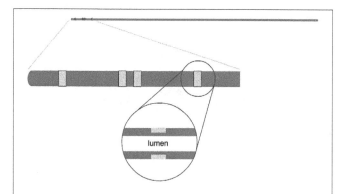

**FIGURE 1 |** An illustration of an impedance catheter where the four electrodes are spaced at the tip (two inner and two outer electrodes) in the top panel; a zoom of the embedded portion of the electrode arrangement is shown in the middle panel; and a further zoom of the wire tunneling is shown in the lower panel.

## Conductivity of Fluid and Stent

A calibration of known CSA was made in four acrylic tubes with sizes ranging from 2.5 mm to 5.0 mm in diameter. The catheter was placed in each of the four tubes. All four tubes were filled with either 0.45 or 0.9% NaCl solutions at room temperature. By using the voltage reading from the catheter, the conductivity, $\sigma$, of both NaCl solutions was determined by plotting the conductance, $G$, against $CSA/L$ ($G = a.CSA/L$ where L is the distance between the inner electrodes). The calibration was then repeated with a stainless steel Jostent (316L stent, Jomed) embedded within each tube. The conductance readings were plotted in order to determine the effect of stent.

## Stent CSA in Tygon Tubing

The CSA measurements were taken with the catheter placed in the lumen of each tube with known CSA containing a stent. The conductivity was determined for each solution as described above and the measured conductance was adjusted to accommodate for the offset caused by the stent. The CSA was then calculated using $CSA = G \cdot L/s$.

## Stent CSA in *ex-vivo* Vessels

The lumped cylindrical model that relates the conductance, $G$ ($G = I/V$, ratio of current to voltage), to the CSA as:

$$G = \sigma \cdot CSA/L \qquad (1)$$

holds if the electrical current is insulated within the cylinder. It is known that the vessel wall and any surrounding tissue are conductive, however, and will cause an offset error from current leakage known as the effective parallel conductance, $G_p$. Since $G_p$ is constant at any given position on a vessel, using two different concentrations of NaCl solutions will result in the desired relation as:

$$CSA(t) = L[G_2(t) - G_1(t)]/[\sigma_2 - \sigma_1] \qquad (2a)$$

where "1" and "2" refers to 0.45% and 0.9% NaCl solutions with specific conductivities $\sigma_1$ and $\sigma_2$. If we assume that the vessel has a circular cross-section, we can compute the diameter as $D = (4CSA/\pi)^{1/2}$; namely,

$$D(t) = \left( \frac{4L}{\pi} \frac{\Delta G(t)}{\Delta \sigma} \right)^{\frac{1}{2}} \qquad (2b)$$

where $\Delta$ represents the difference in a quantity for the two injections.

Five porcine carotid arteries were harvested from a local slaughter house to validate the stent sizing in *ex-vivo* vessels. The isolated carotid vessels were stored in 0.9% saline solution at 4°C. The carotid artery was cannulated with 6 Fr sheaths on both ends with one end connected to a pressure transducer. The stent was first deployed within the vessel and the catheter was then inserted through the sheath into the lumen of the artery as shown in **Figure 2**. The vessel was perfused with approximately 5 ml of 0.9% followed by 0.45% NaCl solutions. Each infusion was used to pressurize the vessel from 20 to 120 mmHg in increments of 20 mmHg for each solution. The pressurization to change the diameter of vessel was done by hand using a syringe connected to the second sheath. During pressurization, the vessel was placed under a camera to measure the outer diameter during inflation. By using the conductivities of different NaCl (0.45 and 0.9%) solutions with and without the stent and the conductance value for each solution, the CSA was determined by Eq. (2a) at each pressure. The diameter of the stented vessel was subsequently computed from Eq. (2b).

At the completion of experiment, a ring of the artery of 1 mm in thickness was obtained at the site of the detection leads of the catheter. A photo of the no-load (zero pressure) ring was taken under a dissection microscope and the no-load CSA of the vessel ($CSA^{nl}$) was measured. Assuming incompressibility, the inner diameter of the vessel during pressurization was obtained from the outer diameter measurements described above. For a cylindrical vessel, the incompressibility assumption can be stated as:

$$D_i = \sqrt{D_o^2 - \frac{4CSA^{nl}}{\pi \lambda_z}} \qquad (3)$$

where $D_o$, $CSA^{nl}$ and $\lambda_z$ are outer radii at the loaded state, wall area in the no-load state, and the axial stretch ratio, respectively. Hence, the lumen diameter or CSA ($CSA = pD^2/4$ for a cylindrical vessel) determined from equation [3] was directly compared with the impedance measurements.

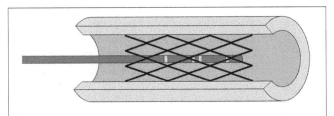

**FIGURE 2 |** A schematic of an impedance catheter in the lumen of a stented vessel.

## CSA for Various Stent Metal Coils

In addition to actual stents, we used several wires to examine different stent metals with varying conductivities. Tungsten and stainless-steel type 316 wires of 0.25 mm diameter were shaped to a 2 cm long coil with approximately one full loop every 5 mm. The diameter of the coil was 3.5 mm for each type of metal and the experiments were repeated similar to those involving stents as described earlier.

## Drug Coated Stents *in vivo*

We also considered 3 drug eluting stents, DES (Xience, Abbott) deployed in swine (n = 2). The 3 mm stents were deployed at nominal pressure as suggested by manufacture's chart as per our previous studies (Chen et al., 2011). These animals were used from other acute studies to maximize animal use. Briefly, normal male swine (60-65 Kg body weight) had expired DES deployed in each of three coronary arteries (RCA, LAD and LCx). The animal studies were approved by the Institutional Animal Care and Use Committee of Indiana University and complied fully with the Guide for the Care and Use of Laboratory Animals published by the National Research Council. After deployment of stent recommended diameter, IVUS was used to measure the diameter of the stent for comparison with the conductance measurements. The procedures and methods were the same as those reported in Ref. 9.

## Statistical Analysis

The relation between phantom (P) or optical (O) and impedance (I) diameter measurements were expressed by $D_{PorO} = \alpha D_I + \beta$ where $\alpha$ and $\beta$ are empirical constants that were determined with linear least squares fit and a corresponding correlation coefficient $R^2$. In a Bland-Altman scatter diagram, we plotted the percent differences between the two measurements of diameter $\left( \frac{D_{PorO} - D_I}{D_{PorO}} \times 100 \right)$ against their means $\left( \frac{D_{PorO} + D_I}{2} \right)$. In the scatter diagram, the precison and bias of the method can be quantified. We also determined the root mean squares (rms) error to further assess the reliability of the technique.

## RESULTS

### Conductivity of Saline and Stent

**Figure 3A** shows the conductance measured by the catheter for each CSA in 0.45% and 0.9% NaCl solutions. A saline only calibration was used as a baseline run to show that the 0.9% saline has a higher (approximately 2 times) conductivity (slope) than the 0.45% saline solution. The NaCl measurements have a nearly zero offset (intercept) in the conductance readings. The calibration of NaCl in the presence of stent showed no change in conductivity (slope) of both solutions but resulted in an offset of about 3 mS for the stainless-steel stent as shown in **Figure 3B**. The two graphs were superimposed to demonstrate that when normalizing for the offset (i.e., subtract the intercepts from **Figures 3A,B**), the stent calibration is nearly identical to the saline calibration (**Figure 3C**).

The saline and stent calibrations were done with four catheters (3Fr and 4Fr) where the conductivity (slope) was unchanged with

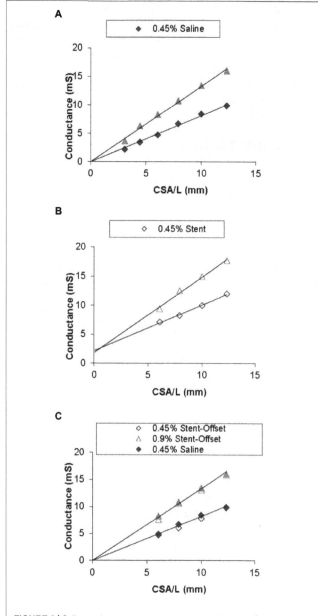

**FIGURE 3 |** Saline and stent calibrations of 0.45 and 0.9% NaCl solutions. Graph **(A)** shows conductance values for each corresponding CSA in acrylic tubes filled with saline only. Graph **(B)** shows the values with the stent embedded in each of the tubes. Graph **(C)** shows both saline only and stent values with normalized offsets. Lines of best fit are shown in Graphs **(A)** and **(B)**.

or without the stent. The conductance offsets of $3.2 \pm 1.2$ and $3.3 \pm 0.72$ for the 0.45% and 0.9% NaCl solutions, respectively, were significantly different from zero in the presence of stent (BMS).

## Stent CSA in Tygon Tubing

Four catheters were placed in five different sized Tygon tubing with the deployed stent to determine the stented diameter. Although the diameter measurements were made with both NaCl

solutions, the difference was not significant and the average from both solutions was used. **Figure 4A** shows the phantom diameter measured by the catheter as compared to the diameter measured with a caliper. To determine the agreement between the two methods, we made a Bland-Altman plot of the percent difference in diameters between the two methods against their mean values. **Figure 4B** shows the Bland-Altman plot where the mean and SD were found to be 0.25 and 4.2, respectively. The upper and lower dotted lines represent mean+2SD (8.6%) and mean-2SD (-8.1%), respectively. The rms error for the impedance measurements was 3.4% of the phantom diameter.

## Stent CSA in *ex vivo* Vessels

**Figure 5A** shows the relationship between carotid vessel diameters measured by impedance and optical methods. The correlation coefficient for the relationship between impedance and optical measurements was 0.946, with a slope and intercept of 1.01 and 0.034, respectively. **Figure 5B** shows the Bland-Altman plot where the mean and SD were found to be 0.37 and 3.4, respectively. The upper and lower dotted lines represent mean+2SD (6.8%) and mean-2SD (-6.0%), respectively. The rms error for the impedance measurements was 3.2% of the vessel diameter.

## CSA for Various Stent Metal Coils

The calibrations with metal (stainless steel and tungsten) coils show that the slopes remain the same (**Table 1**). There were also no differences in the offsets in relation to the NaCl (0.45 or 0.9%) solutions used as shown in **Table 1**. There were differences in the offsets, however, for the two metals. The stainless-steel coil offsets the conductance readings by about 4 mS in four catheters, while the tungsten coil records an offset of 45 mS. Hence, the more conductive tungsten material shows a significantly higher conductance offset (an order of magnitude) than stainless steel ($p < 0.00001$).

## DES Stent CSA in *in-vivo* Vessels

In the stents used, the differences between the conductance catheter measurements and IVUS were 8.2%. We had also confirmed that the drug coated stents were not conductive and did not produce any offset as observed with BMS or stent metal coils. Hence, the two animal studies in 3 coronary arteries were purely confirmatory.

## DISCUSSION

Although stenting reduces acute complications and restenosis as compared to balloon angioplasty, in stent restenosis (ISR) remains an important clinical problem (Chen et al., 2011). Studies suggest that a significant number of ISR lesions contain inadequately expanded stents (Schiele, 2005). Furthermore, stent underexpansion is a significant cause of failure after sirolimus-eluting stent (SES) treatment (Fujii et al., 2004). IVUS studies show that an MSA < 5 mm$^2$ was the optimal threshold to predict target-lesion reascularization after treatment of de novo lesions

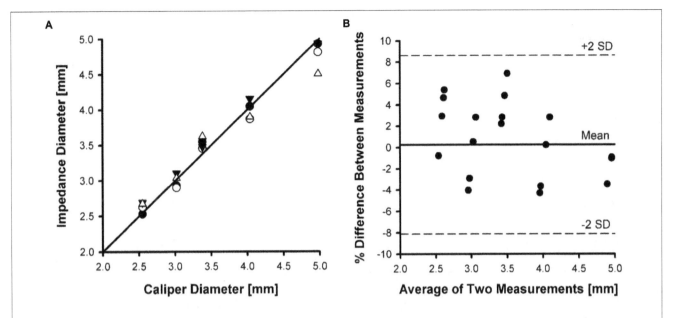

**FIGURE 4 |** Phantom diameter measurements determined using impedance catheters versus a caliper. Four catheters were tested in five different tubing sizes. **(A)** A line of identity shown between caliper diameter and impedance diameter measurements. **(B)** A Bland-Altman plot of mean of diameter measurements versus percent difference in measurements.

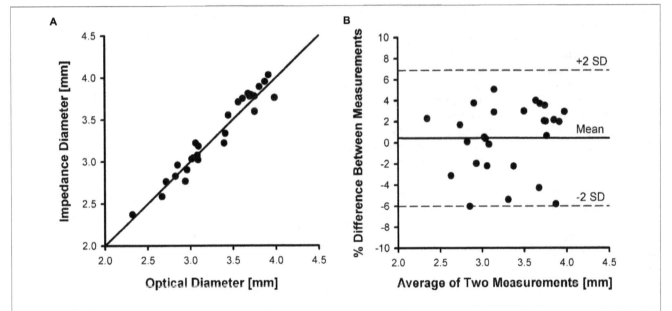

**FIGURE 5 |** Inner diameters of five pig carotid arteries measured by impedance catheters versus diameters measured optically. Each artery was pressurized from 20 to 120 mmHg in increments of 20 mmHg during measurements. **(A)** The line of identity between optical diameter and impedance diameter measurements. **(B)** A Bland-Altman plot of mean of diameter measurements versus percent difference in measurements.

with SES (Fitzgerald et al., 2000). MSA > 5 mm$^2$ predicted long-term patency after treatment of de novo lesions with SES (Fujii et al., 2004, 2005).

Despite the utility of IVUS in the assessment of MSA, it has several shortcomings which limit its routine use in the catheterization laboratory. It requires advancement of a relatively expensive IVUS catheter connected to an expensive apparatus. It also adds longer procedure time and longer fluoroscopic

time, increases the use of contrast material (Chen et al., 2011) and increases the risk of dissection, thrombosis, spasm and acute occlusion during catheter manipulation (Hausmann et al., 1995; Sonoda et al., 2004). Furthermore, it is not unusual that the relatively bulky IVUS catheter cannot be advanced across a lesion due to high grade stenosis, vessel tortuousity or calcification. Finally, since the impedance electrodes can be implanted within a workhorse guidewire (Nair et al., 2018),

**TABLE 1** | The calibration slope and offset of the impedance catheter in NaCl and NaCl plus wire coil (stainless steel and tungsten).

**Stainless Steel (SS)**

|  | 0.45% NaCl | 0.45%NaCl w/ SS | 0.9% NaCl | 0.9%NaCl w/ SS |
|---|---|---|---|---|
| Slope | $1.1 \pm 0.17$ | $1.1 \pm 0.11$ | $1.9 \pm 0.31$ | $1.9 \pm 0.25$ |
| Offset | $-0.47 \pm 0.18$ | $3.8 \pm 1.5$ | $-1.1 \pm 0.71$ | $3.1 \pm 1.8$ |

**Tungsten (T)**

|  | 0.45% NaCl | 0.45%NaCl w/T | 0.9% NaCl | 0.9%NaCl w/T |
|---|---|---|---|---|
| Slope | $1.2 \pm 0.28$ | $1.1 \pm 0.26$ | $1.8 \pm 0.41$ | $1.9 \pm 0.35$ |
| Offset | $-0.78 \pm 0.17$ | $45 \pm 5.6$ | $-0.84 \pm 1.6$ | $46 \pm 6.4$ |

*The values are mean ± SD.*

it is not necessary to change catheters such as with the use of IVUS.

The present device makes easy, accurate and reproducible measurements of the size of stented blood vessels within clinically acceptable error. This enables the determination of MSA with higher accuracy using previously published methods (Kassab et al., 2005, 2009; Hermiller et al., 2011; Nair et al., 2018). The present catheter addresses two key issues that are resolved by modification of the previous device design. First, the four electrodes were exposed at the surface of the catheter where direct contact with stent was possible (Kassab et al., 2005, 2009; Hermiller et al., 2011; Nair et al., 2018). In the present study, a design is implemented where grooves are made into the catheter such that the wires are made sub-surface as shown in **Figure 1**. This design decreases surface contact of wires or electrodes with the stent while allowing the necessary exposure for the conducting electrode in the measurement field.

The second issue addressed here relates to the offset creates by the presence of the stent in the vessel lumen. Previously, it was shown that sizing (cross-sectional area, CSA) is related to the ratio of change in conductance to change in conductivity (slope of the conductivity-conductance relation). **Figure 3A** shows the CSA/L-conductance relationship, which is expected to be linear with zero intercept (Eq. 1). The slope of **Figure 3A** corresponds to the conductivity s. **Figure 3B** shows the same relation in the presence of a stent. It is apparent that the slope of the curve remains unchanged but there is an offset that reflects the conductivity of the stent. Although the conductivity of the metal itself may vary, this will not affect the measurements as the slope which determines the CSA (Eq. 2) remains unchanged. In conclusion, the presence of a stent does not affect the sizing accuracy of the impedance catheter (errors < 5%) as shown in **Figures 4, 5**. The change of offset is inconsequential for the sizing utility of the conductance technology.

Although we used BMS and conductive stent metal to consider the worst-case scenario, current clinical stents are either DES or bio-resorbable stents which, in either case, are not conductive and hence would not present any offset or conductive issues for measurements. Since the strut thickness is relatively small, the sizing measurements is essentially that of lumen area or MSA. Furthermore, although the measurements were made on

a conductance catheter, the methodology presented is completely translatable to a sizing guidewire as shown in peripheral arteries of animals and patients (Svendsen et al., 2014b; Nair et al., 2018). For example, our peripheral guidewire can size the Supera (Abbott) or the Viabahn (Gore) as neither of these devices is electrically conductive.

## Limitations of Study

As with any technology, the conductance method has limitations. First, the electrical conductivity measurements of lumen size cannot confirm stent apposition (i.e., this method is non-tomographic and hence does not allow visualization of relation between struts and vessel wall at the current state). A sizing post-dilation method using the same electrical platform technology can be used to address this issue for coronary or peripheral applications (Svendsen et al., 2014a, 2015). Second, the saline injections (although routine in the clinic) do add steps to the procedure. An injection-less method is possible with the current technology where feasibility has been recently demonstrated (Dabiri and Kassab, 2018). Finally, the comparison of accuracy is made in comparison with IVUS. Ultimately, a clinical outcome study may be necessary to establish the clinical utility of this technology similar to IVUS studies (Zhang et al., 2018).

## SUMMARY

We validated a conductance device that allows accurate sizing of the stent vessel. Undoubtedly, a workhorse guidewire that allows reliable and accurate assessment of coronary and peripheral stent area may provide a powerful treatment tool for the interventionalist. This may improve clinical outcomes by ensuring the desired MSA without over-distension which should lead to better clinical outcome.

## AUTHOR CONTRIBUTIONS

The author confirms being the sole contributor of this work and has approved it for publication.

# REFERENCES

Chen, H. Y., Sinha, A. K., Choy, J. S., Zheng, H., Sturek, M., Bigelow, B., et al. (2011). Mis-sizing of stent promotes intimal hyperplasia: impact of endothelial shear and intramural stress. *Am. J. Physiol. Heart Circ. Physiol.* 301, H2254–H2263. doi: 10.1152/ajpheart.00240.2011

Dabiri, A., and Kassab, G. S. (2018). Injection-less conductance method for vascular sizing. *Front. Physiol.* 9:371. doi: 10.3389/fphys.2018.00371

Di Mario, C., and Karvouni, E. (2000). The bigger, the better: true also for in-stent restenosis? *Eur. Heart J.* 21, 710–711. doi: 10.1053/euhj.1999.2021

Fitzgerald, P. J., Oshima, A., Hayase, M., Metz, J. A., Bailey, S. R., Baim, D. S., et al. (2000). Final results of the can routine ultrasound influence stent expansion (CRUISE) study. *Circulation* 102, 523–530. doi: 10.1161/01.CIR.102.5.523

Fujii, K., Carlier, S. G., Mintz, G. S., Yang, Y. M., Moussa, I., Weisz, G., et al. (2005). Stent underexpansion and residual reference segment stenosis are related to stent thrombosis after sirolimus-eluting stent implantation: an intravascular ultrasound study. *J. Am. Coll. Cardiol.* 45, 995–998. doi: 10.1016/j.jacc.2004.12.066

Fujii, K., Mintz, G. S., Kobayashi, Y., Carlier, S. G., Takebayashi, H., Yasuda, T., et al. (2004). Contribution of stent underexpansion to recurrence after sirolimus-eluting stent implantation for in-stent restenosis. *Circulation* 109, 1085–1088. doi: 10.1161/01.CIR.0000121327.67756.19

Grewal, J., Ganz, P., Selwyn, A., and Kinlay, S. (2001). Usefulness of intravascular ultrasound in preventing stenting of hazy areas adjacent to coronary stents and its support of support spot-stenting. *Am. J. Cardiol.* 87, 1246–1249. doi: 10.1016/S0002-9149(01)01513-2

Hausmann, D., Erbel, R., Alibelli-Chemarin, M. J., Boksch, W., Caracciolo, E., Cohn, J. M., et al. (1995). The safety of intracoronary ultrasound. A multicenter survey of 2207 examinations. *Circulation* 91, 623–630.

Hermiller, J., Choy, J. S., Svendsen, M., Bigelow, B., Fouts, A., Hall, J., et al. (2011). A non-imaging catheter for measurement of coronary artery lumen area: a first in man pilot study. *Catheter. Cardiovasc. Interv.* 78, 202–210. doi: 10.1002/ccd.22842

Kasaoka, S., Tobis, J. M., Akiyama, T., Reimers, B., Di Mario, C., Wong, N. D., et al. (1998). Angiographic and intravascular ultrasound predictors of in-stent restenosis. *J. Am. Coll. Cardiol.* 32, 1630–1635. doi: 10.1016/S0735-1097(98)00404-5

Kassab, G. S., Choy, J. S., Svendsen, M., Sinha, A. K., Alloosh, M., Sturek, M., et al. (2009). A novel system for lumen reconstruction of coronary arteries in real-time: a preclinical validation. *Am. J. Physiol. Heart Circ. Physiol.* 297, H485–H492. doi: 10.1152/ajpheart.01224.2008

Kassab, G. S., Lontis, E. R., Horlyck, A., and Gregersen, H. (2005). Novel method for measurement of medium size arterial lumen area with an impedance catheter: in vivo validation. *Am. J. Physiol. Heart Circ. Physiol.* 288, H2014–H2020. doi: 10.1152/ajpheart.00508.2004

Nair, P. K., Carr, J. G., Bigelow, B., Bhatt, D. L., Berwick, Z. C., and Adams, G. (2018). LumenRECON guidewire: pilot study of a novel, nonimaging technology for accurate vessel sizing and delivery of therapy in femoropopliteal disease. *Circ. Cardiovasc. Interv.* 11:e005333. doi: 10.1161/CIRCINTERVENTIONS.117.005333

Schiele, T. M. (2005). Current understanding of coronary in-stent restenosis. Pathophysiology, clinical presentation, diagnostic work-up, and management. *Z. Kardiol.* 94, 772–790. doi: 10.1007/s00392-005-0299-x

Sonoda, S., Morino, Y., Ako, J., Terashima, M., Hassan, A. H., Bonneau, H. N., et al. (2004). Impact of final stent dimensions on long-term results following sirolimus-eluting stent implantation: serial intravascular ultrasound analysis from the sirius trial. *J. Am. Coll. Cardiol.* 43, 1959–1963. doi: 10.1016/j.jacc.2004.01.044

Svendsen, M. C., Akingba, G., Sinha, A. K., Chattin, B., Turner, A., Brass, M., et al. (2014a). Conductance sizing balloon for measurement of peripheral artery stent area. *J. Vasc. Surg.* 60, 759–766. doi: 10.1016/j.jvs.2013.06.095

Svendsen, M. C., Choy, J. S., Ebner, A., Bigelow, B., Sinha, A., Moussa, I., et al. (2014b). A lumen sizing workhorse guidewire for peripheral vasculature: two functions in one device. *Catheter. Cardiovasc. Interv.* 83, E85–E93. doi: 10.1002/ccd.24950

Svendsen, M. C., Sinha, A. K., Hermiller, J. B., Bhatt, D. L., Jansen, B., Berwick, Z. C., et al. (2015). Accurate conductance-based post-dilation balloon catheter sizing. *JACC Cardiovasc. Imaging* 8, 618–620. doi: 10.1016/j.jcmg.2014.07.021

Wu, Z., McMillan, T. L., Mintz, G. S., Maehara, A., Canos, D., Bui, A. B., et al. (2003). Impact of the acute results on the long-term outcome after the treatment of in-stent restenosis: a serial intravascular ultrasound study. *Catheter. Cardiovasc. Interv.* 60, 483–488. doi: 10.1002/ccd.10715

Zhang, J., Gao, X., Kan, J., Ge, Z., Han, L., Lu, S., et al. (2018). Intravascular ultrasound versus angiography-guided drug-eluting stent implantation: the ULTIMATE trial. *J. Am. Coll. Cardiol.* 72, 3126–3137. doi: 10.1016/j.jacc.2018.09.013

Ziada, K. M., Tuzcu, E. M., De Franco, A. C., Kim, M. H., Raymond, R. E., Franco, I., et al. (1997). Intravascular ultrasound assessment of the prevalence and causes of angiographic "haziness" following high-pressure coronary stenting. *Am. J. Cardiol.* 80, 116–121. doi: 10.1016/S0002-9149(97)00339-1

# 11

# Bond Graph Model of Cerebral Circulation: Toward Clinically Feasible Systemic Blood Flow Simulations

*Soroush Safaei[1]\*, Pablo J. Blanco[2,3], Lucas O. Müller[4], Leif R. Hellevik[4] and Peter J. Hunter[1]*

[1] Auckland Bioengineering Institute, University of Auckland, Auckland, New Zealand, [2] National Laboratory for Scientific Computing, Petrópolis, Brazil, [3] National Institute of Science and Technology in Medicine Assisted by Scientific Computing, Petrópolis, Brazil, [4] Division of Biomechanics, Department of Structural Engineering, Norwegian University of Science and Technology, Trondheim, Norway

**\*Correspondence:**
Soroush Safaei
soroush.safaei@auckland.ac.nz

We propose a detailed CellML model of the human cerebral circulation that runs faster than real time on a desktop computer and is designed for use in clinical settings when the speed of response is important. A lumped parameter mathematical model, which is based on a one-dimensional formulation of the flow of an incompressible fluid in distensible vessels, is constructed using a bond graph formulation to ensure mass conservation and energy conservation. The model includes arterial vessels with geometric and anatomical data based on the ADAN circulation model. The peripheral beds are represented by lumped parameter compartments. We compare the hemodynamics predicted by the bond graph formulation of the cerebral circulation with that given by a classical one-dimensional Navier-Stokes model working on top of the whole-body ADAN model. Outputs from the bond graph model, including the pressure and flow signatures and blood volumes, are compared with physiological data.

Keywords: cardiovascular system, circulation model, bond graph, CellML, OpenCOR, ADAN model, 0D model, blood flow

## 1. INTRODUCTION

Two challenges for biophysically based physiological modeling are to link the model parameters to patient-specific data and to make the models fast enough to become useful and accessible both, to reach a wide community of users, and to fit a clinical setting. For the prediction of pressure and flow in the patient-specific vascular system there is also the need to "close the loop" to ensure continuity of blood flow, and this requires a systems level model that includes arteries, veins and the capillary networks within specified tissue beds. The appropriate level of granularity for a model depends of course on the clinical or scientific question being studied. Available formulations for blood flow include three-dimensional (3D) FSI models (Heil and Hazel, 2011; Brown et al., 2012), rigid domain 3D fluid models (Shojima et al., 2004; Cebral et al., 2005), one-dimensional (1D) models (Reymond et al., 2009; Blanco et al., 2014), and zero-dimensional (0D) or "lumped-parameter" models (Korakianitis and Shi, 2006). In this paper we address the issue of execution time and the question of granularity in the context of a model of the cerebral circulation which will make it possible to model the exchange of solutes between blood and various tissue beds under conditions where vasodilation can also occur.

The analysis of pressure and flow in the vascular system is usually based on the incompressible direct Navier-Stokes (DNS) equations that ensure mass conservation and energy balance. We assume laminar flow since the Reynolds numbers are below the transition to turbulence in our example. The model parameters for the incompressible fluid considered here, blood, viscosity, and density, are both well understood and measurable. The compliance of the vessel wall is described by a constitutive relation that links the vessel diameter (and temporal deformation rate in the case of viscoelastic vessel wall models) to the fluid pressure. 1D blood flow equations are derived from 3D DNS by assuming negligible radial flow and integrating axial fluid velocity over the vessel cross-section. Moreover, an additional assumption must be made about the time-varying radial profile of the axial velocity. For a steady state well developed flow, such profile is of course parabolic, but a more realistic assumption is a flatter-than-parabolic profile, which then requires at least one more empirical parameter to be specified (Hunter, 1972). These empirically determined parameters imply that, given the uncertainty in geometrical and biophysical parameters for the patient specific modeling, there is always uncertainty in the predicted pressure and flow results and the need to include computationally expensive fluid calculations (e.g., solving 3D DNS) must be balanced against this uncertainty.

The primary goal of this paper is to compare flow and pressure waveforms predicted by a 1D blood flow model, consisting of partial differential equations, with the output of a bond graph based model, which generates a system of ordinary differential equations (ODEs) that can be solved approximately 200x faster than the 1D model and at close to real time on a desktop computer. The model used here is based on the ADAN cerebral circulation model (Blanco et al., 2015), along with a relatively simple model of flow through the heart and lungs, as an example. The results show the bond graph solution to be within 5% of the 1D model solution for flow and pressure at every point in the cerebral circulation model.

This paper is organized as follows. In section 2.1, the bond graph method is introduced and various components are presented. In section 2.2, the architecture of the cardiovascular system model is described. The software, model structure and simulation setup are presented in the section 3.1. The simulation results of the bond graph arterial model (open-loop) and comparisons against 1D model are presented in section 3.2 and section 3.3. Then the simulation results for the closed-loop bond graph model of the cardiovascular system are demonstrated in section 3.4. Finally, concluding remarks and future works are outlined in section 4.

# 2. MATERIALS AND METHODS

## 2.1. Bond Graph Approach

The bond graph approach to formulating models dealing with mass and energy transfer was developed by Henry Paynter in the 1960s to represent electro-mechanical control systems (Paynter, 1961). It was later extended to include chemical processes by Breedveld (1984), including concepts from the theory of network thermodynamics by Aharon Katchalsky and colleagues (Oster et al., 1971). Papers by Peter Gawthrop and Edmund

Crampin have brought the approach into the bioengineering domain (Gawthrop and Crampin, 2014; Gawthrop et al., 2015a,b; Gawthrop and Crampin, 2016).

The first key idea, based on recognizing that energy and power are the only quantities that are common across different physical systems, is to separate energy transmission from storage and dissipation, and to provide the concept of *potential* (called "effort" in the engineering literature) with units of Joules per some_quantity as the common driving force behind the *flow* of that some_quantity per second. The product of potential and flow is then always power in units of Joules per second. The "some_quantity" has units of meters, meters³, Coulombs, Candela, moles, or entropy for, respectively, rigid body mechanics, continuum mechanics (including fluid flow), electrical, electromagnetic, chemical, and heat transfer processes. As explained further below, the second key concept is that of a *0-junction*, where potential is defined and mass balance is applied, and a *1-junction*, where flow is defined and energy balance is applied. The extraordinary utility of these concepts is to recognize that Kirchhoff's voltage law in electrical circuits, Newton's force balance in a mechanical system, and stoichiometric balance in a biochemical system, are all just different manifestations of the same underlying principle of energy conservation and can therefore be represented by the same bond graph equation.

### 2.1.1. Units

Many physical systems can be described by a driving *potential* expressed as Joules per unit of some quantity, and a *flow* expressed as that quantity per second. The quantity could be coulomb, meters, moles, etc., in different physical systems. The power is always the product of the driving force and the flow expressed as Joules per second. The seven units of the SI system under the newly proposed definitions are now based on constants that are consistent with the use of Joules and seconds (together covering energy and power), meters, moles, entropy, Coulombs, and Candela. Table 1 in Supplementary Material displays the bond graph concepts in the fluid mechanics domain.

### 2.1.2. Bond Graph Formulation

In bond graph formulation, there are four basic variables. In the fluid mechanics domain these are given by: potential $\mu$ is energy density or *pressure* ($J.m^{-3}$), flow $\upsilon$ is *volumetric flow* ($m^3.s^{-1}$), time integral of potential $p$ is *momentum* ($J.s.m^{-3}$) and time integral of flow $q$ is quantity or *volume* ($m^3$). Product $\mu.\upsilon$ is power ($J.s^{-1}$) which is a generalized coordinate to model the complete systems residing in several energy domains. A bond with covariables $\mu$ and $\upsilon$ is therefore used to represent *transmission of energy*. The bond represents a mechanism for the transmission of energy and power, and the arrow head indicates the assumed direction of power flow (see **Figure 1**). The flow $\upsilon$ and potential $\mu$ must satisfy conservation laws.

There are also the concept of *0-junction* and *1-junction* for conservation laws. The *0-junction* defines a common potential $\mu$ which ensures that the potential is identical at each port and imposes mass conservation constraint based on $\upsilon$. The *1-junction* defines a common flow $\upsilon$ which ensures that the flow is identical at each port and imposes energy conservation constraint based on $\mu$. Since sum of the flows is zero with $\mu$ constant for *0-junction*

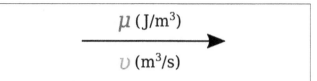

$$\mu \ (\text{J/m}^3)$$

$$\upsilon \ (\text{m}^3/\text{s})$$

**FIGURE 1** | Representation of energy bond.

and sum of the potentials is zero with $\upsilon$ constant for *1-junction*, the transmission of power through junction is conserved for both kinds of junctions, that is:

$$\sum \mu.\upsilon = 0. \tag{1}$$

## 2.1.3. Bond Graph Elements

Bond graph formulation is a graphical notation for the set of linear constraint equations (the conservation laws), but the constitutive relations (to be addressed next) can be nonlinear.

### 2.1.3.1. R-element

Energy $\mu$ can be dissipated by a resistor $R$ in proportion to the flow $\upsilon$ with an empirical relation which can be a simple linear relation such as Equation 2 or a complex nonlinear relation:

$$\mu = \upsilon R. \tag{2}$$

In the fluid mechanics systems, the $R$-element represents the viscous resistance in opposition to the blood flow and for a cylindrical vessel can be analytically calculated using Poiseuille relation:

$$R = \frac{8\nu l}{\pi r^4}, \tag{3}$$

where $\nu$ is the blood viscosity, $l$ is the vessel length and $r$ is the vessel radius.

### 2.1.3.2. C-element

Energy $\mu$ can be stored statically by a capacitor $C$ without any loss. In the bond graph terminology, a one-port capacitor relates energy to the quantity $q$ or time integral of flow by an empirical relation such as Equation 4. The $C$-element stores $q$ by accumulating the net flow $\upsilon$ to the storage element:

$$\mu = \frac{q}{C}, \tag{4}$$

$$\dot{q} = \upsilon, \tag{5}$$

in which the dot stands for time derivative. In the fluid mechanics systems, and particularly in the cardiovascular system, the $C$-element represents the vessel wall compliance and can be calculated from blood vessel properties. For a homogeneous linear elastic material and for a cylindrical vessel, the compliance is characterized as follows:

$$C = \frac{2\pi r^3 l}{hE}, \tag{6}$$

where $E$ is the Young's modulus and $h$ is the vessel thickness.

### 2.1.3.3. I-element

Energy $\mu$ can be stored dynamically by an inductor $I$ without any loss. In bond graph formulation, a one-port inductor relates flow to the momentum $p$ or time integral of potential by an empirical relation such as Equation 7. The $I$ stores $p$ by accumulating the net potential $\mu$ to the storage element.

$$\upsilon = \frac{p}{I}, \tag{7}$$

$$\dot{p} = \mu. \tag{8}$$

In the fluid mechanics systems, the $I$-element is used to model the mass inertial effects in a pipe and can be defined for straight cylindrical vessels as:

$$I = \frac{\rho l}{\pi r^2}, \tag{9}$$

where $\rho$ is the blood density and $l$ is the vessel length.

**Figure 2** shows the relation of the state variables to the constitutive relations.

## 2.1.4. Causality

Causality establishes the cause and the effect relationship. It specifically implies that either the potential or flow variable on that bond is known. Causality is generally indicated by a causal stroke at the end to which the potential receiver is connected. Elements which store or dissipate energy do not impose causality on the system, but they have preferred causality for computational reasons. These elements with their preferred causality are shown in **Figure 3**.

In the bond graph approach, junctions interconnect the corresponding elements and constrain the possible causalities of the element ports connected to it. A *0-junction* can only have one potential output. In a similar way, a *1-junction* can only have one flow output. **Figure 4** illustrates causality in four-port *0-junction* and *1-junction*.

## 2.1.5. Vessel Segments

In this section, we developed a library of bond graph elements for modeling the blood flow in distensible vessels. The modularity of the bond graph approach enables us to develop a wide range of elements and incorporate them into the model based on a set of assumptions. There are four basic types of elements for a vessel segment depending on whether potential or flow BC is prescribed at the inlet and the outlet (see **Figure 5**). Each vessel segment is represented by a parallel combination of one $C$-element and a series combination of one $R$-element and one $I$-element. The $C$, $R$, and $I$ represent the vessel wall compliance, the viscous friction and the inertia of the blood, respectively. These elements are interconnected by a *0-junction* for same blood pressure and a *1-junction* for the same blood flow.

The set of equations for $\mu\upsilon$-*type* (see **Figure 5A**) after rearrangements is:

$$\dot{\mu} = \frac{\upsilon - \upsilon_{out}}{C}, \tag{10}$$

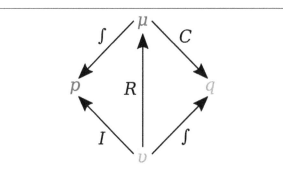

**FIGURE 2 |** State variables and constitutive relations in the bond graph approach.

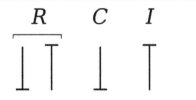

**FIGURE 3 |** Preferred causality for $R$, $C$, and $I$ elements.

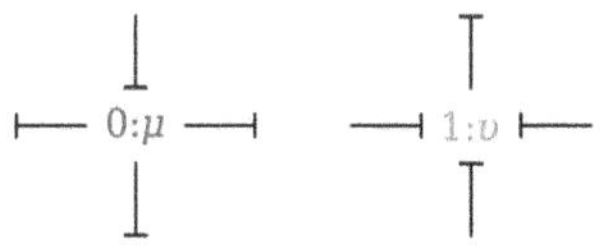

**FIGURE 4 |** Causality in four-port 0-junction and 1-junction.

$$\dot{\upsilon} = \frac{\mu_{in} - \mu - \upsilon R}{I}. \tag{11}$$

Also a similar set of equations can be derived for $\upsilon\mu$-type (see **Figure 5B**). For $\mu\mu$-type (see **Figure 5C**) we have:

$$\dot{\mu} = \frac{\upsilon - \upsilon_d}{C}, \tag{12}$$

$$\dot{\upsilon} = \frac{\mu_{in} - \mu - \upsilon (R/2)}{I/2}, \tag{13}$$

$$\dot{\upsilon}_d = \frac{\mu - \mu_{out} - \upsilon_d (R/2)}{I/2}. \tag{14}$$

In a similar way, we can write the equations for $\upsilon\upsilon$-type (see **Figure 5D**).

### 2.1.6. Viscoelastic Vessel Wall

The bond graph representation makes it very easy to implement the viscoelasticity effect of the vessel wall into the model. Two common existing models in the literature are the Voigt model and the Maxwell model. A more sophisticated model is the generalized model developed by Westerhof and Noordergraaf (1970). However, the generalized model is complex and

computationally expensive to solve, and for this reason we chose the Voigt model to represent the viscoelastic effect of the vessel wall in this work. The classical Voigt model in mechanical symbols is shown in **Figure 6**.

Bond graph representation of the Voigt model is illustrated in **Figure 6**. By taking advantage of the modular nature of the bond graph technique we can easily plug in the Voigt model into any configuration of the vessel elements described before. **Figure 6** shows the viscoelastic $\mu\upsilon$-type element. The governing equations for this element are described below:

$$\mu = \mu_v + (\upsilon - \upsilon_{out})\, R_v, \tag{15}$$

$$\dot{\mu}_v = \frac{\upsilon - \upsilon_{out}}{C}, \tag{16}$$

$$\dot{\upsilon} = \frac{\mu_{in} - \mu - \upsilon R}{I}. \tag{17}$$

As can be seen, by adding only one equation to the basic set of equations we can take into account the viscoelastic effect of the vessel wall. Using a similar approach, other basic elements can also be equipped with the viscoelastic effect accounted for by $C_v$.

### 2.1.7. Junctions

The *0-junction* is a powerful concept in the bond graph approach that allows us to model the splitting or merging flows in blood vessels. It satisfies the conservation of flow and also imposes a common potential on all the branches to make sure pressure is continuous throughout the junction, which is a good approximation of branching in arterial vessels. It is important to know that only $\mu\upsilon$-type and $\upsilon\upsilon$-type elements can be used as the parent vessel in a junction. In a similar way, only $\mu\upsilon$-type and $\mu\mu$-type elements can be implemented as daughter vessels in a junction. These restrictions are due to arranging compatible segment types into a structure, with inlets and outlets coupled appropriately in the sense that BCs are settled by the state of their adjacent compartments.

#### 2.1.7.1. Splitting flow

In the splitting flow junctions, a *0-junction* represents the separation point at the end of the parent vessel and the daughter vessels are connected via this port to the parent vessel (see **Figure 7**).

We created another element specifically for splitting flow junctions and called it $\mu\upsilon$-*split-type*. To implement the splitting flow junction, only the parent vessel element needs to use $\mu\upsilon$-*split-type* and the daughter vessels remain basic $\mu\upsilon$-*type*. The governing equations for this element type are stated below:

$$\dot{\mu} = \frac{\upsilon - \upsilon^1 - \upsilon^2}{C}, \tag{18}$$

$$\dot{\upsilon} = \frac{\mu_{in} - \mu - \upsilon R}{I}, \tag{19}$$

where $\upsilon^1$ and $\upsilon^2$ are the daughter branches flow.

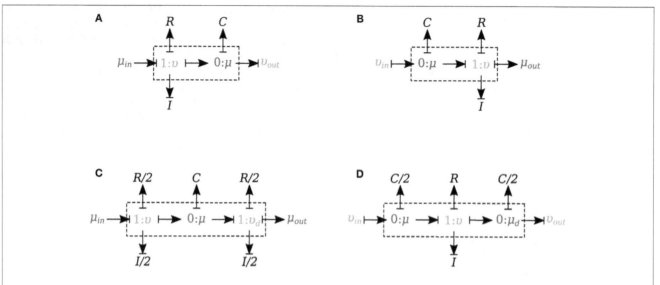

FIGURE 5 | Different configurations of bond graph model for a vessel segment, **(A)** the $\mu\upsilon$-type has inlet pressure BC and outlet flow BC, **(B)** the $\upsilon\mu$-type has the reversed characteristics, **(C)** coupling these two configurations with the $C$ in the middle gives us a $\mu\mu$-type with inlet and outlet pressure BCs. The $R$ and $I$ values are divided equally between the two resistors and two inductors at both ends, **(D)** coupling these two configurations with the $R$ and $I$ in the middle gives us a $\upsilon\upsilon$-type with inlet and outlet flow BCs. The $C$-value is divided equally between the two capacitors at both ends.

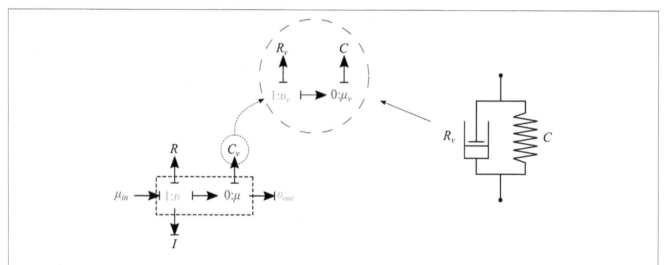

FIGURE 6 | Mechanical representation of the Voigt model consisting of a parallel arrangement of a spring $C$ and a dash pot $R_V$, which represent elastic, and viscous material behavior, respectively.

### 2.1.7.2. Merging flow

In the merging flow junctions, a *0-junction* represents the adjoining point at the beginning of the parent vessel and the daughter vessels are connected via this port to the parent vessel (see **Figure 8**).

We created another element specifically for merging flow junctions and called it $\upsilon\upsilon$-*merge-type*. To implement the merging flow junction, only the parent vessel element needs to use $\upsilon\upsilon$-*merge-type* and the daughter vessels remain basic $\mu\mu$-type. The governing equations for this element type are stated below:

$$\dot{\mu} = \frac{\upsilon_d^1 + \upsilon_d^2 - \upsilon}{C/2}, \quad (20)$$

$$\dot{\upsilon} = \frac{\mu - \mu_d - \upsilon R}{I}, \quad (21)$$

$$\dot{\mu}_d = \frac{\upsilon - \upsilon_{out}}{C/2}, \quad (22)$$

where $\upsilon_d^1$ and $\upsilon_d^2$ are the flows through the daughter branches.

### 2.1.8. Peripheral Circulation

The cumulative effects of all distal vessels (small arteries, arterioles, and capillaries) at terminal locations of the truncated arteries are modeled using *RCR* Windkessel elements (Westerhof et al., 1969; Stergiopulos et al., 1992). For this purpose, a bond graph model of the *RCR* element is developed and attached to a $\mu\upsilon$-*type* element to create a special bond graph element $\mu\mu$-*BC-type* for terminal vessels. *RCR* element contains a proximal terminal resistance $R_{TP}$ in series with a parallel arrangement of a terminal capacitor $C_T$ and a distal terminal resistance, $R_{TD}$ (see **Figure 9**).

The governing equations for the $\mu\mu$-*BC-type* element are:

$$\dot{\mu} = \frac{\upsilon - \upsilon_d}{C}, \tag{23}$$

$$\dot{\upsilon} = \frac{\mu_{in} - \mu - \upsilon R}{I}, \tag{24}$$

$$\dot{\mu}_d = \frac{\upsilon_d - \dfrac{\mu_d}{R_{TD}}}{C_T}, \tag{25}$$

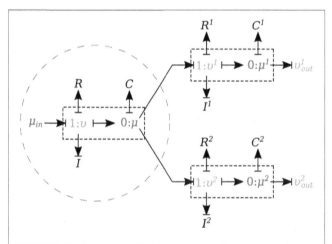

**FIGURE 7 |** Bond graph model for a bifurcating branch.

$$\upsilon_d = \frac{\mu - \mu_d - \mu_{out}}{R_{TP}}. \tag{26}$$

## 2.2. Cardiovascular System

The cardiovascular system is composed of three parts - heart, systemic circulation loop, and pulmonary circulation loop. In this section, we briefly explain how these components are modeled using the bond graph approach. Table 2 in Supplementary Material shows the bond graph elements that have been developed for modeling blood flow in the cardiovascular system. Based on the assumptions and locations, we import vessel segments with the appropriate element type as a new module and connect it to the system.

### 2.2.1. Pulmonary Circulation

The pulmonary circulation is modeled as described in Blanco and Feijóo (2013). We divide it into 2 main compartments, arteries (*par*) and veins (*pvn*). The arteries are highly elastic and the flow is pulsatile in these compartments, so the resistance, compliance and inductance effects must be considered and $\upsilon\mu$-type is the most suitable bond graph element based on the prescribed BCs. Veins also are modeled using the $\upsilon\mu$-type element (see **Figure 10**).

### 2.2.2. Systemic Circulation

The systemic circulation loop consists of a reduced version of the ADAN model Blanco et al. (2014, 2015) and the veins compartment which is similar to the pulmonary veins compartment. Such a reduced version of the ADAN model is composed of a 218-segment arterial model which consisted of the integration between the ADAN-86 model (Safaei et al., 2016) and the anatomically detailed cerebral vasculature of the ADAN model Blanco et al. (2015). **Figure 11** displays the entire model with a detail of the cerebral vasculature.

We constructed a bond graph model using the geometrical properties of the ADAN model (i.e., vessel radius and wall

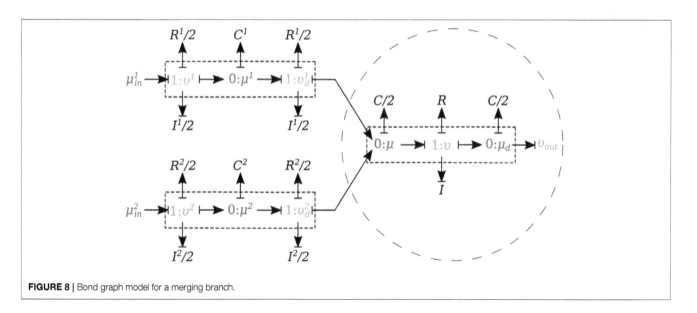

**FIGURE 8 |** Bond graph model for a merging branch.

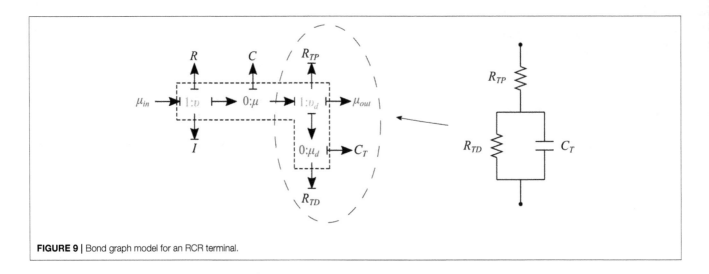

**FIGURE 9 |** Bond graph model for an RCR terminal.

thickness). **Figure 12A,B** illustrate the bond graph model of the systemic arteries and cerebral circulation, respectively.

### 2.2.3. Heart

The heart is modeled as a four-chamber pump with variable elastance and four valves: tricuspid valve, pulmonary valve, mitral valve and aortic valve. The basic pressure-flow relation in each valve is represented with an orifice model which is an advancement over the diode models (Korakianitis and Shi, 2006). The left and right atria and ventricles are modeled as capacitors with time-varying elastance which is a function of the characteristic elastance and an activation function. The activation function represents the contraction and relaxation changes in each cardiac chamber (see **Figure 10**).

#### 2.2.3.1. Ventricles

The left ventricle is represented by a special type of $C$-element which has a time-varying compliance function $C_{lv}(t)$. $v_{la}$ and $v_{lv}$ represent flow through the mitral and aortic valves, respectively, $q_{lv}$ is the blood volume and $\mu_{lv}$ is the blood pressure inside the left ventricle. The differential equations governing the left ventricle model are as follows:

$$\dot{q}_{lv} = v_{la} - v_{lv}, \tag{27}$$

$$\mu_{lv} = \frac{q_{lv} - q_{lv}^o}{C_{lv}(t)}, \tag{28}$$

where $q_{lv}^o$ refers to the dead volume of the chamber. The time-varying compliance function $C_{lv}(t)$ is the inverse of time-varying elastance function $E_{lv}(t)$ and it has been used so as to be consistent with the basic $C$-element constitutive relation:

$$C_{lv}(t) = \frac{1}{E_{lv}(t)}. \tag{29}$$

$E_{lv}(t)$ is a function of the characteristic elastance and an activation function $e_v(t)$:

$$E_{lv}(t) = E_{lv}^B + e_v(t)E_{lv}^A. \tag{30}$$

Here, $E_{lv}^A$ and $E_{lv}^B$ are the amplitude and baseline values of the elastance, and $e_v(t)$ is the ventricle activation function and expresses the contraction and the relaxation changes in the ventricular muscle:

$$e_v(t) = \begin{cases} \frac{1}{2}\left[1 - \cos\left(\pi\frac{t}{T_{vc}}\right)\right], & 0 \le t \le T_{vc} \\ \frac{1}{2}\left[1 + \cos\left(\pi\frac{(t-T_{vc})}{T_{vr}}\right)\right], & T_{vc} < t \le T_{vc} + T_{vr} \\ 0, & T_{vc} + T_{vr} < t \le T \end{cases} \tag{31}$$

where $T$ is the duration of a cardiac cycle. $T_{vc}$ and $T_{vr}$ represent the durations of contraction and relaxation of the ventricles, respectively. The right ventricle is also modeled in a similar manner to the left ventricle model, with different values for system parameters (see Table 3 in Supplementary Material).

#### 2.2.3.2. Atria

The bond graph model of the atrium is also developed in a similar way to that of the ventricle. The only difference is that the atrium activation function which expresses the contraction and the relaxation changes in the atrial muscle. For the left atrium $e_a(t)$ is:

$$e_a(t) = \begin{cases} \frac{1}{2}\left[1 + \cos\left(\pi\frac{(t+T-t_{ar})}{T_{ar}}\right)\right], & 0 \le t \le t_{ar} + T_{ar} - T \\ 0, & t_{ar} + T_{ar} - T < t \le t_{ac} \\ \frac{1}{2}\left[1 - \cos\left(\pi\frac{(t-t_{ac})}{T_{ac}}\right)\right], & t_{ac} < t \le t_{ac} + T_{ac} \\ \frac{1}{2}\left[1 + \cos\left(\pi\frac{(t-t_{ar})}{T_{ar}}\right)\right], & t_{ac} + T_{ac} < t \le T \end{cases} \tag{32}$$

where $T_{ac}$ and $T_{ar}$ are the durations of contraction and relaxation of the atria, and $t_{ac}$ and $t_{ar}$ represent the times when the atria start

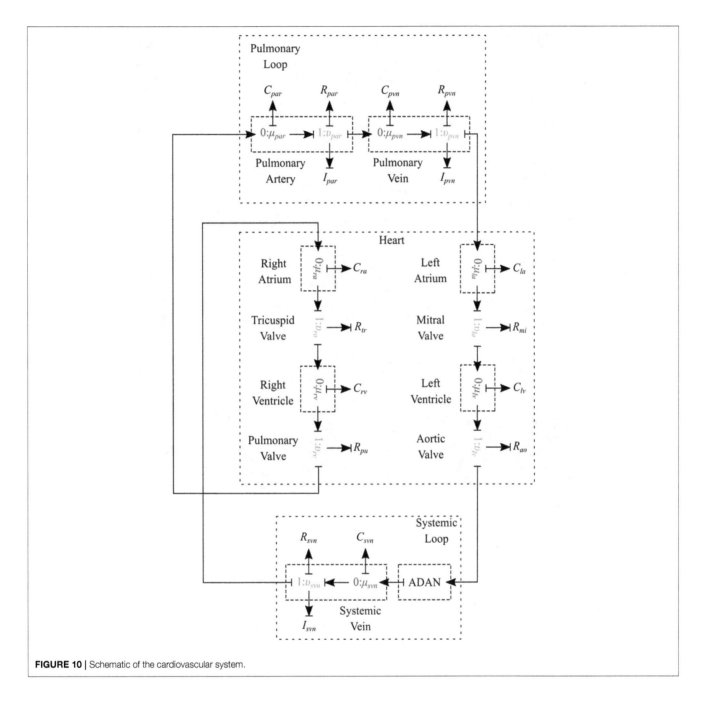

**FIGURE 10 |** Schematic of the cardiovascular system.

to contract and relax, respectively. An analogous relation applies to the right atrium activation function.

### 2.2.3.3. Valves

Heart valves are modeled by a special type of $R$-element which instead of the conventional constitutive relation (Equation 2), uses a nonlinear pressure-flow relation of the orifice model. For the aortic valve we have:

$$\upsilon_{lv} = R_{ao}\alpha_{ao}\sqrt{\lfloor \mu_{lv} - \mu_{root}\rfloor},\qquad(33)$$

where $\upsilon_{lv}$ is the blood flow through the aortic valve, $\mu_{lv}$ is the blood pressure inside the left ventricle, $\mu_{root}$ is the blood pressure

in the aortic root, $R_{ao}$ is the aortic valve resistance, and $\alpha_{ao}$ is the aortic valve opening coefficient. Depending on which side of the valve has higher pressure, the coefficient $\alpha_{ao}$ can switch between fully closed and fully open states:

$$\alpha_{ao} = \begin{cases} 1, & \mu_{lv} > \mu_{root} \\ 0, & \mu_{lv} \le \mu_{root} \end{cases}\qquad(34)$$

The rest of the valves are modeled in the same way with different system parameters (see Table 3 in Supplementary Material).

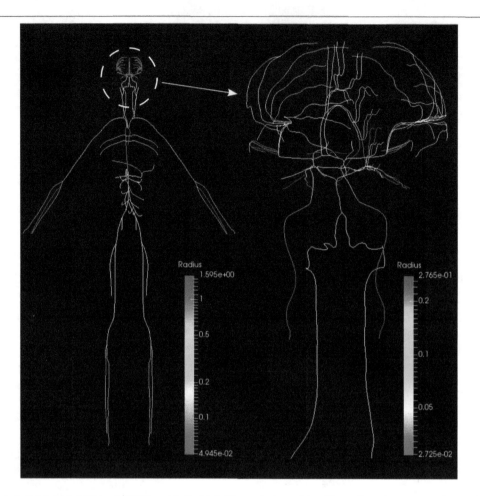

**FIGURE 11 |** Anatomically Detailed Arterial Network (ADAN) model with detail of the cerebral vasculature. The varying colors represent the vessel radii.

### 2.2.4. Physiological Data

The geometrical parameters of the 218 arteries were prescribed based on the data reported in Blanco et al. (2015). Vessel wall thickness $h$ is calculated using the following relation:

$$h = r_o(ae^{br_o} + ce^{dr_o}),$$ (35)

where $r_o$ is the lumen radius. $a$, $b$, $c$, and $d$ are the fitting parameters (see Table 3 in Supplementary Material). The elastic modulus of the arteries were calculated from Blanco et al. (2015). The viscoelastic wall properties are calculated using the relationship between the Voigt model components (Westerhof and Noordergraaf, 1970):

$$R_v = \frac{f}{C},$$ (36)

where $R_v$ is the viscous damping of the wall, $C$ is the vessel wall compliance evaluated using Equation 6, and $f$ is the time constant for stress relaxation (see Table 3 in Supplementary Material). The peripheral resistances ($R_{TP}$ and $R_{TD}$) and compliances ($C_T$) were derived from Blanco et al. (2015). The parameters used in the heart, pulmonary loop and venous system have been assigned or estimated based on the data reported in Liang et al. (2009) and Blanco and Feijóo (2013). The cardiac valve model and the parameters have been adopted from Korakianitis and Shi (2006) (see Table 3 in Supplementary Material).

## 3. SIMULATIONS AND RESULTS

### 3.1. OpenCOR Simulation

OpenCOR (opencor.ws) is an open source modeling environment that works on Windows, Linux and OS X and can be used to organize, edit, simulate and analyse models of ODEs or differential algebraic equations encoded in the CellML format (Garny and Hunter, 2015). It relies on a modular approach, which means that all of its features come in the form of plugins. The bond graph model of the cardiovascular system has been developed using OpenCOR in four separate CellML files:

### 3.1.1. BG_Modules.cellml

This file is the bond graph library and the elements listed in Table 2 in Supplementary Material including all the governing equations exist in this file. The modules defined in this file can be imported into the main file to represent a specific vessel segment or any other element in the fluid mechanics domain.

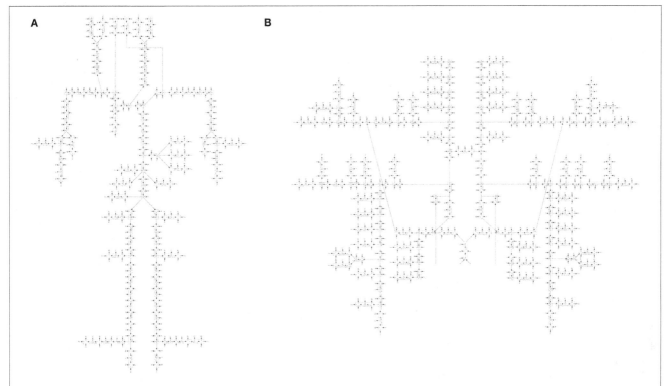

**FIGURE 12 | (A)** The bond graph model of the ADAN-86 model, **(B)** the bond graph model of the ADAN-brain model. These two models are detached in this figure for clarity.

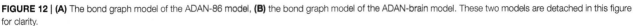

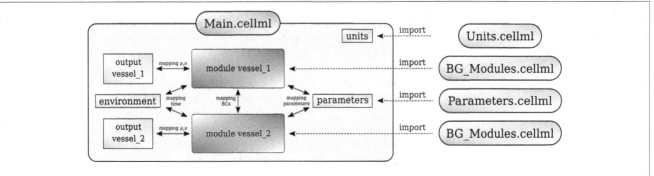

**FIGURE 13 |** Overall structure of the cardiovascular system model showing the CellML model imports and the other key parts (units, components, and mappings) of the top level CellML model.

### 3.1.2. Parameters.cellml

All the parameters have been defined in this file. These parameters include the geometric properties of all the ADAN vessels (length, radius, thickness, Young's modulus), resistance and capacitance at the ADAN terminal locations, and all the system parameters for the heart and the pulmonary circulation path models.

### 3.1.3. Units.cellml

The basic units are implemented in CellML inherently, while any alternative unit system required needs to be constructed. This file contains all the constructed units in the bond graph approach that have been used in the present model.

### 3.1.4. Main.cellml

This is the executable file which runs the simulations using OpenCOR software. It imports all the required modules and contains the information about the model structure, elements connectivity, and mappings between different components.

**Figure 13** shows schematically how components are connected and communicate with each other. The full model is made publicly available at https://models.physiomeproject.org/workspace/4ac.

## 3.2. One-Dimensional ADAN Model

As stated at the beginning of this work, one of the primary goals in this contribution is to provide a comparison of the predictions delivered by the bond graph model and the predictions of the complete ADAN model. The latter is therefore regarded as a reference solution in the present context, and will be referred simply as the "ADAN solution."

The ADAN model incorporates 2, 142 arterial vessels (yielding overall over 4, 000 arterial segments), 1, 598 of which have a well determined name according to the Anatomical Terminology. The disposition of these vessels correspond to a generic male individual of approximately 1.7 m in height. The model supplies blood to 28 specific organs, plus the supply to 116 vascular territories which accommodate the distributed organs. Each of these territories packs the bones, nerves, muscles, fascia and skin. The ADAN model also includes the additional vessels reported in Blanco et al. (2016). As for the calibration, peripheral resistances are determined according to the peripheral blood flow distribution reported in Blanco et al. (2014), while the calibration of arterial vessel behavior (including elastin and collagen constituents as well as viscoelastic phenomena) follow Blanco et al. (2015). The inflow condition is defined below. Finally, blood density and viscosity are taken to be $\mu = 0.004$ J.s.m$^{-3}$ and $\rho = 1040$ J.s$^2$.m$^{-5}$. Finally, the 1D equations for modeling the flow of an incompressible fluid in compliant vessels and the numerical technology employed to solve these 1D equations are reported in Müller and Blanco (2015) and Müller et al. (2016a,b).

The ADAN model was simulated for 10 s, and the results of the last cardiac cycle are considered in the comparisons performed in next section.

### 3.3. Open-Loop Bond Graph Model vs. ADAN Model

In this first case, we are comparing the results of the bond graph arterial model (open-loop) for ADAN (see **Figure 12**) with the reference solution provided by the ADAN 1D model. All the parameters incorporated in the bond graph arterial model for this simulation are adopted from the ADAN 1D model. The inflow BC at the aortic root is prescribed using the flow curve shown in **Figure 14A** acquired from Blanco et al. (2014). Overall, pressure and flow rate waveforms as predicted by the bond graph model aligns closely with the ADAN solution. Qualitative comparisons of pressure and flow waveforms at different arterial locations are given in **Figure 14**. A quantitative assessment of the relative error is performed by computing the root mean square of the error (RMSE) of the predicted waveforms compared with ADAN solution.

In the main aortic segments, the pressure and flow waveforms are very similar to the ADAN solution in the aortic root, thoracic aorta, and proximal abdominal aorta. In the lower and upper limbs, waveform predictions at the femoral and radial arteries are in agreement with ADAN solution, however by refining the model and increasing the number of bond graph modules in the peripheral arteries we would be able to obtain a better match. Regarding the cerebral circulation, the pressure and flow waveforms predicted by the bond graph model are compared with ADAN solution in the internal carotid artery, vertebral artery, prefrontal artery, middle cerebral artery, anterior cerebral artery, posterior cerebral post-communicating artery,

and posterior parietal artery. We observe that, the amplitude and shape of the pressure and flow waveforms in the cerebral arteries are well captured by the bond graph model.

### 3.4. Closed-Loop Bond Graph Model

Now the case in which we have a closed-loop bond graph model is simulated (see **Figure 10**). The model was run for ten cardiac cycles ($T = 1$ s) using a 0.001 s time step, with tolerance $10^{-7}$ and CVODE solver. For the full model with 258 modules (244 modules for ADAN, 8 modules for the heart, 3 modules for pulmonary and systemic circulation loops), the computation took about 23 s, which is near real-time simulation. With a simpler model (only ADAN-86 without ADAN-brain), the same simulation takes 5 s which is faster than real-time simulation. The simulation time has been measured within OpenCOR, running on a Linux Ubuntu 17.10 machine with Intel® Core i7-6820HK Processor @ 2.70 GHz.

One cardiac cycle of the cardiovascular system model already in the periodic state is visualized in **Figure 15**.

## 4. DISCUSSION AND FUTURE WORK

In this paper, we have used the bond graph concept for constructing 0D models. We utilized the bond graph formalism to assemble a system of ODEs in a structured way that satisfies mass and energy conservation for flow in an anatomically detailed model of the cerebral circulation. The most important feature that the bond graph approach provides is the subdivision and reticulation of a network, which is equivalent to the system decomposition or disaggregation, facilitating the introduction/application of hierarchical modeling concepts. We have compared the predicted flow and pressure at a number of points in the vascular model against the solution delivered by a 1D blood flow model and, as an illustrative proof-of-concept, we have shown that the pressure and flow rate waveforms predicted by the bond graph model are within 5% of the 1D model solution at the points of comparison in the cerebral circulation model.

OpenCOR used the CVODE solver which is a solver for stiff and nonstiff ODE systems (initial value problem) given in explicit form $y' = f(t, y)$. The Backward Differentiation Formula (BDF) is employed as the integration method with a dense direct linear solver for Newton iterations. The bond graph model runs approximately 200x faster than the 1D model and at close to real time on a desktop computer for the level of detail we included. The low computational effort is due to the lumped nature of the mathematical representation provided by the ODE system. There are several simplifying assumptions to derive the lumped parameter models from the Navier-Stokes equations. We considered the fluid as Newtonian and applied a flow profile derived for laminar and stationary flow conditions. We also assumed a constant Young's modulus and a uniform circular cross-section along the length of the segment. The assumption of uniform elastic properties over a large pressure range has some disadvantages. While it is desirable to keep the model linear for speed-up, the drawback is that it is unable to represent the complex behavior of the vessel wall accurately, and therefore affects the model's predictive ability for various

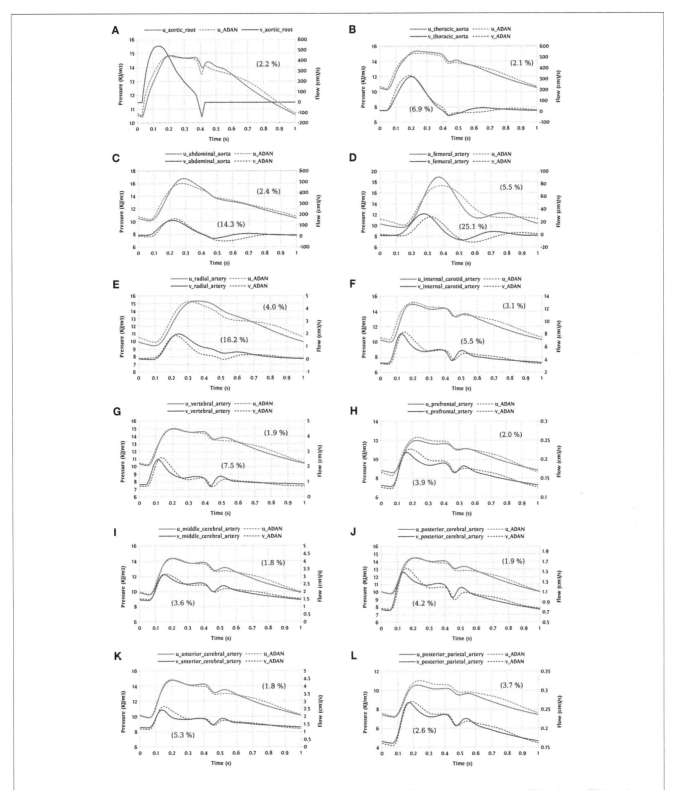

**FIGURE 14 |** Comparison of pressure and flow waveforms between the bond graph model and ADAN solution; u, pressure; v, flow; **(A)** aortic root; **(B)** thoracic aorta; **(C)** abdominal aorta; **(D)** femoral artery; **(E)** radial artery; **(F)** internal carotid artery; **(G)** vertebral artery; **(H)** prefrontal artery; **(I)** middle cerebral artery; **(J)** posterior cerebral post-communicating artery; **(K)** anterior cerebral artery; **(L)** posterior parietal artery. In parentheses are root mean square errors (RMSE) computed between the simulations and ADAN solution and expressed in percentage relative to the ADAN solution systolic values.

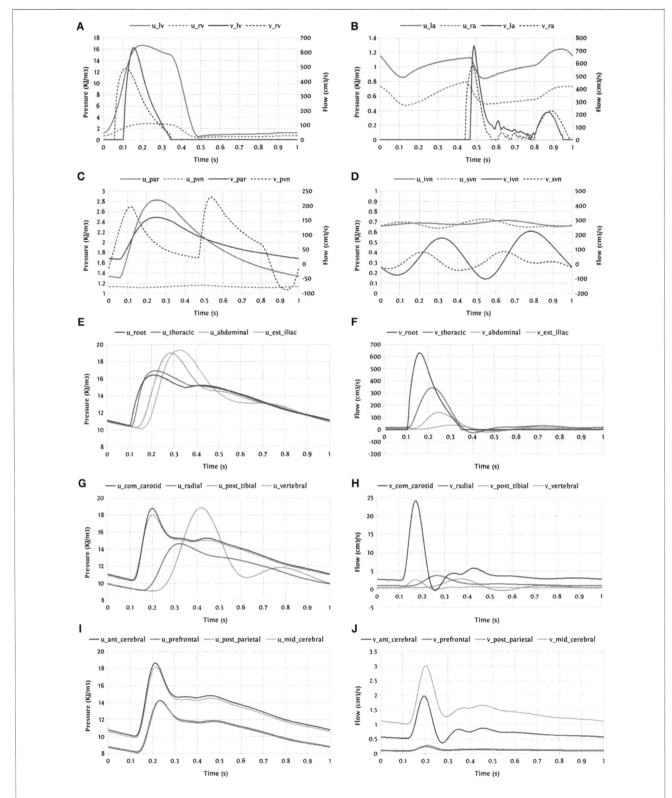

**FIGURE 15 |** Pressure and flow rate in the main segments during one cardiac cycle; u, pressure; v, flow; **(A)** lv, left ventricle; rv, right ventricle; **(B)** la, left atrium; ra, right atrium; **(C)** par, pulmonary arteries; pvn, pulmonary veins; **(D)** ivn, inferior vena-cava; svn, superior vena-cava; **(E,F)** ext, external; **(G,H)** com, common; post, posterior; **(I,J)** ant, anterior; mid, middle.

pressure levels. This problem can be addressed by incorporating a nonlinear elastic material in the *C*-element that provides the pressure-dependent compliance. The current model has only 86 compartments for systemic flow paths outside the head in addition to the heart and lungs (since we were focussing on the cerebral circulation), but we plan to extend the model to include higher resolution models of the rest of the systemic circulation in the future. We will also look into the possibilities of profiling and parallelising the code for optimisation and speed-up.

Our overall goal for this work has been to create an anatomically detailed model of the cardiovascular circulation that can be made patient-specific (at least to some extent) and can be run in real time (Safaei et al., 2016). The model presented here will be made available in the public domain with freely available open source tools, enabling users to examine pressures and flow rates at any point in the circulation under a variety of physiological conditions. The bond graph formulation makes it straightforward to extend the model to include various tissue exchange mechanisms and to incorporate tissue and cellular parameters that characterize various chronic diseases. In the present contribution, this formalism served

to provide a structured and compartmental description of the whole circulatory system including the heart, pulmonary loop and the venous system. This model can also include self-regulating and metabolic dynamics in a simple way and at a low computational cost. Cerebral auto-regulation is a precise system involving vasodilation and vasoconstriction in a network of collateral vessels. By adding metabolic models to the bond graph model we would be able to simulate cerebral auto-regulation, which is a feedback mechanism driving an appropriate blood supply into the cerebral vasculature depending on the oxygen demand by the brain. There are also many other physiological mechanisms that can be added into this system such as baroreflex regulation, respiratory control system, autonomic nervous system, etc.

## AUTHOR CONTRIBUTIONS

SS, PH, and PB contributed conception and design of the study; SS performed the statistical analysis; SS wrote the first draft of the manuscript; SS, PH, PB, LM, and LH wrote sections of the manuscript. All authors contributed to manuscript revision, read and approved the submitted version.

## REFERENCES

Blanco, P., and Feijóo, R. (2013). A dimensionally-heterogeneous closed-loop model for the cardiovascular system and its applications. *Med. Eng. Phys.* 35, 652–667. doi: 10.1016/j.medengphy.2012.07.011

Blanco, P. J., Müller, L. O., Watanabe, S. M., and Feijóo, R. A. (2016). Computational modeling of blood flow steal phenomena caused by subclavian stenoses. *J. Biomech.* 49, 1593–1600. doi: 10.1016/j.jbiomech.2016.03.044

Blanco, P. J., Watanabe, S. M., Dari, E. A., Passos, M. A. R., and Feijóo, R. A. (2014). Blood flow distribution in an anatomically detailed arterial network model: criteria and algorithms. *Biomech. Model. Mechanobiol.* 13, 1303–1330. doi: 10.1007/s10237-014-0574-8

Blanco, P. J., Watanabe, S. M., Passos, M. A. R., Lemos, P. A., and Feijóo, R. A. (2015). An anatomically detailed arterial network model for one-dimensional computational hemodynamics. *IEEE Trans. Biomed. Eng.* 62, 736–753. doi: 10.1109/TBME.2014.2364522

Breedveld, P. C. (1984). *Physical Systems Theory Terms of Bond Graphs.* PhD thesis, University of Twente, Faculty of Electrical Engineering.

Brown, A. G., Shi, Y., Arndt, A., Müller, J., Lawford, P., and Hose, D. R. (2012). Importance of realistic lvad profiles for assisted aortic simulations: evaluation of optimal outflow anastomosis locations. *Comput. Methods Biomech. Biomed. Eng.* 15, 669–680. doi: 10.1080/10255842.2011.556628

Cebral, J. R., Castro, M. A., Burgess, J. E., Pergolizzi, R. S., Sheridan, M. J., and Putman, C. M. (2005). Characterization of cerebral aneurysms for assessing risk of rupture by using patient-specific computational hemodynamics models. *Am. J. Neuroradiol.* 26, 2550–2559.

Garny, A., and Hunter, P. J. (2015). Opencor: a modular and interoperable approach to computational biology. *Front. Physiol.* 6:26. doi: 10.3389/fphys.2015.00026

Gawthrop, P. J., and Crampin, E. J. (2014). Energy-based analysis of biochemical cycles using bond graphs. *Proc. R. Soc. A* 470:20140459. doi: 10.1098/rspa.2014.0459

Gawthrop, P. J., and Crampin, E. J. (2016). Modular bond-graph modelling and analysis of biomolecular systems. *IET Syst. Biol.* 10, 187–201. doi: 10.1049/iet-syb.2015.0083

Gawthrop, P. J., Cursons, J., and Crampin, E. J. (2015a). Hierarchical bond graph modelling of biochemical networks. *Proc. R. Soc. A,* 471:20150642. doi: 10.1098/rspa.2015.0642

Gawthrop, P. J., Siekmann, I., Kameneva, T., Saha, S., Ibbotson, M. R., and Crampin, E. J. (2015b). The energetic cost of the action potential: bond graph

modelling of electrochemical energy transduction in excitable membranes. *arXiv preprint arXiv:1512.00956.*

Heil, M., and Hazel, A. L. (2011). Fluid-structure interaction in internal physiological flows. *Ann. Rev. Fluid Mech.* 43, 141–162. doi: 10.1146/annurev-fluid-122109-160703

Hunter, P. (1972). *Numerical Simulation of Arterial Blood Flow.* Masters thesis, ResearchSpace, Auckland.

Korakianitis, T., and Shi, Y. (2006). A concentrated parameter model for the human cardiovascular system including heart valve dynamics and atrioventricular interaction. *Med. Eng. Phys.* 28, 613–628. doi: 10.1016/j.medengphy.2005.10.004

Liang, F., Takagi, S., Himeno, R., and Liu, H. (2009). Multi-scale modeling of the human cardiovascular system with applications to aortic valvular and arterial stenoses. *Med. Biol. Eng. Comput.* 47, 743–755. doi: 10.1007/s11517-009-0449-9

Müller, L. O., Blanco, P. J., Watanabe, S. M., and Feijóo, R. A. (2016a). A high-order local time stepping finite volume solver for one-dimensional blood flow simulations: application to the ADAN model. *Int. J. Numer. Methods Biomed. Eng.* 32:e02761. doi: 10.1002/cnm.2761

Müller, L. O., and Blanco, P. J. (2015). A high order approximation of hyperbolic conservation laws in networks: application to one-dimensional blood flow. *J. Comput. Phys.* 300, 423–437. doi: 10.1016/j.jcp.2015.07.056

Müller, L. O., Leugering, G., and Blanco, P. J. (2016b). Consistent treatment of viscoelastic effects at junctions in one-dimensional blood flow models. *J. Comput. Phys.* 314, 167–193. doi: 10.1016/j.jcp.2016.03.012

Oster, G., Perelson, A., and Katchalsky, A. (1971). Network thermodynamics. *Nature* 234, 393–399.

Paynter, H. M. (1961). *Analysis and Design of Engineering Systems.* Cambridge, MA: MIT press.

Reymond, P., Merenda, F., Perren, F., Rüfenacht, D., and Stergiopulos, N. (2009). Validation of a one-dimensional model of the systemic arterial tree. *Am. J. Physiol. Heart Circ. Physiol.* 297, H208–H222. doi: 10.1152/ajpheart.00037.2009

Safaei, S., Bradley, C. P., Suresh, V., Mithraratne, K., Muller, A., Ho, H., et al. (2016). Roadmap for cardiovascular circulation model. *J. Physiol.* 594, 6909–6928. doi: 10.1113/JP272660

Shojima, M., Oshima, M., Takagi, K., Torii, R., Hayakawa, M., Katada, K., et al. (2004). Magnitude and role of wall shear stress on cerebral aneurysm. *Stroke* 35, 2500–2505. doi: 10.1161/01.STR.0000144648.89172.0f

Stergiopulos, N., Young, D., and Rogge, T. (1992). Computer simulation of arterial flow with applications to arterial and aortic stenoses. *J. Biomech.* 25, 1477–1488. doi: 10.1016/0021-9290(92)90060-E

Westerhof, N., Bosman, F., De Vries, C. J., and Noordergraaf, A. (1969). Analog studies of the human systemic arterial tree. *J. Biomech.* 2,

121IN1135IN3137IN5139–134136138143. doi: 10.1016/0021-9290(69)90024-4

Westerhof, N., and Noordergraaf, A. (1970). Arterial viscoelasticity: a generalized model: effect on input impedance and wave travel in the systematic tree. *J. Biomech.* 3, 357IN15371–370IN16379.

# 12

# Autonomic Differentiation Map: A Novel Statistical Tool for Interpretation of Heart Rate Variability

*Daniela Lucini[1]\*, Nadia Solaro[2] and Massimo Pagani[1]*

[1] *BIOMETRA Department, University of Milan, Milan, Italy,* [2] *Department of Statistics and Quantitative Methods, University of Milano-Bicocca, Milan, Italy*

**\*Correspondence:**
*Daniela Lucini*
*daniela.lucini@unimi.it*

In spite of the large body of evidence suggesting Heart Rate Variability (HRV) alone or combined with blood pressure variability (providing an estimate of baroreflex gain) as a useful technique to assess the autonomic regulation of the cardiovascular system, there is still an ongoing debate about methodology, interpretation, and clinical applications. In the present investigation, we hypothesize that non-parametric and multivariate exploratory statistical manipulation of HRV data could provide a novel informational tool useful to differentiate normal controls from clinical groups, such as athletes, or subjects affected by obesity, hypertension, or stress. With a data-driven protocol in 1,352 ambulant subjects, we compute HRV and baroreflex indices from short-term data series as proxies of autonomic (ANS) regulation. We apply a three-step statistical procedure, by first removing age and gender effects. Subsequently, by factor analysis, we extract four ANS latent domains that detain the large majority of information (86.94%), subdivided in oscillatory (40.84%), amplitude (18.04%), pressure (16.48%), and pulse domains (11.58%). Finally, we test the overall capacity to differentiate clinical groups vs. control. To give more practical value and improve readability, statistical results concerning individual discriminant ANS proxies and ANS differentiation profiles are displayed through peculiar graphical tools, i.e., significance diagram and ANS differentiation map, respectively. This approach, which simultaneously uses all available information about the system, shows what domains make up the difference in ANS discrimination. e.g., athletes differ from controls in all domains, but with a graded strength: maximal in the (normalized) oscillatory and in the pulse domains, slightly less in the pressure domain and minimal in the amplitude domain. The application of multiple (non-parametric and exploratory) statistical and graphical tools to ANS proxies defines differentiation profiles that could provide a better understanding of autonomic differences between clinical groups and controls. ANS differentiation map permits to rapidly and simply synthesize the possible difference between clinical groups and controls, evidencing the ANS latent domains that have at least a medium strength of discrimination, while the significance diagram permits to identify the single ANS proxies inside each ANS latent domain that resulted in significant comparisons according to statistical tests.

Keywords: autonomic nervous system, heart rate variability, spectral analysis, baroreflex, statistics, chronic conditions, prevention

# INTRODUCTION

The burden of chronic conditions, such as obesity (Christakis and Fowler, 2007) or hypertension (Forouzanfar et al., 2017), is continuously growing worldwide and represents an important barrier to modernization in developing countries. Lifestyle optimization (Ding et al., 2015), focusing on better nutrition, more active life, and management of stress, represents a potentially useful intervention strategy. Advantages may be obtained both organizationally and economically. The extent of the problem and the emergence of new large-scale technologies suggest that novel approaches and types of analysis might provide a fresher point of view to seemingly established conditions, such as obesity or physical activity (Althoff et al., 2017). Lifestyle therapy aims at combating obesity, increasing physical activity, and reducing stress, potentially improving autonomic cardiac regulation. Notably, autonomic regulation can be assessed non-invasively by computer analysis of beat by beat RR interval (more frequently indicated as Heart Rate Variability, HRV) (Task Force of the European Society of Cardiology and the North American Society of Pacing and Electrophysiology, 1996) and arterial pressure variability.

The success of clinical applications heavily depends on the balance between complexity of technique and ease of use (Abraham and Michie, 2008). Thus it should not surprise that HRV (Task Force of the European Society of Cardiology and the North American Society of Pacing and Electrophysiology, 1996) alone gained a broad interest for clinical applications. However, there are several methodological criticalities:

- with protocols (frequently based on laboratory conditions, and relatively small samples), and
- with methods of analysis and interpretation (Billman et al., 2015; Sassi et al., 2015).

Regarding this latter one, we should consider:

- the length of data series (long-term, typically 24 h, or short-term, usually 5–10 min),
- the techniques employed to extract autonomic indices (time or frequency domain, deterministic, or pseudo-stochastic),
- the interpretative codes (Gerstner et al., 1997) of underlying activity and syntax (Buzsáki and Watson, 2012) of autonomic neurons (amplitude, oscillations, coherence, phase, etc.) and of multiple indices that are provided by the analysis of HRV.

For instance, it is well-recognized that to interpret neural activity we must consider a large set of coding modalities. Conversely, the majority of studies on RR interval or its variability give less relevance to the embedded codes of higher order (Pagani and Malliani, 2000).

The usual focus is on the different value of raw and normalized units in assessing the interaction between low- and high-frequency components (LF and HF) of HRV as a proxy of the neural balance between sympathetic and vagal modulation (taken as indices of excitatory/inhibitory influences; Pagani et al., 1986). This latter view is in line with historical models (Hess, 2014) and with electrophysiological studies with single unit recordings of efferent vagal fibers (Schwartz et al., 1973). Overall these studies support a dual antagonistic sympathetic/parasympathetic innervation of SA node. A definite improvement in the strength of clinical prediction, particularly in cardiac conditions, is offered by the addition of the cardiac baroreflex (La Rovere et al., 1998), assessed either in time (baroreflex slope) (Bertinieri et al., 1985) or frequency domain (index alpha) (Pagani et al., 1988).

A more-in-depth understanding of the hidden meaning of various autonomic proxies could be achieved using specific statistical tools. By Principal Component Analysis (Tarvainen et al., 2014) or Factor Analysis (Fukusaki et al., 2000), one can focus on the less explored hypothesis that information distributed across HRV derived variables could be exploited simultaneously, or again, by discriminant analysis (Jeong and Finkelstein, 2015), used for a more efficient separation in clinical groups. In particular, latent factor statistical methods may also help identify homogeneous clusters of few variables capable of exploring the pathophysiology underlying HRV characteristics. For instance, in relatively large groups of participants, mathematical forecasting showed that the major part of information (>80%) predicting the stand induced sympathetic excitation in normal humans is concentrated in only three variables (RR interval, LF and HF in nu; Malliani et al., 1997). Moreover, a logistic regression modeling approach showed that the autonomic information predicting the hypertensive state is concentrated on RR variance, the stand induced increase in LF nu, and the index alpha (Lucini et al., 2014).

Following this rationale, we hypothesize that a data-driven, pragmatic study protocol (Ford and Norrie, 2016), using multiple statistical methods in an integrated way for detecting latent domains (Thompson, 2004), could provide a novel approach to assess which autonomic (ANS) clusters might define profiles with the greatest discriminant capability across different clinical conditions. Specifically, we start from the assumption that groups such as athletes, normal subjects, obese subjects, people with high stress and hypertensives, overall form a physiological-pathological continuum of ANS regulation and dysregulation that could be captured by statistical tools that are not model-based. This is a crucial point. Setting up a statistical model requires specifying a functional form plus a set of conjectures about the data distribution through which a dependent variable, e.g., the probability of membership to a group, is linked to a set of good explicative variables, as, e.g., in the multinomial logistic model. Statistical modeling could, however, carry with it that data be severely forced within a too stringent statistical-mathematical formulation, which could even lead to poor fitting. We argued that this is particularly true in the context of ANS variables (or proxies), where relationships among them are still substantially under investigation (e.g., the difference between the raw and normalized power of LF and HF oscillations; Pagani et al., 1986). Moreover, most ANS proxies are typically not normally distributed, so that application of classical methods of statistical inference could lead to misleading conclusions. Also, it would be useful to provide practical indications about which ANS proxies could help distinguish subjects outside a "normal" ANS condition. In this sense, we treat subjects without pathologies (normal group) as the reference condition and compare, with respect to this, the other states along the ANS continuum (Narkiewicz and Somers, 1998).

All these considerations influenced the choice of the statistical approach where the primary concern was avoiding potential bias in the analyses. We then preferred to rely on non-parametric and multivariate exploratory statistical techniques and use them in an integrated manner rather than refer to statistical modeling (e.g., multinomial logistic regression model) or discriminant analysis (e.g., linear or quadratic discriminant analysis, which requires multivariate normality of data; Jobson, 2012). More specifically, we assess on a relatively large population of ambulant subjects with an expected wide variation of autonomic performance (from good to poor) whether clinical (or test) groups (athletes, obese subjects, people with high stress, and hypertensives) can be differentiated from controls (normal group) according to differences in ANS latent domains. ANS latent domains that prove to be capable of distinguishing clinical groups from controls are the constitutive elements of what we regard as ANS differentiation profiles of the clinical groups. We set up such profiles in a three-step analysis, the first of which is the preliminary handling of the ANS proxies. Since these latter ones are affected by age and gender effects, we first compute adjusted (Adj) ANS proxies, which are free from such effects, and use them throughout the analyses to detect the ANS differentiation profiles for each test group. We use non-parametric statistical procedures (Bowman and Azzalini, 1997; Hollander et al., 2014) to disclose individual Adj-ANS proxies that are capable of recognizing differences between test and normal groups. Then, we employ factor analysis to reduce the ANS proxies into few ANS latent domains (Thompson, 2004) and assess their overall capacity to recognize clinical groups vs. controls by exploiting the results achieved for the individual discriminant ANS proxies. Lastly, to give more practical value and improve readability, statistical results concerning individual discriminant ANS proxies and ANS differentiation profiles are displayed through peculiar graphical tools, i.e., significance diagram and ANS differentiation map, respectively. Implicitly this approach supports novel hypotheses between statistical properties of data clusters and underlying physiological organization (Pagani and Malliani, 2000).

Because of the complexity of the statistical approach and richness of the results, a large part of them is omitted from the text and presented in the Supplementary Material. We will not however make specific reference to it throughout the text.

## METHODS

Data for this study, which is part of an ongoing series of investigations, focused on the use of autonomic indices in cardiovascular prevention. They refer to a population of 1,352 ambulant subjects, who visited our outpatient Exercise Medicine Clinic for reasons varying from a health check-up to cardiovascular prevention (Lucini and Pagani, 2012) for obesity, stress, or hypertension, or the annual pre-participation sport screening (see **Table 1**). Data were excluded from the study if subjects were outside the range of 18–75 years, if they were smokers (any quantity), or affected by acute diseases

**TABLE 1 |** Frequency and percentage distributions of participants within clinical groups.

| Groups | Count | Percentage | Description |
|---|---|---|---|
| Athlete | 149 | 11.0% | Competitive sports, e.g., basket players, football players, badminton players, cyclists, rowers: Years of intense training and participation to competitions |
| Normal | 547 | 40.5% | Non-smoking subjects without pathologies |
| Obese | 102 | 7.5% | Subjects with BMI $\geq$ 30 (kg/m$^2$) |
| Stress | 190 | 14.1% | Psychological dimension of stress: Presence/absence of stress according to self-report of participants who asked advice for stress symptoms lasting more than three months, or referral by their physicians |
| Hypertensive (HT) | 271 | 20.0% | Subjects with Systolic BP $\geq$ 140 mmHg or Diastolic BP $\geq$ 90 mmHg, or both |
| HT-Obese | 55 | 4.1% | Obese subjects with high BP |
| HT-Stress | 38 | 2.8% | Stressed subjects with high BP |
| **Total** | 1352 | 100.0% | |

(within 3 months), or treated with drugs known to interfere with autonomic cardiovascular regulation or performance. The protocol of the study followed the principles of the Declaration of Helsinki and Title 45, US Code of Federal Regulations, Part 46, Protection of Human Subjects, Revised 13 November 2001, effective 13 December 2001 and was approved by the Independent Ethics Committee of IRCCS Humanitas Clinical Institute (Rozzano, IT). All subjects gave their informed consent to participate.

## Autonomic Evaluation

The day of recordings, all individuals arrived at the laboratory at least 2 h after a light breakfast, avoiding caffeinated beverages and heavy physical exercise in the previous 24 h. To account for circadian variations, acquisition of ECG (single thoracic lead) and respiration (piezoelectric belt) (Marazza, Monza, Italy), and arterial pressure waveforms (Finapres, TNO, Netherlands), were always performed between 10.00 and 12.00 h. Following our usual procedure, continuous signal (ECG, respiration, and arterial pressure waveform) acquisition was obtained for at least 5–7 min at rest and 5 min upon standing up. As described previously (Pagani et al., 1986), from the autoregressive spectral analysis of RR interval and systolic arterial pressure (SAP) variability, a series of indices indirectly reflecting cardiovascular autonomic modulation was derived, with minimal operator involvement thanks to a dedicated software (Badilini et al., 2005; see **Table 2**).

We use (Pagani et al., 1986) an autoregressive algorithm to automatically compute power and frequency of spectral components in the bandwidth of interest, discarding components of <5% power that are treated as noise. The software tool

**TABLE 2 |** Definition of the variables (ANS proxies) employed in the study.

| Vars. | Units | Definition |
|---|---|---|
| HR | beat/min | Heart Rate |
| RR Mean | msec | Average of RR interval from tachogram |
| RR TP | $msec^2$ | RR variance from tachogram |
| RR LFa | $msec^2$ | Absolute power(a) of Low Frequency (LF) component of RR variability (V) |
| RR HFa | $msec^2$ | Absolute power(a) of High Frequency (HF) component of RRV |
| RR LFnu | nu | Normalized power(nu) of Low Frequency (LF) component of RRV |
| RR HFnu | nu | Normalized power(nu) of High Frequency (HF) component of RRV |
| RR LF/HF | – | Ratio between absolute values of LF and HF |
| RR LFHz | Hz | Center frequency of LF |
| RR HFHz | Hz | Center frequency of HF, providing a measure of respiratory rate |
| $\Delta$RRLFnu | nu | Difference in LF power in nu between stand and rest |
| $\alpha$ index | msec/mmHg | Frequency domain measure of baroreflex gain |
| SAP | mmHg | Systolic arterial pressure by sphygmomanometer |
| DAP | mmHg | Diastolic arterial pressure by sphygmomanometer |
| SAP Mean | mmHg | Average of systogram (i.e., systolic arterial pressure variability by Finometer) |
| SAP LFa | $mmHg^2$ | Absolute power of LF component of systogram |

(Badilini et al., 2005) is set as to consider components with a center frequency of 0.03–0.14 Hz as Low Frequency, and components within the range 0.15–0.35 Hz as High Frequency, recalling that "the HF component is synchronous with the respiration" (Pagani et al., 1986), using a high coherence between RR variability and respiration as a confirmation. Recordings of subjects with low-frequency breathing are discarded to avoid entrainment, and biased increased LF power (Lucini et al., 2017).

The sensitivity of arterial baroreflex control of RR interval was also assessed by a frequency domain method ($\alpha$ index = average of the square root of the ratio between RR interval and SA Pressure Spectral powers of the low-frequency and high-frequency components; Pagani et al., 1988). In all individuals included in the study, respiratory rate coincided with the high-frequency component of RR variability.

## Statistics

Individuals were divided into 7 clinical groups, from athletes to hypertensive-stressed subjects (see **Table 1**). The majority of individuals (40.5% out of 1,352) fell into the normal group, which was regarded as the reference group. The other groups were treated as test groups to be compared with the normal one. Groups were chosen according to the likelihood of presenting a condition of putative higher vagal drive, as expected in elite athletes at midseason (Iellamo et al., 2002), or of excessive sympathetic drive, as expected in patients (Mancia and Grassi, 2014) with obesity, hypertension or stress (Lucini and Pagani,

2012). That is in line with the study hypothesis that various conditions might show different (possibly specific) differentiation profiles of autonomic (ANS) proxies (**Table 1**). To account for intertwined clinical conditions and carry out statistical analyses *ceteris paribus*, subjects who presented a concurrence of obesity and hypertension, or stress and hypertension, were aggregated into two groups: HT-Obese (4.1%, **Table 1**) and HT-Stress (2.8%, **Table 1**). On the other hand, subjects having either stress, and obesity together, or stress, obesity, and hypertension together, were discarded from the study because of their too exiguous number (5 and 2 subjects only, respectively). Apart from these situations, no other form of concurrence of different status was observed.

The main aim of the study was the detection of ANS profiles capable of distinguishing each test group from the normal one in a "real life" ambulant population (Ford and Norrie, 2016). We refer to these profiles as *ANS differentiation profiles*. **Figure 1** sums up statistical analysis steps carried out for their detection. A crucial issue affected the choice of the statistical approach. Clinical groups were not directly comparable because of their different composition in terms of age and gender. For instance, 71.1% of athletes were male, and 75.6% of obese individuals were female; 98% of athletes were under 34 years of age, while 48% of hypertensive subjects were over 50 years. Setting up ANS differentiation profiles by working within "age-by-gender" classes did not prove to be a convenient solution in this case. This choice would have meant dealing with empty subgroups or subgroups too small in size (e.g., there was no female athlete over 50 years of age). Comparability among the groups was thus attained statistically by removing age and gender effects from the considered ANS proxies. A 2-way full ANOVA model including age and gender main effects plus their interaction was fitted to each ANS proxy, and ANOVA residuals, being free of such effects, were used as so-called *adjusted ANS proxies* (Adj-ANS proxies; **Figure 1**, preliminary step).

ANS differentiation profiles were thus built using the Adj-ANS proxies, instead of the original ANS proxies, through the further two-step analysis outlined in **Figure 1** (steps 1 and 2). The aim was first to detect single ANS proxies capable of distinguishing the test groups from the normal one (step 1), and subsequently, from this knowledge, set up discriminant ANS domains in order to reduce the overlapping information of the ANS proxies to a small number of latent dimensions (step 2). Specifically, in the first step, each within-test-group distribution of the Adj-ANS proxies was compared to the corresponding within-normal-group distribution through the non-parametric testing procedures by (a) Bowman and Azzalini's permutation (BA) test (Bowman and Azzalini, 1997), and (b) Jonckheere-Terpstra's (JT) permutation test (Hollander et al., 2014; Seshan, 2017). The nominal significance level was set at 0.05. Regarding the BA test, rejection of the null hypothesis for a specific ANS proxy in a "test-vs.-reference" comparison indicates, controlling for age and gender effects, that the ANS proxy distribution for that test group in the population has a shape generically different to the normal population. By the permutation JT test, the nature of these shape differences was investigated further. For every "test-vs.-reference" comparison involving each Adj-ANS proxy,

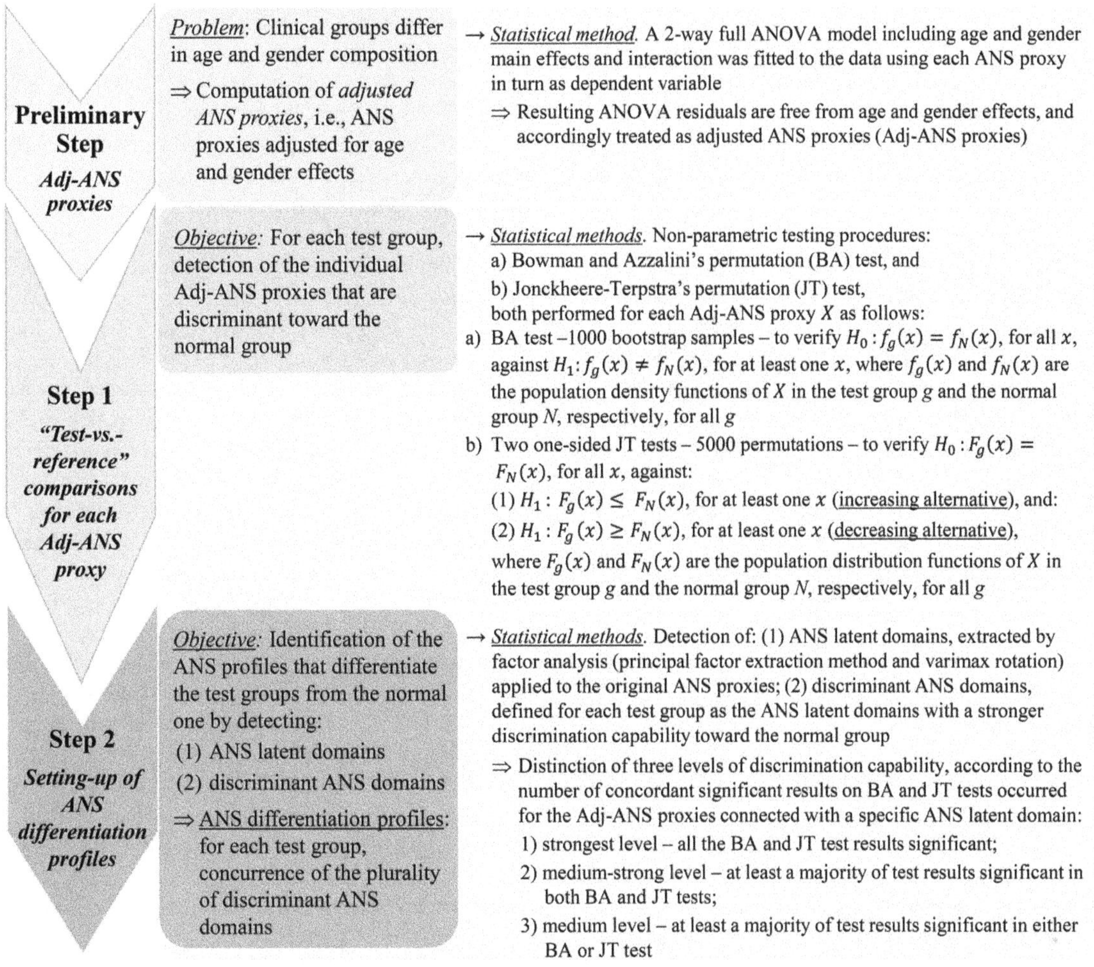

| Preliminary Step<br><br>*Adj-ANS proxies* | *Problem*: Clinical groups differ in age and gender composition<br><br>⇒ Computation of *adjusted ANS proxies*, i.e., ANS proxies adjusted for age and gender effects | → *Statistical method*. A 2-way full ANOVA model including age and gender main effects and interaction was fitted to the data using each ANS proxy in turn as dependent variable<br><br>⇒ Resulting ANOVA residuals are free from age and gender effects, and accordingly treated as adjusted ANS proxies (Adj-ANS proxies) |
|---|---|---|
| Step 1<br><br>*"Test-vs.-reference" comparisons for each Adj-ANS proxy* | *Objective*: For each test group, detection of the individual Adj-ANS proxies that are discriminant toward the normal group | → *Statistical methods*. Non-parametric testing procedures:<br>a) Bowman and Azzalini's permutation (BA) test, and<br>b) Jonckheere-Terpstra's permutation (JT) test,<br>both performed for each Adj-ANS proxy $X$ as follows:<br>a) BA test – 1000 bootstrap samples – to verify $H_0: f_g(x) = f_N(x)$, for all $x$, against $H_1: f_g(x) \neq f_N(x)$, for at least one $x$, where $f_g(x)$ and $f_N(x)$ are the population density functions of $X$ in the test group $g$ and the normal group $N$, respectively, for all $g$<br>b) Two one-sided JT tests – 5000 permutations – to verify $H_0: F_g(x) = F_N(x)$, for all $x$, against:<br>(1) $H_1: F_g(x) \leq F_N(x)$, for at least one $x$ (<u>increasing alternative</u>), and:<br>(2) $H_1: F_g(x) \geq F_N(x)$, for at least one $x$ (<u>decreasing alternative</u>),<br>where $F_g(x)$ and $F_N(x)$ are the population distribution functions of $X$ in the test group $g$ and the normal group $N$, respectively, for all $g$ |
| Step 2<br><br>*Setting-up of ANS differentiation profiles* | *Objective*: Identification of the ANS profiles that differentiate the test groups from the normal one by detecting:<br>(1) ANS latent domains<br>(2) discriminant ANS domains<br>⇒ <u>ANS differentiation profiles</u>: for each test group, concurrence of the plurality of discriminant ANS domains | → *Statistical methods*. Detection of: (1) ANS latent domains, extracted by factor analysis (principal factor extraction method and varimax rotation) applied to the original ANS proxies; (2) discriminant ANS domains, defined for each test group as the ANS latent domains with a stronger discrimination capability toward the normal group<br>⇒ Distinction of three levels of discrimination capability, according to the number of concordant significant results on BA and JT tests occurred for the Adj-ANS proxies connected with a specific ANS latent domain:<br>1) strongest level – all the BA and JT test results significant;<br>2) medium-strong level – at least a majority of test results significant in both BA and JT tests;<br>3) medium level – at least a majority of test results significant in either BA or JT test |

**FIGURE 1 |** Statistical analysis steps for the detection of ANS differentiation profiles.

the null hypothesis of equality between distributions was tested using two separate one-sided JT tests: the first against the so-called increasing alternative, the second against the decreasing alternative (**Figure 1**, step 1). Rejection of the null hypothesis in favor of an increasing (decreasing) alternative would evidence, net of age and gender effects, that the ANS proxy distribution is more highly concentrated around smaller (higher) values in the test rather than the normal population.

In the second step (**Figure 1**), ANS differentiation profiles were set up for each test group in the light of the results achieved separately for the Adj-ANS proxies in step 1. This was accomplished by:

i. detecting latent domains underlying the observed ANS proxies (i.e., *ANS latent domains*), to obtain a limited set of unobserved, uncorrelated dimensions of the ANS system that are practically measured by the plurality of the ANS proxies. This was carried out through factor analysis (Thompson, 2004; principal factor extraction method with varimax rotation) applied to the original ANS proxies. We regard the first common factors each explaining a substantial percentage (i.e.,

at least 10%) of the total communality (i.e., the part of total variance reproducible by common factors) as ANS latent domains. And then:

ii. identifying, for each test group, the ANS latent domains of stronger differentiation capability against the normal group (according to the definition reported in **Figure 1**, step 2) using the BA and JT test results of step 1. We refer to such domains as *discriminant ANS domains*.

Regarding point (ii) above, discrimination capability of an ANS latent domain was appraised for each test group by the number of jointly significant results on BA and JT tests that occurred for the Adj-ANS proxies connected with that specific domain. In this regard, it is worth remarking that BA and JT tests might not lead in general to concordant inferential results because these procedures are based on far different theoretical grounds, and therefore they can capture different aspects in the comparison between two statistical distributions. Nonetheless, a significant BA test followed by a not significant JT test could reveal that two distributions differ in shape, but not in position, because of a major/minor concentration of points in the central part or in the tails of one of the two distributions. The opposite situation (a significant JT test and a not significant BA test) would indeed be less clearly interpretable. From a practical point of view, these situations could indicate weak empirical support toward the alternative hypothesis of difference between distributions.

Statistical analysis ended with the set-up of ANS differentiation profiles for each test group against the normal group. These profiles were given for each test group by the concurrence of the plurality of discriminant ANS domains detected according to the above procedure. To provide a more immediate clinical value, ANS differentiation profiles were visualized through a graphical map (ANS differentiation map) containing different color grades according to the strength of their discrimination capability.

BA test, along with the smoothed density curves appearing in **Figure 2**, and JT permutation test were carried out with software R ver. 3.4.0 (R Core Team, Vienna, Austria, 2017) and the libraries "clinfun" (Seshan, 2017) and "sm" (Bowman and Azzalini, 2014), respectively. Descriptive statistics, construction of Adj-ANS proxies through the 2-way full ANOVA model and factor analysis were carried out with software SAS ver. 9.4.

## RESULTS

Total and within-groups mean and standard deviation of the considered 16 ANS proxies (definitions in **Table 2**) are presented in **Table 3**.

Regarding the "test-vs.-reference" comparisons analysis (step 1, **Figure 1**), **Figure 2** provides a graphical representation of the BA test, which addresses the logic behind it. Empirical density functions of a variable, rather than a usual summary measure (e.g., the mean), are compared in their entirety across two different groups and without assuming a priori hypotheses on the data distribution. In such a way, the overall shape of the distribution, and not only a single value, is considered for comparisons. Pointwise comparisons are expressed by means of a non-parametric 95%-confidence region ("reference band for equality"). If two curves lie both inside it, then they are accepted as equal. Otherwise, they are significantly different. Specifically, in **Figure 2** estimated density curves of the distribution of six selected Adj-ANS proxies in the test groups (red curve) and the normal group (black curve) are depicted, and the reference band for equality (gray region) is juxtaposed to show pointwise equality/difference between the curves (Bowman and Azzalini, 1997). Overall, it is apparent that different clinical conditions translate into diverse profiles of autonomic differentiation from normal group. For instance, the last row of panels in **Figure 2** shows that, after controlling for age and gender effects, the distribution of SAP Mean is different from the normal group in all but athletes (first panel) and stressed individuals (third panel). In these latter two groups, the reference band exactly contains both the red and the black curves (i.e., equality of the curves), while this does not occur for the other groups (i.e., notice the difference between the curves).

**Figure 3** reports the significance diagram concerning the Adj-ANS proxies resulted individually discriminant in each "test-vs.-reference" comparison according to the BA and JT tests jointly considered. Inequality symbol denotes BA significant results. Solid up- and empty down-arrows mark JT significant results (i.e., Adj-ANS proxy values greater/smaller than the normal group, respectively). We regard an Adj-ANS proxy as individually discriminant in a "test-vs.-reference" comparison if both BA and JT test results are significant. In this way, the probability of the overall type I error concerning the null hypothesis of no difference in a "test-vs.-reference" comparison of each Adj-ANS proxy is reduced to $(0.05)^2 = 0.0025$. That is in line with a more conservative approach that makes rejecting the null hypothesis in favor of the alternative of individual discrimination more difficult. A proxy of the level of strength in individual discrimination capability is given here by the magnitude of the BA and JT $p$-values jointly considered and is indicated in the diagram by cells with different background color shades (the darkest/lightest shade denotes the strongest/less strong level of joint significance). On the other hand, blank cells stand for at least a non-significant result and thus denote the absence of individual discrimination capability.

By the significance diagram, it is apparent that, controlling for age and gender effects, athletes tend to have higher values of RR Mean, RR HFa, RR HFnu, ΔRRLFnu, SAP, and DAP than normal individuals (solid up-arrow), and lower values of HR, RR LFa, RR LFnu, RR LF/HF, and RR LFHz (empty down-arrow). Moreover, the most individually discriminant ANS proxies turn out to be RR Mean, RR HFnu, ΔRRLFnu (the darkest yellow cells), and HR, RR LFa, RR LFnu, RR LF/HF, and RR LFHz (the darkest blue cells). On the other hand, hypertensive individuals tend to have higher values of HR, RR HFa, RR LFnu, RR HFHz, SAP, DAP, and SAP Mean (solid up-arrow), and lower values of RR Mean, RR HFnu, ΔRRLFnu, and α index (empty down-arrow), while the most individually discriminant ANS proxies are HR, RR LFnu, SAP, DAP, SAP Mean (the darkest yellow cells), and RR Mean, RR HFnu, and α index (the darkest blue cells).

Regarding setting-up of ANS differentiation profiles (step 2, **Figure 1**), the main results of factor analysis carried out for extracting ANS latent domains are given in **Table 4**. Total communality amounts here to 76.67% of the total variance. In line with the above definition, ANS latent domains are given by the first four common factors, which together account for 86.9% of total communality (**Table 4**). Each factor explains more than 10% of total communality. Specifically, the first factor (40.84% of total communality) represents the Oscillatory Domain (all indices of rhythms are in normalized units), being highly positively correlated with RR HFnu and ΔRRLFnu, and negatively correlated with RR LF/HF and RR LFnu (**Table 4**, first column). The second factor (18.04% of total communality) is the Amplitude Domain because of its highly positive correlations with RR TP, RR HFa, RR LFa, and α index (all indices in raw values, **Table 4**, second column). The third factor (16.48% of total communality) is the Pressure Domain, being highly positively correlated with SAP, DAP, and SAP Mean (**Table 4**, third column). The fourth factor (11.58% of total communality) represents the Pulse (rate) Domain for its highly positive

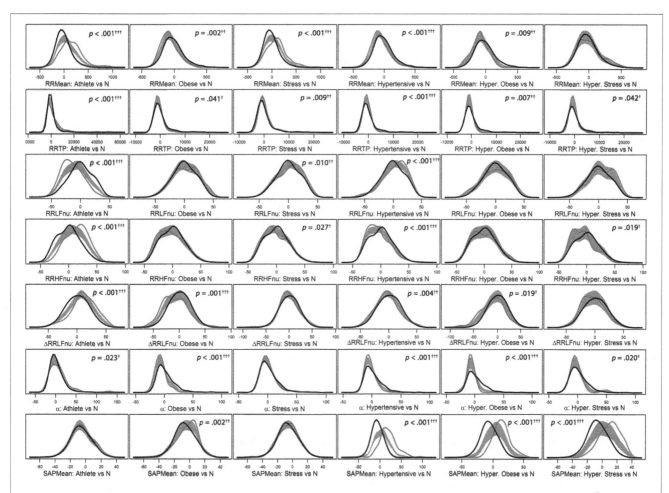

**FIGURE 2** | Panel plot of estimated density curves* of six selected adjusted ANS proxies (i.e., RR Mean, RR TP, RR LFnu, RR HFnu, ΔRRLFnu, α index, and SAP Mean). Gray regions represent reference bands for equality between the curves of each test group against the normal group (N).*Density estimates are obtained through the kernel density method by Bowman and Azzalini (1997). Roughly speaking, histogram of each adjusted ANS proxy is interpolated in order to have a smoothed empirical density curve. Colors in each panel: the black curve refers to the normal group (reference group); the red curve concerns a specific test group (Athlete, Obese, Stress, Hypertensive, HT-Obese, or HT-Stress, resp.) regarded for the comparison with the normal group. The gray region is a reference band for equality between the two curves. Panels with significant results include p-values and significance codes: $0.001^{\dagger\dagger\dagger}$, $0.01^{\dagger\dagger}$, $0.05^{\dagger}$.

correlation with HR and negative correlation with RR Mean (**Table 4**, fourth column). Three of the ANS proxies (i.e., RR HFHz, RR LFHz, and SAP LFa) prove to be linked far weakly with these four factors and then with the ANS latent domains. Accordingly, they are discarded from the analyses subsequently performed to detect discriminant ANS domains (**Figure 1**, step 2).

Finally, **Figure 4** reports the ANS differentiation map, i.e., the graphical map of the ANS differentiation profiles set up for every test group as described in **Figure 1**, step 2. Colored cells represent the discriminant ANS domains, and are shaded differently according to their level of discrimination capability (**Figure 1**, step 2). For example, athletes' ANS differentiation profile consists of all the four domains together. Oscillatory and pulse domains have the strongest discrimination capability, pressure domain has a medium-strong level, and amplitude domain a medium level. Moreover, by the significance diagram (**Figure 3**) it can be seen

that inside the oscillatory domain, controlling for age and gender effects, values of RR HFnu and ΔRRLFnu tend to be higher than in normal individuals, while RR LFnu and RR LF/HF tend to have lower values. Similarly, inside the pulse domain, HR is lower, and RR Mean is higher than in normal individuals (**Figure 3**). In pressure domain, SAP and DAP are higher, while in amplitude domain RR LFa is lower and RR HFa is higher than in normal individuals. ANS differentiation profile of hypertensive subjects is also formed by the four ANS domains together (pressure and pulse domains with the strongest discrimination capability). Obese group differs from the normal group for pulse (strongest discrimination), pressure and amplitude domains, similarly to HT-Obese group (pulse and pressure domains with the strongest discrimination capability). Pulse (strongest discrimination) and amplitude domains characterize Stress group, while pressure (strongest discrimination), oscillatory, and amplitude domains constitute the ANS differentiation profile of HT-Stress.

**TABLE 3 |** ANS proxies: Descriptive data (mean and standard deviation) within clinical groups and over the groups.

| | Groups | | | | | | | | | | | | | | | |
| Vars | Athlete | | Normal | | Obese | | Stress | | Hypertensive | | HT-obese | | HT-stress | | Total | |
| | Mean | SD | Mean | SD | Mean | SD | Mean | SD | Mean | SD | Mean | SD | Mean | SD | Mean | SD |
|---|---|---|---|---|---|---|---|---|---|---|---|---|---|---|---|---|
| HR | 55.54 | 11.22 | 67.02 | 10.39 | 73.85 | 11.05 | 61.27 | 12.40 | 71.83 | 11.39 | 73.82 | 10.66 | 66.39 | 12.01 | 66.69 | 12.31 |
| RR Mean | 1124.00 | 227.53 | 917.62 | 148.68 | 831.11 | 128.45 | 1019.18 | 206.29 | 855.47 | 131.71 | 828.11 | 110.57 | 934.15 | 176.69 | 932.48 | 184.94 |
| RR TP | 6086.07 | 6843.65 | 3184.62 | 3414.38 | 1643.55 | 1689.91 | 2616.41 | 2388.96 | 1507.40 | 1412.89 | 1068.84 | 1189.08 | 1718.37 | 1266.80 | 2844.80 | 3632.93 |
| RR LFa | 1180.54 | 1186.36 | 1022.47 | 1491.71 | 501.45 | 608.27 | 804.60 | 1006.64 | 460.29 | 530.03 | 355.92 | 421.25 | 556.36 | 815.79 | 818.26 | 1170.04 |
| RR HFa | 2672.21 | 3800.57 | 998.40 | 1672.46 | 378.76 | 511.09 | 664.46 | 999.15 | 294.30 | 594.16 | 222.18 | 357.88 | 231.21 | 280.84 | 905.92 | 1878.27 |
| RR LFnu | 34.98 | 17.92 | 51.16 | 20.33 | 53.92 | 21.94 | 54.47 | 22.19 | 58.59 | 20.49 | 54.69 | 22.95 | 61.28 | 20.95 | 51.97 | 21.65 |
| RR HFnu | 59.53 | 19.08 | 41.61 | 20.23 | 37.51 | 21.36 | 37.74 | 21.61 | 31.75 | 18.73 | 36.57 | 20.91 | 29.66 | 18.92 | 40.21 | 21.53 |
| RR LF/HF | 0.82 | 0.91 | 2.28 | 3.24 | 4.29 | 9.87 | 3.34 | 4.97 | 3.99 | 5.82 | 3.18 | 4.59 | 5.98 | 12.33 | 2.90 | 5.31 |
| RR LFHz | 0.10 | 0.02 | 0.10 | 0.02 | 0.09 | 0.03 | 0.09 | 0.02 | 0.10 | 0.03 | 0.09 | 0.03 | 0.09 | 0.02 | 0.10 | 0.03 |
| RR HFHz | 0.27 | 0.06 | 0.27 | 0.06 | 0.30 | 0.07 | 0.25 | 0.06 | 0.28 | 0.06 | 0.30 | 0.08 | 0.23 | 0.06 | 0.27 | 0.06 |
| ΔRRLFnu | 47.57 | 20.92 | 27.44 | 20.54 | 14.45 | 23.40 | 23.05 | 21.90 | 15.44 | 20.21 | 7.95 | 23.12 | 15.85 | 17.76 | 24.55 | 23.20 |
| α index | 34.78 | 22.62 | 24.67 | 16.25 | 12.99 | 9.24 | 20.41 | 14.81 | 11.45 | 8.31 | 8.11 | 4.06 | 15.45 | 14.72 | 20.42 | 16.26 |
| SAP | 112.53 | 15.36 | 113.55 | 11.86 | 119.49 | 9.88 | 117.26 | 12.63 | 147.75 | 16.67 | 149.47 | 15.01 | 140.00 | 11.45 | 123.62 | 19.90 |
| DAP | 68.63 | 7.62 | 70.87 | 7.71 | 75.11 | 6.80 | 74.26 | 8.46 | 93.50 | 9.62 | 93.76 | 11.61 | 91.66 | 5.71 | 77.58 | 12.87 |
| SAP Mean | 108.62 | 12.91 | 114.38 | 12.49 | 120.30 | 12.06 | 119.17 | 13.69 | 150.95 | 19.91 | 144.06 | 12.26 | 140.34 | 14.41 | 123.50 | 20.19 |
| SAP LFa | 4.28 | 4.46 | 4.12 | 5.79 | 4.96 | 6.75 | 4.82 | 6.30 | 5.70 | 8.50 | 6.61 | 8.25 | 6.23 | 8.91 | 4.78 | 6.66 |

# DISCUSSION

This investigation on a relatively large population of ambulant subjects shows that multiple statistical tools used in an integrated way can be profitably applied to the analysis of cardiovascular variability. In particular, it suggests that clustering of ANS proxies according to hidden factors (Thompson, 2004; Lucini et al., 2014) might help differentiate properties of clinical groups (athletes, obese subjects, people with high stress, and hypertensives) from controls. To this end, we employ a three-step statistical analysis. We use 2-way ANOVA residuals instead of raw values of the ANS proxies to account for age and gender effects. We employ non-parametric statistical procedures to identify discriminant Adj-ANS proxies. Finally, we set up ANS differentiation profiles by detecting which ANS latent domains have the highest capacity to discriminate HRV properties of clinical groups vs. controls.

## Statistics: A Novel Tool to Interpret Autonomic Proxies

Usual studies on autonomic innervation representing ANS proxies as raw values must deal with several potential confounders. First, autonomic proxies show an important age (Jandackova et al., 2016) and gender (Dart et al., 2002) dependency, which might hinder clinical applications and affect the capacity to discriminate between clinical groups.

In the present study, we have avoided this possible bias by removing age and gender effects from the considered ANS proxies and obtaining so-called *adjusted ANS proxies* (Adj-ANS proxies), (**Figure 1**, preliminary step). This step permits to assess the discrimination capability (clinical groups against controls) of ANS proxies and ANS latent domains free of age and gender effects. Accordingly, this approach avoids the drawback of the

difficulty of stratifying the subjects within the clinical groups in age and gender classes of adequate size and composition, as already discussed in the Statistics section. In this respect, we argue that resorting to a *de facto* statistical remedy, i.e., the adjustment of the ANS proxies using a statistical model (2-way ANOVA), has the advantage of being applicable in every context where stratification of subjects according to auxiliary characteristics (e.g., age and gender) is not feasible.

Moreover, we are still facing the problem of the redundancy of the measures. In other words, we do not know whether all the individually discriminant ANS proxies carry the same discriminant value (Malliani et al., 1997; Lucini et al., 2014), or which one would be better to employ in practice. In this regard, the significance diagram (**Figure 3**) highlights, with different color shades of the cells, the ANS proxies that result in significant comparisons between clinical groups and control. It should be noticed that these shades represent the empirical significance levels (i.e., the *p*-values) of BA and JT tests jointly considered and not the *pure* discriminant power of the single ANS proxies.

Factor analysis is a statistical tool that helps unravel hidden links between variables (Thompson, 2004). It also provides clusters of variables that carry homogeneous overall meaning. It appears particularly valuable in this context since it permits to formulate hypotheses about the type of information carried by the extracted clusters of ANS proxies. In doing so, it combines statistics with underlying neural physiology. Here we have shown that the information underlying the considered 16 ANS proxies can be represented with a very good degree of approximation by four common factors (whose fraction of information is of sufficient amplitude: at least 10%). The combination of variables strongly linked to the four hidden factors may suggest an underlying meaning and physiological interpretation. More in

| Groups | Athlete | | Obese | | Stress | | Hypertensive | | HT-Obese | | HT-Stress | |
|---|---|---|---|---|---|---|---|---|---|---|---|---|
| Variables | BA | JT | BA | JT | BA | JT | BA | JT | BA | JT | BA | JT |
| HR | ≠ | ↓ | ≠ | ↑ | ≠ | ↓ | ≠ | ↑ | ≠ | ↑ | | |
| RR Mean | ≠ | ↑ | ≠ | ↓ | ≠ | ↑ | ≠ | ↓ | ≠ | ↓ | | |
| RR TP | ≠ | | ≠ | ↓ | ≠ | ↑ | ≠ | | ≠ | | ≠ | |
| RR LFa | ≠ | ↓ | | ↓ | ≠ | ↑ | ≠ | | ≠ | ↓ | ≠ | |
| RR HFa | ≠ | ↑ | ≠ | | ≠ | ↑ | ≠ | ↑ | ≠ | | ≠ | |
| RR LFnu | ≠ | ↓ | | | ≠ | ↑ | ≠ | ↑ | | | | ↑ |
| RR HFnu | ≠ | ↑ | | ↓ | ≠ | | ≠ | ↓ | | | ≠ | ↓ |
| RR LF/HF | ≠ | ↓ | | | | | ≠ | | ≠ | ↓ | ≠ | |
| RR LFHz | ≠ | ↓ | ≠ | ↓ | ≠ | ↓ | | | ≠ | ↓ | | ↓ |
| RR HFHz | | | ≠ | ↑ | ≠ | ↓ | ≠ | ↑ | | ↑ | ≠ | ↓ |
| ΔRRLFnu | ≠ | ↑ | ≠ | ↓ | | | ≠ | ↓ | ≠ | ↓ | | ↓ |
| α index | ≠ | | ≠ | ↓ | | | ≠ | ↓ | ≠ | ↓ | ≠ | |
| SAP | ≠ | ↑ | | ↑ | | | ≠ | ↑ | ≠ | ↑ | ≠ | ↑ |
| DAP | ≠ | ↑ | ≠ | ↑ | ≠ | ↑ | ≠ | ↑ | ≠ | ↑ | ≠ | ↑ |
| SAP Mean | | | ≠ | ↑ | | | ≠ | ↑ | ≠ | ↑ | ≠ | ↑ |
| SAP LFa | ≠ | | | | | | | ↑ | | | | |

**FIGURE 3 |** Significance diagram summing up the results of BA and JT permutation tests applied to the adjusted ANS proxies within each test group. Normal group is the reference term in all the comparisons. <u>Columns with header BA:</u> Two-sided BA permutation test (at 0.05 level) in the comparison between the population density functions $f_g(x)$ of test group $g$ and $f_N(x)$ of normal group, resp.: ≠ stands for significantly different population density functions for at least one $x$, a blank cell denotes equal density curves (**Figure 1**, step 1). <u>Columns with header JT:</u> One-sided JT test (at 0.05 level) in the comparison between the two population distribution functions $F_g(x)$ of test group $g$ and $F_N(x)$ of normal group: ↑ denotes $F_g(x)$ significantly higher than $F_N(x)$ for at least one $x$; ↓ denotes $F_g(x)$ significantly lower than $F_N(x)$ for at least one $x$. A blank cell denotes a non-significant comparison (**Figure 1**, step 1).
Background color shades for joint significance of BA and JT tests:

- JT test with significant alternative ↑

| both $P < .001$ | $P < .001$ and $P < .01$ | $P < .001$ and $P < .05$ | both $P < .01$ | $P < .01$ and $P < .05$ | both $P < .05$ |
|---|---|---|---|---|---|

- JT test with significant alternative ↓

| both $P < .001$ | $P < .001$ and $P < .01$ | $P < .001$ and $P < .05$ | both $P < .01$ | $P < .01$ and $P < .05$ | both $P < .05$ |
|---|---|---|---|---|---|

detail, near 87% of the total communality (**Table 4**) is explained by the first four latent factors. They refer to: (1) oscillatory behavior (oscillatory domain, in nu) (Gerstner et al., 1997; Buzsáki and Watson, 2012); (2) total variance, oscillatory raw values and alpha index (amplitude domain, in absolute units) (La Rovere et al., 1998; Pagani and Malliani, 2000); (3) raw values of arterial pressure (pressure domain), and (4) raw values of heart rate and RR interval (pulse domain). It seems therefore that the major part of information carried by ANS proxies could provide a window on the two principal coding of cardiovascular variability (oscillations and amplitude, i.e., first and second factor) (Pagani and Malliani, 2000) and simple hemodynamic measures (arterial pressure and pulse rate, i.e., third and fourth factor). Importantly this approach might help resolve (at least as a first approximation) the riddle of which autonomic indices should be clinically employed. In fact, it provides information on how hidden factors *govern* major aspects of cardiovascular variability. As a corollary, since all information about HRV and arterial pressure findings can be summarized in four uncorrelated factors, we may propose that this approach could be employed to describe and monitor autonomic regulation and its changes during relevant conditions. Just as an example, we may consider

managing training season in athletes, or monitor the effects of stress and recovery, or of diets interventions in obese individuals.

In this context, the previous report of a strong coherence between RR and ANS rhythms, according to the "concept of common central mechanisms governing sympathetic and parasympathetic rhythmic activity" (Pagani et al., 1997), seem to imply a greater strength of oscillatory (i.e., nu) than amplitude (i.e., raw values) information.

## Individual Discrimination vs. Joint Discrimination, Discrimination Capability vs. Discrimination Power

As already mentioned, a fundamental step in the study was to assess the individual discrimination capability of the Adj-ANS proxies in the comparison between test groups and the reference normal group in order to define the ANS differentiation profiles. On this point, two remarks are worth making. First, we have decided to proceed variable-by-variable and assess what we have denoted as individual discrimination capability. In this way, we intended to give some practical indications directly usable in clinical terms about which ANS proxies could help

**TABLE 4 |** Detection of ANS latent domains by factor analysis: Rotated factor pattern matrix with the varimax method arrested to the first four factors.

| Variables | Factor1 | Factor2 | Factor3 | Factor4 |
|---|---|---|---|---|
| RR HFnu | 92* | 10 | −12 | −14 |
| ΔRRLFnu | 65* | 12 | −22 | −8 |
| RR LF/HF | −57* | −2 | 6 | 11 |
| RR LFnu | −96* | −7 | 8 | 11 |
| RR TP | 15 | 96* | −11 | −17 |
| RR HFa | 40 | 77* | −11 | −9 |
| RR LFa | -21 | 74* | −11 | −15 |
| α index | 17 | 63* | −27 | −25 |
| SAP | −12 | −12 | 96* | 3 |
| SAP Mean | −11 | −13 | 91* | 3 |
| DAP | −19 | −14 | 82* | 8 |
| HR | −15 | −20 | 9 | 96* |
| RR HFHz | −14 | −9 | −3 | 29 |
| RR Mean | 13 | 19 | −7 | −94* |
| RR LFHz | 12 | 6 | −8 | 17 |
| SAP LFa | −14 | 5 | 12 | 3 |
| % of total communality | 40.84% | 18.04% | 16.48% | 11.58% |
| cumulative % of total communality | 40.84% | 58.88% | 75.36% | 86.94% |

*Total communality (i.e., total reproduced variance) = 12.267, total variance = 16, percentage of total variance explained = 76.67%. Printed values are correlation coefficients multiplied by 100 and rounded to the nearest integer. Asterisks flag correlation coefficients greater than, or equal to, 0.4 in absolute value. Interpretation of the first four factors: Factor 1 = Oscillatory domain (variables colored in lilac), Factor 2 = Amplitude domain (variables in pink), Factor 3 = Pressure domain (variables in green), Factor 4 = Pulse domain (variables in blue).*

recognize subjects that are outside the normal group. As an alternative, we could have proceeded by considering the ANS proxies *jointly* and detecting the most discriminant ones *each net of the others*. This would have required us to work within a genuine statistical modeling approach, by specifying a suitable functional form linking the variables along with formulating a set of conjectures about the distribution of the data. Nevertheless, this was outside our objective. At this stage of our exploration, we feel that forcing the data in order that they meet relationships still under investigation may be too premature. As another alternative, we could have tested the discrimination capability of the ANS latent domains produced by factor analysis, rather than the single ANS proxies, thus working indirectly on the clusters of the ANS proxies connected each to a specific HRV domain. However, this approach has two main drawbacks. The common factors representing the ANS latent domains are not observable variables so that any analysis concerning their individual discrimination capability would lead to indications not directly usable in clinical practice. Moreover, the common factors are extracted by the principal factor method, and then from the part of the multidimensional variability shared by all the ANS proxies. Consequently, the specificity of each ANS proxy, which instead is the part of the variability not in common, would have been *de facto* excluded from the discrimination capability analysis.

Accordingly, at this stage, we have chosen to apply the non-parametric BA and JT testing procedures to each single ANS proxy (adjusted for age and gender effects) in order to: (1) carry out "test-vs.-reference" comparisons variable-by-variable without introducing a priori assumptions on the ANS proxy distributions (most ANS proxies, both in original and adjusted units, are not normally distributed), (2) perform the above comparisons by considering the distributions of the ANS proxies in their entirety, (3) draw conclusions about the individual discrimination capability of each ANS proxy using two different statistical testing procedures, to obtain as more robust results as possible.

Second, strictly related to the point above there is the implicit distinction, which ultimately affected the choice of the statistical approach, between discrimination capability and discrimination power. All the analyses we performed were addressed to detecting the potential capability of the ANS proxies of distinguishing a test group from the normal one in a wider population of subjects. As already pointed out, this is not the same as evaluating the discrimination power of the ANS proxies because, in general, it is one thing to assess if a relation exists, quite another to say how strong that relation is. Then, since we are at an exploratory stage of the investigation, we have preferred to focus here on the existence of the discrimination capability of each ANS proxy, and defer any inspection toward their discrimination power in future studies.

## The Differentiation Profile

Traditionally comparison among groups is provided by the difference from controls of various paradigmatic groups. Athletes show, e.g., what could be interpreted as a vagal shift (Iellamo et al., 2002; lower Heart Rate, greater RR variance, smaller LF in nu, higher alpha index), combined with the greatest value of increase LF nu with standing up (suggestive of greatest sympathetic responsiveness, a much valued element in competitive sport; Manzi et al., 2009).

From a practical point of view, we remind that a similar profile can be observed in the distribution of raw and adjusted values. A detailed statistical comparison with BA and JT non-parametric tests suggests that differences between individual paradigmatic groups and controls may be condition specific (Jänig, 2008; **Table 3** and **Figures 2, 3**). Moreover, BA and JT tests may disclose subtle nuances of hidden coding modalities (Gerstner et al., 1997; Buzsáki and Watson, 2012) between different indices that might merit a deeper inquiry, as furnished by factor analysis (Thompson, 2004; **Table 4**) according to a unique approach. In brief, with BA and JT we perform comparisons between the distributions of individual ANS proxies in clinical groups and controls, while with factor analysis we reduce the number of meaningful proxies to only four, and hence we can largely simplify the assessment of the main traits distinguishing clinical groups from controls (**Figure 4**). Instead of dealing with the small portion of information individually distributed across all autonomic indices, we can rely on the strength of the ANS differentiation profiles, i.e., the discriminant ANS latent domains disclosed by combining factor analysis with the test-vs.-reference comparisons based on BA and JT tests. Notably, this approach,

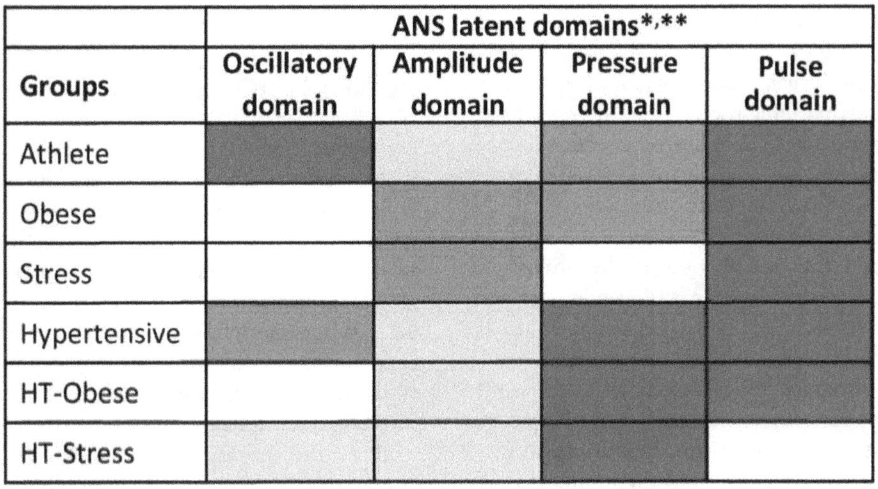

| Groups | ANS latent domains*,** | | | |
|---|---|---|---|---|
| | Oscillatory domain | Amplitude domain | Pressure domain | Pulse domain |
| Athlete | strong | medium | medium-strong | strong |
| Obese | weak | medium-strong | medium-strong | strong |
| Stress | weak | medium-strong | weak | strong |
| Hypertensive | medium-strong | medium | strong | strong |
| HT-Obese | weak | medium | strong | strong |
| HT-Stress | medium | strong | strong | weak |

FIGURE 4 | ANS differentiation map of the test groups toward the normal group. *ANS differentiation profiles are given for each test group by the concurrence of the discriminant ANS domains depicted in red, dark pink and light pink according to their strength of discrimination capability toward the normal group.

| strong | medium-strong | medium | weak (no strength) |
|---|---|---|---|

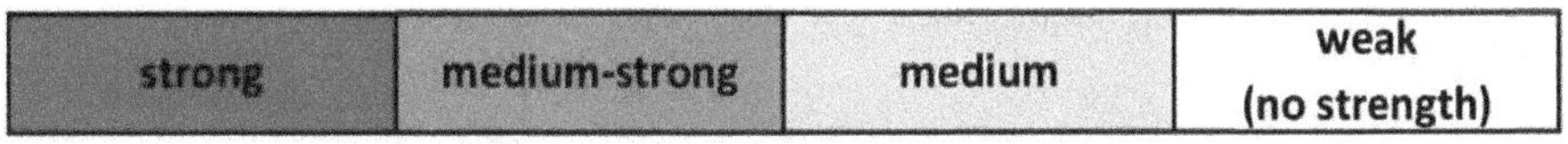

This strength is assessed as the number of jointly significant results on BA and JT tests occurred for the Adj-ANS proxies connected with each specific ANS latent domain. Red cells denote the strongest level of discrimination, where all the tests involving Adj-ANS proxies in that domain are significant. Dark pink cells indicate a medium-strong level of discrimination, in which there is at least a majority of significant results on both BA and JT tests. Light pink cells denote a medium level of discrimination, where there is at least a majority of significant results on either BA or JT tests. Finally, white cells indicate that there are not enough significant test results to regard a specific ANS latent domain as discriminant toward the normal group. **As a result of factor analysis (Table 4), ANS latent domains are connected with the following ANS proxies: Oscillatory domain = RR LFnu, RR HFnu, RR LF/HF, and ΔRRLFnu; Amplitude domain = RR TP, RR LFa, RR HFa, and α index; Pressure domain = SAP, DAP, and SAP Mean; Pulse domain = HR and RR Mean.

which simultaneously uses all available information about the system (Haken, 1977), shows that e.g., athletes (**Figure 4**) differ from controls in all domains, but with a graded strength: maximal in the (normalized) oscillatory and in the pulse domains, slightly less in the pressure domain, and minimal in the amplitude domain.

Also, the hypertensive group differs (Lucini et al., 2014) from control in all the four domains, but with a different grading (maximal strength for pressure and pulse domains, less so for amplitude and oscillatory domains). Obese (Peterson et al., 1988), Ht-Obese and Ht-Stress groups differ in three differentiating domains. The Stress group (Lucini et al., 2002) differs in only two domains (amplitude and pulse). We posit in addition that for clinical applications the ANS differentiation map (as in **Figure 4**) permits to rapidly and simply synthesize the possible difference between clinical groups and controls, evidencing the ANS latent domains that have at least a medium strength of discrimination. While the ANS differentiation map considers, in practice, clusters of ANS proxies, the significance diagram (**Figure 3**) permits to identify the single ANS proxies inside each ANS latent domain that resulted in significant comparisons according to BA and JT tests. This aspect may also help define ANS investigations addressing differences between clinical groups on a more rational basis.

Lastly, it is worth pointing out that the statistical methodology we used here for setting up ANS differentiation profiles is broader in scope. It is given by the integrated use of statistical analysis methods that, from a theoretical point of view, were developed irrespective of specific fields of application. Consequently, we argue that, after due adjustments, this methodology could be as well employed to study ANS differences of other non-normal conditions, or even applied to detect differentiation profiles among groups in other completely different contexts.

## Limitations

Important limitations must be recognized in this pragmatic protocol (Ford and Norrie, 2016). First, this is an indirect study, comparing groups at a one-time point only, but following usual clinical routines. Moreover, the study population is large, and we utilize extensively, we believe for the first time, a set of integrated statistical procedures capable of providing a differentiation map, showing which cluster of variables best indicate the ANS difference between test groups and controls.

In addition, we do not present direct data on activity and syntax of neurovegetative neurons (Buzsáki and Watson, 2012). Indirect is, in particular, the nature of autonomic indices that are employed in this investigation. However, the integrated use of multiple statistical tools permitted to provide empirical support to the hypothesis that autonomic codes are expressed in either amplitude or oscillations (Pagani and Malliani, 2000). Present findings derive from the prevailing use of a data-driven (instead of model-based) approach to the analyses, which allowed us to build the ANS differentiation map directly from the data, without the need for a priori assumptions on the distributions of the ANS proxies and their mutual relationships.

Moreover, given that the composition of the groups was not homogeneous with respect to age and gender, we were forced to rely on a statistical remedy, i.e., performing the analyses on the ANS proxies adjusted for age and gender effects instead of the original ones. Overall, in the "test-vs.-reference" comparisons carried out using the Adj-ANS proxies we have obtained results in line with the literature, e.g., in the hypertensive group results concerning $\Delta$RRLFnu and $\alpha$ index, which are the proxies with the highest informative content for this group, are congruent with what is expected (Lucini et al., 2014). There are, however, few exceptions. Again, in the hypertensive group, net of age and gender effects, RR HFa results significantly greater than in the normal group (**Figure 3**), while we would have expected the opposite situation (**Table 3**). This anomaly could be because we have used the adjusted ANS proxies, with respect to which there is no comparability with the literature yet.

In spite of a relatively large overall population, combined conditions (such as stress, obesity, and hypertension) may lead to very small subgroups, rendering impossible to interpret confounding effects, or generalizing all findings. This would require focused studies, possibly with specific interventions with a longitudinal design.

## CONCLUSIONS

The application of a pragmatic approach (Ford and Norrie, 2016), designed to show the behavior of ANS proxies close to real life rather than in stringent laboratory conditions, and the prevailing use of data-driven statistical methods on a large dataset of several different paradigmatic groups of ambulant subjects indicate that ANS variables cluster in a small number of latent factors. Each factor is strongly linked to few homogeneous proxies of autonomic modulation. The properties of latent factors might therefore suggest a novel way to interpret underlying physiological mechanisms.

Thus the application of multiple (non-parametric and exploratory) statistical and graphical tools to ANS proxies defines differentiation profiles that could pave the way to a better understanding of autonomic differences between clinical groups and controls, with potential beneficial effects on clinical applications.

## AUTHOR CONTRIBUTIONS

DL, NS, and MP contributed to the study design; DL and MP contributed to drafting the manuscript; NS contributed to statistical analysis; DL, NS, and MP contributed to critically revising the text; DL, NS, and MP contributed to and approved the final version of the text.

## REFERENCES

Abraham, C., and Michie, S. (2008). A taxonomy of behavior change techniques used in interventions. *Health Psychol.* 27, 379–387. doi: 10.1037/0278-6133.27.3.379

Althoff, T., Sosic, R., Hicks, J. L., King, A. C., Delp, S. L., and Leskovec, J. (2017). Large-scale physical activity data reveal worldwide activity inequality. *Nature* 547, 336–339. doi: 10.1038/nature23018

Badilini, F., Pagani, M., and Porta, A. (2005). Heartscope: a software tool adressing autonomic nervous system regulation. *Comp. Cardiol.* 32, 259–262. doi: 10.1109/CIC.2005.1588086

Bertinieri, G., di Rienzo, M., Cavallazzi, A., Ferrari, A. U., Pedotti, A., and Mancia, G. (1985). A new approach to analysis of the arterial baroreflex. *J. Hypertens. Suppl.* 3, S79–S81.

Billman, G. E., Huikuri, H. V., Sacha, J., and Trimmel, K. (2015). An introduction to heart rate variability: methodological considerations and clinical applications. *Front. Physiol.* 6:55. doi: 10.3389/fphys.2015.00055

Bowman, A. W., and Azzalini, A. (1997). *Applied Smoothing Techniques for Data Analysis. The Kernel Approach With S-Plus Illustrations.* Oxford, UK: Oxford University Press.

Bowman, A. W., and Azzalini, A. (2014). *R Package "sm": Nonparametric Smoothing Methods.* Version 2.2-5.4. Available online at: https://CRAN.R-project.org/package=sm

Buzsáki, G., and Watson, B. O. (2012). Brain rhythms and neural syntax: implications for efficient coding of cognitive content and neuropsychiatric disease. *Dialog. Clin. Neurosci.* 14, 345.

Christakis, N. A., and Fowler, J. H. (2007). The spread of obesity in a large social network over 32 years. *N. Engl. J. Med.* 357, 370–379. doi: 10.1056/NEJMsa066082

Dart, A. M., Du, X. J., and Kingwell, B. A. (2002). Gender, sex hormones and autonomic nervous control of the cardiovascular system. *Cardiovasc. Res.* 53, 678–687. doi: 10.1016/S0008-6363(01)00508-9

Ding, D., Rogers, K., van der Ploeg, H., Stamatakis, E., and Bauman, A. E. (2015). Traditional and emerging lifestyle risk behaviors and all-cause mortality in middle-aged and older adults: evidence from a large population-based Australian cohort. *PLoS Med.* 12:e1001917. doi: 10.1371/journal.pmed.1001917

Ford, I., and Norrie, J. (2016). Pragmatic trials. *N. Engl. J. Med.* 375, 454–463. doi: 10.1056/NEJMra1510059

Forouzanfar, M. H., Liu, P., Roth, G. A., Ng, M., Biryukov, S., Marczak, L., et al. (2017). Global burden of hypertension and systolic blood pressure of at least 110 to 115 mm Hg, 1990-2015. *JAMA* 317, 165–182. doi: 10.1001/jama.2016.19043

Fukusaki, C., Kawakubo, K., and Yamamoto, Y. (2000). Assessment of the primary effect of aging on heart rate variability in humans. *Clin. Auton. Res.* 10, 123–130. doi: 10.1007/BF02278016

Gerstner, W., Kreiter, A. K., Markram, H., and Herz, A. V. (1997). Neural codes: firing rates and beyond. *Proc. Natl. Acad. Sci. U.S.A.* 94, 12740–12741. doi: 10.1073/pnas.94.24.12740

Haken, H. (1977). Synergetics. *Phys. Bull.* 28:412. doi: 10.1088/0031-9112/28/9/027

Hess, W. R. (2014). *Nobel Lecture: The Central Control of the Activity of Internal Organs.* Nobelprize.org.Nobel Media AB. Available online at: http://www.nobelprize.org/nobel_prizes/medicine/laureates/1949/hess-lecture.html

Hollander, M., Wolf, D. A., and Chicken, E. (ed.). (2014). *Nonparametric Statistical Methods, 3rd Edn.* Hoboken, NJ: John Wiley and Sons.

Iellamo, F., Legramante, J. M., Pigozzi, F., Spataro, A., Norbiato, G., Lucini, D., et al. (2002). Conversion from vagal to sympathetic predominance with strenuous training in high-performance world class athletes. *Circulation* 105, 2719–2724. doi: 10.1161/01.CIR.0000018124.01299.AE

Jandackova, V. K., Scholes, S., Britton, A., and Steptoe, A. (2016). Are changes in heart rate variability in middle-aged and older people normative or caused by pathological conditions? Findings from a large populationΓÇÉbased longitudinal cohort study. *J. Am. Heart Assoc.* 5:e002365. doi: 10.1161/JAHA.115.002365

Jänig, W. (2008). *Integrative Action of the Autonomic Nervous System: Neurobiology of Homeostasis.* Cambridge, UK: Cambridge University Press.

Jeong, I. C., and Finkelstein, J. (2015). Real-time classification of exercise exertion levels using discriminant analysis of HRV data. *Stud. Health Technol. Inform.* 213, 171–174. doi: 10.3233/978-1-61499-538-8-171

Jobson, J. D. (2012). *Applied Multivariate Data Analysis, Vol.* II, *Categorical and Multivariate Methods.* New York, NY: Springer Science and Business Media.

La Rovere, M. T., Bigger, J. T. Jr., Marcus, F. I., Mortara, A., and Schwartz, P. J. (1998). Baroreflex sensitivity and heart-rate variability in prediction of total cardiac mortality after myocardial infarction. ATRAMI (Autonomic Tone and Reflexes After Myocardial Infarction) investigators. *Lancet* 351, 478–484. doi: 10.1016/S0140-6736(97)11144-8

Lucini, D., and Pagani, M. (2012). From stress to functional syndromes: an internist's point of view. *Eur. J. Intern. Med.* 23, 295–301. doi: 10.1016/j.ejim.2011.11.016

Lucini, D., Marchetti, I., Spataro, A., Malacarne, M., Benzi, M., Tamorri, S., et al. (2017). Heart rate variability to monitor performance in elite athletes: criticalities and avoidable pitfalls. *Int. J. Cardiol.* 240, 307–312. doi: 10.1016/j.ijcard.2017.05.001

Lucini, D., Norbiato, G., Clerici, M., and Pagani, M. (2002). Hemodynamic and autonomic adjustments to real life stress conditions in humans. *Hypertension* 39, 184–188. doi: 10.1161/hy0102.100784

Lucini, D., Solaro, N., and Pagani, M. (2014). May autonomic indices from cardiovascular variability help identify hypertension? *J. Hypertens.* 32, 363–373. doi: 10.1097/HJH.0000000000000020

Malliani, A., Pagani, M., Furlan, R., Guzzetti, S., Lucini, D., Montano, N., et al. (1997). Individual recognition by heart rate variability of two different autonomic profiles related to posture. *Circulation* 96, 4143–4145. doi: 10.1161/01.CIR.96.12.4143

Mancia, G., and Grassi, G. (2014). The autonomic nervous system and hypertension. *Circ. Res.* 114, 1804–1814. doi: 10.1161/CIRCRESAHA.114.302524

Manzi, V., Castagna, C., Padua, E., Lombardo, M., D'Ottavio, S., Massaro, M., et al. (2009). Dose-response relationship of autonomic nervous system responses to individualized training impulse in marathon runners. *Am. J. Physiol. Heart Circ. Physiol.* 296, H1733–H1740. doi: 10.1152/ajpheart.00054.2009

Narkiewicz, K., and Somers, V. K. (1998). Chronic orthostatic intolerance: part of a spectrum of dysfunction in orthostatic cardiovascular homeostasis? *Circulation* 98, 2105–2107. doi: 10.1161/01.CIR.98.20.2105

Pagani, M., and Malliani, A. (2000). Interpreting oscillations of muscle sympathetic nerve activity and heart rate variability. *J. Hypertens.* 18, 1709–1719. doi: 10.1097/00004872-200018120-00002

Pagani, M., Lombardi, F., Guzzetti, S., Rimoldi, O., Furlan, R., Pizzinelli, P., et al. (1986). Power spectral analysis of heart rate and arterial pressure variabilities as a marker of sympatho-vagal interaction in man and conscious dog. *Circ. Res.* 59, 178–193. doi: 10.1161/01.RES.59.2.178

Pagani, M., Montano, N., Porta, A., Malliani, A., Abboud, F. M., Birkett, C., et al. (1997). Relationship between spectral components of cardiovascular variabilities and direct measures of muscle sympathetic nerve activity in humans. *Circulation* 95, 1441–1448. doi: 10.1161/01.CIR.95.6.1441

Pagani, M., Somers, V., Furlan, R., Dell'Orto, S., Conway, J., Baselli, G., et al. (1988). Changes in autonomic regulation induced by physical training in mild hypertension. *Hypertension* 12, 600–610. doi: 10.1161/01.HYP.12.6.600

Peterson, H. R., Rothschild, M., Weinberg, C. R., Fell, R. D., McLeish, K. R., and Pfeifer, M. A. (1988). Body fat and the activity of the autonomic nervous system. *N. Engl. J. Med.* 318, 1077–1083. doi: 10.1056/NEJM198804283181701

Sassi, R., Cerutti, S., Lombardi, F., Malik, M., Huikuri, H. V., Peng, C. K., et al. (2015). Advances in heart rate variability signal analysis: joint position statement by the e-Cardiology ESC working group and the European heart rhythm association co-endorsed by the Asia pacific heart rhythm society. *Europace* 17, 1341–1353. doi: 10.1093/europace/euv015

Schwartz, P. J., Pagani, M., Lombardi, F., Malliani, A., and Brown, A. M. (1973). A cardiocardiac sympathovagal reflex in the cat. *Circ. Res.* 32, 215–220. doi: 10.1161/01.RES.32.2.215

Seshan, V. E. (2017). *Clinfun: Clinical Trial Design and Data Analysis Functions.* R package version 1.0.14. Available online at: https://CRAN.R-project.org/package=clinfun

Tarvainen, M. P., Cornforth, D. J., and Jelinek, H. F. (2014). Principal component analysis of heart rate variability data in assessing cardiac autonomic neuropathy. *Conf. Proc. IEEE Eng. Med. Biol. Soc.* 2014, 6667–6670. doi: 10.1109/EMBC.2014.6945157

Task Force of the European Society of Cardiology and the North American Society of Pacing and Electrophysiology. (1996). Heart-rate variability: standards of measurements, physiological interpretation and clinical use. *Circulation* 93, 1043–65. doi: 10.1161/01.CIR.93.5.1043

Thompson, B. (2004). *Exploratory and Confirmatory Factor Analysis: Understanding Concepts and Applications.* Washington, DC: American Psychological Association.

# 13

# Construction and Validation of Subject-Specific Biventricular Finite-Element Models of Healthy and Failing Swine Hearts from High-Resolution DT-MRI

Kevin L. Sack[1,2], Eric Aliotta[3], Daniel B. Ennis[3], Jenny S. Choy[4], Ghassan S. Kassab[4], Julius M. Guccione[2]* and Thomas Franz[1,5]

[1] Division of Biomedical Engineering, Department of Human Biology, University of Cape Town, Cape Town, South Africa, [2] Department of Surgery, University of California, San Francisco, San Francisco, CA, United States, [3] Department of Radiological Sciences, University of California, Los Angeles, Los Angeles, CA, United States, [4] California Medical Innovations Institute, Inc., San Diego, CA, United States, [5] Bioengineering Science Research Group, Engineering Sciences, Faculty of Engineering and the Environment, University of Southampton, Southampton, United Kingdom

*Correspondence:
Julius M. Guccione
Julius.Guccione@ucsf.edu

Predictive computational modeling has revolutionized classical engineering disciplines and is in the process of transforming cardiovascular research. This is particularly relevant for investigating emergent therapies for heart failure, which remains a leading cause of death globally. The creation of subject-specific biventricular computational cardiac models has been a long-term endeavor within the biomedical engineering community. Using high resolution (0.3 × 0.3 × 0.8 mm) ex vivo data, we constructed a precise fully subject-specific biventricular finite-element model of healthy and failing swine hearts. Each model includes fully subject-specific geometries, myofiber architecture and, in the case of the failing heart, fibrotic tissue distribution. Passive and active material properties are prescribed using hyperelastic strain energy functions that define a nearly incompressible, orthotropic material capable of contractile function. These materials were calibrated using a sophisticated multistep approach to match orthotropic tri-axial shear data as well as subject-specific hemodynamic ventricular targets for pressure and volume to ensure realistic cardiac function. Each mechanically beating heart is coupled with a lumped-parameter representation of the circulatory system, allowing for a closed-loop definition of cardiovascular flow. The circulatory model incorporates unidirectional fluid exchanges driven by pressure gradients of the model, which in turn are driven by the mechanically beating heart. This creates a computationally meaningful representation of the dynamic beating of the heart coupled with the circulatory system. Each model was calibrated using subject-specific experimental data and compared with independent in vivo strain data obtained from echocardiography. Our methods produced highly detailed representations of swine hearts that function mechanically in a remarkably similar manner to the in vivo subject-specific strains on a global and regional comparison. The degree of subject-specificity included in the models represents a milestone for modeling efforts that captures realism of the whole heart. This study establishes a foundation for future computational studies that can apply these validated methods to advance cardiac mechanics research.

**Keywords: heart failure, subject-specific, finite element method, realistic simulation, ventricular function**

## 1. INTRODUCTION

For decades researchers have strived to create realistic computational models to represent the mechanical behavior of the heart (Sack et al., 2016a). This challenging endeavor faces difficulties in accounting for the complex geometry, fiber structure and material description of the heart. To further complicate modeling efforts, the circulatory system and the cyclical function of the heart need to be numerically reproduced as heart function is critically coupled to the circulatory system and cannot be modeled in isolation.

The finite element (FE) method is well suited to create computational models as it allows for partial differential equations to be solved over complex geometric domains, as is necessary to investigate the mechanical aspects of heart function, pathology and potential emergent therapies. This is critical as heart failure (HF) is the leading cause of death worldwide (Finegold et al., 2013). Even with optimal modern therapy, the annual mortality rate of patients with HF ranges from 31 to 45% (Chen et al., 2013; Desta et al., 2015), strongly motivating the need for new therapies, and methods that can accelerate their design and development. Modeling HF *in silico* allows the effect of the disease on heart function to be directly quantified (Bogen et al., 1980; Guccione et al., 2001; Kerckhoffs et al., 2007; Fomovsky et al., 2011; Wenk et al., 2011, 2012a,b) while simultaneously collecting critical information such as regional ventricular wall stress, an otherwise unobtainable metric thought to initiate pathological remodeling (Pfeffer and Braunwald, 1990; Sutton and Sharpe, 2000; Matiwala and Margulies, 2004).

Here, we propose a method to combine multiple sources of *in vivo* and *ex vivo* data to produce and validate highly realistic subject-specific FE models of the porcine heart. This process builds on our previously published research on cardiac modeling (Baillargeon et al., 2014, 2015; Sack et al., 2016b) by including subject-specific features into almost every aspect of the model to reduce the number of *ad hoc* modeling assumptions. By incorporating data from high resolution magnetic resonance imaging (MRI) and diffusion tensor magnetic resonance imaging (DT-MRI), we were able to create high-fidelity representations of the biventricular chambers, myofibers and infarcted scar-tissue distribution in the ischemic HF subject. These models include the full ventricular structure, the endocardial papillary structure and all four valve openings. Our modeling techniques simulate heart function by calibrating active and passive material properties of the heart to match measured *in vivo* functional outputs (i.e., volume and pressure measurements). To ensure realistic cardiac function, the mechanical model of the ventricles is coupled to a lumped-parameter circulatory model. This enables closed-loop volume exchange, the modeling of multiple cardiac cycles, and

realistic cyclical pumping akin to the physiological beating heart. The models are validated by comparing predicted regional values of endocardial strain to *in vivo* measurements not used in model creation. This study introduces the first fully subject-specific cardiac models in healthy and failing states.

## 2. METHODS

### 2.1. Experimental Protocol

All animal experiments were performed in accordance with national and local ethical guidelines, including the Guide for the Care and Use of Laboratory Animals, the Public Health Service Policy on Humane Care and Use of Laboratory Animals, the Animal Welfare Act, and an approved California Medical Innovations Institute IACUC protocol regarding the use of animals in research.

Two porcine subjects were used in this study: one normal and one with HF. The description of these animals and the creation of HF has been detailed previously (Choy et al., 2018). The ischemia resulted in decline of the animal's ejection fraction (EF) from 56% at the time of coronary artery occlusion to 32% when the animal was sacrificed, 16 weeks later. Measurements of *in vivo* left ventricular pressure and volume for each subject were recorded at the time of sacrifice (the incorporation of this data is discussed in section 2.5). Excised hearts were arrested in diastole with a saturated solution of potassium chloride and were fixed with buffered formalin (Carson-Millonig formulation).

### 2.2. *Ex Vivo* Imaging

After fixation, the ventricular cavities were filled with a silicone rubber compound (Polyvinylsiloxane, Microsonic Inc., Ambridge, PA) in order to maintain the geometry during imaging. The hearts were then placed in a plastic cylindrical container filled with a susceptibility-matched fluid (Fomblin, Solvay Solexis, West Deptford, NJ) and held in place using open-cell foam. Anatomical MRI was then performed (Magnetom Prisma 3T, Siemens, Erlangen, Germany) with the following parameters: T1-weighted imaging using a 3D Fast Low Angle SHot (FLASH) sequence ($0.3 \times 0.3 \times 0.8$ mm spatial resolution, echo time (TE)/repetition time (TR) = 3.15/12 ms, scan time: 1.5 h); and T2-weighted imaging using a 2D multi-slice Turbo Spin Echo (TSE) sequence ($0.3 \times 0.3 \times 0.8$ mm spatial resolution, TE/TR = 94/15,460 ms, scan time: 2 h).

DT-MRI was performed using a readout-segmented diffusion-weighted spin-echo sequence (Porter and Heidemann, 2009) with b-value = 1,000 s/mm$^2$ along 30 directions and one b-value = 0 s/mm$^2$ reference, TE/TR = 62/18,100 ms and $1.0 \times 1.0 \times 1.0$ mm spatial resolution with 4–6 signal averages to improve signal-to-noise ratio (scan time: 8–12 h). Diffusion tensors were reconstructed from the diffusion-weighted images using linear regression and custom MATLAB (The MathWorks, Inc., Natick, Massachusetts, United States) routines.

## 2.3. Geometric Segmentation and Reconstruction

*Ex vivo* MRI data sets were imported and processed in Simpleware ScanIP (Synopsys, Mountain View, USA). Detailed geometric segmentations of the biventricular structure were created along with segmentations of infarcted tissue in the HF subject. Segmentation relied on a combination of well-established techniques including region growing, level-set thresholding, and morphological smoothing (Vadakkumpadan et al., 2010; Setarehdan and Singh, 2012). Manual intervention was used only if needed to eliminate spurious features.

The full ventricular structure including all four valve openings of the heart was reconstructed from the T2-weighted MRI data sets. The segmented geometry and the cavity morphology are shown in **Figures 1A,B**, respectively. The segmented geometry was meshed with quadratic tetrahedral elements using Simpleware's built in FE meshing suite as shown in **Figure 1C** and the resultant mesh with the cavities enclosed is shown in **Figure 1D**. These meshes were imported into the Abaqus software environment (version 6.14, Dasssult Systèmes, Providence, RI, USA), which was chosen as the FE solver for this research. Since these geometries are constructed from *ex vivo* imaging, they provide the geometry in an unloaded state.

### 2.3.1. Ventricular Chambers

To determine the ventricular cavity volumes, these chambers were enclosed by constructing two-dimensional (2D) triangular surface elements at each valve opening that were adjoined to a center node **Figure 1D**. The degrees of freedom of these center nodes, designated as "slave nodes," were coupled to the average motion of the surrounding nodes on the ventricular structure used to construct these surface elements. These surface elements do not contribute to the stiffness of the valve openings.

## 2.4. 3D Subject-Specific Myofiber Orientations

DT-MRI provides diffusion tensors for each voxel that were decomposed into eigenvalues and corresponding eigenvectors. Primary eigenvectors associated with the largest eigenvalue were identified as the orientation of the myofiber (Scollan et al., 1998; Kung et al., 2011). For practical purposes of computational modeling, a fully continuous 3D field representation of the local material coordinates, derived from diffusion tensors, is needed. This was achieved using a linear invariant interpolation method (Gahm et al., 2012) whereby the diffusion tensor is decomposed into invariants and orientations, which are each interpolated in turn and reconstructed into an interpolated tensor at the point of interest $\mathbf{x} \in \mathbb{R}^3$.

To ensure only voxels containing cardiac tissue (and not fat, air bubbles or voids) were included in the interpolation, the requirements that eigenvalues of each voxel be strictly positive, and that the fractional anisotropy (FA), an invariant of diffusion tensors commonly used for tissue thresholding (FA > 0.12),

were imposed prior to analysis. This value for FA was found experimentally to be the lowest that would fully threshold out non-fibrous tissue and was reasonably different from values of FA for cardiac tissue (Helm et al., 2005; Kung et al., 2011). The inclination angle $\alpha_h$, defined as the angle between the myofiber projected onto the longitudinal-circumferential tangent plane and the circumferential unit vector (Bovendeerd et al., 1992; Scollan et al., 1998; Toussaint et al., 2013), was quantified for each voxel. Results are presented regionally for the left ventricle (LV), partitioned into the 17 regions following the American Heart Association (AHA) guidelines (Cerqueira et al., 2002). This is a commonly reported quantification of myofiber orientation, which allows us to compare our results with literature findings as a source of validation.

## 2.5. Incorporating *in Vivo* Measurements

For the HF pig, *in vivo* pressure and volume measurements were set as target values in the model calibration. For the normal pig, an *in vivo* volume measurement, and pressure derived from the healthy baseline of a larger *in vivo* data set ($n = 5$) (Choy et al., 2018), were similarly used. The complete *in vivo* measurements used for this study are presented in Supplementary Table S1. Measurements of *in vivo* strains were also recorded but deliberately excluded from the calibration process to serve as an independent metric to validate the model.

## 2.6. Constitutive Model

### 2.6.1. Passive Material Description and Parameter Estimation

The passive material response for myocardium follows the structurally motivated constitutive model for anisotropic hyperelastic myocardium introduced by Holzapfel and Ogden (Holzapfel and Ogden, 2009). Descriptions of material parameters are provided in Supplementary Table S2. A modification in the isochoric part of the strain energy density $\Psi_{iso}$, was introduced, allowing for the description of homogenized, pathological tissue:

$$\Psi_{iso} = \frac{\bar{a}}{2b}e^{b(I_1-3)} + \sum_{i=f,s}\frac{\bar{a}_i}{2b_i}\left\{e^{b_i(I_{4i}-1)^2} - 1\right\}$$

$$+ \frac{\bar{a}_{fs}}{2b_{fs}}\left\{e^{b_{fs}(I_{8fs})^2} - 1\right\}, \tag{1}$$

$$\Psi_{vol} = \frac{1}{D}\left(\frac{J^2-1}{2} - \ln(J)\right) \tag{2}$$

where the new parameters $\bar{a}$, $\bar{a}_i$ and $\bar{a}_{fs}$ govern the homogenization of healthy and pathological tissue using a scalar parameter $h$ representing the volume fraction of tissue health. For example $\bar{a}_i$ is defined in the following manner:

$$\bar{a}_i = a_i\left[h + \left(1 - h\right)p\right]. \tag{3}$$

Here, $h$ bound by [0, 1], governs the health of the material point and $p$ scales the passive response according to pathology. The

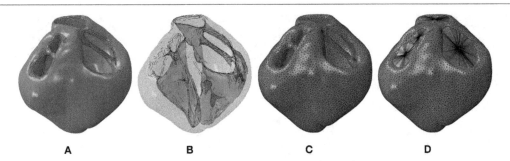

**FIGURE 1 | (A)** Geometric segmentation. **(B)** Transparent geometries revealing the cavity morphology. **(C)** The mesh corresponding to the segmentation. **(D)** The mesh with the cavity structures enclosed using surface elements.

parameters $\bar{a}$ and $\bar{a}_{fs}$ are defined similarly using $h$, $p$, $a$ and $a_{fs}$. Note that the following holds:

$$h = 1 \overset{yields}{\rightarrow} \bar{a}_i = a_i \qquad (4)$$

$$h = 0 \overset{yields}{\rightarrow} \bar{a}_i = a_i p \qquad (5)$$

$\bar{a}_i$ transitions linearly between these values for different values of $h$ bound by $[0, 1]$.

The values of $h$ were determined from *ex vivo* imaging and processed as a regionally varying field, continuous over the domain. This was achieved by interpolating a binary (i.e., infarcted or healthy tissue) segmentation of the high-resolution *ex vivo* data onto regularly spaced nodal points of the biventricular FE mesh, whereby the elemental interpolants populate the domain in a continuous fashion. This allows for regionally detailed descriptions of infarcted tissue and border zone material to be incorporated into the model in a continuous and physiologically reasonable manner (**Figure 2**). Following the above equations, passive material stiffness is determined by the "health" of the material point, $h$; the pathological scaling of infarcted material, $p$, and the material parameters $a_i$ and $b_i$, which govern the linear and exponential response of the cardiac tissue in different modes of deformation.

$h$ is determined *a priori* from the mapping of the segmented infarcted tissue. Without detailed experimental data, we have to rely on literature values to determine the pathological scaling of the material, $p$. Even though multiple studies have investigated the quantification of infarct mechanics, there is no clear consensus on infarct stiffness readily available. Holmes, Borg (Holmes et al., 2005) presents an excellent account of changes in infarct stiffness. The infarct at the remodeling phase (i.e., scar tissue) is relevant to our study, and has been quantified as 2–10 times (Connelly et al., 1985; Gupta et al., 1994; McGarvey et al., 2015; Mojsejenko et al., 2015) as stiff as remote non-infarcted tissue. Particularly relevant is a recent study performed by McGarvey, Mojsejenko (McGarvey et al., 2015) which allows us to narrow this range of infarct stiffness. In that study, the authors quantify the *in vivo* stiffness of infarct and remote tissue of porcine subjects using FE methods and *in vivo* imaging techniques. As they have a similar model of MI and report values for late-stage infarcts (i.e., 12 weeks) their results are

most applicable to our study. Using the ratio of their results for infarcted and remote tissue, we determine a value for $p$ to be 4.56 which we apply throughout our models.

The remaining material parameters, $a_i$ and $b_i$, were found through optimization techniques relying on two stages of determination. Initial values for $a_i$ and $b_i$ were determined from the calibration of normal myocardium specimen samples to experimental tri-axial shear data (Sommer et al., 2015). This is essential to capture the fully orthotropic behavior of cardiac tissue. Calibration was performed using Abaqus as the forward solver, whereby *in silico* cubes of myocardium with edge lengths of 4 mm (i.e. dimensions matching those of the study of interest) were meshed into a uniform 27 linear hex-element mesh. As with Sommer et al. (2015), we assumed an orthonormal coordinate system aligned with the cube dimensions corresponding to the mean fiber, sheet, and sheet-normal directions. Shearing was executed by specifying the translational displacement of a specified cube face, while enforcing zero displacement boundary conditions on the opposite cube face. The optimization was performed in MATLAB using a nonlinear least-square optimization routine with the trust-region-reflective algorithm option.

Here, the minimization between FE model stress $\sigma$ and experimental values $\bar{\sigma}$ can be explicitly defined through the minimization of an objective function $\varphi_1$ by

$$\min \varphi_1(\mathbf{v}_1) = \sum_i \sum_j \left( \sigma_j^i - \bar{\sigma}_j^i \right)^2, \qquad (6)$$

where $i = \{fs, fn, sf, sn, nf, ns\}$ are the six combinations of shear modes, the vector of material parameters is given by $\mathbf{v}_1 = \{a, b, a_f, b_f, a_s, b_s, a_{fs}, b_{fs}\}$ and the index $j$ spans the data points in the shear vector for shear test $i$. The resulting material parameters from shear calibration were identified only once and these formed as the starting set of material parameters for the next stage of calibration, which scales these values to match subject specific left ventricular function.

To adjust the material for each subject, these initial values are scaled consistently to match the "Klotz curve" (Klotz et al., 2006) generated for the diastolic pressure-volume (PV) relation of each subject's LV. Both linear ($a_i$) and exponential ($b_i$) terms were subject to uniform scaling by parameters $A$ and $B$, a scalar

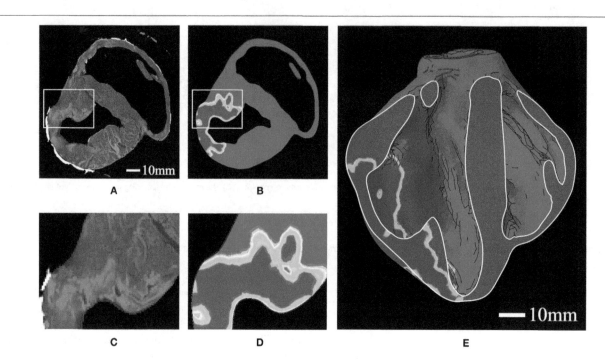

**FIGURE 2 | (A)** Binary segmentation of infarcted tissue (blue) and healthy tissue (red) on a short axis MRI of the porcine subject with HF. **(B)** A short-axis slice of the FE model displaying the interpolated $h$ field with 0 represented as blue and 1 represented as red. Colors in between blue and red represent the "border zone." **(C)** Zoomed-in section corresponding to the box in **(A)**. **(D)** Zoomed-in section corresponding to the box in **(B)**. **(E)** A long-axis cut plane of the FE model displaying the interpolated $h$ field throughout the bisected geometry.

and an exponential multiplier, respectively. These values were found by minimizing the error between the *in silico* diastolic PV course of each subject to the analytical Klotz curve, starting from the unloaded LV volume $V_0$ until the end-diastolic volume (EDV) was reached at the specified end-diastolic pressure (EDP) value given in Supplementary Table S1. The error between the model and predicted *in vivo* pressure-volume relationship was minimized using the same nonlinear least-square optimization routine used in the shear calibration. For the passive filling calibration, we defined our objective function $\varphi_2$ as the difference in pressure values along the pressure volume curve combined with a single measure of EDV, which we found to yield close fits to the PV curve and ensure EDV was met.

$$\min \varphi_2(\mathbf{v_2}) = \sum_j^N \left(P_j - \overline{P_j}\right)^2 + \left(EDV - \overline{EDV}\right)^2, \quad (7)$$

where the vector of material parameters is given by $\mathbf{v_2} = \{A, B\}$, $N$ refers to the total number of data points along the pressure volume curve and values from experimental data are given with the "overbar" notation. To be thorough, the enforcement of incompressibility was investigated by perturbing the parameter $D$ in Eq. (2). We found that at extreme values, i.e., $D < 0.02$ MPa and $D > 20$ MPa, non–physiological deformation was introduced. Within this range ($0.02 < D < 20$ MPa), the effect of incompressibility was minor on material parameter estimation. We chose to set $D = 0.2$, which we found sufficient to enforce incompressibility (99.8% volume retained over passive filling)

and avoid problematic deformations. This value produced a Bulk modulus roughly 1000 times larger than the largest linear terms ($a_i$) – a guideline also used by Göktepe et al. (2011).

To ensure realistic loading of the LV cavity one needs to consider the trans-septal pressure originating from RV filling. To capture this, the RV cavity of the normal subject was also inflated to 4 mmHg for RV EDP during passive filling calibration. This amount was determined from literature values of healthy subjects (Quinn et al., 2006; Mann et al., 2015). As the HF subject had an LV EDP roughly double the LV EDP of the normal subject, we also doubled the RV passive pressure to maintain proportionality.

### 2.6.2. Active Material Description and Parameter Estimation

The description of our time-varying elastance model of active force development (Walker et al., 2005) was also modified to include this description of tissue health:

$$T_a(t, l) = T_{max} \frac{Ca_0^2}{Ca_0^2 + ECa_{50}^2(l)} \frac{\left[1 - \cos\left(\omega\left(\mathrm{mod}(t), l\right)\right)\right]}{2} h, \quad (8)$$

where $T_{max}$, the maximum allowable active tension, is multiplied with a term governing the calcium concentration, and a term governing the timing of contraction (both terms depend on sarcomere length $l$). The timing of contractile function is linked to the heart rate and timing of the cardiac cycle, which is enforced through a modulus function acting on the time variable, $t$. Finally, the entire expression is multiplied by $h$, to ensure tissue contractility is directly proportional to tissue health. This ensures contractile force is zero at the material point of fully infarcted tissue. Further detail of the active tension law is provided in the Supplementary Material.

The total fiber stress, $\sigma_f$, is equal to the passive stress, $\sigma_{pf}$, combined with the active tension in the fiber direction given by:

$$\sigma_f = \sigma_{pf} + T_a\, e_f \otimes e_f \qquad (9)$$

Biaxial investigations on actively contracting rabbit myocardium revealed significant stress development in the cross-fiber direction that could not be completely attributed to fiber dispersion or deformation effects (Lin and Yin, 1998). This has motivated computational efforts to consider a proportion of the active stress developed in the fiber direction to be transferred onto the stress in the sheet direction by a scalar $n_s \in (0, 1)$, such that:

$$\sigma_s = \sigma_{ps} + n_s\, T_a\, e_s \otimes e_s \qquad (10)$$

Using the same nonlinear least-square optimization routine in the passive regime, $T_{max}$ and $n_s$ were subjected to optimization to ensure the correct stroke volume (SV = EDV-ESV) for each subject was achieved. Additionally, to ensure physiological deformation during contraction (and unique values of parameter estimation), left ventricular long-axis shortening (LVLS) was included in the description of error for the optimization routine. Typical values for LVLS are between 15 and 20% for humans (Dumesnil et al., 1979; Carreras et al., 2012), so this was set as a low weighted target in the minimization routine to ensure an LVLS > 0% in our *in silico* porcine model was achieved. This in turn ensures that the optimization routine does not converge on a parameter set that produces ventricular elongation and/or wall thinning. This is defined explicitly in the objective function $\varphi_3$ below:

$$\min \varphi_3(\mathbf{v_3}) = \left(SV - \overline{SV}\right)^2 + 0.2\left(LVLS - \overline{LVLS}\right)^2 \qquad (11)$$

where the vector of active material parameters is given by $\mathbf{v_3} = \{T_{max}, n_s\}$ and target values SV and LVLS are given with the "overbar" notation.

## 2.7. Circulatory System

We introduced a closed loop circulatory model adapted from simple lumped parameter representations (Hoppensteadt and Peskin, 1992; Pilla et al., 2009) of different compartments in the cardiovascular system. The ventricular chambers are defined as fluid-filled cavities fully enclosed by the combined meshed faces of the tetrahedral elements on the cavity surface and the surface elements described in section 2.3.1 that close off the chamber. The coupling of the lumped circulatory system and mechanical function was performed in Abaqus. Details on the numerical underpinnings for this are provided in the Abaqus Theory Guide (2014); here, we provide a brief overview concerning the relation of pressure, volume, compliance, resistance and fluid exchange within a lumped system. The volume $V_i$ and pressure $P_i$ inside a fluid cavity chamber $i$ are related in the following manner:

$$V_i(t) = V_i(0) + \kappa_i P_i(t) \qquad (12)$$

where $\kappa_i$ is the compliance (inverse of stiffness) of the vasculature. For the LV and RV, the compliance is highly nonlinear, depending on both the strain state of the material and time (outlined in sections 2.6.1 and 2.6.2). Following Eq. (12), we define additional

dimensionless compliance vasculature representing key components of the circulatory system. As the FE ventricular model (and not the circulatory circuit) is the central focus of this research, we sought to model a working circulatory system with as few components and assumptions as possible. This resulted in a circulatory system with three compliance vessels representing the systemic arteries (*SA*), systemic veins (*SV*) and the pulmonary circuit (*P*). The FE model of the heart is connected to this lumped representation as illustrated in **Figure 3**.

Unidirectional fluid exchanges governing the flow between compliance vessels are driven by the pressure gradients between these chambers as defined by:

$$Q(t) = \frac{dV}{dt} = \frac{1}{R}\frac{dP}{dt} \qquad (13)$$

In each simulated cardiac cycle, the ventricles contract, increasing the pressure in their chambers until it exceeds the pressure in the connected outflow chamber, driving the flow of blood in the circuit and simulating the physiological circulatory system. Since the total amount of volume in the circulatory system is constant, we have the following:

$$\frac{d}{dt}V_{TOT} = \frac{d}{dt}\sum_i V_i(t) = 0. \qquad (14)$$

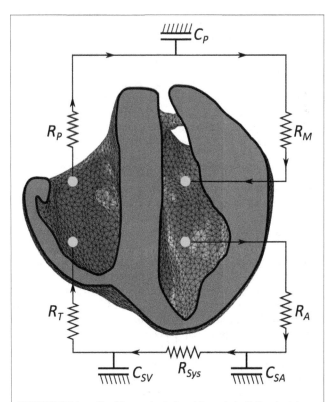

**FIGURE 3** | Schematic of the mechanical model coupled with the circulatory system. $R_M$ is mitral valve resistance, $R_A$ is aortic valve resistance, $C_{SA}$ is systemic arterial compliance, $R_{SYS}$ is systemic arterial resistance, $C_{SV}$ is venous compliance, $R_T$ is tricuspid resistance, $R_P$ is pulmonary valve resistance and $C_P$ is pulmonary system compliance.

This facilitates a stable limit cycle when simulations occur over multiple cardiac cycles.

Resistance and compliance values were based on literature values (Santamore and Burkhoff, 1991; Hoppensteadt and Peskin, 1992; Watanabe et al., 2004; Pilla et al., 2009) and adapted to ensure realistic flow. The values for these parameters are presented in Supplementary Table S3 along with literature values for comparison.

Flows from the pulmonary circuit into the LV and from the systemic circuit into the RV are set to zero during the contractile stages of heart function (i.e., during isovolumetric contraction, ejection, and isovolumetric relation). Outflow from the LV and RV is always permissible but only occurs when the pressures in these cavities exceed the pressures in the chambers they are ejecting into. Combining these restraints with the imposed unidirectional flow of the circuit is sufficient to produce realistic fluid exchanges analogous to the physiological circulatory system.

## 2.8. Boundary Conditions

The physiological heart does not experience rigid constraints on its motion. Boundary conditions are needed in computational models, however, to prevent rigid body motion and ensure the problem is mathematically well posed. To accomplish this without placing overly restrictive constraints on the model motion, we exploited the coupled degrees of freedom introduced by enclosing the ventricular cavities (section 2.3.1). The slave node of the truncated pulmonary trunk was fixed in all directions; this indirectly enforces a weighted average restraint on the nodes it is coupled with; i.e., the valve ring, such that the average deformation is zero. The valve is still able to expand and contract during the heart cycle, but this motion is "centered" on a fixed point in space.

## 2.9. Initial Conditions

In order to initiate the cardiac cycle, each compliance vessel was loaded with fluid until it experienced the physiological pressure at ED. Where possible, pressure catheterization readings from *in vivo* subject-specific measurements were used. The set of initial conditions used in this study is given in Supplementary Table S4.

## 2.10. The *in Silico* Cardiac Cycle

The initial conditions outlined above are sufficient to initiate the dynamic beating of the computational heart model. From the initial conditions (i.e., ED), contraction is initiated, which increases the pressure in the ventricular chambers. These rise until LV and RV pressures exceed the pressures in $C_{SA}$ and $C_p$, respectively. At this stage, fluid exchanges occur and the ventricles empty while the pressures and volumes in $C_{SA}$ and $C_p$ increase. Once LV and RV pressures drop below the pressures in $C_{SA}$ and $C_p$ respectively, the fluid exchanges stop, and the LV and RV pressures decrease with the decline in active tension. The entire duration of these "active contraction" processes is 480 ms, which compares well with literature values for the timing of isovolumetric contraction 66–90 ms (Sengupta et al., 2006), ejection 270–347 ms (Beyar and Sideman, 1984a; Sengupta et al., 2006) and isovolumetric relaxation 64–93 ms (Hanrath et al., 1980; Sengupta et al., 2006), respectively.

At the end of isovolumetric relaxation, all components in the circulatory system behave purely passively. Pressure differences between the compliance chambers in $C_{SV}$ and $C_p$ and the RV and LV, respectively, drive the passive filling of the ventricular chambers. The majority of the volume transferred in the passive filling stage occurs in the early portion of the step when the pressure difference is largest. Passive filling occurs in 300 ms, which is sufficient time for the cavities to inflate to the ED state and results in a heart rate of 77 bpm. Multiple steps of active contraction and passive filling can be simulated in a continuous sequence until convergent behavior over the cardiac cycle is reached.

## 2.11. Damping

Mass proportional Rayleigh damping (i.e., a viscous term introduced in the FE system of equations proportional to the mass matrix; Hughes, 2000) is introduced to dampen unrealistic oscillatory behavior of the low frequency modes. Physiologically, these would be eliminated by the surrounding soft connective tissue in the chest cavity. Similarly, isotropic time-dependent linear viscoelasticity is defined as part of the material constitutive behavior to damp out the high frequency response during active contraction. Whereas cardiac tissue is generally known to exhibit viscoelastic behavior, suitable experimental data on porcine cardiac viscoelasticity were not available. Hence, the model incorporates a small amount of viscoelasticity to eliminate unrealistic transient behavior, which is achieved using a Prony series formulation (Dill, 2006) within the Abaqus material definition (Abaqus Theory Guide, 2014).

## 2.12. Model Validation

*In vivo* strain echo data (TomTec 4D LV-Function, Version 4.6, Build 4.6.3.9, Unterschleißheim, Germany) of the endocardial surface was collected and excluded from calibration to serve as an independent data source to perform model validation. These *in vivo* strains are calculated by partitioning the endocardial surface into 16 segments, and measuring local deformation in longitudinal and circumferential directions (Pedrizzetti et al., 2014). An illustration of this 16-segment partition is shown in Supplementary Figures S1A,B.

These *in vivo* strain measurements reference ED as the initial configuration, and as such, provide relative change in length through a single cardiac cycle compared to the ED state. For purposes of validation, we select ES as the primary point of comparison for measuring heart deformation.

To provide comparable strain measures from our FE model, the endocardial nodes were partitioned into the same 16 segment division as the TomTec strain data. This resulted in 12 quadrilateral segments for the LV trunk and four triangular segments for the apical region. Control nodes placed at the corners and midpoints of the regions were identified. Similarly to the speckle-tracking imaging technique used to determine strain in the *in vivo* case, the nodal deformations of these control points were extracted at different time points in the cardiac cycle. By fitting cubic splines through these control points, longitudinal and circumferential measurements are created. The change in longitudinal and circumferential spline length provides a consistent strain measurement (i.e., engineering strain) analogous to the strain measurements provided by the *in vivo* TomTec strain measurements. The quadrilateral and triangular surfaces, the control nodes, and the fitted cubic splines are illustrated in Supplementary Figures S1C,D.

## 3. RESULTS

## 3.1. Geometric Segmentation

A visualization of the 3D heart structure from T2-weighted MRI data is given in **Figure 4**, along with our ventricular segmentation.

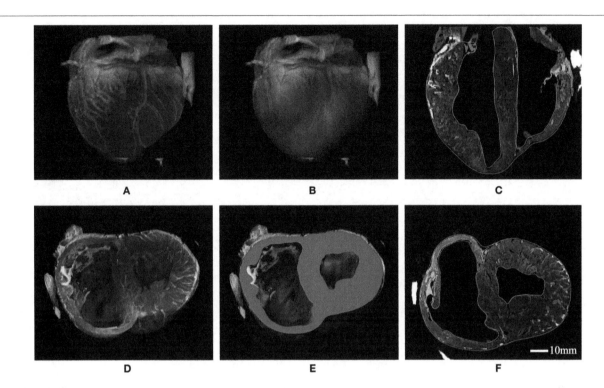

**FIGURE 4 | (A)** 3D constructed visualizations of the full ventricular structure from MRI data. **(B)** Geometric segmentation of the full ventricular structure superimposed over the same background MRI data as **(A)**. **(C)** Long-axis cut plane of the MRI data superimposed with contours (green lines) for the full ventricular segmentation. **(D)** 3D constructed visualizations of the truncated ventricular structure from MRI data, revealing the endocardial ventricular structure. **(E)** Geometric segmentation of truncated ventricular structure superimposed over the same background MRI data in **(D)**. **(F)** Short-axis cut plane of the MRI data superimposed with contours (green lines) for the ventricular segmentation.

Structural details such as wall thickness and trabecular morphology extracted from the MRI data conform to features reported for the porcine heart (Crick et al., 1998). Segmentations of the ventricles were meshed with roughly 85,000 quadratic tetrahedral elements–a refinement determined from a mesh convergence analysis. This analysis identified converged model behavior (i.e., stress, strain, and cavity expansion) over the entire cardiac cycle for mesh resolutions greater than approximately 50,000 elements.

## 3.2. Subject-Specific Myofiber Orientations

Results for the inclinations angles $\alpha_h$ for both porcine LVs are presented graphically in **Figure 5** for each AHA segment. This regional presentation of $\alpha_h$, partitioned by AHA region and further subdivided by transverse wall depth, presents in general with narrow distributions (i.e., small variance). Inclination angles in the normal subject, excluding the apex, vary from $66.5 \pm 16.6°$ on the endocardium to $-37.4 \pm 22.4°$ on the epicardium in a predominantly linear fashion. Similarly, inclination angles in the HF subject vary from $63.0 \pm 18.3°$ on the endocardium to $-43.4 \pm 19.8°$ on the epicardium.

A local orthonormal coordinate system aligned with the myofiber, sheet plane, and sheet normal directions are interpolated to the centroid of each element in the FE mesh. Images revealing the geometry with and without myofiber orientations are presented in **Figure 6**. In addition to the characteristics presented quantitatively above, other qualitative features are as follows. Firstly, myofiber orientations are predominantly tangential with geometric surfaces.

This can be seen in **Figures 6B,D**, by the abundance of myofibers protruding through cut surfaces relative to those seen protruding through natural physiological surfaces. Secondly, myofibers are closely aligned with papillary structure morphology, as can be seen in **Figures 6C–E**. Finally, the distribution in inclination angle in the LV, varying from positive on the endocardium through to negative on the epicardium, is easily identified from the global myofiber arrangement as shown in **Figure 6F**.

## 3.3. Material Parameter Estimation

The calibrated material parameters fit the human shear data (Sommer et al., 2015) with an $R^2 = 0.997$. This excellent fit is illustrated in Supplementary Figure S2 wherein model response (solid lines) is plotted against experimental data (circles). The corresponding material parameters that produced this response are a $= 1.05$ kPa, b $= 7.542$, $a_f = 3.465$(kPa), $b_f = 14.472$, $a_s = 0.481$(kPa), $b_s = 12.548$, $a_{fs} = 0.283$(kPa), and $b_{fs} = 3.088$.

The subject-specific calibration resulted in suitable values for the passive material scaling parameters $A$ and $B$, and active material parameters $T_{MAX}$ and $n_s$. These values are presented in **Table 1** along with the initial unloaded LV cavity volumes $V_0$, as these are fundamental to the resulting material parameters.

To illustrate the efficacy of the optimization routine, the passive filling curve resulting from optimizing is given in **Figure 7A**. These passive filling curves fit the analytical Klotz curves with an $R^2 = 0.967$ for the normal subject and an $R^2 = 0.995$ for the HF subject. The final calibrated EDV also matches closely with target values; i.e., 57.3

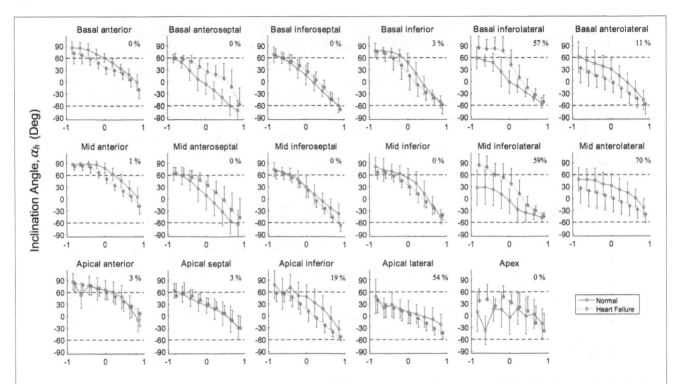

**FIGURE 5 |** Inclination angles $\alpha_h$ in the 17 left ventricle regions (Cerqueira et al., 2002) showing the distribution along the radial depth for the normal (healthy) and diseased (heart failure) subjects. Normalized radial coordinates were used to indicated the endocardium (−1), mid wall (0) and epicardium positions (+1). Dashed lines corresponding to +60° and −60° are plotted for ease of comparison and because a significant number of studies use these bounds when prescribing $\alpha_h$ in LV computational models. Percentage given in top right corner of each panel corresponds to the degree of infarcted tissue in the AHA region for the heart failure model, calculated as 1−mean(h).

vs. 57.8 ml (normal) and 102.4 vs. 103.0 ml (HF). Sample long- and short-axis profiles of the ventricular structure in the unloaded (i.e., initial) and the ED configuration are presented in **Figures 7B,C** for the normal subject.

## 3.4. Coupled Mechanical and Circulatory Model

Cardiac function was simulated for six consecutive cardiac cycles (**Figure 8**) to ensure converged solutions were achieved. All values and results reported in the following sections correspond to the final and converged solution; i.e., these values will differ slightly from the calibrated targets that were acquired for only the first beat simulated, which is visible in **Figure 8**.

LV functional outputs compared reasonably between *in vivo* and *in silico* results. This is seen in SV, which was 32.2 vs. 30.9 ml in the normal subject for *in silico* and *in vivo* respectively, and 34.5 vs. 33.0 ml in the HF subject for *in silico* and *in vivo* respectively. Similarly, ejection fraction (EF) was 54.4 vs. 53.4% in the normal subject for *in silico* and *in vivo* respectively, and 35.0 vs. 32.0% in the HF subject for *in silico* and *in vivo*, respectively. These differences in SV and EF are considered minor when compared to the biological variations that occur from beat to beat.

Using the key parts of the cardiac cycle as presented in **Figure 8**, we assessed myofiber stress and strain values for each ventricle. These values were volumetrically averaged (i.e., normalized by element volume) to remove potential mesh artifacts. The mean volumetrically averaged myofiber stress is at its lowest at the end of relaxation (ER);

it increases during passive filling, reaching a peak passive stress at end diastole (ED) and then rapidly increases during the systolic phase of the heart. By the start of ejection (SE), the myofiber stress is higher (order of magnitude greater than passive stress), which enables the continued contraction of the heart through ejection. While the myofiber stresses are high at end systole (ES), they continuously decline from this point, reaching the lowest values at ER, when the cycle repeats.

The mean volumetrically-averaged myofiber stresses in the LV and RV are presented in **Table 2**. Additionally, myofiber stress contours are presented in **Figure 9** over long-axis cut planes of the ventricular structure. These contour plots reveal qualitative details about the myofiber stress distributions associated with geometric position; e.g., peak stresses are seen on the endocardial surface of the LV.

Since the HF subject had additional geometric information regarding the position and degree of pathological tissue (via the $h$ field variable), we could further analyze stress by tissue health. Considering healthy tissue as regions whereby $h = 1$, infarcted tissue as $h = 0$, and border-zone tissue as values between these, we found mean myofiber stress was significantly different ($p < 0.001$) between all three regions, with substantially increased stress values within the infarcted tissue (**Table 3**).

The differences in stress values between normal and border-zone tissue are muted due to averaging. Analysis of these values as a function of geometric proximity to the fully infarcted/fibrotic tissue reveals more substantial differences (**Figure 10**). Most interestingly, the border-zone tissue experiences peak stresses roughly 1 mm away

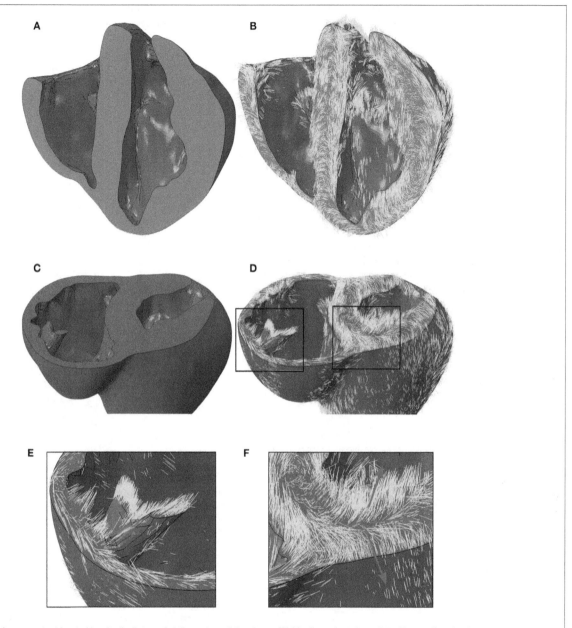

**FIGURE 6 | (A)** Porcine geometry bisected longitudinally to reveal the endocardial surfaces. **(B)** Myofiber orientations plotted in cyan lines for the same geometry revealed in **(A)**. **(C)** Porcine geometry cut along a short axis to reveal cut papillary structures in the RV and the short-axis plane in the LV. **(D)** Myofiber orientations plotted in cyan lines for the same geometry revealed in **(C)**. **(E)** Zoomed-in image of the cut RV papillary structure with fibers from **(D)**. **(F)** Zoomed-in image of the LV short-axis plane from **(D)**. Red arrows aligned with the local myofiber orientation are added for regions in the epicardial, mid wall and endocardial regions. LV, left ventricle; RV, right ventricle.

from the fibrotic tissue, after which they decrease and converge with healthy tissue values (distances >2 mm) for both ED and ES. Overlapping data points were analyzed for statistical significance and are illustrated in (**Figure 10**).

Similar to the analysis of myofiber stress, strain results were analyzed at the same key points in the cardiac cycle. The mean volumetrically averaged myofiber strains in the LV and RV are presented in **Table 4**. A detailed analysis of regional strain in the LV with respect to the local longitudinal and circumferential directions is presented in Section 3.5.

## 3.5. Model Validation

Initial comparison of the endocardial strains revealed strong agreement of global strains (i.e., averaged over the entire surface). For the normal subject, the global circumferential strain (GCS) for the FE simulations was −22.0%, which compares very well with the *in vivo* measurement of −21.9% from TomTec data. Global longitudinal strain (GLS) was −10.3% for the FE model simulation and −14.7% for the *in vivo* measurement. The HF subject produced similar comparisons: GCS for the FE simulations and the *in vivo* measurement were −14.4 and −12.7%, respectively, and GLS for the

FE simulations and the *in vivo* measurement were −4.6 and −8.3%, respectively. In both subjects, circumferential strains were in closer agreement than longitudinal strains, which were both 4% lower than *in vivo* measurements from echocardiograms.

A regional analysis of comparison for FE model results and the *in vivo* measured values for strain on the endocardium surface reveals a very strong agreement in circumferential strains for both subjects, as seen in **Figures 11B,D**. Qualitatively, it is clear that the longitudinal strain behavior from the FE model correlates to the recorded *in vivo* values, with similar regional patterns displayed in both modalities, as seen in **Figures 11A,C**.

## 4. DISCUSSION

The high degree of subject-specificity incorporated into these models vastly reduces the number of model assumptions needed to produce computational cardiac simulations. This has led to realistic mechanical behavior shown in the reported pressure-volume loops, our realistic determination of active tension (i.e., minimal cross-fiber contraction) and the independently reached strain behavior, which matches the measured strains from *in vivo* echocardiography.

### 4.1. Geometric Segmentation
The geometric model construction used in this study is one of the most sophisticated ventricular structures produced for FE modeling of the heart compared to those found in the literature. While biventricular representations of the heart have become popular

geometric choices for FE studies in recent years, most of these models truncate the geometry or exclude the papillary structures. The cardiac model from the Dassault Systèmes Living Heart Project (Baillargeon et al., 2014, 2015; Genet et al., 2016; Sack et al., 2016b) is an exception that does include this level of detail (and atrial structures); however, this heart geometry is not entirely patient-specific.

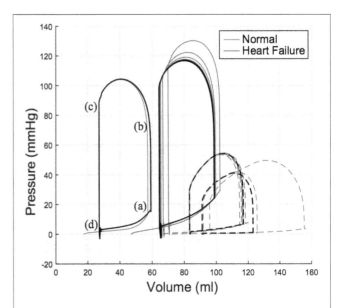

**FIGURE 8 |** Pressure volume relation for the left ventricle (solid lines) and right ventricle (dashed lines) of both subjects over six simulated cardiac cycles with a heart rate of 77 bpm. The 5 and 6th cardiac cycle is plotted in black illustrating convergence. Key parts of the cardiac cycle are labeled on the LV PV loop for the normal (healthy) subject, which correspond to **(a)** end diastole, **(b)** start ejection, **(c)** end systole, and **(d)** end relaxation. LV, left ventricle; PV, pressure volume.

**TABLE 1 |** Initial volumes and calibrated material parameters for the normal and heart failure subjects.

| Pig | $V_0$ | A | B | $T_{MAX}$ | $n_s$ |
|---|---|---|---|---|---|
| Normal | 17.5 | 0.16 | 0.73 | 118.0 | 0.07 |
| Heart failure | 47.1 | 1.69 | 0.87 | 140.6 | 0.14 |

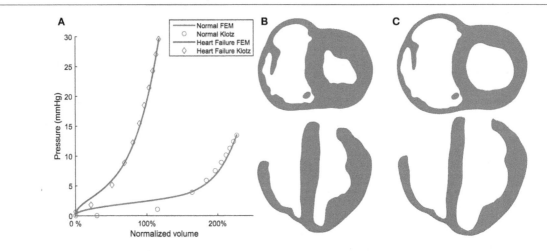

**FIGURE 7 | (A)** Klotz curve (markers) and model response (solid lines) for the normal (healthy) and diseased (heart failure) subjects after calibration whereby the volume is nominalized to $V_0$. **(B)** Long-axis and short-axis views of the ventricular structure at the unloaded configuration. **(C)** Long-axis and short-axis views of the ventricular structure at the end-diastole configuration.

The geometric model of HF used in this study is a novel extension of how infarcted tissue has typically been presented in computational studies. Previously, studies have represented infarcted tissue using discrete concentric zones accounting for infarction and the border-zone as neat self-contained geometric regions (Wenk et al., 2011; Miller et al., 2013; Berberoglu et al., 2014). Our study incorporates subject-specific pathological detail, allowing for the description of infarcted material that ranges from concentrated to diffuse descriptions, as can be seen in **Figure 2**. Moreover, this level of subject-specific geometric detail is coupled with subject-specific fiber detail accounting for regionally precise myofiber detail throughout the ventricular structure, which has never been included in models with HF.

**TABLE 2 |** Volumetric-averaged mean myofiber stress results for the converged hearts presented separately for the LV and RV throughout the cardiac cycle.

| Time point | LV myofiber stress (kPa) | | RV myofiber stress (kPa) | |
| --- | --- | --- | --- | --- |
| | Normal | Heart failure | Normal | Heart failure |
| ED | 2.1 ± 4.2 | 4.7 ± 4.9 | 0.6 ± 0.6 | 3.5 ± 3.6 |
| SE | 23.4 ± 16.9 | 27.1 ± 18.9 | 21.1 ± 14 | 27.1 ± 16.9 |
| ES | 18.6 ± 14.9 | 24.4 ± 18.7 | 25.1 ± 18.3 | 24.8 ± 17.9 |
| ER | 0.0 ± 0.0 | 0.5 ± 0.5 | 0.1 ± 0.1 | 0.3 ± 0.4 |

*Results are presented with standard deviations. ED, end-diastole; SE, start-ejection; ES, end-systole; ER, end-relaxation.*

## 4.2. Subject-Specific Myofiber Orientation

The critical role of myofiber orientation on mechanical and electrical function is well recognized (Beyar and Sideman, 1984b; Bovendeerd et al., 1992; Chen et al., 2005; Bishop et al., 2009; Wang et al., 2013). Fiber orientation, along with a second orthogonal vector within the laminar sheet, provides sufficient information to establish a local orthonormal coordinate system whereby each basis vector

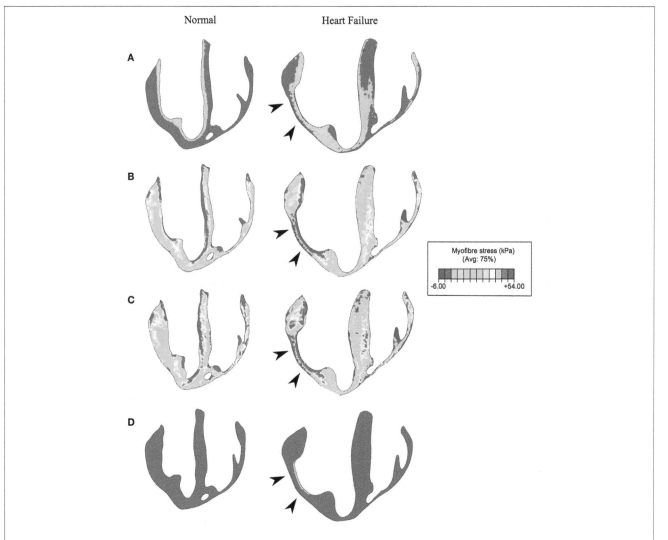

**FIGURE 9 |** Myofiber stress at **(A)**: end-diastole, **(B)** start of ejection, **(C)** end-systole, and **(D)** end-relaxation. Left and right columns reveal the long axis cut planes of the ventricles for the normal (healthy) and diseased (heart failure) subjects respectively. The infarcted/fibrotic region is identified in the heart failure subject by black arrowheads. Non-symmetric contour limits were chosen to allow for a single set of limits to be used across the whole cardiac cycle.

corresponds to a principal anisotropic direction. To the best of our knowledge, the present models are the first mechanical models to include subject-specific local coordinates derived from DTMRI.

The values of $\alpha_h$ in the normal subject conform well to other studies of large animals in terms of mean values (Streeter and Bassett, 1966; Streeter et al., 1969; Nielsen et al., 1991; Geerts et al., 2002; Helm et al., 2005; Ennis et al., 2008) and typical standard deviations expected from regional DTMRI myofiber analysis (Scollan et al., 1998; Lombaert et al., 2012). Our data reveals larger angles (i.e., close alignment with the longitudinal direction) in the anterior and inferior endocardial region when compared to other AHA regions circumferentially. These regions typically contain large papillary muscles on the endocardium, which explain this observation. These endocardial values of $\alpha_h$ in the anterior and inferior regions tend to plateau with values before declining linearly as a position of wall depth. The study of fiber orientation in papillary muscles is relatively unreported in the literature, due to difficulty in segmentation from *in vivo* imaging. In the early experimental work of Streeter et al. (1969), however, the authors also identified a plateau of myofiber angle $\alpha_h$ of roughly 90° in papillary muscles.

Myofiber orientations in the failing heart have striking similarities to the healthy heart in anterior, inferior, and the majority of septal (i.e., excluding basal anteroseptal) regions. Our results show that the largest discrepancies in myofiber angles correspond to regions in the LV free wall (i.e., basal and mid lateral regions), regardless of underlying fibrotic tissue content. This suggests that together with underlying pathology, mechanical factors relating to the position and function of an LV region are linked to its susceptibility to remodel.

Lower values of the myofiber inclination angle $\alpha_h$ in the vulnerable anterolateral regions are consistent with values reported in other studies investigating change in fiber orientation due to infarction (Holmes et al., 1997; Wu et al., 2007, 2009). In contrast, the inferolateral regions in the current HF model present with higher values of $\alpha_h$, especially near the endocardial surface. Here, $\alpha_h$ plateau with values highly aligned longitudinally, indicative that the inferior papillary muscle was segmented within these regions and may be clouding the results. Even with consistent segmentation techniques, biological variance between subjects is an unavoidable challenge when sources of discrepancies are being determined. This likely explains the disagreement seen in regions with little fibrotic content.

## 4.3. Passive Material Estimation

The choice to use human shear experimental data, instead of porcine data from an earlier study (Dokos et al., 2002) was made after we calibrated our model to both and found that the porcine data produced *much* stiffer material behavior, especially in the fiber direction. As the human study was performed over a decade after the porcine study, more sophisticated methods were utilized in preventing contracture of heart muscles in the specimen extraction process, making the results likely more reliable representations of

**TABLE 3 |** ED and ES volumetric-averaged mean myofiber stress results within the LV of the failing.

| Time point | LV myofiber stress (kPa) | | |
|---|---|---|---|
| | Healthy tissue | Border-zone | Infarcted |
| ED | 4.1 ± 4.5 | 4.6 ± 4.9 | 10.5 ± 10 |
| ES | 23.2 ± 19.8 | 24.1 ± 21.1 | 39.4 ± 43.8 |

*Results are presented with standard deviations. ED, end-diastole; ES, end-systole.*

**TABLE 4 |** ED and ES volumetric-averaged mean myofiber strain results for the converged hearts presented separately for the LV and RV.

| Time point | LV myofiber strain (%) | | RV myofiber strain (%) | |
|---|---|---|---|---|
| | Normal | Heart failure | Normal | Heart failure |
| ED | 9.6 ± 6.7 | 6.9 ± 4.3 | 8.3 ± 5.7 | 5.5 ± 5.0 |
| SE | −1.0 ± 10.4 | 1.0 ± 7.4 | −4.3 ± 10 | −2.6 ± 7.4 |
| ES | −9.8 ± 5.0 | −5.4 ± 6.5 | −8.9 ± 6.5 | −8.4 ± 3.7 |
| ER | 0.7 ± 2.0 | 1.9 ± 1.6 | 1.4 ± 2.4 | 1.0 ± 1.8 |

*Results are presented with standard deviations. ED, end-diastole; SE, start-ejection; ES, end-systole; ER, end-relaxation; LV, left ventricle; RV, right ventricle.*

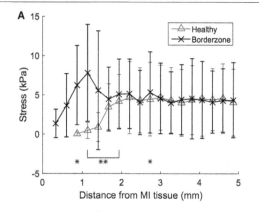
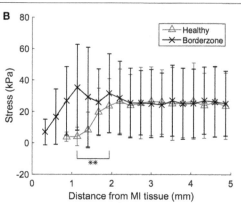

**FIGURE 10 |** Myofiber LV stress within healthy and border-zone (i.e., 0< *h* <1) tissue presented by proximity to pathological tissue (within 5 mm from fully infarcted/fibrotic tissue). **(A)** Results shown for end-diastole and **(B)** end-systole for the failing subject. Error bars correspond to ± SD, *p < 0.05, and **p < 0.01. MI, myocardial infarction.

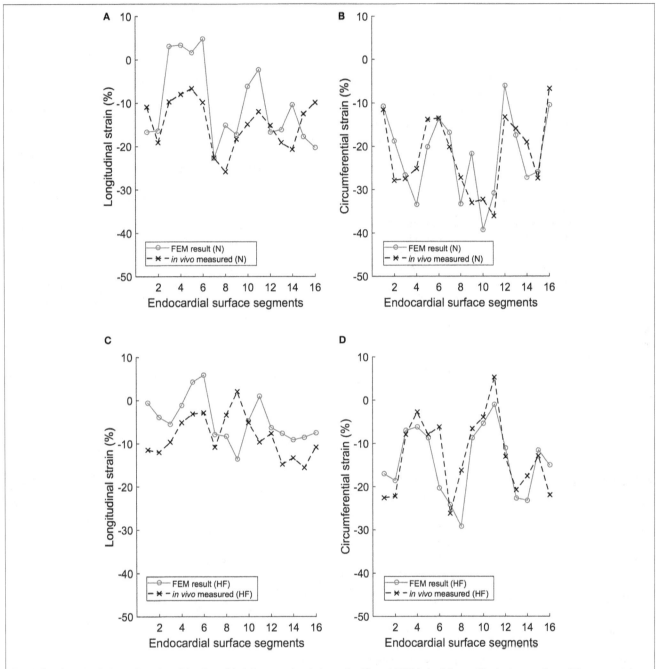

**FIGURE 11 |** Longitudinal and circumferential endocardial strain comparison between the FE model (FEM) simulation and the *in vivo* recordings of the same porcine subject. **(A)** Longitudinal strain results for each of the 16 endocardial surface regions in the normal subject (N). **(B)** Circumferential strain results for each of the 16 endocardial surface regions in the normal subject (N). **(C)** Longitudinal strain results for each of the 16 endocardial surface regions in the heart failure subject (HF). **(D)** Circumferential strain results for each of the 16 endocardial surface regions in the heart failure subject (HF).

*in vivo* material response. Our calibration methods are proficient in capturing experimentally recorded orthotropic material response, as seen in Supplementary Figure S2, and when scaled, match the predicted Klotz curve for passive filling accurately (**Figure 7**). This two-stage method of cardiac tissue calibration, which utilizes small specimen data and pressure-volume data, is becoming a common method for obtaining realistic (and subject-specific) parameters (Krishnamurthy et al., 2013; Gao et al., 2015; Sack et al., 2016c). It

ensures that the resulting material parameters produce a material that conforms to the anisotropy uncovered from mechanical experimentation and realistic *in vivo* function.

The determination of passive material parameters for the myocardial tissue ultimately depends on three factors: (1) the unloaded volumes $V_0$ of the ventricles; (2) the target ED volumes; and (3) the assumption regarding infarct stiffness. Our calibration techniques found that the HF subject yielded material parameters roughly an order of magnitude greater (considering the linear scaling coefficient A) (**Table 1**) than the normal subject, resulting in a much stiffer passive filling curve (**Figure 7**). This increase in remote stiffness is in line with other studies that have found that the remote tissue experiences changes in material properties (Bogaert et al., 2000; McGarvey et al., 2015), as well as the underlying physiological process of adverse remodeling, which results in collagen content, deposition, and cross-linking increasing in both infarcted and remote regions of the heart (Holmes et al., 2005; van den Borne et al., 2008; Fomovsky and Holmes, 2010). Another noteworthy finding is that the unloaded LV cavity in the subject with HF is almost three times as large as that of the healthy counterpart (**Table 1**).

## 4.4. Active Material Estimation

Contraction is initiated by sarcomere shortening in series, which in turn contracts myofibrils. Whereas the mechanical analysis of this multi-scale phenomenon would seem to only occur in the myofiber direction, contraction has also been recorded in cross-fiber directions (Lin and Yin, 1998), which has been linked to the splay and dispersion of myofibers. The active material calibration resulted in $T_{max} = 114.0$ kPa and $n_s = 0.07$ in the normal subject, and $T_{max} = 140.6$ kPa and $n_s = 0.14$ in the HF subject. The value found for $T_{max}$ is in line with the values reported in Genet et al. (2014): 130–155 kPa. These values of $n_s$ are typically lower than those found in cardiac models that use generic fiber descriptions, which typically apply 40% of active stress in this direction (i.e. $n_s = 0.4$) (Lee et al., 2013; Genet et al., 2014; Zhang et al., 2015). Our lower values of $n_s$ are due to the accurate subject-specific fiber orientations incorporated in the model, which naturally reduces the inclusion of unrealistically high (and potentially non-physiological) cross-fiber contraction.

## 4.5. *In Silico* Subject-Specific Heart

The patient-specific metrics used to calibrate the material model of the heart are preserved in the converged cardiac-cycle simulation with an error <5%. This is hardly a shortcoming as a physiological *in vivo* heart operates within a range of values, often experiencing variances in SV, pressure and timing from cardiac cycle to cardiac cycle. Without any subject-specific pressure-volume data for the RV, we assumed the same material properties as the LV and loaded the RV using values derived from the literature. While it appears this initial loading state was far from the converged solution, it had comparatively little impact on the LV function. Rather, the RV experienced the majority of the functional change to ensure hemodynamic equilibrium. It is reassuring to see that despite the lack of appropriate data for the RV, the combined ventricular function converges to a state closely in line with LV *in vivo* targets. This unidirectional ventricular dependence is pronounced in the porcine heart, where the LV is overwhelming the major mechanical component of the heart, and may be less pronounced in human models.

Qualitatively, the strain results conform to expectations. The myofiber elongation is at its greatest at ED, is at its minimum during systole (due to the contractile material behavior), and returns to almost the original length before passive filling starts (**Table 4**). Furthermore, these strain results reveal functional changes due to pathology. The failing heart experiences diminished myofiber strains within the LV at ED ($6.9 \pm 4.3$ vs. $9.6 \pm 6.7$) due to its stiffer material composition, and diminished myofiber strains at ES ($-5.4 \pm 6.5$

vs. $-9.8 \pm 5.0$) due to the loss of contractile function in the infarcted region.

An accurate determination of stress within complex mechanical problems is an unrivaled advantage of computational modeling. This is especially relevant for cardiac mechanics as changes in ventricular wall stress are thought to initiate pathological remodeling (Pfeffer and Braunwald, 1990; Sutton and Sharpe, 2000; Matiwala and Margulies, 2004). A unique problem pertaining to biological materials is that *in vivo* stresses cannot be accurately replicated under *in vitro* experimental protocols and thus, cannot be measured directly (Dorri et al., 2006). Our results show that chronic HF results in increased mean myofiber stresses in both ventricles at ED, and in the LV at ES (**Table 2**). This is interesting in the context of our strain results; i.e., the subject with HF experiences increased stress while simultaneously experiencing reduced strain. Determining stress directly from strain, without accounting for the anatomic features of the infarcted tissue or a proper constitutive characterization of the myocardial tissue (e.g., in Laplace's law), could lead to highly erroneous conclusions about the actual stress state within the failing heart. This has been demonstrated by Zhang et al. (2011), who compared Laplace's law and FE methods to evaluate stress in an infarcted LV. Their analysis showed that the average stress from Laplace's law is significantly different to the comprehensive stress analysis produced through anatomically accurate FE techniques.

While these increases in myofiber stress are prevalent throughout the myocardium, the infarcted region experiences myofiber stress roughly twice as high as in remote regions (**Table 4**). Furthermore, the myocardial wall containing the infarcted region, which is geometrically thinner than other regions, experiences complex stress due to its morphology and stiffer, non-contractile material behavior. Along the endocardium it experiences extremely high tensile stresses and along the epicardium it experiences compression (**Figures 9A–C**). We also discovered that in border-zone regions peak stresses occurred roughly 1 mm from fully infarcted tissue. Since stress is thought to initiate pathological remodeling (Pfeffer and Braunwald, 1990; Sutton and Sharpe, 2000; Matiwala and Margulies, 2004), this may explain the mechanical propagation of infarct expansion.

Due to the lack of comparable porcine computational studies we compared our stress results to available human studies. We found that the LV myofiber stresses in the normal subject compare well with literature values; e.g., our predicted ED stress of $2.1 \pm 4.2$ kPa vs. $1.47 \pm 20.72$ (Sack et al., 2016b) and $2.21 \pm 0.58$ (Genet et al., 2014).

## 4.6. Model Validation

The comparison between *in vivo* and model-predicted strains resulted in very similar qualitatively and quantitative results. For global values, the circumferential strains matched very well (<0.1% error), whereas the longitudinal strains were under-predicted in the FE model by merely 4%. A regional analysis reinforced this–circumferential strains matched extremely well for both subjects (**Figure 11**) and longitudinal strains matched with less accuracy (particularly in HF). The mismatch between longitudinal strain results may be due to simplifications inherent in the derivations of strains from echocardiography or our FE model. One the one hand, the surface resolution of echocardiography is typically low resolution (likely excluding finer morphological features), whereas the FE model has a much higher endocardial surface resolution. Echo-derived strains exclude the papillary muscles, and are often determined "sub-endocardially." These papillary muscles, which pull downward during systole, would clearly alter the longitudinal strain measurement when included in the determination. On the other hand, our FE model excludes the atria and the pericardium. Ventricular motion is likely coupled with the presence (and weight) of the atria and their function (Fritz et al., 2014), which would specifically affect longitudinal strains. To further complicate the comparison, the difficulty in accurately measuring *in vivo* strains from echocardiography is well documented. For example, consistent strain-data reproducibility (intra- and inter-observer) is the subject of multiple medical studies, some showing very poor outcomes (Gayat et al., 2011; Badano et al., 2012). Currently, the reliability of global deformation metrics from echo-derived 3D strain is strong, (i.e., GCS and GLS), but the reliability to accurately quantify regional deformation is not (Lang et al., 2015). The uncertainty regarding the reliability of regional strains (from either modality) requires further study either using full-heart models or a better source of *in vivo* strain data (i.e. MRI-derived).

## 4.7. Clinical Translation

Reliable computational heart models offer the potential to integrate diverse data, produce otherwise unobtainable metrics relating to function, and quantify complex coupled mechanical behavior in an unparalleled manner. This can be especially advantageous as a research modality investigating the efficacy of treatments pre-clinically. Computational models allow for therapeutic parameters to easily be perturbed, whereby various *in silico* experiments can be investigated to determine optimal treatment efficacy.

As computing resources become cheaper and more efficient, computational modeling is increasingly being viewed as a viable complementing modality in the clinic. As shown in this study, reliable subject-specific models are achievable with the proper inclusion of high quality imaging data. As imaging technology becomes more advanced, it will become feasible to replicate the quality of models using purely *in vivo* imaging data. This would enable the ability to investigate potential therapies *in silico* prior to their application to patients–with medical decisions, treatment plans and interventions being highly patient-specific.

Additional techniques are needed to integrate clinical data into the methods presented here. Firstly, methods that can indirectly assess the unloaded geometry from an *in vivo* representation, such as inverse-displacement techniques (Bols et al., 2013; Rausch et al., 2017), will likely be required. Secondly, if pressure catheterization data is not available, methods to approximate or infer patient pressures will be needed. Cuff pressures could be used to identify the pressure range in the systemic arteries and Nagueh's formula (Nagueh et al., 1997), can be employed on echocardiogram data to obtain approximate LV filling pressures.

## 4.8. Model Limitations

While geometrically detailed, our computational model is still lacking physiological features such as the atria, the pericardial sac and the diaphragm. This may be the source of discrepancies seen in longitudinal strains, especially among basal regions. For the normal subject, an average value of EDP had to be used when determining the *in vivo* target. A further shortcoming of this work is that it has only been applied to a single subject for each condition, but our current research is focused on expanding this to a larger cohort and including failing hearts treated with biomaterial injection therapy. Our material model of the heart is limited in that it does not include dispersion, micro-structural mechanics or regional heterogeneity of the tissue. Finally, only the mechanical component of heart function was simulated and excluded electro-chemical-mechanical considerations (i.e., the polarization of tissue, excitation and propagation phenomena).

## 5. CONCLUSIONS

This study introduces subject-specific cardiac models for biventricular porcine heart models in healthy and diseased states. Subject specificity is introduced through geometric features, local myofiber directions, loading conditions, hemodynamics and the distribution of fibrotic tissue in the failing heart. These models were calibrated to *in vivo* subject-specific metrics, and were able to accurately capture functional outputs such as SV and EF. The close global and regional agreement between *in vivo* and *in silico* strains illustrated the success of our methods to create computational models that can serve as *in silico* surrogates for real hearts in healthy and diseased states. This level of agreement, and therefore validation, is a milestone for cardiac computational modeling. As such, stress and strain values presented in this study (for both ventricles and at multiple time points during the cardiac cycle) can serve as a guideline for future studies.

## AUTHOR CONTRIBUTIONS

KS, JG, and TF were involved in the conception and design of study. KS created the computational models. Animal experiments were performed by JC and GK. Acquisition of various data critical to model creation was performed by JC, EA, and DE. The analysis and interpretation of modeling results was performed by all authors. KS wrote the first draft of the manuscript. All authors contributed to manuscript revision, read and approved the submitted version.

## ACKNOWLEDGMENTS

The authors thank Pamela Derish in the Department of Surgery, University of California San Francisco for proofreading the manuscript.

# REFERENCES

Badano, L. P., Cucchini, U., Muraru, D., Al Nono, O., Sarais, C., and Iliceto, S. (2012). Use of three-dimensional speckle tracking to assess left ventricular myocardial mechanics: inter-vendor consistency and reproducibility of strain measurements. *Eur. Heart J. Cardiovasc. Imaging* 14, 285–293. doi: 10.1093/ehjci/jes184

Baillargeon, B., Costa, I., Leach, J. R., Lee, L. C., Genet, M., Toutain, A., et al. (2015). Human cardiac function simulator for the optimal design of a novel annuloplasty ring with a sub-valvular element for correction of ischemic mitral regurgitation. *Cardiovasc. Eng. Technol.* 6, 105–116. doi: 10.1007/s13239-015-0216-z

Baillargeon, B., Rebelo, N., Fox, D. D., Taylor, R. L., and Kuhl, E. (2014). The Living Heart Project: a robust and integrative simulator for human heart function. *Eur. J. Mech. A Solids* 48, 38–47. doi: 10.1016/j.euromechsol.2014.04.001

Berberoglu, E., Solmaz, H. O., and Göktepe, S. (2014). Computational modeling of coupled cardiac electromechanics incorporating cardiac dysfunctions. *Eur. J. Mech. A Solids* 48, 60–73. doi: 10.1016/j.euromechsol.2014.02.021

Beyar, R., and Sideman, S. (1984a). Model for left ventricular contraction combining the force length velocity relationship with the time varying elastance theory. *Biophys. J.* 45, 1167–1177. doi: 10.1016/S0006-3495(84)84265-4

Beyar, R., and Sideman, S. (1984b). A computer study of the left ventricular performance based on fiber structure, sarcomere dynamics, and transmural electrical propagation velocity. *Circ. Res.* 55:358. doi: 10.1161/01.RES.55.3.358

Bishop, M. J., Hales, P., Plank, G., Gavaghan, D. J., Scheider, J., and Grau, V. (2009). "Comparison of rule-based and DTMRI-derived fibre architecture in a whole rat ventricular computational model," in *International Conference on Functional Imaging and Modeling of the Heart* (Berlin; Heidelberg: Springer), 87–96.

Bogaert, J., Bosmans, H., Maes, A., Suetens, P., Marchal, G., and Rademakers, F. E. (2000). Remote myocardial dysfunction after acute anterior myocardial infarction: impact of left ventricular shape on regional function: a magnetic resonance myocardial tagging study. *J. Am. Coll. Cardiol.* 35, 1525–1534. doi: 10.1016/S0735-1097(00)00601-X

Bogen, D. K., Rabinowitz, S. A., Needleman, A., McMahon, T. A., and Abelmann, W. H. (1980). An analysis of the mechanical disadvantage of myocardial infarction in the canine left ventricle. *Circ. Res.* 47, 728–741. doi: 10.1161/01.RES.47.5.728

Bols, J., Degroote, J., Trachet, B., Verhegghe, B., Segers, P., and Vierendeels, J. (2013). A computational method to assess the *in vivo* stresses and unloaded configuration of patient-specific blood vessels. *J. Comput. Appl. Math.* 246, 10–17. doi: 10.1016/j.cam.2012.10.034

Bovendeerd, P. H., Arts, T., Huyghe, J. M., van Campen, D. H., and Reneman, R. S. (1992). Dependence of local left ventricular wall mechanics on myocardial fiber orientation: a model study. *J. Biomech.* 25, 1129–1140. doi: 10.1016/0021-9290(92)90069-D

Carreras, F., Garcia-Barnes, J., Gil, D., Pujadas, S., Li, C. H., Suarez-Arias, R., et al. (2012). Left ventricular torsion and longitudinal shortening: two fundamental components of myocardial mechanics assessed by tagged cine-MRI in normal subjects. *Int. J. Cardiovasc. Imaging* 28, 273–284. doi: 10.1007/s10554-011-9813-6

Cerqueira, M. D., Weissman, N. J., Dilsizian, V., Jacobs, A. K., Kaul, S., Laskey, W. K., et al. (2002). Standardized myocardial segmentation and nomenclature for tomographic imaging of the heart-A statement for healthcare professionals from the Cardiac Imaging Committee of the Council on Clinical Cardiology of the American Heart Association. *Circulation* 105, 539–542. doi: 10.1161/hc0402.102975

Chen, J., Hsieh, A., Dharmarajan, K., Masoudi, F. A., and Krumholz, H. M. (2013). National trends in heart failure hospitalization after acute myocardial infarction for medicare beneficiaries: 1998–2010. *Circulation* 128, 2577–2584. doi: 10.1161/CIRCULATIONAHA.113.003668

Chen, J., Liu, W., Zhang, H., Lacy, L., Yang, X., Song, S. K., et al. (2005). Regional ventricular wall thickening reflects changes in cardiac fiber and sheet structure during contraction: quantification with diffusion tensor MRI. *Am. J. Physiol. Heart Circ. Physiol.* 289, H1898–H1907. doi: 10.1152/ajpheart.000 41.2005

Choy, J. S., Leng, S., Acevedo-Bolton, G., Shaul, S., Fu, L., Guo, X., et al. (2018). Efficacy of intramyocardial injection of Algisyl-LVR for the treatment of ischemic heart failure in Swine. *Int. J. Cardiol.* 255, 129–135. doi: 10.1016/j.ijcard.2017.09.179

Connelly, C. M., Vogel, W. M., Wiegner, A. W., Osmers, E. L., Bing, O. H., Kloner, R. A., et al. (1985). Effects of reperfusion after coronary artery occlusion on post-infarction scar tissue. *Circ. Res.* 57, 562–577. doi: 10.1161/01.RES.57.4.562

Crick, S. J., Sheppard, M. N., HO, S. Y., Gebstein, L., and Anderson, R. H. (1998). Anatomy of the pig heart: comparisons with normal human cardiac structure. *J. Anat.* 193, 105–119. doi: 10.1046/j.1469-7580.1998.19310105.x

Desta, L., Jernberg, T., Löfman, I., Hofman-Bang, C., Hagerman, I., Spaak, J., et al. (2015). Incidence, temporal trends, and prognostic impact of heart failure complicating acute myocardial infarction. The SWEDEHEART Registry (Swedish Web-System for Enhancement and Development of Evidence-Based Care in Heart Disease Evaluated According to Recommended Therapies): a study of 199,851 patients admitted with index acute myocardial infarctions, 1996 to 2008. *JACC Heart Fail.* 3, 234–242. doi: 10.1016/j.jchf.2014.10.007

Dill, E. H. (2006). Continuum *Mechanics: Elasticity, Plasticity, Viscoelasticity*. Boca Raton, FL: CRC press.

Dokos, S., Smaill, B. H., Young, A. A., and LeGrice, I. J. (2002). Shear properties of passive ventricular myocardium. *Am. J. Physiol. Heart Circ. Physiol.* 283, H2650–H2659. doi: 10.1152/ajpheart.00111.2002

Dorri, F., Niederer, P. F., and Lunkenheimer, P. P. (2006). A finite element model of the human left ventricular systole. *Comput. Methods Biomech. Biomed. Engin.* 9, 319–341. doi: 10.1080/10255840600960546

Dumesnil, J., Shoucri, R., Laurenceau, J., and Turcot, J. (1979). A mathematical model of the dynamic geometry of the intact left ventricle and its application to clinical data. *Circulation* 59, 1024–1034. doi: 10.1161/01.CIR.59.5.1024

Ennis, D. B., Nguyen, T. C., Riboh, J. C., Wigström, L., Harrington, K. B., Daughters, G. T., et al. (2008). Myofiber angle distributions in the ovine left ventricle do not conform to computationally optimized predictions. *J. Biomech.* 41, 3219–3224. doi: 10.1016/j.jbiomech.2008.08.007

Finegold, J. A., Asaria, P., and Francis, D. P. (2013). Mortality from ischaemic heart disease by country, region, and age: statistics from World Health Organisation and United Nations. *Int. J. Cardiol.* 168, 934–945. doi: 10.1016/j.ijcard.2012.10.046

Fomovsky, G. M., and Holmes, J. W. (2010). Evolution of scar structure, mechanics, and ventricular function after myocardial infarction in the rat. *Am. J. Physiol. Heart Circ. Physiol.* 298, H221–H228. doi: 10.1152/ajpheart.00495.2009

Fomovsky, G. M., Macadangdang, J. R., Ailawadi, G., and Holmes, J. W. (2011). Model-based design of mechanical therapies for myocardial infarction. *J. Cardiovasc. Transl. Res.* 4, 82–91. doi: 10.1007/s12265-010-9241-3

Fritz, T., Wieners, C., Seemann, G., Steen, H., and Dössel, O. (2014). Simulation of the contraction of the ventricles in a human heart model including atria and pericardium. *Biomech. Model. Mechanobiol.* 13, 627–641. doi: 10.1007/s10237-013-0523-y

Gahm, J. K., Wisniewski, N., Kindlmann, G., Kung, G. L., Klug, W. S., Garfinkel, A., et al. (2012). "Linear invariant tensor interpolation applied to cardiac diffusion tensor MRI," in *Medical Image Computing and Computer-Assisted Intervention-MICCAI 2012. 15th International Conference, Nice, France, October 1-5, 2012, Proceedings, Part II* (Berlin; Heidelberg: Springer), 494–501.

Gao, H., Li, W., Cai, L., Berry, C., and Luo, X. (2015). Parameter estimation in a Holzapfel–Ogden law for healthy myocardium. *J. Eng. Math.* 95, 231–248. doi: 10.1007/s10665-014-9740-3

Gayat, E., Ahmad, H., Weinert, L., Lang, R. M., and Mor-Avi, V. (2011). Reproducibility and inter-vendor variability of left ventricular deformation measurements by three-dimensional speckle-tracking echocardiography. *J. Am. Soc. Echocardiogr.* 24, 878–885. doi: 10.1016/j.echo.2011.04.016

Geerts, L., Bovendeerd, P., Nicolay, K., and Arts, T. (2002). Characterization of the normal cardiac myofiber field in goat measured with MR-diffusion tensor imaging. *Am. J. Physiol. Heart Circ. Physiol.* 283, H139–H145. doi: 10.1152/ajpheart.00968.2001

Genet, M., Lee, L. C., Baillargeon, B., Guccione, J. M., and Kuhl, E. (2016). Modeling pathologies of diastolic and systolic heart failure. *Ann. Biomed. Eng.* 44, 112–127. doi: 10.1007/s10439-015-1351-2

Genet, M., Lee, L. C., Nguyen, R., Haraldsson, H., Acevedo-Bolton, G., Zhang, Z., et al. (2014). Distribution of normal human left ventricular myofiber stress at end diastole and end systole: a target for *in silico* design of heart failure treatments. *J. Appl. Physiol. (1985)* 117, 142–152. doi: 10.1152/japplphysiol.00255.2014

Göktepe, S., Acharya, S. N. S., Wong, J., and Kuhl, E. (2011). Computational modeling of passive myocardium. *Int. J. Numer. Methods Biomed. Eng.* 27, 1–12. doi: 10.1002/cnm.1402

Guccione, J. M., Moonly, S. M., Moustakidis, P., Costa, K. D., Moulton, M. J., Ratcliffe, M. B., et al. (2001). Mechanism underlying mechanical dysfunction in the border zone of left ventricular aneurysm: a finite element model study. *Ann. Thorac. Surg.* 71, 654–662. doi: 10.1016/S0003-4975(00)02338-9

Gupta, K. B., Ratcliffe, M. B., Fallert, M. A., Edmunds, L. H. Jr., and Bogen, D. K. (1994). Changes in passive mechanical stiffness of myocardial tissue with aneurysm formation. *Circulation* 89, 2315–2326. doi: 10.1161/01.CIR.89.5.2315

Hanrath, P., Mathey, D. G., Kremer, P., Sonntag, F., and Bleifeld, W. (1980). Effect of verapamil on left ventricular isovolumic relaxation time and regional left ventricular filling in hypertrophic cardiomyopathy. *Am. J. Cardiol.* 45, 1258–1264. doi: 10.1016/0002-9149(80)90487-7

Helm, P. A., Tseng, H. J., Younes, L., McVeigh, E. R., and Winslow, R. L. (2005). *Ex vivo* 3D diffusion tensor imaging and quantification of cardiac laminar structure. *Magn. Reson. Med.* 54, 850–859. doi: 10.1002/mrm.20622

Holmes, J. W., Borg, T. K., and Covell, J. W. (2005). Structure and mechanics of healing myocardial infarcts. *Annu. Rev. Biomed. Eng.* 7, 223–253. doi: 10.1146/annurev.bioeng.7.060804.100453

Holmes, J. W., Nuñez, J. A., and Covell, J. W. (1997). Functional implications of myocardial scar structure. *Am. J. Physiol. Heart Circ. Physiol.* 272, H2123–H2130. doi: 10.1152/ajpheart.1997.272.5.H2123

Holzapfel, G. A., and Ogden, R. W. (2009). Constitutive modelling of passive myocardium: a structurally based framework for material characterization. *Philos. Trans. A Math. Phys. Eng. Sci.* 367, 3445–3475. doi: 10.1098/rsta.2009.0091

Hoppensteadt, F. C., and Peskin, C. S. (1992). *Mathematics in Medicine and The Life Sciences*. New York, NY: Springer-Verlag.

Hughes, T. J. (2000). *The Finite Element Method: Linear Static and Dynamic Finite Element Analysis*. Englewood Cliffs, NJ: Courier Corporation.

Kerckhoffs, R. C., Neal, M. L., Gu, Q., Bassingthwaighte, J. B., Omens, J. H., and McCulloch, A. D. (2007). Coupling of a 3D finite element model of cardiac ventricular mechanics to lumped systems models of the systemic and pulmonic circulation. *Ann. Biomed. Eng.* 35, 1–18. doi: 10.1007/s10439-006-9212-7

Klotz, S., Hay, I., Dickstein, M. L., Yi, G. H., Wang, J., Maurer, M. S., et al. (2006). Single-beat estimation of end-diastolic pressure-volume relationship: a novel method with potential for noninvasive application. *Am. J. Physiol. Heart Circ. Physiol.* 291, H403–H412. doi: 10.1152/ajpheart.01240.2005

Krishnamurthy, A., Villongco, C. T., Chuang, J., Frank, L. R., Nigam, V., Belezzuoli, E., et al. (2013). Patient-specific models of cardiac biomechanics. *J. Comput. Phys.* 244, 4–21. doi: 10.1016/j.jcp.2012.09.015

Kung, G. L., Nguyen, T. C., Itoh, A., Skare, S., Ingels, N. B., Miller, D. C., et al. (2011). The presence of two local myocardial sheet populations confirmed by diffusion tensor MRI and histological validation. *J. Magn. Reson. Imaging* 34, 1080–1091. doi: 10.1002/jmri.22725

Lang, R. M., Badano, L. P., Mor-Avi, V., Afilalo, J., Armstrong, A., Ernande, L., et al. (2015). Recommendations for cardiac chamber quantification by echocardiography in adults: an update from the American Society of Echocardiography and the European Association of Cardiovascular Imaging. *J. Am. Soc. Echocardiogr.* 28, 1.e14–39.e14. doi: 10.1016/j.echo.2014.10.003

Lee, L. C., Wenk, J. F., Zhong, L., Klepach, D., Zhang, Z., Ge, L., et al. (2013). Analysis of patient-specific surgical ventricular restoration: importance of an ellipsoidal left ventricular geometry for diastolic and systolic function. *J. Appl. Physiol. (1985)* 115, 136–144. doi: 10.1152/japplphysiol.00662.2012

Lin, D., and Yin, F. (1998). A multiaxial constitutive law for mammalian left ventricular myocardium in steady-state barium contracture or tetanus. *J. Biomech. Eng.* 120, 504–517. doi: 10.1115/1.2798021

Lombaert, H., Peyrat, J. M., Croisille, P., Rapacchi, S., Fanton, L., Cheriet, F., et al. (2012). Human atlas of the cardiac fiber architecture: study on a healthy population. *IEEE Trans. Med. Imaging* 31, 1436–1447. doi: 10.1109/TMI.2012.2192743

Mann, D. L., Zipes, D. P., Libby, P., Bonow, R. O., and Braunwald, E. (2015). *Braunwald's Heart Disease*. Philidelphia, PA: Elsevier-Saunders.

Matiwala, S., and Margulies, K. B. (2004). Mechanical approaches to alter remodeling. *Curr. Heart Fail. Rep.* 1, 14–18. doi: 10.1007/s11897-004-0012-9

McGarvey, J. R., Mojsejenko, D., Dorsey, S. M., Nikou, A., Burdick, J. A., Gorman, J. H. III, et al. (2015). Temporal changes in infarct material properties: an *in vivo* assessment using magnetic resonance imaging and finite element simulations. *Ann. Thorac. Surg.* 100, 582–590. doi: 10.1016/j.athoracsur.2015.03.015

Miller, R., Davies, N. H., Kortsmit, J., Zilla, P., and Franz, T. (2013). Outcomes of myocardial infarction hydrogel injection therapy in the human left ventricle dependent on injectate distribution. *Int. J. Numer. Methods Biomed. Eng.* 29, 870–884. doi: 10.1002/cnm.2551

Mojsejenko, D., McGarvey, J. R., Dorsey, S. M., Gorman, J. H. III., Burdick, J. A., Pilla, J. J., et al. (2015). Estimating passive mechanical properties in a myocardial infarction using MRI and finite element simulations. *Biomech. Model Mechanobiol.* 14, 633–647. doi: 10.1007/s10237-014-0627-z

Nagueh, S. F., Middleton, K. J., Kopelen, H. A., Zoghbi, W. A., and Quiñones, M. A. (1997). Doppler tissue imaging: a noninvasive technique for evaluation of left ventricular relaxation and estimation of filling pressures. *J. Am. Coll. Cardiol.* 30, 1527–1533. doi: 10.1016/S0735-1097(97)00344-6

Nielsen, P. M., Le Grice, I. J., Smaill, B. H., and Hunter, P. J. (1991). Mathematical model of geometry and fibrous structure of the heart. *Am. J. Physiol.* 260(4 Pt 2), H1365–H1378. doi: 10.1152/ajpheart.1991.260.4.H1365

Pedrizzetti, G., Sengupta, S., Caracciolo, G., Park, C. S., Amaki, M., Goliasch, G., et al. (2014). Three-dimensional principal strain analysis for characterizing subclinical changes in left ventricular function. *J. Am. Soc. Echocardiogr.* 27, 1041.e1–1050.e1. doi: 10.1016/j.echo.2014.05.014

Pfeffer, M. A., and Braunwald, E. (1990). Ventricular remodeling after myocardial infarction. Experimental observations and clinical implications. *Circulation* 81, 1161–1172. doi: 10.1161/01.CIR.81.4.1161

Pilla, J. J., Gorman, J. H. III., and Gorman, R. C. (2009). Theoretic Impact of Infarct Compliance on Left Ventricular Function. *Ann. Thorac. Surg.* 87, 803–810. doi: 10.1016/j.athoracsur.2008.11.044

Porter, D. A., and Heidemann, R. M. (2009). High resolution diffusion-weighted imaging using readout-segmented echo-planar imaging, parallel imaging and a two-dimensional navigator-based reacquisition. *Magn. Reson. Med.* 62, 468–475. doi: 10.1002/mrm.22024

Quinn, T. A., Berberian, G., Cabreriza, S. E., Maskin, L. J., Weinberg, A. D., Holmes, J. W., et al. (2006). Effects of sequential biventricular pacing during acute right ventricular pressure overload. *Am. J. Physiol. Heart Circ. Physiol.* 60, H2380–H2387. doi: 10.1152/ajpheart.00446.2006

Rausch, M. K., Genet, M., and Humphrey, J. D. (2017). An augmented iterative method for identifying a stress-free reference configuration in image-based biomechanical modeling. *J. Biomech.* 58, 227–231. doi: 10.1016/j.jbiomech.2017.04.021

Sack, K. L., Baillargeon, B., Acevedo-Bolton, G., Genet, M., Rebelo, N., Kuhl, E., et al. (2016b). Partial LVAD restores ventricular outputs and normalizes LV but not RV stress distributions in the acutely failing heart *in silico*. *Int. J. Artif. Organs* 39, 421–430. doi: 10.5301/ijao.5000520

Sack, K. L., Davies, N. H., Guccione, J. M., and Franz, T. (2016a). Personalised computational cardiology: patient-specific modelling in cardiac mechanics and biomaterial injection therapies for myocardial infarction. *Heart Fail. Rev.* 21, 815–826. doi: 10.1007/s10741-016-9528-9

Sack, K. L., Skatulla, S., and Sansour, C. (2016c). Biological tissue mechanics with fibres modelled as one-dimensional Cosserat continua. Applications to cardiac tissue. *Int. J. Solids Struct.* 81, 84–94. doi: 10.1016/j.ijsolstr.2015.11.009

Santamore, W. P., and Burkhoff, D. (1991). Hemodynamic consequences of ventricular interaction as assessed by model analysis. *Am. J. Physiol. Heart Circ. Physiol.* 260, H146–H157. doi: 10.1152/ajpheart.1991.260.1.H146

Scollan, D. F., Holmes, A., Winslow, R., and Forder, J. (1998). Histological validation of myocardial microstructure obtained from diffusion tensor magnetic resonance imaging. *Am. J. Physiol.* 275(6 Pt 2), H2308–H2318. doi: 10.1152/ajpheart.1998.275.6.H2308

Sengupta, P. P., Khandheria, B. K., Korinek, J., Wang, J., Jahangir, A., Seward, J. B., et al. (2006). Apex-to-base dispersion in regional timing of left ventricular shortening and lengthening. *J. Am. Coll. Cardiol.* 47, 163–172. doi: 10.1016/j.jacc.2005.08.073

Setarehdan, S. K., and Singh, S. (2012). *Advanced Algorithmic Approaches to Medical Image Segmentation: State-of-the-Art Applications in Cardiology, Neurology, Mammography and Pathology*. London: Springer Science & Business Media.

Sommer, G., Schriefl, A. J., Andrä, M., Sacherer, M., Viertler, C., Wolinski, H., et al. (2015). Biomechanical properties and microstructure of human ventricular myocardium. *Acta Biomater.* 24, 172–192. doi: 10.1016/j.actbio.2015. 06.031

Streeter, D. D., and Bassett, D. L. (1966). An engineering analysis of myocardial fiber orientation in pig's left ventricle in systole. *Anat. Rec.* 155, 503–511. doi: 10.1002/ar.1091550403

Streeter, D. D., Spotnitz, H. M., Patel, D. P., Ross, J., and Sonnenblick, E. H. (1969). Fiber orientation in the canine left ventricle during diastole and systole. *Circ. Res.* 24, 339–347. doi: 10.1161/01.RES.24.3.339

Sutton, M. G., and Sharpe, N. (2000). Left ventricular remodeling after myocardial infarction pathophysiology and therapy. *Circulation* 101, 2981–2988. doi: 10.1161/01.CIR.101.25.2981

Abaqus Theory Guide. (2014). Version 6.14. Providence, RI: Dassault Systèmes, Simulia Corp.

Toussaint, N., Stoeck, C. T., Schaeffter, T., Kozerke, S., Sermesant, M., and Batchelor, P. G. (2013). *In vivo* human cardiac fibre architecture estimation using shape-based diffusion tensor processing. *Med. Image Anal.* 17, 1243–1255. doi: 10.1016/j.media.2013.02.008

Vadakkumpadan, F., Arevalo, H., Prassl, A. J., Chen, J. J., Kickinger, F., Kohl, P., et al. (2010). Image-based models of cardiac structure in health and disease. *Wiley Interdiscip. Rev. Syst. Biol. Med.* 2, 489–506. doi: 10.1002/wsbm.76

van den Borne, S. W., Isobe, S., Verjans, J. W., Petrov, A., Lovhaug, D., Li, P., et al. (2008). Molecular imaging of interstitial alterations in remodeling myocardium after myocardial infarction. *J. Am. Coll. Cardiol.* 52, 2017–2028. doi: 10.1016/j.jacc.2008.07.067

Walker, J. C., Ratcliffe, M. B., Zhang, P., Wallace, A. W., Fata, B., Hsu, E. W., et al. (2005). MRI-based finite-element analysis of left ventricular aneurysm. *Am. J. Physiol. Heart Circ. Physiol.* 289, H692–H700. doi: 10.1152/ajpheart.01226.2004

Wang, H. M., Gao, H., Luo, X. Y., Berry, C., Griffith, B. E., Ogden, R. W., et al. (2013). Structure-based finite strain modelling of the human left ventricle in diastole. *Int. J. numer. method. biomed. eng.* 29, 83–103. doi: 10.1002/cnm.2497

Watanabe, H., Sugiura, S., Kafuku, H., and Hisada, T. (2004). Multiphysics simulation of left ventricular filling dynamics using fluid-structure interaction finite element method. *Biophys. J.* 87, 2074–2085. doi: 10.1529/biophysj.103.035840

Wenk, J. F., Ge, L., Zhang, Z., Soleimani, M., Potter, D. D., Wallace, A. W., et al. (2012a). A coupled biventricular finite element and lumped-parameter circulatory system model of heart failure. *Comput. Methods Biomech. Biomed. Engin.* 16, 807–818. doi: 10.1080/10255842.2011.641121

Wenk, J. F., Klepach, D., Lee, L. C., Zhang, Z. H., Ge, L., Tseng, E. E., et al. (2012b). First evidence of depressed contractility in the border zone of a human myocardial infarction. *Ann. Thorac. Surg.* 93, 1188–1194. doi: 10.1016/j.athoracsur.2011.12.066

Wenk, J. F., Sun, K., Zhang, Z., Soleimani, M., Ge, L., Saloner, D., et al. (2011). Regional left ventricular myocardial contractility and stress in a finite element model of posterobasal myocardial infarction. *J. Biomech. Eng.* 133:044501. doi: 10.1115/1.4003438

Wu, E. X., Wu, Y., Nicholls, J. M., Wang, J., Liao, S., Zhu, S., et al. (2007). MR diffusion tensor imaging study of postinfarct myocardium structural remodeling in a porcine model. *Magn. Reson. Med.* 58, 687–695. doi: 10.1002/mrm.21350

Wu, Y., Chan, C. W., Nicholls, J. M., Liao, S., Tse, H. F., and Wu, E. X. (2009). MR study of the effect of infarct size and location on left ventricular functional and microstructural alterations in porcine models. *J. Magn. Reson. Imaging* 29, 305–312. doi: 10.1002/jmri.21598

Zhang, X., Haynes, P., Campbell, K. S., and Wenk, J. F. (2015). Numerical evaluation of myofiber orientation and transmural contractile strength on left ventricular function. *J. Biomech. Eng.* 137:044502. doi: 10.1115/1.4028990

Zhang, Z., Tendulkar, A., Sun, K., Saloner, D. A., Wallace, A. W., Ge, L., et al. (2011). Comparison of the Young-Laplace law and finite element based calculation of ventricular wall stress: implications for postinfarct and surgical ventricular remodeling. *Ann. Thorac. Surg.* 91, 150–156. doi: 10.1016/j.athoracsur.2010.06.132

# 14

# Relationship of Transmural Variations in Myofiber Contractility to Left Ventricular Ejection Fraction: Implications for Modeling Heart Failure Phenotype with Preserved Ejection Fraction

*Yaghoub Dabiri[1], Kevin L. Sack[1], Semion Shaul[1], Partho P. Sengupta[2] and Julius M. Guccione[1*]*

[1] Department of Surgery, University of California, San Francisco, San Francisco, CA, United States, [2] Section of Cardiology, West Virginia University Heart and Vascular Institute, West Virginia University, Morgantown, WV, United States

**\*Correspondence:**
*Julius M. Guccione*
*julius.guccione@ucsf.edu*

The pathophysiological mechanisms underlying preserved left ventricular (LV) ejection fraction (EF) in patients with heart failure and preserved ejection fraction (HFpEF) remain incompletely understood. We hypothesized that transmural variations in myofiber contractility with existence of subendocardial dysfunction and compensatory increased subepicardial contractility may underlie preservation of LVEF in patients with HFpEF. We quantified alterations in myocardial function in a mathematical model of the human LV that is based on the finite element method. The fiber-reinforced material formulation of the myocardium included passive and active properties. The passive material properties were determined such that the diastolic pressure-volume behavior of the LV was similar to that shown in published clinical studies of pressure-volume curves. To examine changes in active properties, we considered six scenarios: (1) normal properties throughout the LV wall; (2) decreased myocardial contractility in the subendocardium; (3) increased myocardial contractility in the subepicardium; (4) myocardial contractility decreased equally in all layers, (5) myocardial contractility decreased in the midmyocardium and subepicardium, (6) myocardial contractility decreased in the subepicardium. Our results indicate that decreased subendocardial contractility reduced LVEF from 53.2 to 40.5%. Increased contractility in the subepicardium recovered LVEF from 40.5 to 53.2%. Decreased contractility transmurally reduced LVEF and could not be recovered if subepicardial and midmyocardial contractility remained depressed. The computational results simulating the effects of transmural alterations in the ventricular tissue replicate the phenotypic patterns of LV dysfunction observed in clinical practice. In particular, data for LVEF, strain and displacement are consistent with previous clinical observations in patients with HFpEF, and substantiate the hypothesis that increased subepicardial contractility may compensate for subendocardial dysfunction and play a vital role in maintaining LVEF.

Keywords: heart failure and preserved ejection fraction, left ventricle, myocardial contractility, finite element method, simulation

## INTRODUCTION

Heart Failure (HF) is the only cardiovascular disease for which incidence, prevalence, morbidity, mortality, and costs are not decreasing. According to the 2017 Update (Benjamin et al., 2017), the prevalence of HF has increased from 5.7 million (2009 to 2012) to 6.5 million (2011 to 2014) in Americans >20 years of age and projections show prevalence will increase 46% by 2030, resulting in over 8 million adults with HF (Heidenreich et al., 2013). In 2012, the total cost for HF was estimated to be $31 billion and projections show that by 2030, the total cost will increase to $70 billion or roughly ~$244 for every US adult (Heidenreich et al., 2013). Among patients hospitalized for an HF incident, 47% had HF with preserved ejection fraction (HFpEF) or systolic function, which is the focus of this paper.

The mechanism of the development of HFpEF is not well-understood (Aurigemma and Gaasch, 2004; Shah and Solomon, 2012; Steinberg et al., 2012; Sengupta and Marwick, 2018), and optimal treatment options remain unclear (Vasan et al., 1995; Bhuiyan and Maurer, 2011). Recent studies have suggested that HFpEF is associated with transmural changes in myocardial deformation (Shah and Solomon, 2012; Omar et al., 2016, 2017). Understanding the transmural variations in left ventricular (LV) mechanics associated with HFpEF may offer pathophysiological insights for developing potential therapeutic targets. We therefore explored a physics-based mathematical [finite element (FE)] model of the normal human LV to test the hypothesis that reduced subendocardial contractility combined with compensatory high subepicardial contractility may help in preserving LVEF independent of changes in myocardial geometry and material properties. We used our established computational framework in this paper. To the best of our knowledge, this is the first study that quantifies the development of HFpEF based on transmural variation in contractility, using patient-specific parameters.

## METHODS
### Patient Data
*In vivo* echocardiographic recordings were obtained under a protocol approved by our institutional review board. Individual patients provided informed consent and anonymized data were sent to a core laboratory for analysis.

### Geometry Considerations
The ventricle model pertains to a normal human subject. The LV was modeled as a truncated thick-walled ellipsoid (Mercier et al., 1982; LeGrice et al., 2001). Based on echocardiography recordings for end diastolic volume (EDV), LV diameter and wall thicknesses for the posterior and septal wall, we back-calculated ellipsoidal surfaces for the endocardium and epicardium at end diastole (ED).

Using a linearly regressed estimation of the unloaded LV cavity volume V0 (Klotz et al., 2006) we scaled the dimensions of the endocardium surface to match the calculated volume V0. The epicardium dimensions were then scaled to maintain the

same myocardial wall volume ascertained at the ED configuration (preservation of mass).

TruGrid (XYZ Scientific Applications Inc, Pleasant Hill, California, USA) was used to mesh LV surfaces. The ventricle was meshed to produce eight layers through the radial direction (**Figure 1**). Finite element calculations were performed in ABAQUS (SIMULIA, Providence, RI, USA). The FE meshes are shown in **Figure 1**.

We used a rule-based approach coded in MATLAB 2012b (The MathWorks, Inc., Natick, Massachusetts, United States) to assign myofiber orientations to the centroid of each element in the meshed LV geometry. The aggregated myofiber orientation was assumed to present with an angle of $-60°$ from the local circumferential direction on the epicardium surface that varies linearly through the LV wall thickness to an angle of $+60°$ on the endocardial surface. This assumption is well-established in LV modeling studies (Carrick et al., 2012; Lee et al., 2013, 2015; Genet et al., 2014), and based on histological studies (Streeter et al., 1969), and diffusion tensor MRI studies (Lombaert et al., 2011).

## Constitutive Equation and Material Parameters
The material formulation of the LV tissue includes passive and active properties. The passive behavior of the tissue was described using the model introduced by Holzapfel and Ogden (Holzapfel and Ogden, 2009; Göktepe et al., 2011). Briefly, the strain energy function used to compute passive stresses is composed of

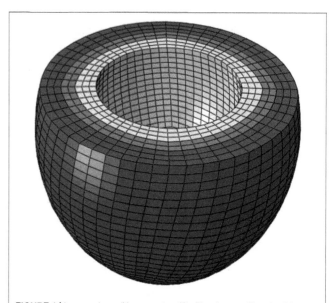

**FIGURE 1 |** In normal conditions, contractility ($T_{max}$) was uniform in all layers (scenario 1). To simulate no contraction in the subendocardial region, contractility in three layers in white was set to zero (scenario 2). The three layers in red were used to simulate alterations in subepicardial contractility (scenario 3). The three white layers, the two green layers, and the three red layers comprise subendocardial, midmyocardial, and subepicardial regions, respectively.

deviatoric ($\Psi_{dev}$) and volumetric ($\Psi_{vol}$) parts as follows:

$$\Psi_{dev} = \frac{a}{2b}e^{b(l_1-3)} + \sum_{i=f,s} \frac{a_i}{2b_i}\left\{ e^{b_i(l_{4i}-1)^2} - 1 \right\}$$
$$+ \frac{a_{fs}}{2b_{fs}}\left\{ e^{b_{fs}(l_{8fs})^2} - 1 \right\} \tag{1}$$

$$\Psi_{vol} = \frac{1}{D}\left(\frac{J^2-1}{2} - \ln(J)\right)$$

where $a$ and $b$ represent isotropic stiffness of the tissue, $a_f$ and $b_f$ represent tissue stiffness in the fiber direction, and $a_{fs}$ and $b_{fs}$ represent the stiffness resultant from connection between fiber and sheet directions; $l_1$, $l_{4i}$, and $l_{8fs}$ are invariants, defined as follows:

$$l_1 := tr(\boldsymbol{C})$$
$$l_{4i} := \boldsymbol{C}:(\boldsymbol{f}_0 \otimes \boldsymbol{f}_0)$$
$$l_{8fs} := \boldsymbol{C}:sym(\boldsymbol{f}_0 \otimes \boldsymbol{s}_0)$$

where $\boldsymbol{C}$ is the right Cauchy-Green tensor, and $\boldsymbol{f}_0$ and $\boldsymbol{s}_0$ are vectors specifying the fiber and sheet directions, respectively. $J$ is the deformation gradient invariant, and $D$ is a multiple of the Bulk Modulus $K$ (i.e., $D = 2/K$).

The material constants $a$, $a_i$, and $a_{fs}$ scale the strain-stress curve, whereas material constants $b$, $b_i$, and $b_{fs}$ determine the shape of the strain-stress curve. To determine these parameters we used the End Diastolic Pressure Volume (ED PV) curve as described by Klotz et al. who reported an analytical expression for the ED PV curve based on a single PV point that is applicable for multiple species, including humans (Klotz et al., 2006). The LV EDV of 53 ml was recorded using echocardiography and the LV EDP of 14.3 mmHg was approximated from echocardiography data using Nagueh's formula (Nagueh et al., 1997).

The optimized material properties were found using an in-house Python script that minimized the error between the ED PV curve from the FE model and the analytical expression (Klotz et al., 2006). The sequential least squares (SLSQP) algorithm (Jones et al., 2001) was used in the Python script, and ABAQUS was used for the FE modeling, as the forward solver (**Table 1** and **Figure 2**).

The formulation for the active stress has been described extensively in the literature (Guccione and McCulloch, 1993; Walker et al., 2005; Genet et al., 2014; Sack et al., 2016). In short, the active stress in the myofiber direction was calculated as:

$$T_0 = T_{max}\frac{Ca_0^2}{Ca_0^2 + ECa_{50}^2}C_t \tag{2}$$

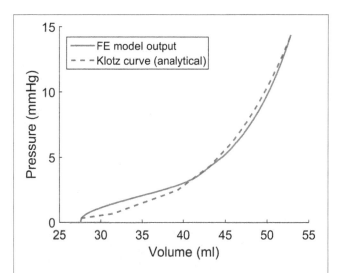

**FIGURE 2** | The passive material properties were determined such that the end diastolic pressure volume (ED PV) curve from finite element model was close to the experimental ED PV curve determined by Klotz et al. (2006).

where $T_{max}$ is the isometric tension at the largest sarcomere length and highest calcium concentration, $Ca_0$ is the peak intracellular calcium concentration, and

$$C_t = \frac{1}{2}(1 - cos\omega),$$

$$\omega = \begin{cases} \pi\frac{t}{t_0} & when\ 0 \leq t \leq t_0 \\ \pi\frac{t-t_0+t_r}{t_r} & when\ t_0 \leq t \leq t_0 + t_r' \\ 0 & when\ t \geq t_0 + t_r \end{cases}$$

$$t_r = ml + b$$

$m$, $b$ = constants that govern the shape of the linear relaxation duration and sarcomere length relaxation.

Also,

$$ECa_{50} = \frac{(Ca_0)_{max}}{\sqrt{\exp\left[B\left(l-l_0\right)\right] - 1}}, l = l_R\sqrt{2E_{ff} + 1}$$

where $E_{ff}$ is the Lagrangian strain in the fiber direction, $B$ is a constant that governs the shape of the peak isometric tension-sarcomere length relation, $l_0$ is the sarcomere length that does not produce active stress, $l_R$ is the sarcomere length with the stress-free condition, and $(Ca_0)_{max}$ is the maximum peak intracellular calcium concentration.

The active stress was added to the passive stress to compute total stress:

$$S = S_{Passive} + T \tag{3}$$

where $S$ is the total stress.

The boundary and load conditions generally follow the ABAQUS Living Heart Model (Baillargeon et al., 2014,

---

**TABLE 1** | Passive material properties that produced a pressure-volume curve close to the experimental pressure-volume curve (**Figure 2**).

| $a$ (MPa) | $b$ | $a_f$ (MPa) | $b_f$ | $a_s$ (MPa) | $b_s$ | $a_{fs}$ (MPa) | $b_{fs}$ |
|---|---|---|---|---|---|---|---|
| $6.832e^{-4}$ | 7.541 | $2.252e^{-3}$ | 14.471 | $3.127e^{-4}$ | 12.548 | $1.837e^{-4}$ | 3.088 |

166 Cardiovascular Systems: Mathematical and Numerical Modeling

2015; Sack et al., 2016). In particular, the center of the LV proximal cross-section (base) was fixed. The average rotation and translation of nodes of the endocardial annulus were coupled to the center of the LV base. This boundary condition prevents rigid body rotation, but allows inflations and contractions of the annulus. The nodes of the base were fixed in the longitudinal direction. A pressure load was applied to the LV surface to simulate diastole, whereas the contraction of the LV muscles caused systole. Surface-based fluid cavities and fluid exchanges were used to model blood flow (ABAQUS Analysis User's Guide).

When $T_{max}$ is changed in Equation (2), the total contractile force of the tissue is altered, and other parameters related to the passive and active material formulations (Equations 1, 2) either do not change or change in a consistent way. We can prescribe different values of $T_{max}$ in transmural layers to introduce regionally varying contractility throughout the LV. We considered six scenarios with different contractile properties, as explained in **Table 2**. Homogenous contractile properties were considered in scenario 1, which also served to establish a baseline value for normal $T_{max}$. $T_{max}$ was calibrated to produce the echocardiogram-recorded value for end- systolic volume (ESV) for this patient (24.8 ml). To simulate the diseased condition, subendocardial contractility was set to zero by setting $T_{max} = 0$ (scenario 2). To recover ESV, a scenario was considered in which $T_{max}$ was increased in the subepicardial layers (scenario 3). To further assess the effects of transmural contractility, three more scenarios with different contractility in the transmural layers were created. In scenario 4, $T_{max}$ in all regions was reduced by 50%. In scenario 5, $T_{max}$ was set to zero in subepicardial and midmyocardial regions. In scenario 6, $T_{max}$ was set to zero in the subepicardial region.

To calculate LV torsion, we use the following formula (Aelen et al., 1997; Rüssel et al., 2009).

$$\tau = \frac{(\emptyset_{apex} - \emptyset_{base}) \times (\rho_{apex} + \rho_{base})}{2D} \quad (4)$$

Where $\tau$ is normalized LV torsion; $\emptyset_{apex}$ and $\emptyset_{base}$ are rotations in the apex and base, respectively; $\rho_{apex}$ and $\rho_{base}$ are the radius of the apex and base, respectively; and $D$ is the distance between the apex and base (**Figure 3**).

## RESULTS

The EF decreased from 53.2 to 40.5% when $T_{max}$ was set to zero in the subendocardial layers (**Table 2** and **Figure 4**: scenario 2 vs. 1: 23.9% reduction in EF). The depressed contractility in the subendocardial region was enough to drop EF below 50%, producing HF with reduced EF (HFrEF). The EF normalized

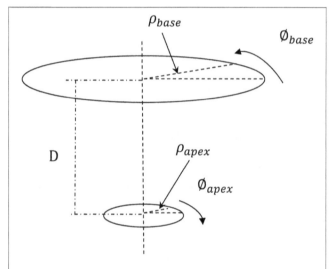

**FIGURE 3 |** The torsion of the LV was computed based on the apical and basal rotations, the apical and basal radius, and the distance between the apex and base. The formula used to compute the LV torsion (Equation 4) makes the LV torsion comparable for hearts of different sizes (Aelen et al., 1997; Rüssel et al., 2009). The positive rotation is counterclockwise when seen from apex.

**TABLE 2 |** Six scenarios were created to examine effects of contractility ($T_{max}$) on EF.

| Scenario | $T_{max}$ (MPa) | | | EF (%) | ESV (ml) | ESP (mmHg) | Torsion (degrees) | Strain (%) | | |
|---|---|---|---|---|---|---|---|---|---|---|
| | Three inner layers (subendocardium) | Two middle layers (midmyocardium) | Three outer layers (subepicardium) | | | | | $E_l$ | $E_c$ | $E_r$ |
| 1 | 0.086 | 0.086 | 0.086 | 53.2 | 24.7 | 88.9 | 24.7 | −8.5 | −29.7 | 44 |
| 2 | 0.0 | 0.086 | 0.086 | 40.5 | 31.4 | 94.5 | 26.7 | −4.5 | −15.8 | 25.3 |
| 3 | 0.0 | 0.086 | 0.117 | 53.2 | 24.7 | 92.8 | 30.2 | −6.1 | −28.1 | 39.9 |
| 4 | 0.043 | 0.043 | 0.043 | 13.3 | 45.8 | 82.6 | 18.6 | −5.7 | −0.6 | 12.9 |
| 5 | 0.086 | 0.0 | 0.0 | 0.3 | 52.6 | 63.2 | −7.6 | −7.6 | 2.7 | 4.9 |
| 6 | 0.086 | 0.086 | 0.0 | 12.7 | 46.0 | 80.1 | −13.0 | −5 | −4.4 | 7.15 |

*Scenario 1 represents the normal condition; scenario 2 represents zero subendocardial contractility; scenario 3 represents zero subendocardial contractility and increased subepicardial contractility (an HFpEF condition); scenario 4 represents decreased contractility in all regions; scenario 5 represents zero midmyocardial and subepicardial contractility, and scenario 6 represents zero subepicardial contractility. For scenario 1, the computational EF matched the experimental EF. For all scenarios, EDV = 53 ml, EDP = 14.3 mmHg. El, Ec, and Er are, respectively, ES strain in longitudinal, circumferential and radial directions. The circumferential and radial strains were computed using the nodes located at the endocardial annulus (base of the LV).*

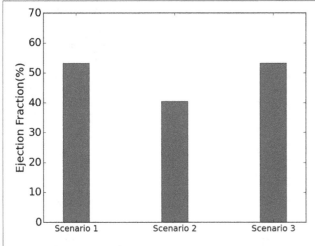

FIGURE 4 | When the subendocardial contractility was zero, EF reduced by 23.9% relative to scenario 1 (scenarios 1 and 2). Increased subepicardial contractility recovered EF to scenario 1 (scenarios 1 and 3).

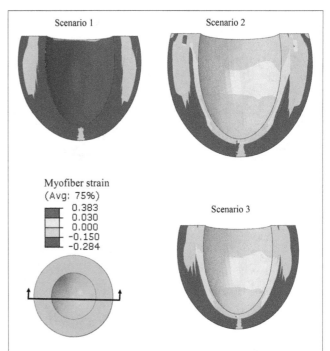

FIGURE 5 | A long-axis view showing that at end systole, with uniform $T_{max}$ (scenario 1), all layers experienced compressive strain in myofiber directions. When subendocardial contractility was zero, the strain pattern was altered (scenarios 1 and 2), but it partially recovered when subepicardial contractility increased (scenarios 1 and 3).

when $T_{max}$ was increased in the subepicardial layers (**Table 2** and **Figure 4**: scenario 3 vs. 1). This increased subepicardial contractility was enough to recover EF from the failing value of 40.5% and reach 53.2% (vs. 53.2% in the normal scenario). End-systolic pressure (ESP) and ESV increased when subendocardial contractility was zero. After subepicardial contractility increased, ESV and ESP decreased (**Table 2**, scenario 3 vs. 1 and 2).

The EF decreased by 75% when contractility decreased by 50% in all layers (**Table 2**: scenario 4 vs. 1). When subepicardial and midmyocardial contractility was zero, EF became almost zero (0.3% in scenario 5, **Table 2**). Similarly, when subepicardial contractility was zero, EF decreased dramatically compared to the normal scenario (12.7% in scenario 6 vs. 53.2% in scenario 1, **Table 2**). ESV noticeably increased and ESP decreased in scenarios 4, 5, and 6 vs. scenario 1.

When subendocardial contractility was zero, LV torsion increased (scenario 2 vs. 1). The torsion further increased after contractility in a remaining region was increased to compensate (scenario 3 vs. 1 and 2). The torsion decreased when contractility in all transmural regions decreased by 50% (scenario 4 vs. 1). The torsion reversed when midmyocardial and subepicardial contractility were decreased to zero (scenario 5 vs. 1). The reversed torsion increased when only subepicardial contractility was zero (scenario 6 vs. 5).

Strains (which are independent of displacement boundary conditions) were altered in diseased conditions. The global longitudinal, circumferential, and radial strains decreased in HFpEF, but recovered after subepicardial contractility increased (**Table 2**, scenarios 2 and 3 vs. scenario 1). In addition, the global strains decreased when contractility decreased by half in all layers, and when subepicardial and midmyocardial contractility were zero, and also when subepicardial contractility was zero (**Table 2**, scenarios 4, 5, and 6 vs. scenario 1). The direction of circumferential strain changed when midmyocardial and subepicardial contractility were both zero (Scenario 5 vs. 1, **Table 2**). With normal homogenous contractility (scenario 1),

all layers experienced contractile strains (**Figures 5–7**). Regional changes in contractility to simulate HFrEF (scenario 2) and HFpEF (scenario 3) both presented with tensile strains in the subendocardial regions where contractility was set to zero (**Figures 5–7**). However, the increased subepicardial contractility in HFpEF had a global effect on strains throughout all layers, reducing the strains in all regions. Qualitatively, the transmural strain curve of the HFpEF case (scenario 3) replicated the pathological HFrEF curve (scenario 2), albeit with strains that were 23.8% lower on average.

ES stress in the myofiber direction was noticeably reduced when subendocardial contractility decreased (scenarios 1 and 2, **Figure 8**). A trend to recovery in the stress distribution was observed when subepicardial contractility increased (scenarios 1 and 3, **Figure 8**).

The ES-shortening longitudinal displacement of the LV was profoundly decreased when subendocardial contractility was zero (scenarios 1 and 2, **Figure 9**). The longitudinal displacement was partially recovered when subepicardial contractility increased (scenarios 1 and 3, **Figure 9**).

The ES sphericity index (defined as the ratio between the lengths of the LV long axis and the short axis) was approximated as 1.1, 1.0, and 1.1 for scenarios 1, 2, and 3, respectively. In the HFrEF case (scenario 2), the ES sphericity index decreased compared to scenario 1. However, the ES sphericity index in the HFpEF scenario normalized toward the normal scenario. In other words, when the subendocardial contractility was zero, the LV shape became more spherical, compared to scenario 1. The

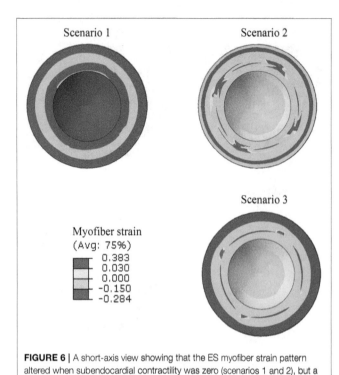

**FIGURE 6 |** A short-axis view showing that the ES myofiber strain pattern altered when subendocardial contractility was zero (scenarios 1 and 2), but a partial recovery in strain pattern was observed when subepicardial contractility increased (scenarios 1 and 3).

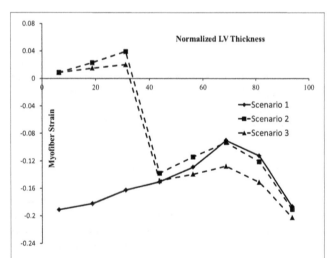

**FIGURE 7 |** The ES myofiber strain at various points along LV thickness. In the horizontal axis, 0% represents the endocardium and 100% represents the epicardium. The alterations in strains in scenario 2 are noticeable, compared to scenario 1. In scenario 3, the tensile strains decreased compared to scenario 2.

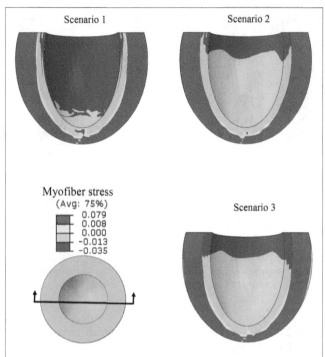

**FIGURE 8 |** A long-axis view showing the ES myofiber compressive stress decreased when the subendocardial contractility was zero (scenarios 1 and 2). The stress pattern became partially similar to the normal case when subepicardial contractility increased (scenarios 1 and 3).

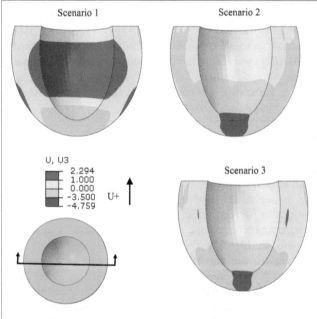

**FIGURE 9 |** The ES longitudinal deformation was altered when subendocardial contractility was zero (scenarios 1 and 2). Deformation partially recovered when subepicardial contractility increased (scenarios 1 and 3).

shape of the LV recovered toward the normal scenario when subepicardial contractility increased.

## DISCUSSION

In this study, we used a realistic FE model of the human LV to examine the role of altered LV systolic mechanics as a mechanism

of HFpEF. Our findings support the hypothesis that HFpEF could be a result of lower subendocardial contractility linked with increased subepicardial contractility (Sengupta and Narula,

2008; Shah and Solomon, 2012; Omar et al., 2016, 2017). When subendocardial contractility was zero, LVEF decreased by 23.9% (**Table 2**: 53.2% in scenario 1 vs. 40.5% in scenario 2). The EF normalized when subepicardial contractility increased (**Table 2**: 53.2% in scenario 3 vs. 53.2% in scenario 1). The change in subepicardial contractility (less than a 40% increase from normal values) resulted in a 31.4% improvement in EF. Unlike scenario 1, scenarios 2 and 3 experienced abnormal strains within the subendocardial region (**Figures 5–7**), even though scenario 3 experienced normal EF. The ES sphericity index decreased in scenario 2 (1.0) compared to scenario 1 (1.1), but it recovered in scenario 3 (1.1). The LV torsion increased in scenario 2 (26.7°) compared to scenario 1 (24.7°), and it further increased in scenario 3 (30.2°).

The subendocardial region played an important role in the LV systolic mechanics, as our results showed. In particular, when subendocardial contractility was zero, the EF was reduced below 50%. A scenario with EF below 50% and zero subendocardial contractility corresponds to HFrEF (Vasan et al., 1999; Owan and Redfield, 2005; Yancy et al., 2013). Also, reducing EF below 50% by zeroing subendocardial contractility is in line with previous studies that reported the important role of the subendocardial region in the mechanics of the LV (Sabbah et al., 1981; Algranati et al., 2011). Based on our adopted definition of end-systolic elastance ($E_{ES}$) (Chen et al., 2001), our results imply that $E_{ES}$ decreased after subendocardial contractility was zero, but $E_{ES}$ recovered when subepicardial contractility increased (**Table 2**, scenarios 2 and 3 vs. scenario 1). Increased ESP in HFpEF could be due to alterations in the ejection period of the LV (scenario 2). After subendocardial contractility was lost, the ejection period shortened and ended with a higher pressure.

The EF decreased by 75% when contractility decreased by 50% in all layers (scenario 4 vs. scenario 1, **Table 2**). On the other hand, setting subepicardial and midmyocardial contractility to zero affected EF more than subendocardial contractility (0.3% in scenario 5 and 12.7% in scenario 6 vs. 40.5% in scenario 2, **Table 2**). This result illustrates the important role of subepicardial and midmyocardial regions and confirms previous experimental (Haynes et al., 2014) and computational (Wang et al., 2016) studies that indicated the important roles of the epicardium and midmyocardium in systolic mechanics of the LV. Also, based on our adopted definition of $E_{ES}$, this parameter decreased when contractility decreased in all layers by 50%, and when subepicardial and midmyocardial contractility were zero, and also when subepicardial contractility was set to zero (**Table 2**, scenarios 4, 5, and 6 vs. scenario 1).

Quantifying changes in torsional deformation related to changes in transmural contractility revealed an interesting relationship between the two. Abnormally high torsion could be a useful index of pathology, as we showed when subendocardial contractility was lost (**Table 2**, scenarios 2 and 3 vs. 1). This result confirms previous reports according to which the LV torsion increases in subendocardial ischemia (Prinzen et al., 1984), which has been related to the counter torque applied by the subendocardial region against the subepicardial region (Aelen et al., 1997). Also, this counter torque effect between subendocardium and subepicarium can be seen in scenarios

5 and 6 (**Table 2**). In these scenarios a negative torsion was seen after midmyocardium and subepicardium contractility was set to zero. The torsion of the LV is strongly coupled to the LV contractility and the inability to complete ejection properly (**Table 2**).

The longitudinal strain has been reported as a criterion to diagnose normal and diseased hearts (Henein and Gibson, 1999; Takeda et al., 2001; Yu et al., 2002; Vinereanu et al., 2005). The decreased longitudinal strain in our results (**Table 2**) corresponds to clinical studies that reported longitudinal strains decrease in HFpEF (Mizuguchi et al., 2010). Also, the contour of ES longitudinal displacement, which is directly related to longitudinal strain, was noticeably altered in the diseased scenario compared to the normal scenario (**Figure 9**, scenarios 1 and 2). However, when subepicardial contractility increased, the pattern of longitudinal displacement became more similar to the normal scenario (**Figure 9**, scenarios 1 and 3). The ES strain pattern across the regional layers of the LV wall (**Figure 7**) also supported the hypothesis that increased subepicardial contractility in HFpEF improves function globally (Sengupta and Narula, 2008). Moreover, the alterations in circumferential and radial strains are in line with clinical studies that reported these strains decrease in HFpEF (Wang et al., 2008; Mizuguchi et al., 2010). Yet, our results should be interpreted with caution. The circumferential and radial strains for normal conditions (scenario 1) were in line with clinical data reported in the literature, whereas the longitudinal strain was smaller than reported clinical data (Moore et al., 2000; Yingchoncharoen et al., 2013). The methodology of our study is similar to previous computational models of LV in our group. The longitudinal strain results of these previous models have been validated against experimental strain data (for example, Genet et al., 2014).

It has been well-documented that the shape of the LV changes in HF (Grossman et al., 1975; Carabello, 1995; Gaasch and Zile, 2011). In particular, LV concentric hypertrophy is seen in patients with HFpEF (Melenovsky et al., 2007), and exercise capacity is correlated with the sphericity index of the LV (Tischler et al., 1993). In line with previous studies, in our simulations, the shape of the LV was altered when the subendocardial contractility was zero. The ES sphericity index decreased in scenario 2 (1.0) compared to scenario 1 (1.1). When subepicardial contractility increased, the shape of the LV recovered toward the normal case, as seen in the ES sphericity index in scenario 3 (1.1) compared to scenario 2 (1.0). Thus, the increased subepicardial contractility may prevent LV dilatation in HFpEF, and help preserve the LV shape. This phenomenon will further support the normalization of LVEF due to the direct interplay between the LV shape and function (Grossman et al., 1975; Stokke et al., 2017).

In this study we used tissue-level load-independent properties ($T_{max}$) to alter myocardium contractility. This approach is more appropriate than using the LV strains. In fact, the popular notion of equating myocardial contractility with strain measurements (that are load dependent) is "off the mark [and] if contractility means anything, it is as an expression of the ability of a given piece of myocardium to generate tension and shortening under any loading conditions" (Reichek, 2013). Therefore, our approach to alter transmural contractility, which might not be feasible using current experimental methods, could lead to a better understanding of the development of HFpEF.

Novel physics-based mathematical modeling was used in this study to examine a possible mechanism underlying preservation of LVEF in HFpEF. The results from the simulations provide evidence of the potential role of myocardial contractility in the genesis of preserved EF in the HFpEF phenotype. Previous studies on HFpEF were mostly based on experimental data (for example, Phan et al., 2009), where the contribution of a single feature like myocardial contractility could not be varied in isolation of other parameters. However, we used FE modeling to simulate and isolate transmural contractility as a feature and study its effect on LV systolic mechanics. Our results provide important first steps toward eventual development of a computational model of HFpEF.

## Study Limitations and Future Directions

The simulation addressed only the relationship between transmural myocardial contractility and LV systolic mechanics. Modeling all aspects of HFpEF was beyond the scope of this paper. In clinical conditions, several factors contribute to the development of HFpEF (Bench et al., 2009; Shah and Solomon, 2012; Sengupta and Marwick, 2018). These factors include abnormalities in both the systolic and the diastolic mechanics of the LV (MacIver and Townsend, 2008; MacIver, 2009; Shah and Solomon, 2012), the LV hypertrophy and geometric changes (Aurigemma et al., 1995; Vasan et al., 1999; Adeniran et al., 2015) and material properties of the LV (stiffness). A recent study employed computational models with heterogeneous transmural distributions of $T_{max}$ (Wang et al., 2016). In our investigation, only in one scenario (scenario 1) did we assume $T_{max}$ to be uniform in the transmural direction. Also, since this study focused on the LV, we assumed timing and activation of contractility are homogenous. A more realistic assumption would be to consider the sequence of electrical stimulations in the tissue (Chabiniok et al., 2012; Villongco et al., 2014; Crozier et al., 2016; Giffard-Roisin et al., 2017), particularly in the septum. However, a heterogeneous distribution of $T_{max}$ would be more important if atria were also included in the model. Moreover, we only modeled LV data from one human subject in our study. Modeling data from multiple subjects is the goal of a subsequent study. Here, our intent was to document our modeling methodology and demonstrate its utility.

Alterations in strain distributions might lead to remodeling in the LV tissue (**Figures 5–7**). The response of myocardial tissue to an altered mechanical environment will likely lead to changes in tissue properties that will in turn affect the LV inflation, contraction, and relaxation. It is well-documented that diastolic LV tissue stiffness becomes abnormally high in HFpEF (Zile et al., 2004). Our study focused on the systolic mechanics of the LV. As a future direction, integration of tissue response in diastole and systole will provide a more realistic and informative model to understand the mechanisms involved during the onset and development of HFpEF. Integration of cell-based cross-bridge cycling and contractility could provide more realistic information about the tissue alterations over the course of HFpEF development (Adeniran et al., 2015; Shavik et al., 2017).

Although our study explored a simplified representation of HFpEF (appropriately so, to isolate mechanical effects), the clinical definition and diagnosis of HFpEF and HFrEF are more complex than just calculations of EF (Borlaug and Paulus, 2011). In fact, HFpEF lacks a clear validated diagnostic guideline (Lam, 2010; Oghlakian et al., 2011). In this hypothesis-generating study, we simply assumed EF < 50% represents HFrEF. This assumption is in line with some definitions used for HFrEF in the literature (Vasan et al., 1999; Paulus et al., 2007). However, an EF = 40.5% (scenario 2) might also be defined as borderline HFpEF (for example, Yancy et al., 2013). These points may be considered semantic because they do not affect the conclusions of our study, which quantified alterations in contractility with changes in EF, torsion and strain. It would be interesting to apply these methods to personalized models derived from patients diagnosed clinically with HFpEF and HFrEF.

Several other scenarios need to be investigated, including more graded loss of subendocardial contractility, and graded decrease of subendocardial contractility, with both coupled to a graded increase in subepicardial contractility. Moreover, the definitions of subendocardium, midmyocardium, and subepicardium regions were arbitrary in this study because exact definitions are not available. A more realistic imaging approach might better delineate transmural layers and their related contractility. Furthermore, exercise intolerance has been reported as a key factor in HFpEF (Roh et al., 2017), and could be implemented in our modeling methodology to better understand the mechanisms of HFpEF development. Despite these limitations, this paper reports instructive quantitative information about development of HFpEF, as we could change one aspect of the model (contractility at a particular location) and determine its effects alone.

## CONCLUSIONS

The results of this study support the hypothesis that preservation of LVEF in patients with HFpEF could be explained on the basis of reduced subendocardial contractility with a compensatory increase in subepicardial contractility. These findings underscore the roles of regional LV myocardial contractility in HF syndromes and emphasize the importance of computational models in understanding pathophysiological mechanisms underlying complex phenotypic presentations like HFpEF.

## AUTHOR CONTRIBUTIONS

PS and JG designed the study. KS developed the constitutive model. YD and KS created the computational models. YD ran simulations, compiled results, and wrote the initial draft of the paper. SS helped with the modeling process. YD, KS, JG, and PS contributed to analysis of the results, and manuscript writing.

## ACKNOWLEDGMENTS

We thank Pamela Derish in the Department of Surgery, University of California San Francisco, for assistance with proofreading the manuscript.

# REFERENCES

Adeniran, I., MacIver, D. H., Hancox, J. C., and Zhang, H. (2015). Abnormal calcium homeostasis in heart failure with preserved ejection fraction is related to both reduced contractile function and incomplete relaxation: an electromechanically detailed biophysical modeling study. *Front. Physiol.* 6:78. doi: 10.3389/fphys.2015.00078

Aelen, F. W., Arts, T., Sanders, D. G., Thelissen, G. R., Muijtjens, A. M., Prinzen, F. W., et al. (1997). Relation between torsion and cross-sectional area change in the human left ventricle. *J. Biomech.* 30, 207–212. doi: 10.1016/S0021-9290(96)00147-9

Algranati, D., Kassab, G. S., and Lanir, Y. (2011). Why is the subendocardium more vulnerable to ischemia? A new paradigm. *Am. J. Physiol. Heart Circ. Physiol.* 300, H1090–H1100. doi: 10.1152/ajpheart.00473.2010

Aurigemma, G. P., and Gaasch, W. H. (2004). Clinical practice. Diastolic heart failure. *N. Engl. J. Med.* 351, 1097–1105. doi: 10.1056/NEJMcp022709

Aurigemma, G. P., Silver, K. H., Priest, M. A., and Gaasch, W. H. (1995). Geometric changes allow normal ejection fraction despite depressed myocardial shortening in hypertensive left ventricular hypertrophy. *J. Am. Coll. Cardiol.* 26, 195–202. doi: 10.1016/0735-1097(95)00153-Q

Baillargeon, B., Costa, I., Leach, J. R., Lee, L. C., Genet, M., Toutain, A., et al. (2015). Human cardiac function simulator for the optimal design of a novel annuloplasty ring with a sub-valvular element for correction of ischemic mitral regurgitation. *Cardiovasc. Eng. Technol.* 6, 105–116. doi: 10.1007/s13239-015-0216-z

Baillargeon, B., Rebelo, N., Fox, D. D., Taylor, R. L., and Kuhl, E. (2014). The living heart project: a robust and integrative simulator for human heart function. *Eur. J. Mech. A Solids* 48, 38–47. doi: 10.1016/j.euromechsol.2014.04.001

Bench, T., Burkhoff, D., O'Connell, J. B., Costanzo, M. R., Abraham, W. T., St John Sutton, M., et al.(2009). Heart failure with normal ejection fraction: consideration of mechanisms other than diastolic dysfunction. *Curr. Heart Fail. Rep.* 6, 57–64. doi: 10.1007/s11897-009-0010-z

Benjamin, E. J., Blaha, M. J., Chiuve, S. E., Cushman, M., Das, S. R., Deo, R., et al. (2017). American heart association statistics committee and stroke statistics Subcommittee. heart disease and stroke statistics-2017 update: a report from the American Heart Association. *Circulation* 135, e146–e603. doi: 10.1161/CIR.0000000000000485

Bhuiyan, T., and Maurer, M. S. (2011). Heart failure with preserved ejection fraction: persistent diagnosis, therapeutic enigma. *Curr. Cardiovasc. Risk Rep.* 5, 440–449. doi: 10.1007/s12170-011-0184-2

Borlaug, B. A., and Paulus, W. J. (2011). Heart failure with preserved ejection fraction: pathophysiology, diagnosis, and treatment. *Eur. Heart J.* 32, 670–679. doi: 10.1093/eurheartj/ehq426

Carabello, B. A. (1995). The relationship of left ventricular geometry and hypertrophy to left ventricular function in valvular heart disease. *J. Heart Valve Dis.* 4(Suppl. 2), S132–S138.

Carrick, R., Ge, L., Lee, L. C., Zhang, Z., Mishra, R., Axel, L., et al. (2012). Patient-specific finite element-based analysis of ventricular myofiber stress after Coapsys: importance of residual stress. *Ann. Thorac. Surg.* 93, 1964–1971. doi: 10.1016/j.athoracsur.2012.03.001

Chabiniok, R., Moireau, P., Lesault, P. F., Rahmouni, A., Deux, J. F., and Chapelle, D. (2012). Estimation of tissue contractility from cardiac cine-MRI using a biomechanical heart model. *Biomech. Model. Mechanobiol.* 11, 609–630. doi: 10.1007/s10237-011-0337-8

Chen, C. H., Fetics, B., Nevo, E., Rochitte, C. E., Chiou, K. R., Ding, P. A., et al. (2001). Noninvasive single-beat determination of left ventricular end-systolic elastance in humans. *J. Am. Coll. Cardiol.* 38, 2028–2034. doi: 10.1016/S0735-1097(01)01651-5

Crozier, A., Blazevic, B., Lamata, P., Plank, G., Ginks, M., Duckett, S., et al.,(2016). The relative role of patient physiology and device optimisation in cardiac resynchronisation therapy: a computational modelling study. *J. Mol. Cell. Cardiol.* 96, 93–100. doi: 10.1016/j.yjmcc.2015.10.026

Gaasch, W. H., and Zile, M. R. (2011). Left ventricular structural remodeling in health and disease: with special emphasis on volume, mass, and geometry. *J. Am. Coll. Cardiol.* 58, 1733–1740. doi: 10.1016/j.jacc.2011.07.022

Genet, M., Lee, L. C., Nguyen, R., Haraldsson, H., Acevedo-Bolton, G., Zhang, Z., et al. (2014). Distribution of normal human LV myofiber stress at end diastole and end systole: a target for in silico design of heart failure treatments. *J. Appl. Physiol.* 117, 142–152. doi: 10.1152/japplphysiol.00255.2014

Giffard-Roisin, S., Jackson, Th, Fovargue, L., Lee, J., Delingette, H., Razavi, R., et al. (2017). Noninvasive personalization of a cardiac electrophysiology model from body surface potential mapping. *IEEE Trans. Biomed. Eng.* 64, 2206–2218. doi: 10.1109/TBME.2016.2629849

Göktepe, S., Acharya, S. N. S., Wong, J., and Kuhl, E. (2011). Computational modeling of passive myocardium. *Int. J. Numer. Methods Biomed. Eng.* 27, 1–12. doi: 10.1002/cnm.1402

Grossman, W., Jones, D., and McLaurin, L. P. (1975). Wall stress and patterns of hypertrophy in the human left ventricle. *J. Clin. Invest.* 56, 56–64. doi: 10.1172/JCI108079

Guccione, J. M., and McCulloch, A. D. (1993). Mechanics of active contraction in cardiac muscle. I. Constitutive relations for fiber stress that describe deactivation. *J. Biomech. Eng.* 115, 72–81. doi: 10.1115/1.2895473

Haynes, P., Nava, K. E., Lawson, B. A., Chung, C. S., Mitov, M. I., Campbell, S. G., et al. (2014). Transmural heterogeneity of cellular level power output is reduced in human heart failure. *J. Mol. Cell Cardiol.* 72, 1–8. doi: 10.1016/j.yjmcc.2014.02.008

Heidenreich, P. A., Albert, N. M., Allen, L. A., Bluemke, D. A., Butler, J., Fonarow, G. C., et al. (2013). Forecasting the impact of heart failure in the United States: a policy statement from the American Heart Association. *Circ. Heart Fail.* 6, 606–619. doi: 10.1161/HHF.0b013e318291329a

Henein, M. Y., and Gibson, D. G. (1999). Long axis function in disease. *Heart* 81, 229–231. doi: 10.1136/hrt.81.3.229

Holzapfel, G. A., and Ogden, R. W. (2009). Constitutive modelling of passive myocardium: a structurally based framework for material characterization. *Philos. Trans. A Math. Phys. Eng. Sci.* 367, 3445–3475. doi: 10.1098/rsta.2009.0091

Jones, E., Oliphant, T., and Peterson, P. (2001). *SciPy: Open Source Scientific Tools for Python.* Available online at: http://www.scipy.org

Klotz, S., Hay, I., Dickstein, M. L., Yi, G. H., Wang, J., Maurer, M. S., et al. (2006). Single-beat estimation of end-diastolic pressure-volume relationship: a novel method with potential for noninvasive application. *Am. J. Physiol. Heart Circ. Physiol.* 291, H403–H412. doi: 10.1152/ajpheart.01240.2005

Lam, C. S. (2010). Heart failure with preserved ejection fraction: invasive solution to diagnostic confusion? *J. Am. Coll. Cardiol.* 55, 1711–1712. doi: 10.1016/j.jacc.2009.12.034

Lee, L. C., Genet, M., Acevedo-Bolton, G., Ordovas, K., Guccione, J. M., and Kuhl, E. (2015). A computational model that predicts reverse growth in response to mechanical unloading. *Biomech. Model. Mechanobiol.* 14, 217–229. doi: 10.1007/s10237-014-0598-0

Lee, L. C., Zhihong, Z., Hinson, A., and Guccione, J. M. (2013). Reduction in left ventricular wall stress and improvement in function in failing hearts using Algisyl-LVR. *J. Vis. Exp.* 74:50096. doi: 10.3791/50096

LeGrice, I., Hunter, P., Young, A., and Small, B. (2001). The architecture of the heart: a data-based model. *Philos. Trans. R. Soc. Lond. Ser. A Math. Phys. Eng. Sci.* 359, 1217–1232. doi: 10.1098/rsta.2001.0827

Lombaert, H., Peyrat, J.-M., Croisille, P., Rapacchi, S., Fanton, L., Clarysse, P., et al. (2011). "Statistical analysis of the human cardiac fiber architecture from DT-MRI," in *Functional Imaging and Modeling of the Heart* (Berlin; Heidelberg: Springer), 171–179.

MacIver, D. H. (2009). Heart failure with preserved ejection fraction: is it due to contractile dysfunction? *Circ. J.* 73:1169. doi: 10.1253/circj.CJ-09-0190

MacIver, D. H., and Townsend, M. (2008). A novel mechanism of heart failure with normal ejection fraction. *Heart* 94, 446–449. doi: 10.1136/hrt.2006.114082

Melenovsky, V., Borlaug, B. A., Rosen, B., Hay, I., Ferruci, L., Morell, C. H., et al. (2007). Cardiovascular features of heart failure with preserved ejection fraction versus nonfailing hypertensive left ventricular hypertrophy in the urban Baltimore community: the role of atrial remodeling/dysfunction. *J. Am. Coll. Cardiol.* 49, 198–207. doi: 10.1016/j.jacc.2006.08.050

Mercier, J. C., DiSessa, T. G., Jarmakani, J. M., Nakanishi, T., Hiraishi, S., Isabel-Jones, J., et al. (1982). Two-dimensional echocardiographic assessment of left ventricular volumes and ejection fraction in children. *Circulation* 65, 962–969. doi: 10.1161/01.CIR.65.5.962

Mizuguchi, Y., Oishi, Y., Miyoshi, H., Iuchi, A., Nagase, N., and Oki, T. (2010). Concentric left ventricular hypertrophy brings deterioration of systolic longitudinal, circumferential, and radial myocardial deformation in hypertensive patients with preserved left ventricular pump function. *J. Cardiol.* 55, 23–33. doi: 10.1016/j.jjcc.2009.07.006

Moore, C. C., Lugo-Olivieri, C. H., McVeigh, E. R., and Zerhouni, E. A. (2000). Three-dimensional systolic strain patterns in the normal human left ventricle: characterization with tagged MR imaging. *Radiology* 214, 453–466. doi: 10.1148/radiology.214.2.r00fe17453

Nagueh, S. F., Middleton, K. J., Kopelen, H. A., Zoghbi, W. A., and Quiñones, M. A. (1997). Doppler tissue imaging: a noninvasive technique for evaluation of left ventricular relaxation and estimation of filling pressures. *J. Am. Coll. Cardiol.* 30, 1527–1533. doi: 10.1016/S0735-1097(97)00344-6

Oghlakian, G. O., Sipahi, I., and Fang, J. C. (2011). Treatment of heart failure with preserved ejection fraction: have we been pursuing the wrong paradigm? *Mayo Clin. Proc.* 86, 531–539.

Omar, A. M., Bansal, M., and Sengupta, P. P. (2016). Advances in echocardiographic imaging in heart failure with reduced and preserved ejection fraction. *Circ. Res.* 119, 357–374. doi: 10.1161/CIRCRESAHA.116.309128

Omar, A. M. S., Narula, S., Abdel Rahman, M. A., Pedrizzetti, G., Raslan, H., Rifaie, O., et al. (2017). Precision phenotyping in heart failure and pattern clustering of ultrasound data for the assessment of diastolic dysfunction. *JACC Cardiovasc. Imaging* 10, 1291–1303. doi: 10.1016/j.jcmg.2016.10.012

Owan, T. E., and Redfield, M. M. (2005). Epidemiology of diastolic heart failure. *Prog. Cardiovasc. Dis.* 47, 320–332.

Paulus, W. J., Tschöpe, C., Sanderson, J. E., Rusconi, C., and Flachskampf, F. A. (2007). How to diagnose diastolic heart failure: a consensus statement on the diagnosis of heart failure with normal left ventricular ejection fraction by the Heart Failure and Echocardiography Associations of the European Society of Cardiology. *Eur. Heart J.* 28, 2539–2550. doi: 10.1093/eurheartj/ehm037

Phan, T. T., Abozguia, K., Nallur Shivu, G., Mahadevan, G., Ahmed, I., Williams, L., et al. (2009). Heart failure with preserved ejection fraction is characterized by dynamic impairment of active relaxation and contraction of the left ventricle on exercise and associated with myocardial energy deficiency. *J. Am. Coll. Cardiol.* 54, 402–409. doi: 10.1016/j.jacc.2009.05.012

Prinzen, F. W., Arts, T., van der Vusse, G. J., and Reneman, R. S. (1984). Fiber shortening in the inner layers of the left ventricular wall as assessed from epicardial deformation during normoxia and ischemia. *J. Biomech.* 17, 801–811.

Rüssel, I. K., Götte, M. J., Bronzwaer, J. G., Knaapen, P., Paulus, W. J., and van Rossum, A. C. (2009). Left ventricular torsion: an expanding role in the analysis of myocardial dysfunction. *JACC Cardiovasc. Imaging* 2, 648–655. doi: 10.1016/j.jcmg.2009.03.001

Reichek, N. (2013). Right ventricular strain in pulmonary hypertension: flavor du jour or enduring prognostic index? *Circul. Cardiovasc. Imaging* 6, 609–611. doi: 10.1161/CIRCIMAGING.113.000936

Roh, J., Houstis, N., and Rosenzweig, A. (2017). Why Don't we have proven treatments for HFpEF? *Circ. Res.* 120, 1243–1245. doi: 10.1161/CIRCRESAHA.116.310119

Sabbah, H. N., Marzilli, M., and Stein, P. D. (1981). The relative role of subendocardium and subepicardium in left ventricular mechanics. *Am. J. Physiol.* 240, H920–H926.

Sack, K. L., Baillargeon, B., Acevedo-Bolton, G., Genet, M., Rebelo, N., Kuhl, E., et al. (2016). Partial LVAD restores ventricular outputs and normalizes LV but not RV stress distributions in the acutely failing heart in silico. *Int. J. Artif. Organs.* 39, 421–430. doi: 10.5301/ijao.5000520

Sengupta, P. P., and Marwick, T. H. (2018). The many dimensions of diastolic function: a curse or a blessing? *JACC Cardiovasc. Imaging.* 11, 409–410. doi: 10.1016/j.jcmg.2017.05.015

Sengupta, P. P., and Narula, J. (2008). Reclassifying heart failure: predominantly subendocardial, subepicardial, and transmural. *Heart Fail. Clin.* 4, 379–382. doi: 10.1016/j.hfc.2008.03.013

Shah, A. M., and Solomon, S. D. (2012). Phenotypic and pathophysiological heterogeneity in heart failure with preserved ejection fraction. *Eur. Heart J.* 33, 1716–1717. doi: 10.1093/eurheartj/ehs124

Shavik, S. M., Wall, S. T., Sundnes, J., Burkhoff, D., and Lee, L. C. (2017). Organ-level validation of a cross-bridge cycling descriptor in a left ventricular finite element model: effects of ventricular loading on myocardial strains. *Physiol. Rep.* 5:e13392. doi: 10.14814/phy2.13392

Steinberg, B. A., Zhao, X., Heidenreich, P. A., Peterson, E. D., Bhatt, D. L., Cannon, C. P., et al. (2012). Trends in patients hospitalized with heart failure and preserved left ventricular ejection fraction: prevalence, therapies, and outcomes. *Circulation* 126, 65–75. doi: 10.1161/CIRCULATIONAHA.111.080770

Stokke, T. M., Hasselberg, N. E., Smedsrud, M. K., Sarvari, S. I., Haugaa, K. H., Smiseth, O. A., et al. (2017). Geometry as a confounder when assessing ventricular systolic function: comparison between ejection fraction and strain. *J. Am. Coll. Cardiol.* 70, 942–954. doi: 10.1016/j.jacc.2017.06.046

Streeter, D. D., Spotnitz, H. M., Patel, D. P., Ross, J., and Sonnenblick, E. H. (1969). Fiber orientation in the canine left ventricle during diastole and systole. *Circ. Res.* 24, 339–347.

Takeda, S., Rimington, H., Smeeton, N., and Chambers, J. (2001). Long axis excursion in aortic stenosis. *Heart* 86, 52–56. doi: 10.1136/heart.86.1.52

Tischler, M. D., Niggel, J., Borowski, D. T., and LeWinter, M. M. (1993). Relation between left ventricular shape and exercise capacity in patients with left ventricular dysfunction. *J. Am. Coll. Cardiol.* 22, 751–757.

Vasan, R. S., Benjamin, E. J., and Levy, D. (1995). Prevalence, clinical features and prognosis of diastolic heart failure: an epidemiologic perspective. *J. Am. Coll. Cardiol.* 26, 1565–1574.

Vasan, R. S., Larson, M. G., Benjamin, E. J., Evans, J. C., Reiss, C. K., and Levy, D. (1999). Congestive heart failure in subjects with normal versus reduced left ventricular ejection fraction: prevalence and mortality in a population-based cohort. *J. Am. Coll. Cardiol.* 33, 1948–1955.

Villongco, C. T., Krummen, D. E., Stark, P., Omens, J. H., and McCulloch, A. D. (2014). Patient-specific modeling of ventricular activation pattern using surface ECG-derived vectorcardiogram in bundle branch block. *Prog. Biophys. Mol. Biol.* 115, 305–313. doi: 10.1016/j.pbiomolbio.2014.06.011

Vinereanu, D., Nicolaides, E., Tweddel, A. C., and Fraser, A. G. (2005). "Pure" diastolic dysfunction is associated with long-axis systolic dysfunction. Implications for the diagnosis and classification of heart failure. *Eur. J. Heart Fail.* 7, 820–828. doi: 10.1016/j.ejheart.2005.02.003

Walker, J. C., Ratcliffe, M. B., Zhang, P., Wallace, A. W., Fata, B., Hsu, E. W., et al. (2005). MRI-based finite-element analysis of left ventricular aneurysm. *Am. J. Physiol. Heart Circ. Physiol.* 289, H692–H700. doi: 10.1152/ajpheart.01226.2004

Wang, H., Zhang, X., Dorsey, S. M., McGarvey, J. R., Campbell, K. S., Burdick, J. A., et al. (2016). Computational investigation of transmural differences in left ventricular contractility. *ASME J. Biomech. Eng.* 138:114501. doi: 10.1115/1.4034558

Wang, J., Khoury, D. S., Yue, Y., Torre-Amione, G., and Nagueh, S. F. (2008). Preserved left ventricular twist and circumferential deformation, but depressed longitudinal and radial deformation in patients with diastolic heart failure. *Eur. Heart J.* 29, 1283–1289. doi: 10.1093/eurheartj/ehn141

Yancy, C. W., Jessup, M., Bozkurt, B., Butler, J., Casey, D. E. Jr, Drazner, M. H., et al. (2013). ACCF/AHA guideline for the management of heart failure: a report of the American College of Cardiology Foundation/American Heart Association task force on practice guidelines. *J. Am. Coll. Cardiol.* 62, e147–e239. doi: 10.1016/j.jacc.2013.05.019

Yingchoncharoen, T., Agarwal, S., Popović, Z. B., and Marwick, T. H. (2013). Normal ranges of left ventricular strain: a meta-analysis. *J. Am. Soc. Echocardiogr.* 26, 185–191. doi: 10.1016/j.echo.2012.10.008

Yu, C. M., Lin, H., Yang, H., Kong, S. L., Zhang, Q., and Lee, S. W. (2002). Progression of systolic abnormalities in patients with "isolated" diastolic heart failure and diastolic dysfunction. *Circulation.* 105, 1195–1201. doi: 10.1161/hc1002.105185

Zile, M. R., Baicu, C. F., and Gaasch, W. H. (2004). Diastolic heart failure–abnormalities in active relaxation and passive stiffness of the left ventricle. *N. Engl. J. Med.* 350, 1953–1959. doi: 10.1056/NEJMoa032566

# 15

# Biomechanical Material Characterization of Stanford Type-B Dissected Porcine Aortas

Aashish Ahuja[1], Jillian N. Noblet[2], Tony Trudnowski[2], Bhavesh Patel[1], Joshua F. Krieger[2], Sean Chambers[2] and Ghassan S. Kassab[1*]

[1] Cardiovascular Mechanics and Diseases, California Medical Innovations Institute, San Diego, CA, United States, [2] Cook Medical Inc., Bloomington, IN, United States

*Correspondence:
Ghassan S. Kassab
gkassab@calmi2.org

Aortic dissection (AD) involves tearing of the medial layer, creating a blood-filled channel called false lumen (FL). To treat dissections, clinicians are using endovascular therapy using stent grafts to seal the FL. This procedure has been successful in reducing mortality but has failed in completely re-attaching the torn intimal layer. The use of computational analysis can predict the radial forces needed to devise stents that can treat ADs. To quantify the hyperelastic material behavior for therapy development, we harvested FL wall, true lumen (TL) wall, and intimal flap from the middle and distal part of five dissected aortas. Planar biaxial testing using multiple stretch protocols were conducted on tissue samples to quantify their deformation behavior. A novel non-linear regression model was used to fit data against Holzapfel–Gasser–Ogden hyperelastic strain energy function. The fitting analysis correlated the behavior of the FL and TL walls and the intimal flap to the stiffness observed during tensile loading. It was hypothesized that there is a variability in the stresses generated during loading among tissue specimens derived from different regions of the dissected aorta and hence, one should use region-specific material models when simulating type-B AD. From the data on material behavior analysis, the variability in the tissue specimens harvested from pigs was tabulated using stress and coefficient of variation (CV). The material response curves also compared the changes in compliance observed in the FL wall, TL wall, and intimal flap for middle and distal regions of the dissection. It was observed that for small stretch ratios, all the tissue specimens behaved isotropically with overlapping stress–stretch curves in both circumferential and axial directions. As the stretch ratios increased, we observed that most tissue specimens displayed different structural behaviors in axial and circumferential directions. This observation was very apparent in tissue specimens from mid FL region, less apparent in mid TL, distal FL, and distal flap tissues and least noticeable in tissue specimens harvested from mid flap. Lastly, using mixed model ANOVAS, it was concluded that there were significant differences between mid and distal regions along axial direction which were absent in the circumferential direction.

Keywords: aortic dissection, material behavior, Holzapfel–Gasser–Ogden, planar biaxial testing, layered model

## INTRODUCTION

Aortic dissection (AD) is the most common life-threatening disorder affecting the aorta (Hagan et al., 2000). AD is classified as Stanford type-B if it originates distal to the left subclavian artery and does not involve ascending aorta. In type-B dissection, there is separation and propagation between the intima–media where blood enters the layers of the aortic wall to create a false channel, known as the false lumen (FL) in addition to the normal endothelialized channel referred to as the true lumen (TL). The layer of the aorta dissected from its wall is called the intimal flap. The primary pathological changes in the aortic wall leading to AD is attributed to two major theories (Mann et al., 2015). The first ascribes primacy to the development of an intimal tear, followed by penetration of blood from the aortic lumen into a weakened, susceptible medial space (characterized by elastic degeneration of the vessel). The second hypothesis is that initial rupture of the vasa vasorum leads to hemorrhage within the aortic wall and subsequent intimal disruption and propagation of a dissection flap. The dynamics of the intimal flap and the dilation of the FL during the cardiac cycle can cause malperfusion of the vital organs (usually kidneys) and can lead to adverse life-threatening events. AD has been linked with clinical complications such as aneurysmal formation, aortic wall rupture, aortic wall regurgitation, pericardial effusion causing tamponade, hypotension/shock, and malperfusion syndromes leading to end organ ischemia (Erbel et al., 2001; Greenberg et al., 2003; Nienaber and Eagle, 2003; Golledge and Eagle, 2008; Juang et al., 2008; Patel et al., 2014). The two most important acquired risk factors related to the development of AD include hypertension and atherosclerosis. Hypertension has been linked with Stanford Type B dissections in 70% of cases. This is almost twice as many as the number of incidences with type A dissections where hypertension was found to be the leading cause (36%; Hagan et al., 2000). The propensity to AD is also amplified due to genetic diseases and connective tissue disorders. Syndromes such Marfan, Ehlers-Danlos, Loeys-Dietz, familial AD, and annulo-aortic ectasia are all implicated in the development of thoracic aortic aneurysm and dissection (Halme et al., 1985).

The incidence of AD in the United States is approximately 2,000 cases per year and early mortality is as high as 1% per hour if untreated (Vecht et al., 1980; Roberts, 1981). Currently, there are three modes of treating patients suffering from AD: medical management, open surgery, and endovascular treatment. While medical management is suggested for patients that have uncomplicated dissections, for complicated dissections, open surgery or endovascular grafting is recommended. The design and use of endovascular grafts or bare metal stents can provide sufficient radial forces on the intimal flap to push it back against the FL wall and allow reconstitution of the aorta without imposing high mechanical stresses on the FL wall. The research and development of effective mechanical devices for endovascular grafting would require the use of computational techniques to analyze the structural interaction between the rigid stents (usually composed of Stainless steel or Nitinol alloy) and different tissue segments of the dissected aorta (i.e., Intimal flap, FL wall, and TL wall). Unfortunately, the "building

elements" for computational model such as a suitable constitutive model that characterizes the mechanical behavior of a dissected aorta by providing a mathematical formulation for the stress–strain relation is currently lacking (Babu et al., 2015). Structural continuum constitutive models of the different layers of aorta integrate information about the tissue morphology and therefore assess the interrelation between the structure and response to mechanical loading. Fiber-reinforced structural models of different layers of aorta, namely media and adventitia, have been presented in Holzapfel et al. (2000) and Holzapfel and Gasser (2001), but material characterization of intima–media and media–adventitia layers from porcine aortas suffering from dissection is not available. The current Finite Element Analysis (FEA) and Fluid–Structure Interaction models for dissected aorta assume linear elasticity or simplified hyperelasticity for different regions of the dissected aorta (Alimohammadi et al., 2015). The goal of this paper was to develop a novel non-linear regression material model using data from planar biaxial testing on dissected porcine aortas and empirically fit it to a five parameter form of Holzapfel–Gasser–Ogden hyperelastic strain energy function (Gasser et al., 2006). It was also hypothesized that there was a variability in the stresses generated due to loading among tissue specimens derived from different regions of the dissected aorta and hence, one should use region-specific material models when simulating type-B AD. To test the hypothesis, the variability in the tissue specimens harvested from ($n = 5$) pigs was tabulated using stress as the variable and coefficient of variation (CV) as the statistical method. Also, the analysis compared the changes in the compliance and regional variability observed in the TL wall, FL wall, and intimal flap harvested from middle and distal regions of the dissection. The passive behavior was the focus of this work, while the active response will be studied in a subsequent work once the passive foundation is established here. It is hopeful that the biomechanical characterization of a layered model for dissected aorta will expedite the development of endovascular therapy for successfully sealing the FL thereby reducing mortality and future reinterventions.

## MATERIALS AND METHODS

### Materials

The data for the material behavior was collected from five porcine aortas obtained from a slaughterhouse. The aortas were obtained from ~100 kg swine that had been raised on a farm (Sierra for medical sciences, Whittier, CA, USA). The descending thoracic part of the aortas was harvested, cleaned, and flushed with 0.9% NaCl physiological saline solution and later stored in saline at 4°C to slow down any enzymatic tissue breakdown (Rashid et al., 2013). The mechanical testing of the samples were completed within 16 h of tissue harvest.

### Dissection

A healthy porcine aorta was inverted exposing the intima and dissections were created ~5–6 cm from the vessel start (~6–8 cm from the left subclavian artery). Dissections in healthy descending thoracic aorta represented the case of acute Type-B AD. The percent circumferential length of the entry tear was

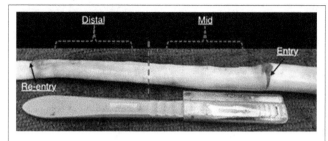

**FIGURE 1 |** An inverted aorta with dissection. An entry was initially created carefully in the descending thoracic aorta and propagated using forceps to the distal region of the aorta where a pocket of re-entry is created. Tissue specimens from two regions (mid and distal) are extracted and tested on planar biaxial testing machine for material characterization.

calculated as 100X (perimeter of the flap/circumference of the vessel). The perimeter of the flap was calculated by measuring the average length of the two edges of the flap in an ultrasound image representing cross-section of the entry tear (Peelukhana et al., 2016; Canchi et al., 2017). Using a surgical blade, a cut was made in the inner lining of the vessel. The layers were separated using the surgical blade and advanced using a fine-tip forceps to the desired axial length. A resulting intimal flap of about ∼10–13 cm in length was created due to surgical dissection as shown in **Figure 1**. At the end of dissection, a reentry was created and the flap separated the TL from the FL in the vessel.

## Mechanical Experiments on Dissected Tissues Using Displacement Controlled Biaxial Protocols

The planar mechanical biaxial experiments were performed using a custom-built planar biaxial testing machine shown in **Figure 2**. The instrument consisted of four motors with attached encoders and each motor had a maximum displacement of 12 mm. The force on the tissue was measured using 1,000-g submersible load cells installed in both x- and y-directions. The strain was measured with the "Bose® digital video extensometer," and the entire system was controlled and monitored using WinTest® version 7 software. The extensometer had a sampling rate of up to 200 Hz. The experiments were conducted at a sampling rate of 0.02 Hz to achieve quasi-static loading conditions. Tissue specimens were oriented in the circumferential and longitudinal directions and attached to the linear arms using clamps. The specimens were immersed in 0.9% NaCl physiological saline solution maintained at 37°C. Several previous studies such as Rassoli et al. (2014), Zemánek et al. (2009), and Jhun et al. (2009) had also used 0.9% saline solution for biaxial testing on soft tissue and bioartificial tissue specimens but did not report any deteriorating effects on their structural integrity. Each specimen was cut into a cruciform shape of 15 × 15 mm cross-sectional area such that the arm width, $w$, was 5 mm. Four graphite markers were applied to the central region (away from corners and arms to avoid errors due to end effects) of the cruciform specimen and the marker positions during deformation were recorded. Using a dedicated proprietary software (prepackaged with Bose® digital video extensometer), the displacements of the

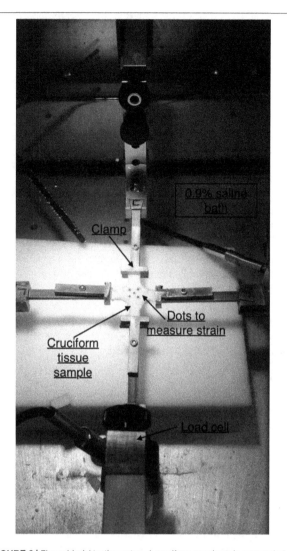

**FIGURE 2 |** Planar biaxial testing setup. A cruciform specimen is suspended using clamps which is stretched along x- and y-axes. The x-axis represents the circumferential direction while y-axis represents the axial direction.

four markers were tracked and the recorded data was used to calculate the circumferential ($\epsilon_\theta$) and longitudinal ($\epsilon_z$) strains in the tissue specimen.

The mechanical testing showed that preconditioning of 10 loading–unloading cycles on specimens could eliminate the viscoelastic response and provide reproducible curves. An additional 10 cycles were done to ensure there was no load cell drift during mechanical testing. For each specimen, enzymatic degradation was not induced as the tissue was tested within 16 h (Rashid et al., 2013). The strains and loads along the two axes were recorded for each of the five different displacement protocols (1:1[1], 1.5:1, 2:1, 1:1.5, 1:2). After completing the preconditioning and reproducibility of force-displacement curves, the loading curves from succeeding three cycles were chosen for the determination of material parameters.

---

[1]1:1 displacement protocol is also referred to as equibiaxial displacement protocol.

The Cauchy stress was computed for both circumferential and longitudinal directions. It is defined as:

$$\sigma_{\theta\theta} = \left(\frac{F_\theta}{tw}\right)\lambda_\theta \qquad (1)$$

$$\sigma_{zz} = \left(\frac{F_z}{tw}\right)\lambda_z \qquad (2)$$

where stresses along circumferential and longitudinal directions were given as $\sigma_{\theta\theta}$ and $\sigma_{zz}$, respectively. $F_\theta$ and $F_z$ were loads registered by the load cells of ElectroForce TestBench instrument along the two directions. The variables $t$ and $w$ (=5 mm) were the initial thickness and width of the tissue sample, respectively and $\lambda_\theta$ (= $\epsilon_\theta + 1$) and $\lambda_z$ (= $\epsilon_z + 1$) were the stretches in circumferential and longitudinal directions which were measured using the CCD camera mounted over the specimen. The thickness of the sample was measured using a Mitutoyo Absolute Digimatic caliper-type micrometer. For each specimen, thickness was measured at four locations using the micrometer. The average measurement for each specimen was recorded and provided in **Table 1**. The shear strains were measured by the data acquisition system and were small and not accounted for in the constitutive model.

## Theory

Using the displacements recorded on the planar biaxial tests, we computed the Green strains (E) in the principal material directions. Strains were represented in terms of the in-plane deformation gradient tensor, F, as:

$$E = \frac{1}{2}(F^T F - I) \qquad (3)$$

where I was the identity tensor and $F^T$ was the transpose of deformation gradient tensor F. The strain-energy function (SEF) proposed on Gasser et al. (2006) was used to represent the inherent hyperelasticity of the aortic tissue. It was given as an additive split of the isochoric SEF into a part associated with isotropic deformations and a part associated with the anisotropic deformations as given by:

$$\Psi = \Psi_{iso} + \Psi_{aniso} \qquad (4)$$

The isotropic component ($\Psi_{iso}$) was associated with the mechanical response of elastin and smooth muscle cells in the passive state (Gundiah et al., 2009) and was described as:

$$\Psi_{iso} = C_{10}(I_1 - 3) \qquad (5)$$

where $C_{10}$ was a material constant and $I_1$ represented the first invariant of the Cauchy-Green tensor (Spencer, 1971). The anisotropic component ($\Psi_{aniso}$) was related to the response of collagen fibers to loading of the tissue specimen. The collagen fibers were crimped at low stretches of the tissue and are not involved in its extension. At higher stretches, the fibers were elongated and were responsible in reinforcing the tissues. An

**TABLE 1** | Specifications of tissue sample and test protocols used for its material characterization.

| Pig number | Region of thoracic aorta and displacement-controlled protocols |
|---|---|
| Pig 1 | Mid TL wall (1:1), |
| | Mid Flap (1:1, 1:1.5, 1:2, 1.5:1, 2:1), |
| | Mid FL wall (1:1, 1:1.5, 1:2, 1.5:1, 2:1), |
| | Distal FL wall (1:1, 1.5:1, 2:1), |
| | Distal Flap (1:1, 1:1.5, 1:2, 1.5:1, 2:1) |
| Pig 2 | Mid TL wall (1:1, 1:1.5, 1:2, 1.5:1, 2:1), |
| | Mid Flap (1:1, 1:1.5, 1:2, 1.5:1, 2:1), |
| | Mid FL wall (1:1, 1:1.5, 1:2, 1.5:1, 2:1), |
| | Distal FL wall (1:1, 1:2, 1.5:1, 2:1), |
| | Distal Flap (1:1, 1:1.5, 1:2, 1.5:1, 2:1) |
| Pig 3 | Mid TL wall (1:1, 1:1.5, 1:2, 1.5:1, 2:1), |
| | Mid Flap (1:1, 1:1.5, 1:2), |
| | Mid FL wall (1:1, 1:1.5, 1:2, 1.5:1, 2:1), |
| | Distal FL wall (1:1), |
| | Distal Flap (1:1, 1:1.5, 1:2, 1.5:1, 2:1) |
| Pig 4 | Mid TL wall (1:1, 1:1.5, 1:2, 1.5:1, 2:1), |
| | Mid Flap (1:1, 1:1.5, 1:2), |
| | Mid FL wall (1:1), |
| | Distal FL wall (1:1, 1:1.5, 1:2, 1.5:1, 2:1), |
| | Distal Flap (1:1, 1:1.5, 1:2, 1.5:1, 2:1) |
| Pig 5 | Mid TL wall (1:1, 1:1.5, 1:2, 1.5:1), |
| | Mid Flap (1:1), |
| | Mid FL wall (1:1), |
| | Distal FL wall (1:1, 1.5:1, 2:1), |
| | Distal Flap (1:1, 1:1.5, 1:2, 1.5:1, 2:1) |

exponential function was used to describe the strain energy stored in the collagen fibers:

$$\Psi_{aniso} = \frac{k_1}{2k_2}\left(\exp\left\{k_2\left[\kappa I_1 + (1 - 3\kappa) I_4 - 1\right]^2\right\}\right)$$
$$+ \frac{k_3}{2k_4}\left(\exp\left\{k_4\left[\kappa I_1 + (1 - 3\kappa) I_6 - 1\right]^2\right\}\right) \qquad (6)$$

where $I_4$, $I_6 \geq 1$ characterized the mechanical response in the preferential directions of the fibers. $k_1 > 0$ and $k_3 > 0$ were stress like parameters while $k_2 > 0$ and $k_4 > 0$ were dimensionless. The parameter $\kappa \in [0, 1/3]$ was also dimensionless and accounted for fiber dispersion. The preferred directions for the fibers contributing to the SEF was represented by invariants $I_4$ and $I_6$. The anisotropy directions in tissues were assumed to be helically oriented at $\pm\theta$ degrees with respect to the longitudinal direction (Holzapfel et al., 2000). Therefore, invariants $I_4$ and $I_6$ became equal and were given as:

$$I_4, I_6 = \lambda_\theta^2 \cos^2\theta + \lambda_z^2 \sin^2\theta \qquad (7)$$

A value of $\kappa$ close to 0 indicated concentration of the fibers along the preferred orientation $\theta$ while a value closer to 1/3 suggested dispersion of the fibers. Also, since each family of fibers represented the main direction we assumed same mechanical response along $\theta$ degrees, therefore, $k_1 = k_3$ and $k_2 = k_4$. The value of $\Psi_{aniso}$ was only valid when the tissue was stretched and became zero when $I_4, I_6 < 1$.

The vascular wall layers, namely TL wall, intimal flap, and FL wall, were incompressible. This meant that the volume of these tissue specimens remained conserved after deformation. As a result, the Jacobian of the deformation gradient, represented as $J = \det(F)$ and defined as the product of stretches in the principal directions, $\lambda_\theta \lambda_z \lambda_r$ was equal to 1. The vessel wall layers were regarded to be composed of elastin, smooth muscle cells and collagen fibers. In a planar biaxial testing experiment of tissue specimen with the axes aligned with the longitudinal and circumferential directions, the deformation gradient, $F$ and corresponding Cauchy stress tensor, $\sigma$ were given as:

$$
F = \begin{bmatrix} \lambda_\theta & 0 & 0 \\ 0 & \lambda_z & 0 \\ 0 & 0 & 1/\lambda_\theta\lambda_z \end{bmatrix}, \ \sigma = \begin{bmatrix} \sigma_{\theta\theta} \\ \sigma_{zz} \\ 0 \end{bmatrix} = \begin{bmatrix} \lambda_\theta \dfrac{\partial\Psi}{\partial\lambda_\theta} \\ \lambda_z \dfrac{\partial\Psi}{\partial\lambda_z} \\ 0 \end{bmatrix}
\tag{8}
$$

The values of stresses along circumferential and axial directions were obtained using Equation (9):

$$
\sigma_{\theta\theta} = \lambda_\theta \left[ 2C_{10} \left( \lambda_\theta - \frac{1}{\lambda_\theta^3 \lambda_z^2} \right) + 4k_1 \left( \kappa I_1 + (1-3\kappa) I_4 - 1 \right) \right.
$$

$$
\left. e^{\{k_2(\kappa I_1 + (1-3\kappa)I_4 - 1)^2\}} \left( \kappa \left( \lambda_\theta - \frac{1}{\lambda_\theta^3 \lambda_z^2} \right) + \lambda_\theta (1-3\kappa) \cos^2\alpha \right) \right]
$$

$$
\sigma_{zz} = \lambda_z \left[ 2C_{10} \left( \lambda_z - \frac{1}{\lambda_\theta^2 \lambda_z^3} \right) + 4k_1 \left( \kappa I_1 + (1-3\kappa) I_4 - 1 \right) \right.
$$

$$
\left. e^{\{k_2(\kappa I_1 + (1-3\kappa)I_4 - 1)^2\}} \left( \kappa \left( \lambda_z - \frac{1}{\lambda_\theta^2 \lambda_z^3} \right) + \lambda_z (1-3\kappa) \cos^2\alpha \right) \right]
\tag{9}
$$

## Statistical Methods

The coefficient of determination $R^2 \in [0, 1]$ and the root square of the reduced chi-square $\varepsilon \in [0, 1]$ were used as a measure of correlation between the model-derived values and the experimental data. They were defined as:

$$
R^2(A) = \frac{\sum_{f=zz,\theta\theta} \sum_{q=1}^{n} \left( A_{q,f}^m - A_{q,f}^{exp} \right)^2}{\sum_{f=zz,\theta\theta} \sum_{q=1}^{n} \left( A_{avg,f}^{exp} - A_{q,f}^{exp} \right)^2}
\tag{10}
$$

$$
\varepsilon(A) = \sqrt{\frac{1}{n - n_v} \sum_{f=zz,\theta\theta} \sum_{q=1}^{n} \left( \frac{A_{q,f}^m - A_{q,f}^{exp}}{A_{avg,f}^{exp}} \right)^2}
\tag{11}
$$

where $A = \sigma_{zz}, \ \sigma_{\theta\theta}$, the subscript "$avg$" indicated the average of the experimental values over all $n$ data points, and

$n_v = 5$ referred to the number of unknown parameters for the model. A high value of $R^2$ indicated that a good fit was globally obtained. A low value of $\varepsilon$ revealed that the differences between model predicted and experimental values were not significant for each data point. The model was fitted to all protocols. Fitting was considered acceptable for $R^2 > 0.8$ and $\varepsilon < 0.25$ over all data points, and $R^2 > 0.9$ with $\varepsilon < 0.2$ for data from equibiaxial protocol. A particular importance was given to data from equibiaxial protocol since equibiaxial displacement conditions were typically favored for model fitting and, in some cases, only data from equibiaxial conditions were retained. This was justified by the fact that, generally, smoother deformation data was captured under equibiaxial conditions. Regardless, we still considered other protocols to inform the model with more data about the material, albeit a particular focus was given to the equibiaxial-displacement data.

A statistically independent mixed model ANOVAS were conducted on the data representing differences in the material behavior of the specimens from middle and distal regions of the dissected aortas. A $p < 0.05$ was considered to be significant.

## Algorithm for Non-linear Regression Modeling

The non-linear regression techniques for determining the parameters of the HGO model were written in Python script. The data from multiple stretching protocols (1:1, 1:1.5, 1:2, 1.5:1, 2:1, with 1:1 being an equibiaxial loading condition) were used in the testing of tissues (**Table 1**). The following algorithm was proposed to select the best data to optimize the parameters for the HGO constitutive model:

1) Import the excel (or.csv) file that contained the load vs. displacement data recorded from the planar biaxial testing of the specimen.
2) Select the protocols (i.e., 1:1, 1:1.5, 1:2, 1.5:1, 2:1 or all of them) which were utilized in curve fitting.
3) For each of the protocols, only select the region in the recorded data that correspond to tensile loading.
4) Since the planar biaxial data may contain noise while recording, it should be filtered. We used the Locally Weighted Scatterplot Smoothing (LOWESS) algorithm (Cleveland, 1979) available in the statistical module of Python to remove noise from data.
5) After filtering the data for each protocol, we made several sets which covered data from each protocol as well as combinations of protocols. As an example, when we considered protocols (1:1, 1:1.5, 1:2, 1.5:1, 2:1), we ended up having 31 different data sets that contained 5 data sets considering each protocol, 10 data sets containing filtered data from a combination of two protocols (i.e., 1:1 and 1.5:1, 1:1 and 1:2, 2:1 and 1:1.5, etc.), 10 data sets containing filtered data from combination of three protocols (i.e., [1:1, 1:1.5, 1:2], [1:1.5, 1.5:1, 2:1], etc.), 5 data sets containing filtered data from combination of four protocols, and 1 data set containing filtered data from all protocols.
6) Using Nelder-Mead minimization algorithm (Nelder and Mead, 1965), we defined the objective function (Equation 12) considering isochoric tissue. In this function, $\sigma_{\theta\theta}$ and $\sigma_{zz}$ were

**TABLE 2 |** Parameter estimation for mid true lumen wall.

| Pig number | Thickness (mm) | C10 (Pa) | $k_1$ (Pa) | $k_2$ | $\alpha$ (deg) | $\kappa$ |
|---|---|---|---|---|---|---|
| 1 | 1.76 | 78,219 | 201,440 | 1.52 | 87.09 | 0.2 |
| 2 | 1.75 | 60,707 | 230,300 | 3.2 | 89.95 | 0.29 |
| 3 | 1.70 | 53,816 | 117,670 | 3.02 | 0 | 0.28 |
| 4 | 1.75 | 51,191 | 188,950 | 1.11 | 2.86 | 0.32 |
| 5 | 1.86 | 54,702 | 110,450 | 2.32 | 61.31 | 0.22 |

**TABLE 3 |** Parameter estimation for mid false lumen wall.

| Pig number | Thickness (mm) | C10 (Pa) | $k_1$ (Pa) | $k_2$ | $\alpha$ (deg) | $\kappa$ |
|---|---|---|---|---|---|---|
| 1 | 1.3 | 53,456 | 952,380 | 4.94 | 7.45 | 0.3 |
| 2 | 1.06 | 88,823 | 94,663 | 18.665 | 0.00 | 0.165 |
| 3 | 1.04 | 72,082 | 32,735 | 14.9 | 21.20 | 0.11 |
| 4 | 1.10 | 19,657 | 45,520 | 2.022 | 49.85 | 0 |
| 5 | 1.33 | 53,316 | 53,787 | 6.0417 | 0.80 | 0.22 |

**TABLE 4 |** Parameter estimation for mid flap.

| Pig number | Thickness (mm) | C10 (Pa) | $k_1$ (Pa) | $k_2$ | $\alpha$ (degrees) | $\kappa$ |
|---|---|---|---|---|---|---|
| 1 | 0.58 | 92,963 | 230,290 | 13.90 | 87.1 | 0.33 |
| 2 | 0.59 | 73,144 | 235,075 | 7.86 | 68.7 | 0.3 |
| 3 | 0.54 | 64,042 | 212,120 | 4.99 | 23.5 | 0.32 |
| 4 | 0.70 | 52,072 | 125,430 | 5.87 | 53.9 | 0.26 |
| 5 | 0.47 | 45,588 | 149,880 | 1.42 | 55.6 | 0.21 |

**TABLE 5 |** Parameter estimation for distal false lumen wall.

| Pig number | Thickness (mm) | C10 (Pa) | $k_1$ (Pa) | $k_2$ | $\alpha$ (degrees) | $\kappa$ |
|---|---|---|---|---|---|---|
| 1 | 1.24 | 72,996 | 20,894 | 9.01 | 66.5 | 0 |
| 2 | 1.17 | 31,299 | 64,299 | 5.44 | 66.5 | 0.25 |
| 3 | 0.87 | 44,479 | 229,920 | 5.02 | 22.3 | 0.3 |
| 4 | 0.85 | 45,167 | 200,820 | 9.84 | 87.7 | 0.27 |
| 5 | 1.01 | 58,489 | 90,846 | 4.78 | 48.1 | 0.21 |

**TABLE 6 |** Parameter estimation for distal flap.

| Pig number | Thickness (mm) | C10 (Pa) | $k_1$ (Pa) | $k_2$ | $\alpha$ (degrees) | $\kappa$ |
|---|---|---|---|---|---|---|
| 1 | 0.4 | 103,140 | 61,969 | 4.1 | 62.4 | 0.1 |
| 2 | 0.34 | 171,740 | 661,830 | 8.05 | 86.5 | 0.3 |
| 3 | 0.43 | 78,686 | 239,090 | 3.18 | 89.9 | 0.3 |
| 4 | 0.29 | 63,554 | 77,013 | 4.76 | 83.4 | 0.11 |
| 5 | 0.47 | 55,960 | 78,560 | 2.86 | 89.9 | 0.19 |

the Cauchy (true) stress data obtained from the experiments, $\sigma_{\theta\theta}^{\Psi}$ and $\sigma_{zz}^{\Psi}$ were the Cauchy stresses for the $i^{th}$ point computed using Equation (9) and $n$ was the number of data points. The minimization algorithm optimized the five parameters for the HGO constitutive model, namely $C_{10}$, $k_1$, $k_2$, $\alpha$, and $\kappa$, using the objective function given as:

$$\chi^2 = \sum_{i=1}^{n} [(\sigma_{\theta\theta} - \sigma_{\theta\theta}^{\Psi})_i^2 + (\sigma_{zz} - \sigma_{zz}^{\Psi})_i^2] \qquad (12)$$

The minimization problem is ill-conditioned and thus, has several solutions for given limits on parameters. To achieve a global minimum, the algorithm was repeated for 200 different initial values of the parameters. Only the parameter estimates corresponding to the lowest chi-square value was selected.

7) For every feasible solution we imposed conditions of $R^2 \geq 0.9$ and a mean square root error, $\epsilon \leq 0.2$ that needed to be satisfied.
8) Performing steps 1–7, we obtained parameter values for each considered combination of protocols. If the parameter values from each combination could fit the data given by the original protocols (i.e., 1:1, 1:1.5, 1:2, 1.5:1, 2:1) with a $R^2 \geq 0.8$ and a mean error value, $\epsilon \leq 0.25$, those parameter values were chosen.
9) Finally, the median of the parameter values from combinations of protocols satisfying Step 8 was computed. The median values for $C_{10}$, $k_1$, $k_2$, and $\kappa$ were used to plot stress-strain curves for hyperelastic tissues.
10) In case the median of the parameter values obtained from Step 9 did not fulfill the criterion laid out in Step 8, we used the parameter values for the combination that considered data points from maximum number of protocols. This combination of protocols had already fulfilled the criterion in Step 8.

The code used to compute material parameters was included as **Supplementary Material**, The estimated parameter values for the different regions of the dissected aortas were recorded in **Tables 2–6**. The data in the tables were published in Ahuja et al. (2018) and reused as part of current research.

## RESULTS

The specimens and their corresponding material testing results from displacement protocols listed in **Table 1** were utilized by the non-linear regression algorithm for parameter estimation. The

estimation for each sample returned a $R^2 \geq 0.8$ and a mean error, $\epsilon \leq 0.25$ for every protocol that was used during the planar biaxial test measurement. The planar biaxial testing of different tissue specimens yielded the results summarized in **Tables 2–6**. The results in **Figure 3** presented stress-stretch curves along the circumferential and axial directions for tissue samples tested with an equibiaxial (1:1) displacement-controlled protocol. It could be observed that there were differences in the mechanical response of the tissues harvested from different animals.

From **Tables 2–6**, the material parameters were used in Equation (9) to give the stress values for all the different stretches i.e., $\lambda_\theta$ and $\lambda_z$. The average computed results as well as the standard errors for all the different tissue specimens were presented in **Figures 4, 5**. Specifically in **Figure 4**, the variation in the stiffnesses of TL wall, FL wall, and flap harvested from the same region were compared. In **Figure 5**,

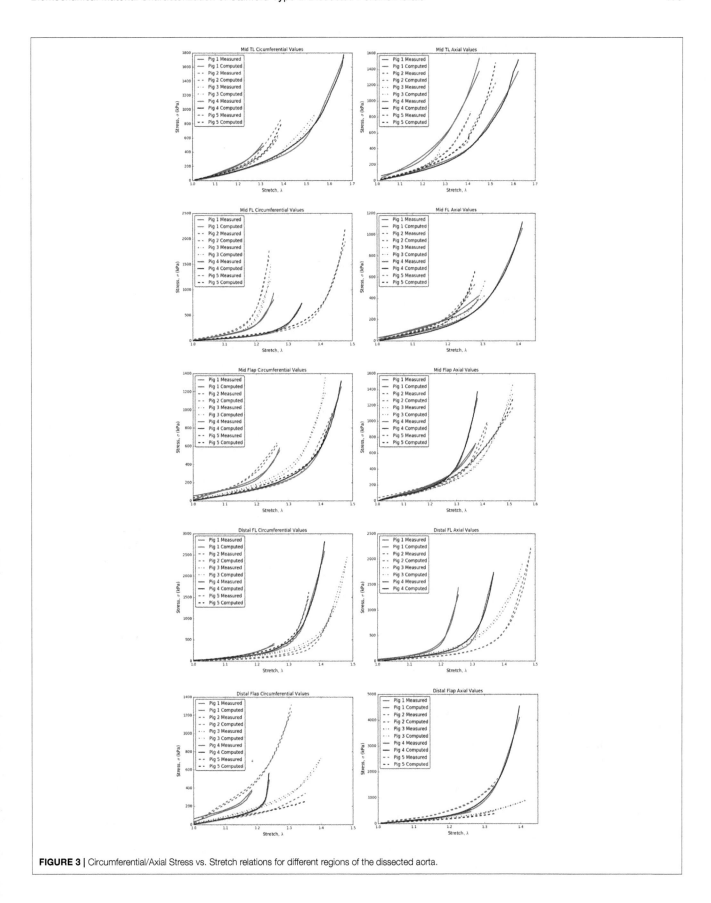

**FIGURE 3 |** Circumferential/Axial Stress vs. Stretch relations for different regions of the dissected aorta.

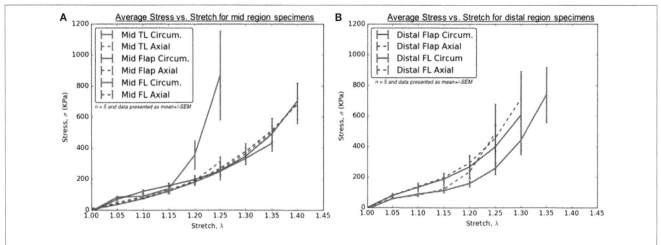

**FIGURE 4 | (A)** Average Stress vs. Stretch for the different specimens harvested from the mid region **(B)** Average Stress vs. Stretch for the different specimens harvested from distal region of thoracic aorta.

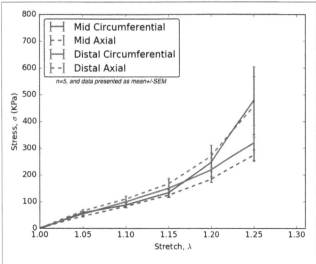

**FIGURE 5 |** For all stretches, $\lambda_\theta$, $\lambda_z \leq 1.25$, the axial and circumferential stresses generated in the mid and distal regions.

we plotted the differences in material behaviors of specimens as one advanced from mid to distal region. The axial and circumferential stresses generated in mid and distal regions were analyzed separately using a mixed-model analyses of variance (ANOVA) using IBM SPSS Statistics (v25, IBM corporation). To accomplish it, the mid TL, mid FL, and mid flap regions were grouped into one section called "Mid" and the remaining distal regions were grouped as another section called "Distal." For both axial and circumferential ANOVAs, mean stresses over the five stretch values (1.05, 1.10, 1.15, 1.20, 1.25) were analyzed with location (Mid vs. Distal) as the between-group variable and stretch value as the within-group (repeated measures) variable. In both axial and circumferential stress ANOVAs, the assumption of sphericity was violated and thus, the Greenhouse–Geisser correction was utilized for the stretch values.

In the ANOVA on axial stretches, results revealed a significant main effect of location [$F_{(1, 22)} = 5.80$, $p = 0.025$] with the distal region showing higher mean stresses than the mid region. There was a significant main effect of the stretch value [$F_{(1.09, 23.99)} = 43.85$, $p < 0.001$] i.e., mean stresses increased with stretch values. The location vs. stretch value interaction was not significant [$F_{(1.09, 23.99)} = 3.24$, $p > 0.05$] suggesting a similar rate of increase in stresses over the increasing stretch ratios in the mid and distal region. In the ANOVA on circumferential stretches, there was no significant main effect of location [$F_{(1, 21)} = 0.31$, $p > 0.05$], while the main effect of stretch value was significant [$F_{(1.02, 21.43)} = 13.90$, $p = 0.001$], again suggesting a similar rate of increase in stresses over the increasing stretch ratios. The location vs. stretch value interaction was not significant in the circumferential ANOVA [$F_{(1.02, 21.43)} = 1.00$, $p > 0.05$]. The comparison between mid and distal regions for axial and circumferential directions were given in **Figure 5**.

The variation in the material behavior of tissues were compared for a range of stretch values, $1 \leq \lambda_z$, $\lambda_\theta \leq 1.4$, and the dimensionless statistic, coefficient of variation ($COV = \sigma/\mu$, where $\sigma$ is the standard deviation and $\mu$ is the mean at a specific stretch value) was calculated from computational values to indicate the extent of variability in relation to the mean. Since standard errors only reflected absolute variability among specimens, we chose $CV$ to give us a relative insight into the variation in material behavior for every considered stretch value. **Tables 7A–J** lists the $CV$ for stresses generated in tissue samples stretched to different values as well as the corresponding mean and standard deviation results. $CV$ has been used to measure dispersion of critical parameter for a number of applications e.g., to measure precision and reproducibility in biological samples/assays, variability in soil compositions, etc. As there is no single $CV$-value to categorize a data series as less or more dispersive, we assumed a $COV > 0.3$ in this research as a measure of greater variation across stress data.

The following inferences were proposed based on the analysis of data in **Tables 7A–J**:

**TABLE 7A |** Statistical data for circumferential region of mid TL.

| Stretch value, $\lambda_\theta$ | CV |
| --- | --- |
| 1.05 | 0.10 |
| 1.10 | 0.13 |
| 1.15 | 0.18 |
| 1.2 | 0.17 |
| 1.25 | 0.19 |
| 1.3 | 0.26 |
| 1.35 | 0.25 |

**TABLE 7B |** Statistical data for axial region of mid TL.

| Stretch value, $\lambda_z$ | CV |
| --- | --- |
| 1.05 | 0.39 |
| 1.10 | 0.34 |
| 1.15 | 0.35 |
| 1.2 | 0.36 |
| 1.25 | 0.34 |
| 1.3 | 0.37 |
| 1.35 | 0.37 |
| 1.4 | 0.38 |

**TABLE 7C |** Statistical data for circumferential region of mid FL.

| Stretch value, $\lambda_\theta$ | CV |
| --- | --- |
| 1.05 | 0.36 |
| 1.10 | 0.38 |
| 1.15 | 0.46 |
| 1.2 | 0.66 |
| 1.25 | 0.73 |

**TABLE 7D |** Statistical data for axial region of mid FL.

| Stretch value, $\lambda_z$ | CV |
| --- | --- |
| 1.05 | 0.30 |
| 1.10 | 0.20 |
| 1.15 | 0.19 |
| 1.2 | 0.17 |
| 1.25 | 0.25 |

**TABLE 7E |** Statistical data for circumferential region of mid flap.

| Stretch value, $\lambda_\theta$ | CV |
| --- | --- |
| 1.05 | 0.32 |
| 1.10 | 0.28 |
| 1.15 | 0.27 |
| 1.2 | 0.33 |
| 1.25 | 0.42 |
| 1.3 | 0.16 |
| 1.35 | 0.20 |
| 1.4 | 0.28 |

**TABLE 7F |** Statistical data for axial region of mid flap.

| Stretch value, $\lambda_z$ | CV |
| --- | --- |
| 1.05 | 0.12 |
| 1.10 | 0.09 |
| 1.15 | 0.10 |
| 1.2 | 0.12 |
| 1.25 | 0.11 |
| 1.3 | 0.15 |
| 1.35 | 0.30 |
| 1.4 | 0.11 |

**TABLE 7G |** Statistical data for circumferential region of distal FL.

| Stretch value, $\lambda_\theta$ | CV |
| --- | --- |
| 1.05 | 0.07 |
| 1.10 | 0.24 |
| 1.15 | 0.28 |
| 1.2 | 0.27 |
| 1.25 | 0.33 |
| 1.3 | 0.33 |
| 1.35 | 0.48 |

**TABLE 7H |** Statistical data for axial region of distal FL.

| Stretch value, $\lambda_z$ | CV |
| --- | --- |
| 1.05 | 0.26 |
| 1.10 | 0.26 |
| 1.15 | 0.32 |
| 1.2 | 0.47 |
| 1.25 | 0.89 |

1. The *CVs* for mid TL wall (circumferential direction; **Table 7A**), mid FL wall (axial direction; **Table 7D**), and mid flap wall (axial direction; **Table 7F**) were <0.3 for all stretch values. Thus, there was less variation in tissue data for all stretches.
2. In the axial direction, the *CVs* for mid TL wall was >0.3 for all stretches, indicating dispersion in data. A large variation was observed between data from pig 1 and data from all other pigs (**Table 7B** and **Figure 3**).
3. In mid FL wall (**Table 7C**) and distal flap (**Table 7I**), the stresses along circumferential direction led to *CV*-values

>0.3. We observed a greater dispersion behavior between all specimens.
4. The circumferential direction of mid flap (**Table 7E**) resulted in *CVs* >0.3. The variation is shown in **Figure 6** and is attributed to differences between (Pigs 1 and 2) and (Pigs 3, 4, and 5).
5. The data analysis on circumferential directions for distal FL (**Table 7G**) yielded *CVs* > 0.3 only for stretches, $\lambda_\theta \geq 1.25$. Hence, at higher stretch values, there was variation among

**TABLE 7I** | Statistical data for circumferential region of distal flap.

| Stretch value, $\lambda_\theta$ | CV |
|---|---|
| 1.05 | 0.55 |
| 1.10 | 0.51 |
| 1.15 | 0.49 |
| 1.2 | 0.57 |
| 1.25 | 0.64 |
| 1.3 | 0.74 |

**TABLE 7J** | Statistical data for axial region of distal flap.

| Stretch value, $\lambda_z$ | CV |
|---|---|
| 1.05 | 0.22 |
| 1.10 | 0.26 |
| 1.15 | 0.29 |
| 1.2 | 0.39 |
| 1.25 | 0.42 |
| 1.3 | 0.51 |

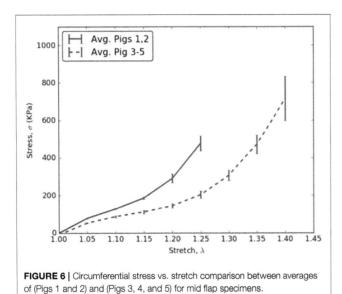

**FIGURE 6** | Circumferential stress vs. stretch comparison between averages of (Pigs 1 and 2) and (Pigs 3, 4, and 5) for mid flap specimens.

tissue specimens. In terms of mathematical formulation, $\Psi_{aniso}$ dictated the differences in the distribution of collagen fibers which led to variation in the stress responses at higher stretch values.

6. Similarly, stretching distal flap along axial direction (**Table 7J**) resulted in CV-values > 0.3 for stretch values, $\lambda_z \geq 1.20$.

## DISCUSSION

AD is the most common life-threatening disorder affecting the aorta. The literature is replete with material behavior characterization of thoracic and abdominal aortic aneurysm wall (Raghavan and Vorp, 2000; Thubrikar et al., 2001; Vorp, 2007; Speelman et al., 2009) but the data on mechanics of dissected aortic wall and intimal flap is incomplete (Pasta et al., 2012).

A better understanding of this critical condition is warranted since greater number of patients are undergoing endovascular treatments which requires interaction between the walls, the intimal flap of the dissection and endograft, or bare metal stent. This will allow us to assess the design and long-term utilization of aortic grafts. Thus, characterizing the material response of the different regions of dissected aorta using a structure based form of strain energy function will be useful in constructing well-informed computational models (e.g., FEA and FSI) which will expedite the development of endovascular therapy for successfully sealing the FL and thereby reducing mortality and future reinterventions.

## Non-linear Regression Analysis for Constitutive Modeling

The present study created artificial dissections in porcine aortas, conducted planar biaxial testing on tissue segments from different regions and then used a novel non-linear regression modeling interface to fit the five parameter HGO model for hyperelastic materials against measured data. The constitutive modeling for soft tissues has been widely utilized to understand its mechanical response and perform computational modeling for developing virtual therapies for treating diseases (Raghavan and Vorp, 2000; Holzapfel et al., 2004; Speelman et al., 2009; Patel et al., 2018). The algorithm introduced in this study utilized data from various protocols (i.e., 1:1, 1:1.5, 1:2, 1.5:1, 2:1) to develop an enriched HGO constitutive model relation that was trained on larger data set for achieving higher stress-stretch predictive capabilities (**Table 1**). The algorithm was validated by ensuring that the parameters selected for the HGO constitutive model could fit the measured data from each protocol with a $R^2 \geq 0.8$ and a mean error value of $\epsilon \leq 0.25$. This was in contrast with the approaches followed traditionally in literature (Zeinali-Davarani et al., 2013; Babu et al., 2015), where data collected from only equibiaxial protocol was considered or parameters were estimated from entire data set (Billiar and Sacks, 2000) without validating the constitutive model response to new data. This study proposed a rigorous algorithm for considering multiple combinations of material testing protocols. The resultant parameters estimated from different combinations were pooled together and the median values for $C_{10}$, $k_1$, $k_2$, $\alpha$, and $\kappa$ were computed. Only in the case when median values did not fit the data (Step 8 in section Algorithm for Non-linear Regression Modeling), the parameter values for the combination that considered data points from maximum number of protocols were used. The implementation of this novel algorithm was undertaken to propose a well-informed constitutive model that would allow development of a better computational model for understanding the mechanics of the aortic tissue in health and disease.

The material parameters, $C_{10}$, $k_1$, $k_2$, $\alpha$, and $\kappa$, for all tissue specimens from different regions of the dissected aorta were presented in **Tables 2–6**. These material parameters were used, as it is, for developing specimen-specific computational models for reproducing AD and analyzing the effects of therapy on the treatment of the disease (Ahuja et al., 2018).

## Clinical Relevance

A healthy aorta is pre-stretched axially to carry the pulse pressure with minimal variation in its length (Van Loon, 1977; Schulze-Bauer and Holzapfel, 2003; Sommer and Holzapfel, 2012). In the circumferential direction, the aorta resists distensibility by stiffening at higher stretches. With the creation of FL due to AD, two new regions, namely FL wall and intimal flap are created. It becomes important to highlight the importance of material response with respect to the circumferential and axial directions to support therapy as well as predict potential complications.

Patients with AD suffer from hypertension, which significantly adds to the existing longitudinal stresses in aorta leading to circumferential tearing along this orientation. As the dissected aorta dilates, the circumferential stresses on mid and distal FL wall increases according to Laplace's law. The weakened wall of distal FL has higher propensity to dilate at lower stresses along circumferential direction (**Figure 4B**) and as a result, there is a risk of aneurysm formation in patients (Lopera et al., 2003; Won et al., 2006). Furthermore, the blood flow induces additional normal and shear stresses on the compromised distal FL wall. Future simulations utilizing region-specific material properties would be required to understand the relationship between hemodynamics and structural loading and the formation of aneurysms in distal FL walls.

For treatment of AD, an endograft is first deployed to exclude the proximal entry tear to redirect blood flow toward the TL and then a stent graft is used to push the intimal flap against the FL wall such that the aorta is reconstituted by sealing the FL. The deployment of stents/graft will be dependent on circumferential stiffnesses of mid and distal flaps. According to our results in **Figure 5**, significant differences were not observed in circumferential stresses between mid and distal regions. This observation will be an important factor in sizing stents (Ahuja et al., 2018).

## Stiffness of TL Wall, FL Wall, and Flap Harvested From the Same Region

In the mid region, the stress-stretch plots for each region were superimposed and shown in **Figure 4A**. It was observed that the mid FL region was the stiffest when tested biaxially in both the circumferential and axial directions. A slightly higher stiffness was observed along the circumferential direction in the mid region of the flap for small stretch values ($\lambda_\theta$ < 1.2). At higher stretch values, the curves for mid region of flap overlapped indicating similar material behavior along the two principal directions. Lower stress values in the circumferential direction of the mid TL region indicated higher density of collagen fibers along axial direction.

In the distal region, a different trend was observed for the flap and the FL wall. The flap tissue was stiffest in the axial direction as shown by high stresses in **Figure 4B**. On the contrary, the FL wall was the least stiff along the circumferential direction but eventually became stiffer and showed asymptotic material behavior in the axial direction for $\lambda_z$ > 1.2.

## Differences Between Mid and Distal Regions

The results in **Figure 5** showed that the mid region tissue was stiffer along circumferential direction at higher stretches ($\lambda_\theta \geq 1.2$) which decreased as one advanced toward the distal region. The axial direction was stiffer in the distal region suggesting greater presence of collagen fibers along that direction. Thus, a change in the distribution and orientation of the collagen fibers as one moved from mid to distal region of dissected aorta was observed.

## Variability Between Tissue Specimens From Different Pigs

The results showed that CVs > 0.3 were obtained for all studied tissue regions (i.e., mid TL, mid FL, mid flap, distal FL, distal flap). In all tissue regions except mid TL, the CV-values were larger along circumferential direction as compared to axial direction. This could be attributed to the differences in the collagen fiber content and their orientations, which led to higher variability between specimens. Consequentially, it becomes imperative to perform patient-specific measurements and computations for choosing the accurate therapy to treat AD patients.

## LIMITATIONS OF STUDY

The planar biaxial testing methodology assumed aortic tissue samples as incompressible because of the presence of high water content. As a result, the stretch of tissue along the radial direction was given as $\lambda_r = 1/\lambda_1\lambda_2$. A small error was introduced in our calculations because of this assumption (Taghizadeh et al., 2015). Moreover, the experimental studies conducted for this research did not include the effects of in-plane shear as we assumed the x- and y-directions for the specimens to be oriented along the principal directions; i.e., circumferential and axial. A method proposed in Sacks (2000) oriented specimens at specific angles to produce a state of simultaneous in-plane shear and normal strains. This method would be explored and incorporated in future studies if the in-plane shear strains are comparable to the normal strains. Our current approach optimized the five parameters for the HGO constitutive model, namely $C_{10}$, $k_1$, $k_2$, $\alpha$, and $\kappa$, using an objective function. The orientation and distribution of fibers in the tissue specimens, represented by $\alpha$ and $\kappa$, respectively, were calculated numerically. An alternative approach would be to conduct histology on the dissected aorta specimens to visualize the collagen fibers using fluorescence microscope. The histological measurements of $\alpha$ and $\kappa$ can then be incorporated into the HGO constitutive model for optimizing the remaining parameters, $C_{10}$, $k_1$, $k_2$. Even though the biaxial measurements were conducted on tissue specimens within 16 h of harvesting, there is a concern regarding swelling of these samples. In future, biaxial tests would be undertaken on fresh samples and compared with samples that have been stored over certain number of hours. This would allow in precisely predicting the enzymatic degradation of tissue samples over a range of time span.

Further, it was realized that the use of healthy tissues could be a limitation in comparing with an actual dissection where the aortic wall is diseased and weak. The presented mathematical model was developed to compare with our developed acute *in-vivo* porcine animal model which is out of the scope of current paper. Nonetheless, these results provided insight into type B dissections occurring, for example, as a result of blunt chest trauma from motor accidents (Turhan et al., 2004).

## CONCLUSIONS

From the results presented above, it was shown that there were significant differences in the mechanical responses of tissue specimens harvested from different regions of a dissected aorta. Hence, the null hypothesis was true, and it was suggested that one should use region-specific material properties when simulating the structural and hemodynamic response of a dissected aorta to external loading. In future, accurate simulations would allow in advancing the development of properly sized grafts for

treating AD and thereby, reducing patient reinterventions during followups.

## AUTHOR CONTRIBUTIONS

AA is the first author of this research and contributed to this manuscript extensively. JN prepared the samples and supervised the bench testing. TT conducted bench testing and saved the data in.csv files. BP assisted AA with the biomechanical characterization of tissues. JK provided expert insight into the material behavior of tissues and assisted with the calibration and functioning of bench testing machine. BP, JN, SC, and GK contributed to critical sections of the paper, the protocol, and revision of the drafts.

## ACKNOWLEDGMENTS

The authors thank Dr. Amy Spilkin for providing expertise in statistical analysis.

## REFERENCES

Ahuja, A., Guo, X., Noblet, J. N., Krieger, J. F., Roeder, B., Haulon, S., et al. (2018). Validated computational model to compute re-apposition pressures for treating type-B aortic dissections. *Front. Physiol.* 9:513. doi: 10.3389/fphys.2018.00513

Alimohammadi, M., Sherwood, J. M., Karimpour, M., Agu, O., Balabani, S., and Díaz-Zuccarini, V. (2015). Aortic dissection simulation models for clinical support: fluid-structure interaction vs. rigid wall models. *Biomed. Eng.* 14:34. doi: 10.1186/s12938-015-0032-6

Babu, A. R., Byju, A. G., and Gundiah, N. (2015). Biomechanical properties of human ascending thoracic aortic dissections. *J. Biomech. Eng.* 137:081013. doi: 10.1115/1.4030752

Billiar, K. L., and Sacks, M. S. (2000). Biaxial mechanical properties of the native and glutaraldehyde-treated aortic valve cusp: part II—a structural constitutive model. *J. Biomech. Eng.* 122, 327–335. doi: 10.1115/1.1287158

Canchi, S., Guo, X., Phillips, M., Berwick, Z., Kratzberg, J., Krieger, J., et al. (2017). Role of re-entry tears on the dynamics of type B dissection flap. *Ann. Biomed. Eng.* 46, 186–196. doi: 10.1007/s10439-017-1940-3

Cleveland, W. S. (1979). Robust locally weighted regression and smoothing scatterplots. *J. Am. Stat. Assoc.* 74, 829–836. doi: 10.1080/01621459.1979.10481038

Erbel, R., Alfonso, F., Boileau, C., Dirsch, O., Eber, B., Haverich, A., et al. (2001). Diagnosis and management of aortic dissection. *Eur. Heart J.* 22, 1642–1681. doi: 10.1053/euhj.2001.2782

Gasser, T. C., Ogden, R. W., and Holzapfel, G. A. (2006). Hyperelastic modelling of arterial layers with distributed collagen fibre orientations. *J. R. Soc. Interf.* 3, 15–35. doi: 10.1098/rsif.2005.0073

Golledge, J., and Eagle, K. A. (2008). Acute aortic dissection. *Lancet* 372, 55–66. doi: 10.1016/S0140-6736(08)60994-0

Greenberg, R., Khwaja, J., Haulon, S., and Fulton, G. (2003). Aortic dissections: new perspectives and treatment paradigms. *Eur. J. Vasc. Endovasc. Surg.* 26, 579–586. doi: 10.1016/S1078-5884(03)00415-5

Gundiah, N., Ratcliffe, M. B., and Pruitt, L. A. (2009). The biomechanics of arterial elastin. *J. Mech. Behav. Biomed. Mater.* 2, 288–296. doi: 10.1016/j.jmbbm.2008.10.007

Hagan, P. G., Nienaber, C. A., Isselbacher, E. M., Bruckman, D., Karavite, D. J., Russman, P. L., et al. (2000). International Registry of Acute Aortic Dissection (IRAD): new insights from an old disease. *JAMA* 283, 897–903. doi: 10.1001/jama.283.7.897

Halme, T., Savunen, T., Aho, H., Vihersaari, T., and Penttinen, R. (1985). Elastin and collagen in the aortic wall: changes in the Marfan

syndrome and annuloaortic ectasia. *Exp. Mol. Pathol.* 43, 1–12. doi: 10.1016/0014-4800(85)90050-4

Holzapfel, G. A., and Gasser, T. C. (2001). A viscoelastic model for fiber-reinforced composites at finite strains: continuum basis, computational aspects and applications. *Comput. Methods Appl. Mech. Eng.* 190, 4379–4403. doi: 10.1016/S0045-7825(00)00323-6

Holzapfel, G. A., Gasser, T. C., and Ogden, R. W. (2000). A new constitutive framework for arterial wall mechanics and a comparative study of material models. *J. Elast.* 61, 1–48. doi: 10.1023/A:1010835316564

Holzapfel, G. A., Sommer, G., and Regitnig, P. (2004). Anisotropic mechanical properties of tissue components in human atherosclerotic plaques. *J. Biomech. Eng.* 126, 657–665. doi: 10.1115/1.1800557

Jhun, C. S., Evans, M. C., Barocas, V. H., and Tranquillo, R. T. (2009). Planar biaxial mechanical behavior of bioartificial tissues possessing prescribed fiber alignment. *J. Biomech. Eng.* 131:081006. doi: 10.1115/1.3148194

Juang, D., Braverman, A. C., and Eagle, K. (2008). Cardiology patient page. Aortic dissection. *Circulation* 118, e507–e510. doi: 10.1161/CIRCULATIONAHA.108.799908

Lopera, J., Patiño, J. H., Urbina, C., García, G., Alvarez, L. G., Upegui, L., et al. (2003). Endovascular treatment of complicated type-B aortic dissection with stent-grafts: midterm results. *J. Vasc. Interv. Radiol.* 14, 195–203. doi: 10.1097/01.RVI.0000058321.82956.76

Mann, D. L., Zipes, D. P., Libby, P., Bonow, R. O., and Braunwald, E. (2015). *Braunwald's Heart Disease A Textbook of Cardiovascular Medicine, 10th Edn.* Philadelphia, PA: Elsevier; Saunders.

Nelder, J. A., and Mead, R. (1965). A simplex method for function minimization. *Comput. J.* 7, 308–313. doi: 10.1093/comjnl/7.4.308

Nienaber, C. A., and Eagle, K. A. (2003). Aortic dissection: new frontiers in diagnosis and management: part I: from etiology to diagnostic strategies. *Circulation* 108, 628–635. doi: 10.1161/01.CIR.0000087009.16755.E4

Pasta, S., Phillippi, J. A., Gleason, T. G., and Vorp, D. A. (2012). Effect of aneurysm on the mechanical dissection properties of the human ascending thoracic aorta. *J. Thorac. Cardiovasc. Surg.* 143, 460–467. doi: 10.1016/j.jtcvs.2011.07.058

Patel, A. Y., Eagle, K. A., and Vaishnava, P. (2014). Acute type B aortic dissection: insights from the International Registry of Acute Aortic Dissection. *Ann. Cardiothorac. Surg.* 3:368. doi: 10.3978/j.issn.2225-319X.2014.07.06

Patel, B., Chen, H., Ahuja, A., Krieger, J. F., Noblet, J., Chambers, S., et al. (2018). Constitutive modeling of the passive inflation-extension behavior of the swine colon. *J. Mech. Behav. Biomed. Mater.* 77, 176–186. doi: 10.1016/j.jmbbm.2017.08.031

Peelukhana, S. V., Wang, Y., Berwick, Z., Kratzberg, J., Krieger, J., Roeder, B., et al. (2016). Role of pulse pressure and geometry of primary entry tear in acute type B dissection propagation. *Ann. Biomed. Eng.* 45, 592–603. doi: 10.1007/s10439-016-1705-4

Raghavan, M. L., and Vorp, D. A. (2000). Toward a biomechanical tool to evaluate rupture potential of abdominal aortic aneurysm: identification of a finite strain constitutive model and evaluation of its applicability. *J. Biomech.* 33, 475–482. doi: 10.1016/S0021-9290(99)00201-8

Rashid, B., Destrade, M., and Gilchrist, M. D. (2013). Influence of preservation temperature on the measured mechanical properties of brain tissue. *J. Biomech.* 46, 1276–1281. doi: 10.1016/j.jbiomech.2013.02.014

Rassoli, A., Shafigh, M., Seddighi, A., Seddighi, A., Daneshparvar, H., and Fatouraee, N. (2014). Biaxial mechanical properties of human ureter under tension. *Urol. J.* 11, 1678–1686. doi: 10.22037/uj.v11i3.2472

Roberts, W. C. (1981). Aortic dissection: anatomy, consequences, and causes. *Am. Heart J.* 101, 195–214. doi: 10.1016/0002-8703(81)90666-9

Sacks, M. S. (2000). Biaxial mechanical evaluation of planar biological materials. *J. Elast.* 61, 199. doi: 10.1023/A:1010917028671

Schulze-Bauer, C. A., and Holzapfel, G. A. (2003). Determination of constitutive equations for human arteries from clinical data. *J. Biomech.* 36, 165–169. doi: 10.1016/S0021-9290(02)00367-6

Sommer, G., and Holzapfel, G. A. (2012). 3D constitutive modeling of the biaxial mechanical response of intact and layer-dissected human carotid arteries. *J. Mech. Behav. Biomed. Mater.* 5, 116–128. doi: 10.1016/j.jmbbm.2011.08.013

Speelman, L., Bosboom, E. M., Schurink, G. W., Buth, J., Breeuwer, M., Jacobs, M. J., et al. (2009). Initial stress and nonlinear material behavior in patient-specific AAA wall stress analysis. *J. Biomech.* 42, 1713–1719. doi: 10.1016/j.jbiomech.2009.04.020

Spencer, A. J. M. (1971). "Theory of invariants," in *Continuum Physics*, ed A. C. Eringen (New York, NY: Academic Press), 239–253. doi: 10.1016/B978-0-12-240801-4.50008-X

Taghizadeh, H., Tafazzoli-Shadpour, M., Shadmehr, M. B., and Fatouraee, N. (2015). Evaluation of biaxial mechanical properties of aortic media based on the lamellar microstructure. *Materials (Basel).* 8, 302–316. doi: 10.3390/ma8010302

Thubrikar, M. J., Labrosse, M., Robicsek, F., Al-Soudi, J., and Fowler, B. (2001). Mechanical properties of abdominal aortic aneurysm wall. *J. Med. Eng. Technol.* 25, 133–142. doi: 10.1080/03091900110057806

Turhan, H., Topaloglu, S., Cagli, K., Sasmaz, H., and Kutuk, E. (2004). Traumatic type B aortic dissection causing near total occlusion of aortic lumen and diagnosed by transthoracic echocardiography: a case report. *J. Am. Soc. Echocardiogr.* 17, 80–82. doi: 10.1016/j.echo.2003.09.011

Van Loon, P. (1977). Length-force and volume-pressure relationships of arteries. *Biorheology* 14, 181–201. doi: 10.3233/BIR-1977-14405

Vecht, R. J., Besterman, E. M., Bromley, L. L., Eastcott, H. H., and Kenyon, J. R. (1980). Acute dissection of aorta: long-term review and management. *Lancet* 1, 109–111. doi: 10.1016/S0140-6736(80)90601-7

Vorp, D. A. (2007). Biomechanics of abdominal aortic aneurysm. *J. Biomech.* 40, 1887–1902. doi: 10.1016/j.jbiomech.2006.09.003

Won, J. Y., Suh, S. H., Ko, H. K., Lee, K. H., Shim, W. H., Chang, B. C., et al. (2006). Problems Encountered during and after Stent-Graft Treatment of Aortic Dissection. *J. Vasc. Interv. Radiol.* 17 (2): 271–281. doi: 10.1097/01.RVI.0000195141.98163.30

Zeinali-Davarani, S., Chow, M. J., Turcotte, R., and Zhang, Y. (2013). Characterization of biaxial mechanical behavior of porcine aorta under gradual elastin degradation. *Ann. Biomed. Eng.* 41, 1528–1538. doi: 10.1007/s10439-012-0733-y

Zemánek, M., Burša, J., and Děták, M. (2009). Biaxial tension tests with soft tissues of arterial wall. *Eng. Mech.* 16, 3–11. Available online at: http://dlib.lib.cas.cz/5251/

# 16

# Evaluation of a Novel Finite Element Model of Active Contraction in the Heart

*Xiaoyan Zhang[1], Zhan-Qiu Liu[1], Kenneth S. Campbell[2] and Jonathan F. Wenk[1,3]\**

[1] *Department of Mechanical Engineering, University of Kentucky, Lexington, KY, United States, [2] Department of Physiology, University of Kentucky, Lexington, KY, United States, [3] Department of Surgery, University of Kentucky, Lexington, KY, United States*

*\*Correspondence:*
*Jonathan F. Wenk*
*wenk@engr.uky.edu*

Finite element (FE) modeling is becoming a widely used approach for the investigation of global heart function. In the present study, a novel model of cellular-level systolic contraction, which includes both length- and velocity-dependence, was implemented into a 3D non-linear FE code. To validate this new FE implementation, an optimization procedure was used to determine the contractile parameters, associated with sarcomeric function, by comparing FE-predicted pressure and strain to experimental measures collected with magnetic resonance imaging and catheterization in the ventricles of five healthy rats. The pressure-volume relationship generated by the FE models matched well with the experimental data. Additionally, the regional distribution of end-systolic strains and circumferential-longitudinal shear angle exhibited good agreement with experimental results overall, with the main deviation occurring in the septal region. Moreover, the FE model predicted a heterogeneous distribution of sarcomere re-lengthening after ventricular ejection, which is consistent with previous *in vivo* studies. In conclusion, the new FE active contraction model was able to predict the global performance and regional mechanical behaviors of the LV during the entire cardiac cycle. By including more accurate cellular-level mechanisms, this model could provide a better representation of the LV and enhance cardiac research related to both systolic and diastolic dysfunction.

**Keywords: cross-bridge kinetics, velocity-dependence, relaxation, sarcomere lengthening, left ventricle**

## INTRODUCTION

Cardiac muscle constitutes the histological foundation of the heart. The contraction of cardiac muscle cells (i.e., myocytes) generates force and propels blood out of the heart chambers into the circulatory system. In general, the active contraction of myocytes involves complex mechanisms. Briefly, upon activation, the influx of $Ca^{2+}$ ions promotes their binding to the troponin C molecules, altering the shape of the troponin complex and exposing the binding sites on the actin monomers to myosin heads. Once attached to the binding sites, the myosin heads undergo conformational changes and generate force, leading to shortening of the sarcomeres, the contractile units of myocytes (Gordon et al., 2000; Kobayashi and Solaro, 2005). *In vitro* cellular experiments have shown that the force generated during myocyte contraction depends on the intracellular concentration of free $Ca^{2+}$ and the length, as well as the shortening velocity, of sarcomeres (ter Keurs et al., 1980; Daniels et al., 1984; Keurs et al., 1988).

Computational modeling is an important approach for studying the function of the heart, especially the left ventricle (LV). Previously, several finite element (FE) models have been established to investigate the muscle contraction of the LV during cardiac systole (Guccione and McCulloch, 1993; Guccione et al., 1993; Hunter et al., 1998). Among those widely used FE models is the simple but computationally efficient time-varying "elastance" model, in which the active fiber stress is computed from a function of peak intracellular $Ca^{2+}$ concentration, time and sarcomere length (Guccione et al., 1993; Kerckhoffs et al., 2007). This model has been used to successfully assess the effects of apical torsion on heart function (Trumble et al., 2011), as well as predict decreased contractility in the border zone myocardium of ovine and human hearts with myocardial infarction (Wenk et al., 2011, 2012). However, this modeling approach does not include the force-velocity relation of cardiac muscle contraction, and neglects to represent the processes occurring at the cellular level.

In addition to the global-level FE models, there are several cellular-level models of myocyte contraction (Trayanova and Rice, 2011). These models were developed based on the Huxley 2-state cross-bridge model (Huxley, 1957), and have been shown to reproduce the typical mechanical features of myocyte contraction under certain experimental conditions (Schneider et al., 2006; Campbell et al., 2008; Rice et al., 2008). Recently, a more flexible myocyte contraction model (called MyoSim) has been developed by Campbell (2014). MyoSim extends the Huxley model by incorporating $Ca^{2+}$ activation, cooperative effects and the effects of interfilamentary movement, which implicitly depend on the length and velocity of sarcomeres during contraction (Campbell, 2014). Moreover, the use of cross-bridge distribution techniques allows MyoSim to predict the mechanical behavior of myocytes under a wider range of experimental conditions as compared to the deformation-based methods (Razumova et al., 1999; Rice et al., 2008). However, cellular-level models are unable to predict the global function of the heart. In this regard, a deformation-based myocyte contraction model (Rice et al., 2008) has been previously adapted into a FE model of the LV to investigate the mechanical properties of a mouse heart (Land et al., 2012). This suggests that the incorporation of an enhanced cellular-level contraction model, i.e., MyoSim, may further improve the behavior of a global-level FE model of ventricular function.

Along this line, the present work introduces a 3D FE implementation of cardiac muscle contraction that was developed based on MyoSim. This allows for the coupling of cellular-level mechanisms into a ventricle-level model. The new method was then validated using animal-specific FE models of the whole LV in rats. Specifically, the results of the models were fit to experimental measures of myocardial strain and ventricular hemodynamics, in order to determine the sarcomeric parameters that govern contraction.

## MATERIALS AND METHODS
### Experimental Measurements
In order to assess regional wall deformation in the LVs of healthy rats, 3D cine displacement encoding with stimulated echoes (DENSE) cardiovascular magnetic resonance (CMR) imaging was performed on 5 female Sprague-Dawley rats (~6 months; Harlan, Indianapolis, IN, USA) using a 7T Bruker ClinScan system (Bruker, Ettlingen, Germany; Zhong et al., 2011; Haggerty et al., 2013; Zhang et al., 2017), followed by LV pressure measurements using a pressure transducer (SPR-903, Millar Instruments, Houston, TX, USA; Pacher et al., 2008). End systolic (ES) strains, relative to end diastole (ED), were calculated using the software DENSEanalysis (Spottiswoode et al., 2007). ES LV torsion, represented as the circumferential-longitudinal (CL) shear angle $\alpha_{CL}$, was calculated as follows (Rüssel et al., 2009; Zhang et al., 2017):

$$\alpha_{CL} = sin^{-1} \frac{2E_{cl}}{\sqrt{(1 + 2E_{cc})(1 + 2E_{ll})}} \tag{1}$$

In order to generate animal-specific FE models, at a minimally loaded state, the LV myocardium was contoured from the CMR images at early-diastolic filling. These contours where then converted into 3D geometric surfaces. All animal procedures were approved by the Institutional Animal Care and Use Committee at the University of Kentucky and were in agreement with the guidelines by the National Institutes of Health for the care and use of laboratory animals (NIH Publication 85–23, revised 1996).

### Ventricular FE Model
Each animal-specific LV FE model was created based on the geometric surface data and size of the corresponding rat LV at early diastole (**Figure 1**). The FE mesh was produced by filling the myocardial wall with 8-node hexahedral brick elements incorporating a trilinear interpolation scheme (TrueGrid; XYZ Scientific, Inc., Livermore, CA, USA). The myocardium was evenly divided into 3 layers (i.e., epicardium, mid-myocardium, and endocardium; **Figure 1**; Zhang et al., 2015). The initial sarcomere lengths in each of the three layers, defined in the unloaded reference state of the model, were epi: 1,910 nm, mid: 1,850 nm, and endo: 1,780 nm (Guccione et al., 1993). The helical fiber angles in the epicardium, mid-myocardium, and endocardium were assigned as −60, 0, and 60°, respectively, relative to the circumferential direction. The boundary conditions of the LV were assigned to allow the base to expand/contract radially within the plane, with movement in the direction normal to the plane fully constrained. To simulate the passive filling and ejection of the LV, the volumetric flowrate into and out of the LV was estimated from CMR images (**Figures 2A,B**) and used to drive the entire cardiac cycle.

The myocardium of the LV was assumed to be nearly incompressible, transversely isotropic, and hyperelastic. The passive stresses were derived from the following strain energy function:

$$W = \frac{C}{2} \left\{ exp \left[ b_f E_{11}^2 + b_t \left( E_{22}^2 + E_{33}^2 + E_{23}^2 + E_{32}^2 \right) \right. \right.$$
$$\left. \left. + b_{fs}(E_{12}^2 + E_{21}^2 + E_{13}^2 + E_{31}^2) \right] - 1 \right\} \tag{2}$$

where $E_{11}$ is fiber strain, $E_{22}$ is cross-fiber strain, $E_{33}$ is radial strain, and the remaining terms are shear strains (Guccione et al.,

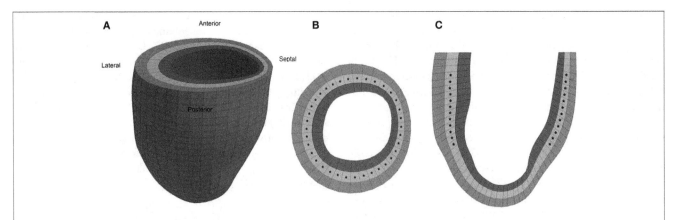

**FIGURE 1 |** Representative animal-specific FE model of a rat LV. **(A)** Full view of the LV model with the four segments labeled, **(B)** Short axis view of a mid-ventricular slice, and **(C)** Long axis view of a longitudinal slice. Stars represent the points in the model where strain was compared to experimental measurements during the optimization.

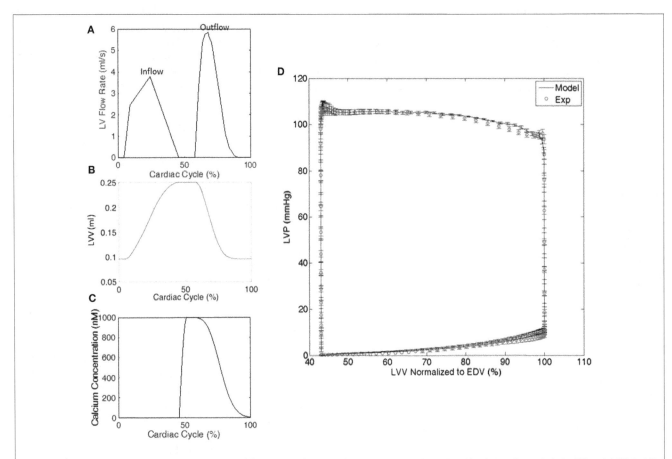

**FIGURE 2 |** Representative examples from a single rat of **(A)** the volumetric flowrate into and out of the LV used to drive the cardiac cycle in the FE model, **(B)** the LV volume (LVV) generated by the FE model, and **(C)** the calcium transient in the LV model. **(D)** The LV pressure-volume relationship generated by all of the FE models and experiments. LV pressure (LVP) data are mean ± standard error (SE); $n = 5$. LVV data shown in **(D)** were normalized to end diastolic volume (EDV).

1993; Wenk et al., 2011). Values for the material constants $b_f$, $b_t$, and $b_{fs}$ were chosen as 18.48, 3.58, and 1.627, respectively, based on previous studies (Guccione et al., 2001; Zhang et al., 2015). The material constant $C$ was adjusted until the LV ED pressure matched the experimentally measured value for each rat. The

value was found to be $C = 0.262 ± 0.082$ kPa (mean ± standard error).

The active material properties were derived from the 2-state MyoSim model of striated muscle (Campbell, 2014). Briefly, the myosin heads can switch between detached and attached states, and can form cross-bridges with different lengths ranging from −10 to 10 nm (**Figure 3**). Particularly, when a myosin head is bound to a directly opposed binding site, the length of the cross-bridge was assigned a value of $x_{ps}$ (**Figure 3**). In the current model, the cross-bridges were classified, based on their lengths, into 21 bins with bin-width of 1 nm (i.e., $x_1$ to $x_n$, $n = 21$; **Figure 3**). 21 bins were used to maintain an appropriate balance between accuracy and computational efficiency. The population distribution of cross-bridges in the $i$th bin, i.e., the number of myosin heads attached to the thin filament with a cross-bridge length of $x_i$ at time $t$, which is defined as $A(x_i, t)$, was calculated with the following set of 21 coupled ordinary differential equations (ODE) using an explicit 4th-order Runge-Kutta method with adaptive time-step size:

$$\frac{\partial A(x_i, t)}{\partial t} = k_1(x_i) D(t) - k_{-1}(x_i) A(x_i, t) \ (i = 1, 2, 3, ..., 21)$$

$$(3)$$

where $k_1(x_i)$ and $k_{-1}(x_i)$ are the strain-dependent rate constants for the attachment and detachment transitions, respectively. $D(t)$ is the number of myosin heads in the detached state and is determined by the following equation:

$$D(t) = N(t) - N_{bound} \qquad (4)$$

where $N(t)$ is the total number of sites that are activated and available for myosin heads to attach to, and $N_{bound}$ is the number of sites that have already been occupied by myosin heads and is equivalent to the total number of myosin heads in the attached state (i.e., $\sum_{i=1}^{21} A(x_i, t)$). To compute the total number of activated sites, $N(t)$, a forward Euler method was used to solve the following equation:

$$\frac{dN(t)}{dt} = a_{on} \left[ Ca^{2+} \right] \left( N_{overlap} - N(t) \right) - a_{off} \left( N(t) - N_{bound} \right)$$

$$+ k_{plus} N_{bound} - k_{minus}(N_{overlap} - N(t)) \qquad (5)$$

where $a_{on}$ and $a_{off}$ are rate constants, $k_{plus}$ and $k_{minus}$ are constants defining cooperative effects, and $N_{overlap}$ is the maximum number of binding sites that heads could potentially interact with and was defined by the relative positions of the thick and thin filaments within each half of a sarcomere, as previously reported (Campbell, 2009). A calcium transient $\left[ Ca^{2+} \right]$, which was based on experimentally recorded transients from intact rabbit hearts (Laurita and Singal, 2001), was temporally scaled according to each animal-specific heart rate and used in all 5 FE models in the present study (**Figure 2C**). The beginning of the transient was synchronized to the beginning of the isovolumic phase in each FE model. To include the effects of interfilamentary movement, linear interpolation was used to displace the population distributions $A(x_i, t)$ by $(1/2)\Delta x$, yielding $A_s(x_i, t)$, where $\Delta x$ is the half-sarcomere length change between time steps (Huxley et al., 1994; Tajima et al., 1994; Campbell, 2014). Since $\Delta x$ is highly influenced by the velocity of sarcomere shortening/lengthening, the incorporation of interfilamentary movement accounts for, at least in part, the velocity-dependence of force generation.

Finally, the active stress along the fiber direction ($T$) produced by cross-bridges was calculated as follows:

$$T(t) = \sum_{i=1}^{21} \rho k_{cb} A_s(x_i, t)(x_i + x_{ps}) \qquad (6)$$

where $\rho$ is the number of myosin heads in a hypothetical half-sarcomere with a cross-sectional area of 1 m$^2$, and $k_{cb}$ is the stiffness of the cross-bridges. To ensure that the FE model generates realistic active stress throughout the entire cardiac cycle, the following conditions were applied within the model framework: (i) $N(t) \geq 0$ at any time; (ii) $N(t) \geq N_{bound}$ at any time point; (iii) $D(t) \geq 0$ at any time; (iv) active fiber stress $T = 0$ when the sarcomere length was shortened to 1.20 µm. These conditions are necessary in order to maintain a physiological response, i.e., not allowing $N(t)$ to attain a negative value. A summary of parameters used for the active stress calculation is shown in **Table 1**, which are related to the MyoSim model (Campbell, 2014). In addition, stress components equivalent to 25% of the fiber stress were added to the two cross-fiber directions.

Both the passive and active material laws were implemented as a user defined material subroutine in the explicit non-linear FE solver LS-DYNA (Livermore Software Technology Corporation, Livermore, CA, USA).

## Optimization Procedure

In order to determine the active material parameters used for the 2-state contraction model, numerical optimization was

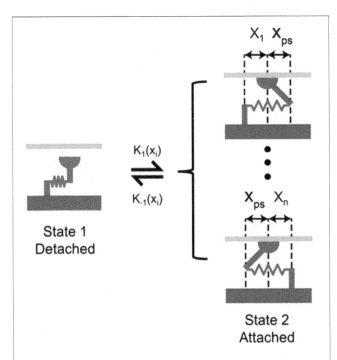

**FIGURE 3** | Schematic of the 2-state contraction model based on MyoSim. $x_1$ to $x_n$ are different lengths of cross-bridges ($n = 21$ in the proposed FE model); $x_{ps}$ is the cross-bridge length when the myosin head is bound to a directly opposed binding site; $k_1(x_i)$ and $k_{-1}(x_i)$ are the strain-dependent rate constants for the attachment and detachment transitions, respectively.

**TABLE 1 |** Parameters for active stress calculation with 2-state model.

| Parameter | Definition | Value | Unit |
|---|---|---|---|
| $\rho$ | Number of myosin heads in a hypothetical half-sarcomere with a cross-sectional area of 1 m$^2$ | $6.9 \times 10^{16}$ | m$^{-2}$ |
| $k_{cb}$ | Stiffness of the cross-bridges | 0.001 | N/m |
| $x_{ps}$ | Cross-bridge length when a myosin head is bound to a directly opposed binding site | 5 | nm |
| $a_{on}$ | Rate constant | DO* | s$^{-1}$nM$^{-1}$ |
| $a_{off}$ | Rate constant | DO* | s$^{-1}$ |
| $k_{plus}$ | Constant defining positive cooperative effects | DO* | s$^{-1}$ |
| $k_{minus}$ | Constant defining negative cooperative effects | DO* | s$^{-1}$ |
| $k_1(x_i)$ | Attachment rate constant | $C_k e^{\frac{-k_{cb}x_i^2}{2BT}}$ (DO*) | s$^{-1}$nm$^{-1}$ |
| $k_{-1}(x_i)$ | Detachment rate constant | $k_d + k_{db}x_i^4$ (DO*) | s$^{-1}$ |

$x_i$, cross-bridge length as defined in **Figure 3** in nm. B, Boltzmann constant (1.381 $\times 10^{-23}$ JK$^{-1}$). T, the experimental temperature (288 K).
DO*, Determined by optimization.

performed with the software LS-OPT (Livermore Software Technology Corporation, Livermore, CA) as previously described (Wenk et al., 2012; Wang et al., 2016). In the current study, a hybrid technique was employed, which utilized global and local search algorithms. Specifically, simulated annealing was used as a global optimizer to locate the region of the parameter space with the highest probability of containing the best set of parameters. Once this region was identified, the sequential response surface method, which is a gradient-based method, was employed to find the local minimum by iteratively reducing the size of the parameter space until the optimal set of parameters was achieved. A total of 10 parameters were optimized within the ranges initially set according to the values used for unloaded twitch contraction (**Table 2**) (Campbell, 2014). The goal of the optimization was to minimize the objective function ($\Phi$), which was taken to be the sum of the squared error between experimentally measured data and FE predicted results, and was defined as follows:

$$\Phi = \sum_{n=1}^{N} \sum_{i,j=1,2,3} (E_{ij,n} - \bar{E}_{ij,n})^2 + \sum_{m=1}^{6} (\frac{P_m - \bar{P}_m}{\bar{P}_m})^2$$

(7)

The first term of the objective function represents the errors induced by ES strains, where n is the strain point within the myocardium, N is the total number of strain points (N $\geq$ 250 points evenly distributed throughout the mid-layer of the FE model), and $E_{ij}$ and $\bar{E}_{ij}$ are FE-predicted and experimentally measured ES strains, respectively. The second term represents the errors due to LV pressures. In this study, 6 pressure points were compared, including pressure at the end of isovolumetric contraction (IVC), three points during systolic ejection (including the peak pressure), ES pressure, and the end of isovolumetric relaxation (IVR). $P_m$ and $\bar{P}_m$ are the FE-predicted and experimentally measured LV pressures, respectively.

**TABLE 2 |** Optimization results.

| | | Initial range | Case 1 | Case 2 | Case 3 | Case 4 | Case 5 |
|---|---|---|---|---|---|---|---|
| $a_{on}$ | | (0.001, 0.04) | 0.019 | 0.020 | 0.028 | 0.024 | 0.021 |
| $a_{off}$ | | (100, 1,000) | 211 | 348 | 309 | 460 | 206 |
| $C_k$ | $x_i > 0$ | (0, 2,100) | 1,544 | 1,735 | 1,885 | 2,085 | 2,015 |
| | $x_i < 0$ | (0, 2,100) | 264 | 1,345 | 1,166 | 1,113 | 529 |
| $k_d$ | $x_i > 0$ | (0, 400) | 293 | 343 | 280 | 190 | 247 |
| | $x_i < 0$ | (0, 400) | 195 | 74 | 51 | 290 | 267 |
| $k_{db}$ | $x_i > 0$ | (0, 50) | 26 | 49 | 47 | 42 | 36 |
| | $x_i < 0$ | (0, 50) | 47 | 19 | 28 | 18 | 19 |
| | $k_{plus}$ | (0, 100) | 54 | 50 | 40 | 72 | 35 |
| | $k_{minus}$ | (0, 20) | 12 | 14 | 19 | 18 | 13 |
| $\Phi$/element (strain) | | N/A | 0.077 | 0.078 | 0.055 | 0.080 | 0.076 |

$x_i$: cross-bridge length as defined in **Figure 1** in nm.

## Single Element FE Model

In order to confirm that the optimized parameters, which were determined by fitting organ level data, result in reasonable *in vivo* cellular level function, a single element FE model was employed. Specifically, the model was subjected to boundary conditions and calcium levels that replicate the following cellular experiments (de Tombe and Stienen, 2007):

1. Maximum tension generation ($T_{max}$) at a fixed sarcomere length of 2,300 nm and maximal calcium concentration.
2. Force-calcium relationship, in terms of Calcium sensitivity ($pCa_{50}$) and Hill coefficient, at a fixed sarcomere length of 2,300 nm.
3. Maximum and minimum tension redevelopment ($k_{tr}$) at a sarcomere length of 2,300 nm with 20% length release for 20 ms followed by restretch to 2,300 nm.

## RESULTS

The optimizations for all 5 animal cases displayed good convergence, and the values of the 10 active parameters optimized for each case are shown in **Table 2**. The mean of squared errors between experimentally measured strains and FE predicted data, i.e., $\Phi$/element (strain), is also shown for each case with values <0.1. Using optimized values for the active parameters, the FE models generated a LV pressure-volume (PV) loop that showed strong agreement with experimental results over the entire cardiac cycle, especially during systole (**Figure 2D**).

In order to assess the accuracy of the FE modeling approach for capturing regional variations in LV wall deformation, all 6 components of ES strain (i.e., $E_{rr}$, $E_{cc}$, $E_{ll}$, $E_{cl}$, $E_{rl}$, and $E_{cr}$) were analyzed within 4 wall segments (i.e., Anterior, Lateral, Posterior, and Septal) in the mid-ventricular region. In terms of the axial components of strain, the FE model predicted similar ES circumferential and radial ($E_{cc}$ and $E_{rr}$) strain distributions in the majority of the mid-myocardium,

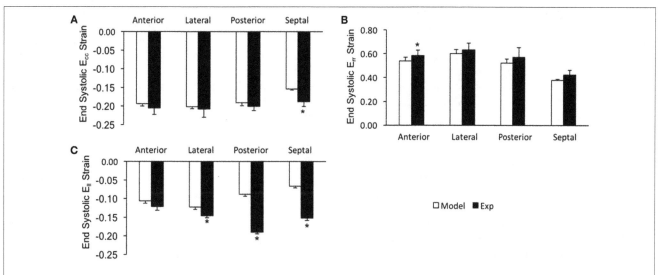

FIGURE 4 | End systolic axial strain components (A: $E_{cc}$, B: $E_{rr}$, and C: $E_{ll}$) averaged at the mid-LV in the mid-myocardial layer. Data are mean ± SE; $n = 5$; *$p < 0.05$ for comparisons between model-predicted and experiment-derived strains using paired two-tailed $t$-test.

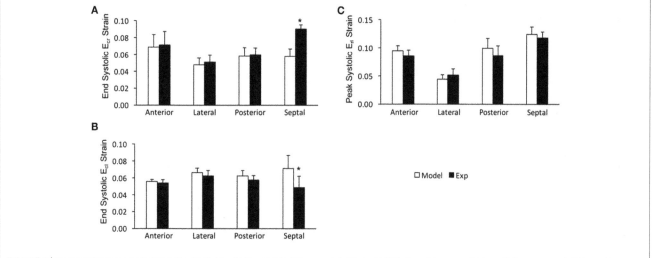

FIGURE 5 | End systolic shear strain components (A: $E_{cr}$, B: $E_{cl}$, and C: $E_{rl}$) averaged at the mid-LV in the mid-myocardial layer. Data are mean ± SE; $n = 5$; *$p < 0.05$ for comparisons between model-predicted and experiment-derived strains using paired two-tailed $t$-test.

when compared to the experimental measures, with significant ($p < 0.05$) deviation seen only in the septal and anterior segments, respectively (**Figures 4A,B**). The FE model, however, significantly ($p < 0.05$) underestimated systolic longitudinal strain ($E_{ll}$) in the lateral, posterior and septal segments of the mid-myocardium (**Figure 4C**). This could be due to the assumed longitudinal myofiber angle distribution. While there existed some significant ($p < 0.05$) differences between FE predicted values and experimental measures for ES shear strains $E_{cr}$ and $E_{cl}$ (only in the septal segment of the mid-myocardium), the shear strain $E_{rl}$ predicted by the model was comparable with experimental data throughout the entire mid-myocardium (**Figure 5**). Moreover, the mid-ventricular torsion at ES, represented as CL shear angle, was similar to that estimated from experimental measures over the entire mid-myocardium (**Figure 6**).

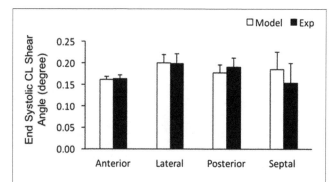

FIGURE 6 | End systolic circumferential-longitudinal (CL) shear angles averaged at the mid-LV in the mid-myocardial layer. Data are mean ± SE; $n = 5$. No significant differences between model-predicted and experiment-derived results using paired two-tailed $t$-test.

The FE model predicted sequential relaxation throughout the entire LV myocardium. Specifically, in contrast to the prompt sarcomere re-lengthening that occurred at the base, both the mid-ventricle and apex exhibited prolonged post-systolic shortening (PSS) and delayed re-lengthening and relaxation in the epicardial layer (**Figure 7**, arrows indicate the beginning of re-lengthening). This sequential re-lengthening and relaxation was mitigated in the mid-myocardium, and eventually reversed in the endocardium (data not shown). At the mid-ventricle, the onset of sarcomere re-lengthening was sequential in the 3 transmural layers. Namely, re-lengthening first occurred in the epicardium, followed by the mid-myocardium and then the endocardium (**Figure 8**, arrows indicate the beginning of re-lengthening).

The single element FE model results, which utilized the animal-specific parameters determined from the optimization of the five cases, are shown in **Table 3**. The maximum tension generation ($T_{max}$) was found to be 135.3 ± 2.3 kPa. The calcium sensitivity, indicated by the level of calcium at which 50% of the maximum tension is developed ($pCa_{50}$), was found to be 6.46 ± 0.024 and the Hill coefficient was 2.41 ± 0.057. The force-pCa curve for Case 1 is shown in **Figure 9**. The maximum tension redevelopment ($k_{tr-max}$) at saturated calcium was 96.1 ± 1.91 $s^{-1}$ and the minimum tension redevelopment ($k_{tr-min}$) at low calcium was 16.1 ± 1.80 $s^{-1}$.

## DISCUSSION

In the present study, a novel FE model of active contraction was developed by incorporating a 2-state myocyte contraction model (i.e., MyoSim) into animal-specific ventricle models. This new model includes both length- and velocity-dependence of force generation, and, therefore, has the potential to provide a more accurate representation of cardiac function

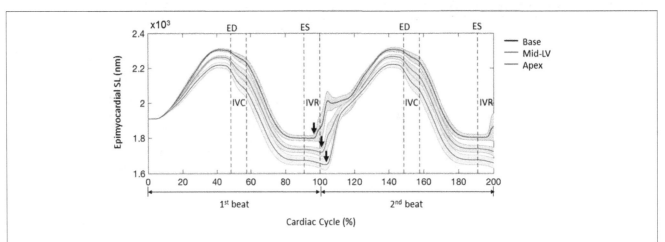

**FIGURE 7** | Profiles of sarcomere length (SL) over 2 cardiac cycles obtained from 3 representative elements located at the base, mid-LV, and apex in the lateral epicardium. Data are mean (thick solid lines) ± SE (shaded area); $n = 5$. Note that the simulations start from the unloaded state. Arrows indicate the beginning of re-lengthening.

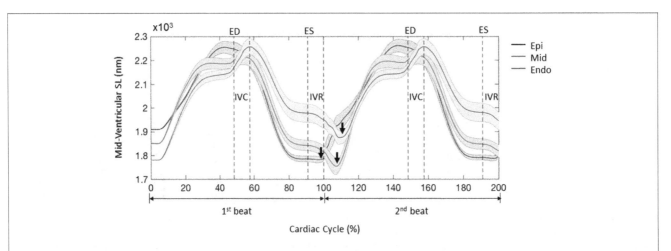

**FIGURE 8** | Profiles of sarcomere length (SL) over 2 cardiac cycles obtained from 3 representative elements located in the lateral epicardium (epi), mid-myocardium (mid), and endocardium (endo) at the mid-LV. Data are mean (thick solid lines) ± SE (shaded area); $n = 5$. Note that the simulations start from the unloaded state. Arrows indicate the beginning of re-lengthening.

**TABLE 3 |** Results of the single element simulations of maximum tension generation, calcium sensitivity, and tension redevelopment.

|  | Case 1 | Case 2 | Case 3 | Case 4 | Case 5 |
|---|---|---|---|---|---|
| $T_{max}$ (kPa) | 139.5 | 135.1 | 126.5 | 138.5 | 137 |
| $pCa_{50}$ | 6.53 | 6.42 | 6.39 | 6.48 | 6.47 |
| Hill coefficient | 2.51 | 2.25 | 2.29 | 2.53 | 2.45 |
| $k_{tr-max}$ (s$^{-1}$) | 89.5 | 98.4 | 101.0 | 96.3 | 95.4 |
| $k_{tr-min}$ (s$^{-1}$) | 10.3 | 17.6 | 21.3 | 16.5 | 14.8 |

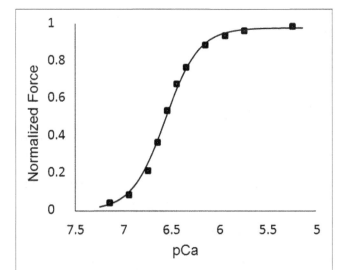

**FIGURE 9 |** Force-pCa curve for Case 1. The square markers represent the values from the single element simulations, while the curve fit is the Hill equation with a value of $pCa_{50} = 6.53$ and a Hill coefficient = 2.51.

at the global level, since it is embedded into the 3D FE framework.

Among the several improvements of the new FE contraction model is the inclusion of cooperative effects in dynamic coupling of binding sites and myosin heads. In real muscles, the status of the binding sites influences the status of the myosin heads, and vice versa. This dynamic coupling is further influenced by the status of near neighbor molecules, which is referred to as cooperative effects and is determined by the values of $k_{plus}$ and $k_{minus}$. Incorporation of this molecular effect allows the proposed FE model to simulate cardiac muscles with altered $Ca^{2+}$ sensitivity, for example, due to a disease state. This could be assessed by optimizing related parameters (i.e., $a_{on}$, $a_{off}$, $k_{plus}$ and $k_{minus}$) using experimental data from a diseased animal model, which is beyond the scope of the current study. Moreover, a cross-bridge distribution approach is employed in the proposed FE model to solve the kinetics of binding sites and myosin heads. This approach provides greater control on the strain-dependence of myosin kinetics, enabling the proposed model to mimic the contractile properties of muscles under a wider range of conditions. In addition, the proposed model incorporates the effects of interfilamentary movement. According to Huxley (1957), the length of the cross-bridges changes when the

filaments move. The interfilamentary movement, especially at a higher speed relative to the rate of cross-bridge cycling, can perturb the normal cross-bridge distributions, and thus impact the production of active force. This incorporation accounts, at least in part, for the velocity-dependency in the FE model of muscle contraction. Since all of the parameters can be adjusted to fit cellular-level experimental data, this FE contraction model is directly linked to cellular mechanical properties. This is critical, especially when the model is used to relate changes in the mechanical properties of cardiac muscle at the cellular level to variations in the global function of the LV.

In order to validate this new FE contraction model, parameters were optimized to match the experimental data from normal healthy rats. Overall, the proposed model demonstrated strong agreement with the experimental results in terms of LV global function (i.e., PV loop) and regional deformation (i.e., systolic strains and ventricular torsion), although there existed some deviations from experimental measures of strain, mainly in the septal region. Particularly, the notable underestimation of systolic $E_{ll}$ may be due to the assumption of constant fiber angle distribution along the longitudinal direction and could be improved by using more realistic distributions of fiber angles (from DT-MRI for example). The proposed FE model was able to capture the heterogeneity of ventricular relaxation, which has been observed in experiments of intact ventricles *in vivo* (Sengupta et al., 2006; Ashikaga et al., 2007). This is important particularly because the observed delay of sarcomere re-lengthening in the epicardial apex has been associated with pressure drop during early diastole (Sengupta et al., 2006), and therefore may impact diastolic filling. As such, the proposed FE contraction model was able to match experimental PV measurements of not only the systolic phase, but also the diastolic filling phase. This capability could be beneficial in facilitating research related to diastolic dysfunction (Sugiura et al., 2012). Moreover, pilot studies using the time-varying elastance model, a commonly used FE model which does not include a force-velocity relation, failed to optimize the material properties using the same optimization procedure to match the experimental pressure measurements. In addition, these models exhibited synchronized relaxation throughout the entire ventricle. These observations lend further support for the improvement of this new FE model implementation in providing a more accurate representation of LV global function.

It should be noted that some of the optimized values for the active parameters varied from animal to animal, particularly for those used to calculate attachment/detachment rate constants. However, the sensitivity studies previously conducted by Campbell showed that the contraction model (MyoSim) was less sensitive to changes in the strain-dependence of myosin kinetics, as compared to changes in calcium sensitivity which is mediated predominantly by $a_{on}$ (Campbell, 2014). In line with this, the present study showed similar calcium sensitivity in healthy rats with a narrow range of $a_{on}$ values. Moreover, although there existed some differences between the optimized values in the present study and those used for unloaded twitch contraction, the maximum proportions of total available binding sites (N: 0.15~0.25) and bound myosin heads ($N_{bound}$:

0.13∼0.23) were comparable to the results reported for unloaded twitch contraction (Campbell, 2014). In terms of the single element FE models, which were used to assess *in vivo* cellular-level function, the values for $pCa_{50}$ were found to be greater than those typically measured with *in vitro* permeabilized cell preparations. However, it has been shown in several studies that intact cells, which are evaluated at *in vivo* temperatures, exhibit greater calcium sensitivity (de Tombe and Stienen, 2007; Chung et al., 2016). Thus, the values found in the present study provide a reasonable representation of *in vivo* values. Additionally, the maximum tension redevelopment ($k_{tr-max}$) at saturated calcium was found to be greater than those measured with *in vitro* experiments. But, it has been shown (de Tombe and Stienen, 2007) that as the temperature of these experiments is increased, the value of $k_{tr-max}$ also increases. Thus, it can be inferred from de Tombe and Stienen (2007) that the values found in the current study are a reasonable estimate of *in vivo* function. The value of the Hill coefficient was found to be lower than those measured from *in vitro* studies (Dobesh et al., 2002; de Tombe and Stienen, 2007), but was still in a range that indicates cooperativitly is in effect. Finally, the maximum tension generated in the current study is in agreement with values found in previous studies (Land et al., 2012).

One limitation of the proposed FE contraction model is the use of a simpler 2-state cross-bridge myosin scheme rather than a more complex 6-state model (Campbell, 2014). However, the 2-state scheme was chosen for a balance between computational efficiency and accuracy. Enhancements to the 2-state model will be pursued in future work. Moreover, the proposed model did not include the effects of cellular shortening on $Ca^{2+}$ transient. But, this effect is relatively small, and the proposed model includes the shortening effects on the total number of binding sites activated by $Ca^{2+}$ as a compensating method. When comparing the FE model strain to the experimental strain, only $n = 5$ samples were used. Finally, the FE models did not include the right ventricle

(RV). This likely caused the deformation in the septal region of the FE models to deviate from the experimental measurements from CMR. To overcome this limitation, the RV will be included in future models.

In conclusion, the proposed FE contraction model successfully predicted both the global function and regional deformation of the LV. The capability of the proposed model to capture an important feature of ventricular relaxation makes it a powerful tool for the future investigation of diastolic dysfunction. Moreover, the incorporation of cellular-level mechanisms may enable the proposed model to assess how pharmaceutical treatments that target cellular function influence global ventricular function.

## AUTHOR CONTRIBUTIONS

XZ wrote the finite element code, performed the computational analysis, collected the experimental data, and wrote most of the manuscript. Z-QL analyzed the experimental data in terms of 3D surface generation and regional strain. KC developed the cellular-level code and helped implement it into the finite element framework. JW helped implement the finite element code, analyze both the experimental/computational results, write the manuscript, and developed the conceptual design of the work.

## ACKNOWLEDGMENTS

The authors wish to thank Hua Wang and Amir Nikou for their help with CMR scans. This study was supported by an award from the American Heart Association 14BGIA18850020 (JW), a grant from the National Science Foundation CMMI-1538754 (JW), grants from the National Institutes of Health R01 HL090749 (KC) and P30 GM110787 (LH), and a postdoctoral fellowship from the University of Kentucky Center for Computational Sciences (XZ).

## REFERENCES

Ashikaga, H., Coppola, B. A., Hopenfeld, B., Leifer, E. S., Mcveigh, E. R., and Omens, J. H. (2007). Transmural dispersion of myofiber mechanics: implications for electrical heterogeneity *in vivo. J. Am. Coll. Cardiol.* 49, 909–916. doi: 10.1016/j.jacc.2006.07.074

Campbell, K. S. (2009). Interactions between connected half-sarcomeres produce emergent mechanical behavior in a mathematical model of muscle. *PLoS Comput. Biol.* 5:e1000560. doi: 10.1371/journal.pcbi.1000560

Campbell, K. S. (2014). Dynamic coupling of regulated binding sites and cycling myosin heads in striated muscle. *J. Gen. Physiol.* 143, 387–399. doi: 10.1085/jgp.201311078

Campbell, S. G., Flaim, S. N., Leem, C. H., and Mcculloch, A. D. (2008). Mechanisms of transmurally varying myocyte electromechanics in an integrated computational model. *Philos. Trans. A Math. Phys. Eng. Sci.* 366, 3361–3380. doi: 10.1098/rsta.2008.0088

Chung, J. H., Biesiadecki, B. J., Ziolo, M. T., Davis, J. P., and Janssen, P. M. (2016). Myofilament calcium sensitivity: role in regulation of *in vivo* cardiac contraction and relaxation. *Front. Physiol.* 7:562. doi: 10.3389/fphys.2016.00562

Daniels, M., Noble, M. I., Ter Keurs, H. E., and Wohlfart, B. (1984). Velocity of sarcomere shortening in rat cardiac muscle: relationship to force, sarcomere length, calcium and time. *J. Physiol.* 355, 367–381. doi: 10.1113/jphysiol.1984.sp015424

de Tombe, P. P., and Stienen, G. J. (2007). Impact of temperature on cross-bridge cycling kinetics in rat myocardium. *J. Physiol.* 584, 591–600. doi: 10.1113/jphysiol.2007.138693

Dobesh, D. P., Konhilas, J. P., and De Tombe, P. P. (2002). Cooperative activation in cardiac muscle: impact of sarcomere length. *Am. J. Physiol. Heart Circ. Physiol.* 282, H1055–H1062. doi: 10.1152/ajpheart.00667.2001

Gordon, A. M., Homsher, E., and Regnier, M. (2000). Regulation of contraction in striated muscle. *Physiol. Rev.* 80, 853–924. doi: 10.1152/physrev.2000.80.2.853

Guccione, J. M., and McCulloch, A. D. (1993). Mechanics of active contraction in cardiac muscle: Part I–Constitutive relations for fiber stress that describe deactivation. *J. Biomech. Eng.* 115, 72–81. doi: 10.1115/1.2895473

Guccione, J. M., Moonly, S. M., Moustakidis, P., Costa, K. D., Moulton, M. J., Ratcliffe, M. B., et al. (2001). Mechanism underlying mechanical dysfunction in the border zone of left ventricular aneurysm: a finite element model study. *Ann. Thorac. Surg.* 71, 654–662. doi: 10.1016/S0003-4975(00)02338-9

Guccione, J. M., Waldman, L. K., and McCulloch, A. D. (1993). Mechanics of active contraction in cardiac muscle: Part II–Cylindrical models of the systolic left ventricle. *J. Biomech. Eng.* 115, 82–90. doi: 10.1115/1.2895474

Haggerty, C. M., Kramer, S. P., Binkley, C. M., Powell, D. K., Mattingly, A. C., Charnigo, R., et al. (2013). Reproducibility of cine displacement encoding with stimulated echoes (DENSE) cardiovascular magnetic resonance for measuring left ventricular strains, torsion, and synchrony in mice. *J. Cardiovasc. Magn. Reson.* 15:71. doi: 10.1186/1532-429X-15-71

Hunter, P. J., McCulloch, A. D., and Ter Keurs, H. E. (1998). Modelling the mechanical properties of cardiac muscle. *Prog. Biophys. Mol. Biol.* 69, 289–331. doi: 10.1016/S0079-6107(98)00013-3

Huxley, A. F. (1957). Muscle structure and theories of contraction. *Prog. Biophys. Biophys. Chem.* 7, 255–318.

Huxley, H. E., Stewart, A., Sosa, H., and Irving, T. (1994). X-ray diffraction measurements of the extensibility of actin and myosin filaments in contracting muscle. *Biophys. J.* 67, 2411–2421. doi: 10.1016/S0006-3495(94)80 728-3

Kerckhoffs, R. C., Neal, M. L., Gu, Q., Bassingthwaighte, J. B., Omens, J. H., and Mcculloch, A. D. (2007). Coupling of a 3D finite element model of cardiac ventricular mechanics to lumped systems models of the systemic and pulmonic circulation. *Ann. Biomed. Eng.* 35, 1–18. doi: 10.1007/s10439-006-9 212-7

Kobayashi, T., and Solaro, R. J. (2005). Calcium, thin filaments, and the integrative biology of cardiac contractility. *Annu. Rev. Physiol.* 67, 39–67. doi: 10.1146/annurev.physiol.67.040403.114025

Land, S., Niederer, S. A., Aronsen, J. M., Espe, E. K., Zhang, L., Louch, W. E., et al. (2012). An analysis of deformation-dependent electromechanical coupling in the mouse heart. *J. Physiol.* 590, 4553–4569. doi: 10.1113/jphysiol.2012.2 31928

Laurita, K. R., and Singal, A. (2001). Mapping action potentials and calcium transients simultaneously from the intact heart. *Am. J. Physiol. Heart Circ. Physiol.* 280, H2053–H2060. doi: 10.1152/ajpheart.2001.280.5.H2053

Pacher, P., Nagayama, T., Mukhopadhyay, P., Batkai, S., and Kass, D. A. (2008). Measurement of cardiac function using pressure-volume conductance catheter technique in mice and rats. *Nat. Protoc.* 3, 1422–1434. doi: 10.1038/nprot.2008.138

Razumova, M. V., Bukatina, A. E., and Campbell, K. B. (1999). Stiffness-distortion sarcomere model for muscle simulation. *J. Appl. Physiol.* 87, 1861–1876. doi: 10.1152/jappl.1999.87.5.1861

Rice, J. J., Wang, F., Bers, D. M., and De Tombe, P. P. (2008). Approximate model of cooperative activation and crossbridge cycling in cardiac muscle using ordinary differential equations. *Biophys. J.* 95, 2368–2390. doi: 10.1529/biophysj.107.119487

Rüssel, I. K., Tecelao, S. R., Kuijer, J. P., Heethaar, R. M., and Marcus, J. T. (2009). Comparison of 2D and 3D calculation of left ventricular torsion as circumferential-longitudinal shear angle using cardiovascular magnetic resonance tagging. *J. Cardiovasc. Magn. Reson.* 11:8. doi: 10.1186/1532-429X-11-8

Schneider, N. S., Shimayoshi, T., Amano, A., and Matsuda, T. (2006). Mechanism of the Frank-Starling law–a simulation study with a novel cardiac muscle contraction model that includes titin and troponin I. *J. Mol. Cell. Cardiol.* 41, 522–536. doi: 10.1016/j.yjmcc.2006.06.003

Sengupta, P. P., Khandheria, B. K., Korinek, J., Wang, J., Jahangir, A., Seward, J. B., et al. (2006). Apex-to-base dispersion in regional timing of left ventricular shortening and lengthening. *J. Am. Coll. Cardiol.* 47, 163–172. doi: 10.1016/j.jacc.2005.08.073

Spottiswoode, B. S., Zhong, X., Hess, A. T., Kramer, C. M., Meintjes, E. M., Mayosi, B. M., et al. (2007). Tracking myocardial motion from cine DENSE images using spatiotemporal phase unwrapping and temporal fitting. *IEEE Trans. Med. Imaging* 26, 15–30. doi: 10.1109/TMI.2006.884215

Sugiura, S., Washio, T., Hatano, A., Okada, J., Watanabe, H., and Hisada, T. (2012). Multi-scale simulations of cardiac electrophysiology and mechanics using the University of Tokyo heart simulator. *Prog. Biophys. Mol. Biol.* 110, 380–389. doi: 10.1016/j.pbiomolbio.2012.07.001

Tajima, Y., Makino, K., Hanyuu, T., Wakabayashi, K., and Amemiya, Y. (1994). X-ray evidence for the elongation of thin and thick filaments during isometric contraction of a molluscan smooth muscle. *J. Muscle Res. Cell Motil.* 15, 659–671. doi: 10.1007/BF00121073

Keurs, H. E., Bucx, J. J., De Tombe, P. P., Backx, P., and Iwazumi, T. (1988). The effects of sarcomere length and Ca++ on force and velocity of shortening in cardiac muscle. *Adv. Exp. Med. Biol.* 226, 581–593.

ter Keurs, H. E., Rijnsburger, W. H., Van Heuningen, R., and Nagelsmit, M. J. (1980). Tension development and sarcomere length in rat cardiac trabeculae. Evidence of length-dependent activation. *Circ. Res.* 46, 703–714. doi: 10.1161/01.RES.46.5.703

Trayanova, N. A., and Rice, J. J. (2011). Cardiac electromechanical models: from cell to organ. *Front. Physiol.* 2:43. doi: 10.3389/fphys.2011.00043

Trumble, D. R., McGregor, W. E., Kerckhoffs, R. C., and Waldman, L. K. (2011). Cardiac assist with a twist: apical torsion as a means to improve failing heart function. *J. Biomech. Eng.* 133:101003. doi: 10.1115/1.4005169

Wang, H., Zhang, X., Dorsey, S. M., McGarvey, J. R., Campbell, K. S., Burdick, J. A., et al. (2016). Computational investigation of transmural differences in left ventricular contractility. *J. Biomech. Eng.* 138, 114501. doi: 10.1115/1.4034558

Wenk, J. F., Klepach, D., Lee, L. C., Zhang, Z., Ge, L., Tseng, E. E., et al. (2012). First evidence of depressed contractility in the border zone of a human myocardial infarction. *Ann. Thorac. Surg.* 93, 1188–1193. doi: 10.1016/j.athoracsur.2011.12.066

Wenk, J. F., Sun, K., Zhang, Z., Soleimani, M., Ge, L., Saloner, D., et al. (2011). Regional left ventricular myocardial contractility and stress in a finite element model of posterobasal myocardial infarction. *J. Biomech. Eng.* 133:044501. doi: 10.1115/1.4003438

Zhang, X., Haynes, P., Campbell, K. S., and Wenk, J. F. (2015). Numerical evaluation of myofiber orientation and transmural contractile strength on left ventricular function. *J. Biomech. Eng.* 137:044502. doi: 10.1115/1.4028990

Zhang, X., Liu, Z. Q., Singh, D., Wehner, G. J., Powell, D. K., Campbell, K. S., et al. (2017). Regional quantification of myocardial mechanics in rat using 3D cine DENSE cardiovascular magnetic resonance. *NMR Biomed.* 30:e3733. doi: 10.1002/nbm.3733

Zhong, X., Gibberman, L. B., Spottiswoode, B. S., Gilliam, A. D., Meyer, C. H., French, B. A., et al. (2011). Comprehensive cardiovascular magnetic resonance of myocardial mechanics in mice using three-dimensional cine DENSE. *J. Cardiovasc. Magn. Reson.* 13:83. doi: 10.1186/1532-429X-13-83

# 17

# Scaling Laws of Flow Rate, Vessel Blood Volume, Lengths and Transit Times with Number of Capillaries

Mohammad S. Razavi [1,2], Ebrahim Shirani [3] and Ghassan S. Kassab [4*]

[1] The George W. Woodruff School of Mechanical Engineering, Georgia Institute of Technology, Atlanta, GA, United States,
[2] The Petit Institute for Bioengineering and Bioscience, Georgia Institute of Technology, Atlanta, GA, United States,
[3] Department of Engineering, Foolad Institute of Technology, Isfahan, Iran, [4] California Medical Innovations Institute,
San Diego, CA, United States

**\*Correspondence:**
Ghassan S. Kassab
gkassab@calmi2.org

The structure-function relation is one of the oldest hypotheses in biology and medicine; i.e., form serves function and function influences form. Here, we derive and validate form-function relations for volume, length, flow, and mean transit time in vascular trees and capillary numbers of various organs and species. We define a vessel segment as a "stem" and the vascular tree supplied by the stem as a "crown." We demonstrate form-function relations between the number of capillaries in a vascular network and the crown volume, crown length, and blood flow that perfuses the network. The scaling laws predict an exponential relationship between crown volume and the number of capillaries with the power, $\lambda$, of $4/3 < \lambda < 3/2$. It is also shown that blood flow rate and vessel lengths are proportional to the number of capillaries in the entire stem-crown systems. The integration of the scaling laws then results in a relation between transit time and crown length and volume. The scaling laws are both intra-specific (i.e., within vasculatures of various organs, including heart, lung, mesentery, skeletal muscle and eye) and inter-specific (i.e., across various species, including rats, cats, rabbits, pigs, hamsters, and humans). This study is fundamental to understanding the physiological structure and function of vascular trees to transport blood, with significant implications for organ health and disease.

Keywords: vascular design, transport, blood flow, structure-function relation, scaling laws, intraspecific scaling

## SIGNIFICANCE STATEMENT

The present study reveals the simplicity of nature's proportionality laws between the form and function of a biological transport system. The mean transit time to transport blood, oxygen, nutrients, hormones, and cellular waste within the vasculature (which is fundamental to the maintenance of physiological homeostasis) is shown to scale with morphological parameters (e.g., length and diameter of blood vessels) of vascular networks. It is found that the flow needed to nourish an organ is linearly proportional to the number of capillaries needed to distribute such flow to the tissue of the organ and organism. The scaling laws hold for all organs (e.g., heart, lung, mesentery, skeletal muscle and eye) and species (e.g., rats, cats, rabbits, pigs, hamsters, humans) throughout the range of vascular dimensions (from $\mu$m to cm) for which there exist morphometric data.

# INTRODUCTION

The major role of vascular networks in the circulatory system is to transport blood, oxygen, nutrients, hormones, and cellular waste in various organs to maintain biological homeostasis. Physiological trees play a key role to transport flow to the capillary beds to support tissue demands. The tissue metabolic needs and the minimization of some specific costs for growth to maintain the delivery of nutrients and elimination of waste products generally guides the vascular development (LaBarbera, 1990).

Allometric scaling illustrates how biologic parameters vary with shape and size, regardless of the variations between organisms. Scaling laws are independent of the specific nature of an organism and originate from common underlying mechanisms. A study of the circulation requires an understanding between hemodynamic (blood flow), morphological (e.g., diameter, length, volume, etc.), and topological (e.g., connectivity patterns) information of the vasculature and any potential structure-function relations thereof. Functionally, the vascular structure serves metabolism where there is an intimate structure-function relation (LaBarbera, 1990). The vascular patterns have been used as a basis to elucidate the origin of biological allometric scaling laws (e.g., metabolic rate scaling law, West et al., 1997) and various intraspecific scaling laws (e.g., volume-diameter, flow-length, length-volume, and scaling law of flow resistance (Kassab, 2006;

Huo and Kassab, 2012). For example, it is widely accepted that animal's basal metabolic rate and body mass scale to the power 3/4, known as Kleiber's law. West, Brown, and Enquist used a hemodynamic analysis of vascular networks to derive the 3/4 scaling law. Although a great majority of available empirical data comply with the 3/4 exponent, there is also statistical evidence that the 2/3 power rather 3/4 provides a better fit (Dodds et al., 2001; White and Seymour, 2003). Based on the minimum energy hypothesis, several form-form and form-function scaling relations such as volume-diameter, length-diameter, flow-length, and flow- diameter have been previously proposed and validated (Huo and Kassab, 2012). Yet, there is a need to develop scaling relations for the number of capillaries to various morphological and functional parameters based on laws of physics.

The mean transit time (MTT), which is the time required to transport blood within the vascular network, plays a vital role in the physiological function of the circulatory system (Crumrine and LaManna, 1991; Derdeyn et al., 1999). The vascular network has structural heterogeneity, the complexity of spatial arrangement of vessels and adaptation of vascular anatomy in response to hemodynamic and metabolic stimuli (Pries and Secomb, 2009). Hence, development of structure-function relations which relate the MTT to vascular morphology are fundamental to understanding the interplay between vascular form and function, and thus provide a better rationale for clinical diagnostics and therapies.

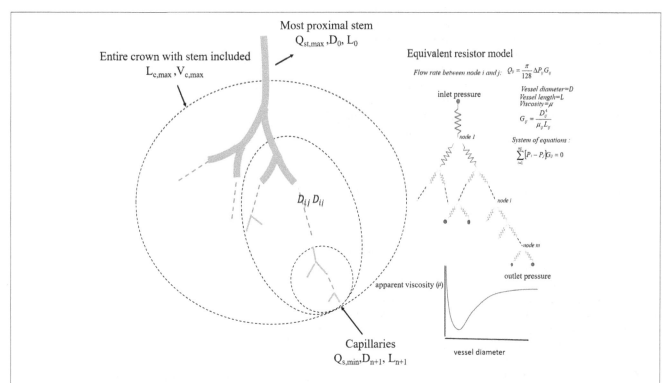

**FIGURE 1** | A schematic illustration of the definition of stem-crown units and the equivalent resistor model. The corresponding parameters. D, L, Q, and V are the diameter, length, flow rate, and volume, respectively. Subscriptst' "s" and "c" corresponding to stem and crown, respectively, in a stem-crown unit and subscripts "max" represent the most proximal stem-crown unit in a vascular tree.

**TABLE 1 |** Variables and respective descriptions.

| Symbol | | Description |
| --- | --- | --- |
| $V_C$ | Crown volume | Cumulative volume of vessels within a stem-crown system |
| $L_C$ | Crown length | Cumulative length of vessels within a stem-crown system |
| $N_C$ | Crown capillary number | Number of capillaries within a stem-crown system |
| $T_C$ | Crown transit time | Time required for blood to travel from a stem to capillaries |
| $Q_{st}$ | Stem flow rate | Flow rate corresponding to a stem |
| $Q_{cp}$ | Capillary flow rate | Flow rate corresponding to capillaries |
| $T_c$ | Segment transit time | Time required for blood to travel within a vessel |
| $T_{sg}$ | Segment length | Length of a vessel in stem-crown system |
| $L_{cp}$ | Capillary length | The average length of capillaries |
| $Br$ | Branching ratio | Ratio of vessel numbers in two consecutive branching levels |

An adequate tissue perfusion (volumetric blood flow per unit mass of tissue) through a transport structure to match metabolic requirements of an organ is essential for normal function of an organism across all species. Too low of tissue perfusion may cause hypoxia, ischemia, cell death, and ultimate loss of organ function. Histological assessment of biopsy tissues, including capillary density measurements, are common but invasive and the connection with the flow and hence function is empirical and qualitative. Since there is no equivalent relation between flow and capillarity (i.e., number or density of capillaries), deriving such a relation would be of significant importance.

Here, we hypothesize the existence of scaling relations between volume, length, and flow through a branch (i.e., stem flow) of an organ's vascular system and the respective number of capillaries through which the blood distributes. Based on the scaling law of metabolic rate and fractal nature of blood vasculature, we propose and test scaling of blood volume and cumulative length of vascular networks with the respective number of terminal capillaries. We employ a one-dimensional hemodynamic analysis of an entire network incorporating the variation in blood viscosity with vessel's size (Fåhræus–Lindqvist effect) to compute blood flow. The scaling relations between capillaries, flow and cumulative length of vascular trees, in conjunction with the definition of mean transit time, provide yet another link between structure (number of capillaries) and function (mean transit time). Ultimately, we provide a form-function relation for an analytical determination of transit time based on the cumulative length and volume of vascular systems in various species and organs throughout the vasculature. The scaling laws were formulated and validated in different vascular trees (e.g., coronary, pulmonary, mesenteric vessels, skeletal muscle vasculature, and conjunctiva vessels) of various species (e.g., rats, cats, rabbits, pigs, hamsters, humans) and organs (e.g., heart, lung, mesentery, skeletal muscle, and eye) for which there exist morphometric data. The implications of the

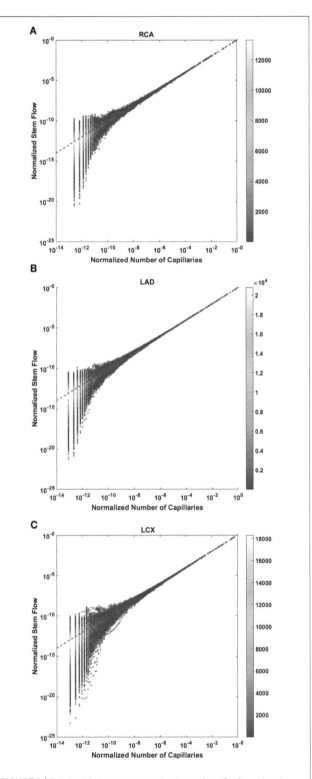

**FIGURE 2 |** Relationship between normalized stem flow ($Q_S/Q_{S,max}$) and normalized number of capillaries ($N_C/N_{C,max}$) for the full asymmetric porcine arterial tree shown in a log-log density plot: **(A)** RCA, right coronary artery; **(B)** LAD, left anterior descending artery; **(C)** LCx, left circumflex artery. The total number of data points shown in **(A–C)** are 838,462, 950,014, and 575,868; respectively. The dash lines correspond to the theoretical exponent of unity. The values of exponents, the confidence interval and $R^2$ for each species and organs are summarized in **Table 2**.

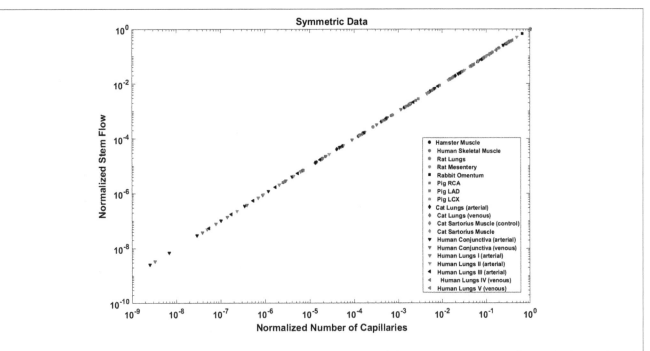

**FIGURE 3** | Relationship between normalized stem flow ($Q_s/Q_{s,max}$) and normalized number of capillaries ($N_c/N_{c,max}$) for the symmetric trees of various species and organs shown in a log-log scatter plot. RCA, right coronary artery; LAD, left anterior descending artery; LCx, left circumflex artery; PA, pulmonary artery; PV, pulmonary vein; SMA, sartorius muscle arteries; MA, mesentery arteries; OV, omentum veins; BCA, bulbar conjunctiva arteries; BCV, bulbar conjunctiva veins; RMA, retractor muscle artery. The values of exponents are consistent with the theoretical value of unity. The values of scaling exponents, the confidence interval and $R^2$ for various species and organs are summarized in **Table 2**.

remarkably simple scaling laws are discussed in health and disease.

## MATERIALS AND METHODS

We define a vessel segment as a "stem" and the vascular tree supplied by the stem as a "crown," (see **Figure 1**). A stem-crown system in which the volume of the crown (Vc) is defined as the sum of the intravascular volume of vessel segments in the entire stem-crown system (arterial or venous trees proximal or distal to the capillaries, respectively). Similarly, the crown length (Lc) is defined as the cumulative vascular lengths in the entire arterial or venous crown. Blood flow (Q) and the number of capillaries (N) correspond to the stem and the respective network. The subscripts *c, st,* and *cp* stand for crown, stem and capillary respectively. To derive and test the existence of various scaling laws, morphometric data based on the full asymmetric and simplified symmetric vascular system were used. The entire tree consists of many stem-crown units down to the capillary vessels (Sho et al., 2004; Huo and Kassab, 2012). At each bifurcation, there is a unique stem-crown unit which continues down to the smallest unit: an arteriole with two capillaries for an arterial tree or a venule and two capillaries for a venous tree. Functionally, each stem supplies or collects blood from the crown for an arterial or venous tree, respectively. The present analysis applies strictly to a tree structure (arterial or venous) down to the first capillary bifurcation. The entire arterial network was reconstructed down

to the first capillaries ($<8\,\mu m$). Missing data from the cast were reconstructed based on histological data ($<40\,\mu m$) using a computational algorithm. Details of reconstruction algorithm can be found in Mittal et al. (2005). To obtain blood flow, each vessel is modeled as a resistor (**Figure 1**). Based on this assumption, blood vessel resistance is a function of vessel's geometry and viscosity that takes into account the Fåhræus effect. Boundary conditions were prescribed by assigning an inlet pressure of 120 mmHg and a uniform pressure of 25 mmHg at the outlet of the first capillary segment. Subsequently, a system of simultaneous linear algebraic equations for the nodal pressures is obtained. Once the vessel resistances are evaluated from the geometry, and suitable boundary conditions are prescribed, flow rate is simulated to estimate the transit time within the vascular trees (please see the Supplementary Information for details).

### Existing Vascular Morphometric Data

Singhal S. et al. (1973); Singhal S. S. et al. (1973) and Horsfield and Gordon (1981) studied the morphometry of the pulmonary arteries and veins of humans, whereas Yen et al. (1983, 1984) used it to study the cat pulmonary arterial and venous trees. The microvasculatures of cat sartorius muscle (Koller et al., 1987), hamster retractor muscle (Ellsworth et al., 1987), hamster skin muscle (Bertuglia et al., 1991), rat mesenteric microvessels (Ley et al., 1986), rabbit omentum (Fenton and Zweifach, 1981), and human bulbar conjunctiva microvessels (Fenton and Zweifach, 1981) have also been reconstructed. Kassab et al. (Mittal et al., 2005) reconstructed the porcine right coronary

TABLE 2 | The validation of scaling relations in the entire stem-crown system of various – square fits.

**Species and organ**

| Asymmetric data | $Q \propto Nc^\lambda$ | | $Lc \propto Nc^\lambda$ | | $Vc \propto Nc^\lambda$ | | $Tc*Lc \propto Vc^\lambda$ | | References |
|---|---|---|---|---|---|---|---|---|---|
| | Exponent | $R^2$ | Exponent | $R^2$ | Exponent | $R^2$ | Exponent | $R^2$ | |
| Pig RCA | 1.005 (1.004, 1.005) | 0.9919 | 1.029 (1.029, 1.029) | 0.9992 | 1.481 (1.481, 1.481) | 0.9995 | 0.9814 (0.9814, 0.9814) | 0.9966 | Mittal et al., 2005 |
| Pig LAD | 1.002 (1.002, 1.002) | 0.9937 | 1.031 (1.031, 1.031) | 0.9993 | 1.453 (1.453, 1.453) | 0.9995 | 0.9883 (0.9883, 0.9883) | 0.9973 | Mittal et al., 2005 |
| Pig LCX | 1.005 (1.005, 1.005) | 0.9937 | 1.031 (1.031, 1.031) | 0.9992 | 1.479 (1.479, 1.479) | 0.9995 | 0.9891 (0.9891, 0.9891) | 0.9972 | Mittal et al., 2005 |
| **SYMMETRIC DATA** | | | | | | | | | |
| Hamster Muscle | 1 (1, 1) | 1 | 1.235 (1.063, 1.407) | 0.9943 | 1.622 (1.435, 1.808) | 0.9961 | 0.8052 (0.693, 0.9174) | 0.9093 | Bertuglia et al., 1991 |
| Rat Lungs | 1 (1, 1) | 1 | 1.033 (1.016, 1.05) | 0.998 | 1.441 (1.418, 1.464) | 0.9995 | 1.023 (1.012, 1.035) | 0.9997 | Jiang et al., 1994 |
| Rat Mesentery | 1 (1, 1) | 1 | 1.137 (1.064, 1.211) | 0.9988 | 1.306 (1.221, 1.391) | 0.9987 | 1.106 (1.057, 1.156) | 0.9994 | Ley et al., 1986 |
| Rabbit Omentum | 1 (1, 1) | 1 | 1.179 (1.123, 1.236) | 0.9993 | 1.448 (1.152, 1.745) | 0.9877 | 1.125 (1.11, 1.139) | 0.9999 | Fenton and Zweifach, 1981 |
| Pig RCA | 1 (1, 1) | 1 | 1.021 (1.009, 1.032) | 0.9997 | 1.447 (1.428, 1.467) | 0.9996 | 1.014 (1.006, 1.022) | 0.9999 | Mittal et al., 2005 |
| Pig LAD | 1 (1, 1) | 1 | 1.022 (1.009, 1.034) | 0.9997 | 1.44 (1.408, 1.473) | 0.9999 | 1.015 (1.007, 1.024) | 0.9990 | Mittal et al., 2005 |
| Pig LCX | 1 (1, 1) | 1 | 1.028 (1.013, 1.043) | 0.9996 | 1.506 (1.473, 1.539) | 0.9991 | 1.019 (1.009, 1.029) | 0.9998 | Mittal et al., 2005 |
| Cat Lungs (arterial) | 1 (1, 1) | 1 | 1.03 (1.02, 1.04) | 0.9998 | 1.401 (1.339, 1.463) | 0.9966 | 1.022 (1.016, 1.028) | 0.9999 | Yen et al., 1983 |
| Cat Lungs (venous) | 1 (1, 1) | 1 | 1.029 (1.01, 1.048) | 0.994 | 1.44 (1.414, 1.465) | 0.9994 | 1.021 (1.008, 1.034) | 0.9997 | Yen et al., 1984 |
| Cat Sartorius Muscle | 1 (1, 1) | 1 | 1.092 (1.074, 1.109) | 0.9999 | 1.174 (1.161, 1.187) | 1.0000 | 1.078 (1.063, 1.093) | 0.9999 | Koller et al., 1987 |
| Cat Sartorius Muscle | 1 (1, 1) | 1 | 1.092 (1.074, 1.109) | 0.9999 | 1.196 (1.176, 1.216) | 0.9999 | 1.077 (1.061, 1.092) | 0.9999 | Koller et al., 1987 |
| Human Skeletal Muscle | 1 (1, 1) | 1 | 1.43 (0.9181, 1.943) | 0.9634 | 1.731 (1.087, 2.375) | 0.9607 | 1.27 (1.075, 1.466) | 0.9930 | Ellsworth et al., 1987 |
| Human Conjunctiva (arterial) | 1 (1, 1) | 1 | 1.105 (1.063, 1.146) | 0.9993 | 1.227 (1.181, 1.273) | 0.9993 | 1.086 (1.055, 1.117) | 0.9996 | Fenton and Zweifach, 1981 |
| Human Conjunctiva (venous) | 1 (1, 1) | 1 | 1.113 (1.056, 1.17) | 0.9986 | 1.406 (1.337, 1.476) | 0.9987 | 1.081 (1.043, 1.119) | 0.9994 | Fenton and Zweifach, 1981 |
| Human Lungs I (arterial) | 1 (1, 1) | 1 | 1.006 (1.001, 1.011) | 0.9999 | 1.123 (1.114, 1.132) | 0.9998 | 1.013 (1.009, 1.017) | 0.9999 | Singhal S. S. et al., 1973 |
| Human Lungs II (arterial) | 1.01 (1.003, 1.016) | 0.9999 | 1.01 (1.003, 1.016) | 0.9999 | 1.152 (1.124, 1.18) | 0.9982 | 1.009 (1.004, 1.014) | 0.9999 | Huang et al., 1996 |
| Human Lungs III (arterial) | 1 (1, 1) | 1.0000 | 1.002 (1.001, 1.003) | 1.0000 | 1.197 (1.187, 1.207) | 0.9998 | 1.005 (1.004, 1.005) | 1.0000 | Singhal S. et al., 1973 |
| Human Lungs IV (venous) | 1 (1, 1) | 1 | 1.033 (1.019, 1.046) | 0.9995 | 1.294 (1.24, 1.349) | 0.9947 | 1.026 (1.017, 1.036) | 0.9997 | Huang et al., 1996 |
| Human Lungs V (venous) | 1 (1, 1) | 1 | 1.011 (1.004, 1.019) | 0.9998 | 1.215 (1.204, 1.225) | 0.9998 | 1.01 (1.003, 1.016) | 0.9999 | Horsfield and Gordon, 1981 |
| Mean | 1.0010 | | 1.0765 | | 1.3723 | | 1.0347 | | |
| SD | 0.0024 | | 0.1022 | | 0.1659 | | 0.0819 | | |

The morphometric data were obtained from the full asymmetric arterial tree and simplified symmetric trees. The data were normalized using the maximum values in the respective tree. The least-square fit was used to obtain scaling exponent of lambda ($Y = X^\lambda$). $R^2$ is correlation coefficient; RCA, right coronary artery; LCx, left circumflex artery; LAD, left anterior descending artery; PA, pulmonary artery; PV, pulmonary vein; SMA, sartorius muscle arteries; MA, mesentery arteries; OV, omentum veins; BCA, bulbar conjunctiva arteries; BCV, bulbar conjunctiva veins; RMA, retractor muscle artery. $R^2 = 1 - \frac{\sum (\log(y_{data}) - \log(y_{fit}))^2}{\sum (\log(y_{data}))^2}$.

**TABLE 3 |** The r-squared values for the hypothesized exponent λ = 1, corresponding to flow-length, length-capillary, and transit time scaling relations in stem-crown systems of symmetric data at each branching level of various species and organs, the morphometric data were obtained from the symmetric trees.

| Branching level | | 0 | 1 | 2 | 3 | 4 | 5 | 6 | 7 | 8 | 9 | 10 | 11 | 12 | 13 | 14 | 15 |
|---|---|---|---|---|---|---|---|---|---|---|---|---|---|---|---|---|---|
| Human Lungs I (arterial) | Flow-Capillary | 1.000 | 1.000 | 1.000 | 1.000 | 1.000 | 1.000 | 1.000 | 1.000 | 1.000 | 1.000 | 1.000 | 1.000 | 1.000 | 1.000 | 1.000 | 1.000 |
| | Length-Capillary | 1.000 | 1.000 | 1.000 | 1.000 | 1.000 | 1.000 | 1.000 | 1.000 | 1.000 | 1.000 | 1.000 | 1.000 | 1.000 | 1.000 | 0.997 | 0.956 |
| | Transit Time | 0.988 | 0.999 | 0.998 | 0.997 | 0.998 | 0.999 | 0.999 | 0.999 | 0.999 | 0.999 | 0.999 | 0.998 | 0.997 | 0.995 | 0.986 | 0.873 |
| Human Lungs II (arterial) | Flow-Capillary | 1.000 | 1.000 | 1.000 | 1.000 | 1.000 | 1.000 | 1.000 | 1.000 | 1.000 | 1.000 | 1.000 | 1.000 | 1.000 | 1.000 | | |
| | Length-Capillary | 1.000 | 1.000 | 1.000 | 1.000 | 1.000 | 1.000 | 1.000 | 1.000 | 1.000 | 1.000 | 1.000 | 0.998 | 0.995 | 0.987 | | |
| | Transit Time | 1.000 | 1.000 | 0.998 | 0.999 | 0.998 | 0.998 | 0.998 | 0.996 | 0.986 | 0.974 | 0.979 | 0.937 | 0.946 | 0.931 | | |
| Human Lungs III (arterial) | Flow-Capillary | 1.000 | 1.000 | 1.000 | 1.000 | 1.000 | 1.000 | 1.000 | 1.000 | 1.000 | 1.000 | 1.000 | 1.000 | 1.000 | 1.000 | 1.000 | 1.000 |
| | Length-Capillary | 1.000 | 1.000 | 1.000 | 1.000 | 1.000 | 1.000 | 1.000 | 1.000 | 1.000 | 1.000 | 1.000 | 1.000 | 1.000 | 1.000 | 1.000 | 1.000 |
| | Transit Time | 0.976 | 0.994 | 0.999 | 0.996 | 0.993 | 0.996 | 0.995 | 0.991 | 0.995 | 0.994 | 0.994 | 0.994 | 0.994 | 0.993 | 0.994 | 1.000 |
| Human Lungs IV (venous) | Flow-Capillary | 1.000 | 1.000 | 1.000 | 1.000 | 1.000 | 1.000 | 1.000 | 1.000 | 1.000 | 1.000 | 1.000 | 1.000 | 1.000 | 1.000 | | |
| | Length-Capillary | 1.000 | 1.000 | 1.000 | 1.000 | 1.000 | 1.000 | 1.000 | 1.000 | 1.000 | 1.000 | 0.999 | 0.990 | 0.998 | 0.992 | | |
| | Transit Time | 0.996 | 0.997 | 0.996 | 0.989 | 0.994 | 0.995 | 0.990 | 0.996 | 0.995 | 0.993 | 0.992 | 0.946 | 0.963 | 0.959 | | |
| Human Lungs V (venous) | Flow-Capillary | 1.000 | 1.000 | 1.000 | 1.000 | 1.000 | 1.000 | 1.000 | 1.000 | 1.000 | 1.000 | 1.000 | 1.000 | 1.000 | 1.000 | | |
| | Length-Capillary | 1.000 | 1.000 | 1.000 | 1.000 | 1.000 | 1.000 | 1.000 | 1.000 | 1.000 | 1.000 | 1.000 | 0.999 | 0.994 | 0.970 | | |
| | Transit Time | 0.991 | 0.995 | 0.992 | 0.991 | 0.993 | 0.999 | 0.996 | 0.996 | 0.996 | 0.993 | 0.989 | 0.980 | 0.958 | 0.900 | | |
| Pig RCA | Flow-Capillary | 1.000 | 1.000 | 1.000 | 1.000 | 1.000 | 1.000 | 1.000 | 1.000 | 1.000 | 1.000 | | | | | | |
| | Length-Capillary | 1.000 | 1.000 | 1.000 | 1.000 | 1.000 | 1.000 | 0.999 | 0.997 | 0.991 | 0.969 | | | | | | |
| | Transit Time | 0.996 | 0.984 | 0.983 | 0.978 | 0.972 | 0.979 | 0.939 | 0.966 | 0.952 | 0.896 | | | | | | |
| Pig LAD | Flow-Capillary | 1.000 | 1.000 | 1.000 | 1.000 | 1.000 | 1.000 | 1.000 | 1.000 | 1.000 | 1.000 | | | | | | |
| | Length-Capillary | 1.000 | 1.000 | 1.000 | 1.000 | 1.000 | 1.000 | 0.999 | 0.997 | 0.994 | 0.955 | | | | | | |
| | Transit Time | 0.997 | 0.991 | 0.980 | 0.977 | 0.967 | 0.977 | 0.945 | 0.943 | 0.968 | 0.865 | | | | | | |
| Pig LCX | Flow-Capillary | 1.000 | 1.000 | 1.000 | 1.000 | 1.000 | 1.000 | 1.000 | 1.000 | 1.000 | | | | | | | |
| | Length-Capillary | 1.000 | 1.000 | 1.000 | 1.000 | 1.000 | 0.999 | 0.996 | 0.994 | 0.955 | | | | | | | |
| | Transit Time | 0.997 | 0.984 | 0.966 | 0.978 | 0.957 | 0.943 | 0.938 | 0.969 | 0.865 | | | | | | | |
| Cat Lungs (arterial) | Flow-Capillary | 1.000 | 1.000 | 1.000 | 1.000 | 1.000 | 1.000 | 1.000 | 1.000 | 1.000 | | | | | | | |
| | Length-Capillary | 1.000 | 1.000 | 1.000 | 1.000 | 1.000 | 0.998 | 0.995 | 0.999 | 0.998 | | | | | | | |
| | Transit Time | 0.995 | 0.994 | 0.993 | 0.988 | 0.973 | 0.946 | 0.910 | 0.984 | 0.980 | | | | | | | |
| Cat Lungs (venous) | Flow-Capillary | 1.000 | 1.000 | 1.000 | 1.000 | 1.000 | 1.000 | 1.000 | 1.000 | 1.000 | | | | | | | |
| | Length-Capillary | 1.000 | 1.000 | 1.000 | 1.000 | 1.000 | 1.000 | 0.999 | 0.993 | 0.959 | | | | | | | |
| | Transit Time | 0.975 | 0.989 | 0.987 | 0.987 | 0.973 | 0.964 | 0.975 | 0.955 | 0.873 | | | | | | | |
| Rat Lungs | Flow-Capillary | 1.000 | 1.000 | 1.000 | 1.000 | 1.000 | 1.000 | 1.000 | 1.000 | 1.000 | 1.000 | | | | | | |
| | Length-Capillary | 1.000 | 1.000 | 1.000 | 1.000 | 1.000 | 1.000 | 0.999 | 0.996 | 0.987 | 0.994 | | | | | | |
| | Transit Time | 0.981 | 0.970 | 0.976 | 0.982 | 0.982 | 0.977 | 0.969 | 0.957 | 0.889 | 0.968 | | | | | | |
| Human Conjunctiva (arterial) | Flow-Capillary | 1.000 | 1.000 | 1.000 | 1.000 | | | | | | | | | | | | |
| | Length-Capillary | 0.999 | 0.997 | 0.994 | 0.981 | | | | | | | | | | | | |
| | Transit Time | 0.991 | 0.979 | 0.972 | 0.933 | | | | | | | | | | | | |
| Human Conjunctiva (venous) | Flow-Capillary | 1.000 | 1.000 | 1.000 | 1.000 | | | | | | | | | | | | |
| | Length-Capillary | 0.999 | 0.996 | 0.985 | 0.970 | | | | | | | | | | | | |
| | Transit Time | 0.982 | 0.955 | 0.898 | 0.911 | | | | | | | | | | | | |
| Cat Sartorius Muscle | Flow-Capillary | 1.000 | 1.000 | 1.000 | | | | | | | | | | | | | |
| | Length-Capillary | 0.999 | 0.997 | 0.998 | | | | | | | | | | | | | |
| | Transit Time | 0.988 | 0.982 | 0.992 | | | | | | | | | | | | | |
| Cat Sartorius Muscle | Flow-Capillary | 1.000 | 1.000 | 1.000 | | | | | | | | | | | | | |
| | Length-Capillary | 0.999 | 0.997 | 0.998 | | | | | | | | | | | | | |
| | Transit Time | 0.990 | 0.984 | 0.992 | | | | | | | | | | | | | |
| Human Skeletal Muscle | Flow-Capillary | 1.000 | 1.000 | 1.000 | | | | | | | | | | | | | |
| | Length-Capillary | 0.997 | 0.974 | 0.815 | | | | | | | | | | | | | |
| | Transit Time | 0.977 | 0.954 | 0.770 | | | | | | | | | | | | | |

(Continued)

**TABLE 3 |** Continued

| Branching level | | 0 | 1 | 2 | 3 | 4 | 5 | 6 | 7 | 8 | 9 | 10 | 11 | 12 | 13 | 14 | 15 |
|---|---|---|---|---|---|---|---|---|---|---|---|---|---|---|---|---|---|
| Rat Mesentery | Flow-Capillary | 1.000 | 1.000 | 1.000 | | | | | | | | | | | | | |
| | Length-Capillary | 0.999 | 0.993 | 0.976 | | | | | | | | | | | | | |
| | Transit Time | 0.989 | 0.958 | 0.925 | | | | | | | | | | | | | |
| Rabbit Omentum | Flow-Capillary | 1.000 | 1.000 | 1.000 | | | | | | | | | | | | | |
| | Length-Capillary | 0.983 | 0.996 | 0.993 | | | | | | | | | | | | | |
| | Transit Time | 0.000 | 0.000 | 0.000 | | | | | | | | | | | | | |
| Hamster Muscle | Flow-Capillary | 1.000 | 1.000 | 1.000 | | | | | | | | | | | | | |
| | Length-Capillary | 0.998 | 0.988 | 0.935 | | | | | | | | | | | | | |
| | Transit Time | 0.970 | 0.940 | 0.869 | | | | | | | | | | | | | |

*The order number "0" corresponds to the main stem in the entire stem-crown systems and the last level includes terminal stem-crown system one pre-capillary branching. RCA, right coronary artery; LAD, left anterior descending artery; LCx, left circumflex artery; PA, pulmonary artery; PV, pulmonary vein; SMA, sartorius muscle arteries; MA, mesentery arteries; OV, omentum veins; BCA, bulbar conjunctiva arteries; BCV, bulbar conjunctiva veins; RMA, retractor muscle artery.*

artery (RCA), left anterior descending (LAD) artery, and left circumflex (LCx) arterial trees. Huang et al. (1996) measured the human pulmonary arterial and venous trees, while Jiang et al. measured the rat pulmonary arterial tree (Jiang et al., 1994).

## Data Analysis

For the symmetric and asymmetric data, full tree data were presented as log-log scatter plots and log-log density plots, respectively, showing the density of data because of the enormity of data points (Huo et al., 2007). We utilized a nonlinear regression based on the least-square method and a log-log transformation to perform curve fitting of morphometric data in MATLAB, at 95% confidence level to obtain the model coefficients and confidence bounds for the fitted coefficients. R-squared and the standard error of the regression were calculated to evaluate the goodness of fit. Additionally, a nonparametric bootstrap method was used for estimating the standard error and the confidence interval of estimated parameters and correlation coefficients using repeated samples from the original data. This method was based on the sampling with replacement (Wu, 1986). A number of 1,000 bootstrap sample was used to obtain the confidence intervals of estimated parameters. Hemodynamic analyses were performed to obtain network flow based on two different models: (1) Asymmetric full model and (2) Simplified symmetric model as described in the Supplementary Information.

## Theoretical Scaling Laws

In this section, we propose and test different scaling relations for the crown volume (Vc), crown length (Lc), blood flow (Q), and the number of capillaries (N) in the respective network. The subscriptions $c$, $st$, and $cp$ stand for the crown, stem and capillary respectively (please see **Table 1**).

## Flow Perfusion Scales With Capillary Numbers

Since the structure-function relation is pervasive in biology, we hypothesize the existence of a direct relation between flow through a branch (i.e., stem flow) of an organ vascular system

and the respective number of capillaries through which the blood flow distributes.

The formulation invokes the law of conservation of mass which requires the flow at the inlet of the tree or crown ($Q_{st}$ stem flow) to be equal to the sum of the flows at the first capillary segments, $Q_{cp}$; namely:

$$Q_{st} = \sum_{i=1}^{N} Q_{cp,i} \qquad (1)$$

where $N$ is the number of capillaries perfused by a given stem. Using the average capillary flow rate ($\overline{Q}_{cp} = \sum_i^N Q_{cp,i}/N$), Equation (1) reduces to:

$$Q_{st} = kN_c \qquad (2)$$

where $k$ is the average capillary flow and approximately constant across the various stem-crown systems. Hence, the inlet flow is proportional to the total number of capillary vessels. If we normalize the flow and capillarity with respect to an entire tree, we obtain the following:

$$\frac{Q_{st}}{Q_{st,max}} = \left(\frac{N_c}{N_{c,max}}\right) \qquad (3)$$

where $Q_{st,max}$ and $N_{c,max}$ are the inlet flow and the total number of capillaries in a vascular system, respectively.

## Crown Volume Scales With Capillary Number

Crown volume is cumulative blood volume within the network ($Vc = \sum n_i(\pi L_i D_i^2)$, a derivation based on the average branching ratio ($n_i = Br^i, i = 0,.., m$; where n and i are number of vessels and branching level respectively) and scaling of vessel diameters and lengths in each branching level results in a relationship between crown volume and number of capillaries as follows (please see Supplementary Information):

$$V_c = K_{VN} (N_c)^\lambda \qquad (4)$$

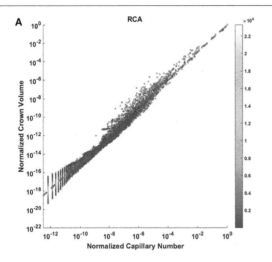

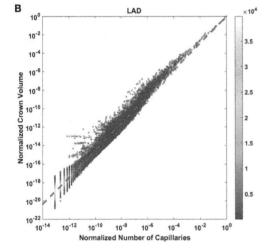

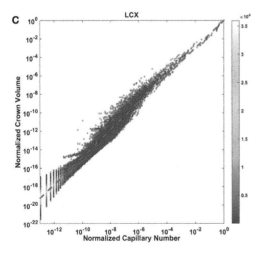

**FIGURE 4** | Relationship between normalized crown volume ($V_c/V_{c,max}$) and normalized number of capillaries ($N_c/N_{c,max}$) for the full asymmetric porcine arterial tree shown in a log-log density plot: **(A)** RCA, right coronary artery; **(B)** LAD, left anterior descending artery; **(C)** LCx, left circumflex artery. The total number of data points shown in **(A–C)** are 838,462, 950,014, and 575,868; respectively. The scaling exponents obtained from the least square fit of each data set are close to 3/2. The values of exponents, the confidence interval and $R^2$ for each species and organs are summarized in **Table 2**.

where $K_{VN}$ is a constant. If we normalize the above equation with respect to maximum crown volume and number of capillaries in the entire vascular network, a general form of scaling relationship is obtained as:

$$\frac{V_c}{V_{c,max}} = \left(\frac{N_c}{N_{c,max}}\right)^{\lambda} \tag{5}$$

## Crown Length Scales With Capillary Number

Since crown length is simply cumulative length of blood vessels of all branching levels within the network ($Lc = \sum n_i L_i$), a derivation based on the average branching ratio ($n_i = Br^i$, $i = 0,..,m$; where n and i are number of vessels and branching level respectively) and scaling of average length of blood vessels in each level of branching $L_i = (Br^{\gamma})^{m-i} L_{cap}$; where Lcap is the average length of capillaries and $\gamma$ is an empirical exponent (Huo and Kassab, 2012), results in a direct relationship between crown length and number of capillaries (please see Supplementary Information), namely:

$$L_c = K_{LN} N_c \tag{6}$$

where $K_{LN} = L_{cap} \sum_{i=o}^{m} Br^{(i-m)(1-\gamma)}$ is approximately a constant. A general form of normalized crown length and number of capillaries with respect to an entire tree is given as:

$$\frac{L_c}{L_{c,max}} = \left(\frac{N_c}{N_{c,max}}\right)^{\lambda} \tag{7}$$

where $L_{c,max}$ and $N_{c,max}$ are the maximum crown length and the number of capillaries in the entire tree. We shall confirm the hypothesis that $\lambda$ is equal to 1 and hence the form of Equation (7) can be described by Equation (6).

## Mean Transit Time Scales With Crown Volume and Length

Because of the structural heterogeneity of vascular networks and hence heterogeneous perfusions, the particles traverse various paths in the network. Hence, the mean transit time (MTT) is the average time required for blood to travel through the vascular network over a period of time. Based on the assumption that blood particles travel with the mean velocity of bulk flow and that the total number of blood particles passing through a vessel segment is proportional to the time-averaged flow rate in the segment, the MTT in the vascular network ($T_c$) can be written as:

$$T_c = \sum_{i=1}^{N} FF_i * T_{sg,i} \tag{8}$$

where $FF$ is the flow fraction (ratio of segment flow to stem flow) and $*T_{sg}$ is the average transit time in a specific segment where $i = 1,2,.., n$; and $n$ is the total number of segments in the entire network. It is well known that transit time can be determined by the ratio of blood volume and blood flow (Meier and Zierler, 1954). An elementary derivation by replacing the definition of the flow fraction (FFi = Qi/Qmax), transit time in a segment (Ti = Vi/Qi) and Equation (8) results in:

$$T_c * N_c = K_{TN} V_c \tag{9}$$

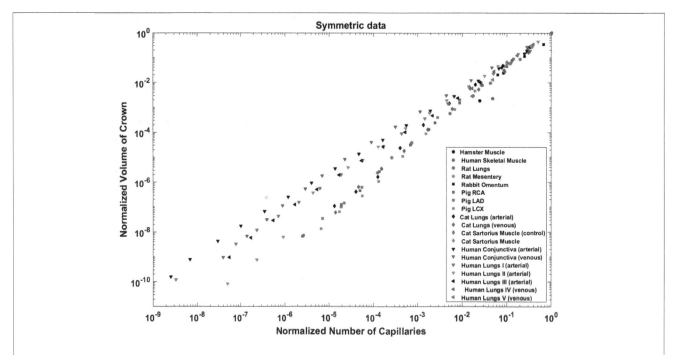

**FIGURE 5** | Relationship between normalized crown volume ($V_c/V_{c,max}$) and normalized number of capillaries ($N_c/N_{c,max}$) for the symmetric trees of various species and organs shown in a log-log scatter plot. RCA, right coronary artery; LAD, left anterior descending artery; LCx, left circumflex artery; PA, pulmonary artery; PV, pulmonary vein; SMA, sartorius muscle arteries; MA, mesentery arteries; OV, omentum veins; BCA, bulbular conjunctiva arteries; BCV, bulbular conjunctiva veins; RMA, retractor muscle artery. The scaling exponent (Equation 6) and $R^2$ for each species and organs summarized in **Table 2** are consistent with 3/2 or 4/3 exponent. The values of exponents, the confidence interval and $R^2$ for each species and organs are summarized in **Table 2**.

where $K_{TN}$ is a proportionality constant in unit of time/volume. A combination of Equations (6) and (9) relates mean transit time to crown volume and length, namely:

$$T_c * L_c = K_{TL} V_c \tag{10}$$

where the parameter $K_{TL}$ is a proportionality constant in unit of time/area. A general normalized form of the above equation can be written as:

$$\left(\frac{T_c}{T_{c,max}}\right) * \left(\frac{L_c}{L_{c,max}}\right) = \left(\frac{V_c}{V_{c,max}}\right)^\lambda \tag{11}$$

where $T_{c,max}$, $L_{c,max}$, and $V_{c,max}$ are the crown time, crown length and crown volume in the entire tree, respectively.

## RESULTS

### Flow Rate Scales With Number of Capillaries

The normalized flow and number of capillaries for all stem-crown units of the full asymmetric coronary arterial trees obeys a power law (**Figure 2**). The values of scaling exponent λ obtained from nonlinear regression were 1.005 ($R^2 = 1$), 1.002 ($R^2 = 1$), and 1.005 ($R^2 = 1$) for the porcine RCA, LAD, and LCx, respectively. The total number of data points shown in **Figures 2A–C** are 838,462, 950,014, and 575,868, respectively.

Analysis of normalized stem flow-crown capillaries for symmetric trees for various vascular trees of various species including the coronary arterial trees shows a linear relation between perfusion flow and the respective number of crown capillaries (**Figure 3**). The exponents in the symmetric analysis for all species and organs are equal to a theoretical value of unity; which is due to neglecting heterogeneity in the symmetric analysis and assumption that all vessel in each branching level has the same length and diameter. **Table 2** summarizes the least squares power law relation for each of the vascular trees, including the coefficient, exponent, and $R^2$. The exponents are nearly unity and the $R^2$ is highly significant. **Table 3** provides the $R^2$ values have been for lambda = 1.

### Crown Volume Scales With Number of Capillaries

The crown volume obeys a power law (Equation 5) as evident by morphometric data of full asymmetric arterial trees of porcine RCA, LAD, and LCx (**Figure 4**). The scaling exponents were 1.481 ($R^2 = 0.9261$), 1.453 ($R^2 = 0.9358$), and 1.479 ($R^2 = 0.9325$). The total number of data points shown in **Figures 4A–C** are 838,462, 950,014, and 575,868; respectively.

The exponents in the symmetric analysis for the RCA, LAD, and LCx is 1.447 ($R^2 = 0.9985$), 1.44 ($R^2 = 0.9962$), and 1.506 ($R^2 = 0.9966$), respectively; which are similar to the asymmetric tree analysis and close to the theoretical value of 3/2 (**Figure 5**). The mean exponent across various species

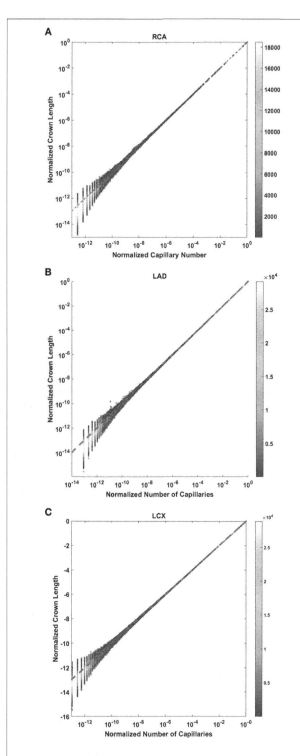

**FIGURE 6 |** Relationship between the normalized crown length ($L_c/L_{c,max}$) and normalized number of capillaries ($N_c/N_{c,max}$) for the full asymmetric porcine arterial tree shown in a log-log scatter plot: **(A)** RCA, right coronary artery; LAD, left anterior descending artery; LCx, left circumflex artery. The total number of data points shown in **(A–C)** are 838,462, 950,014, and 575,868; respectively. The dash lines correspond to the theoretical value of 1 predicted by Equation (7). The scaling exponents obtained from the least square fit of each data set are close to the theoretical value of unity. The values of exponents, the confidence interval and $R^2$ for each species and organ are summarized in **Table 2**.

and organs are $1.3723 \pm 0.1659$ ($R^2 > 0.92$). The scaling exponents, confidence intervals and $R^2$ associated with scaling exponent for various species and organs are summarized in **Table 2**.

## Crown Length Linearly Scales With Number of Capillaries

The crown length linearly scales with the number of capillaries for all stem-crown units of the full asymmetric coronary arterial trees (**Figure 6**). The values of scaling exponent λ (Equation 7) obtained from **Figures 6A–C** were 1.029 ($R^2 = 0.9169$), 1.031 ($R^2 = 0.9225$), and 1.031 ($R^2 = 0.9225$) for the porcine RCA, LAD and LCx, respectively (as compared to a theoretical value of unity, Equation 6). The total number of data points shown in **Figures 4A–C** are 838,462, 950,014, and 575,868, respectively.

The exponents in the symmetric analysis for the RCA, LAD, and LCx is 1.021 ($R^2 = 0.9989$), 1.022 ($R^2 = 0.9988$), and 1.028 ($R^2 = 0.9985$), respectively); which are similar to the asymmetric tree analysis and close to the theoretical unity (**Figure 7**). The average scaling exponent (Equation 7) for all species and organs is $1.0765 \pm 0.1022$ ($R^2 > 0.9$). **Table 2** summarizes the least squares power law relation for each of the vascular trees, including exponent, confidence interval, and $R^2$. The exponents are nearly unity and the $R^2$ is highly significant.

## Transit Time Scales With the Ratio of Crown Volume and Length

The crown volume and the product of crown length and mean transit time of asymmetric coronary arterial trees follows a scaling relationship (**Figure 8**). The scaling exponent λ (Equation 11) were 0.9814 ($R^2 = 1$), 0.9883 ($R^2 = 1$), and 0.9891 ($R^2 = 1$) for the porcine RCA, LAD and LCx, respectively as compared to a theoretical value of unity hypothesized by Equation (10). Similarly, the exponents in the symmetric analysis were 1.014 ($R^2 = 0.9995$), 1.015 ($R^2 = 0.9995$), 1.019 ($R^2 = 0.9994$) for RCA, LAD, LCx, respectively; which are close to the exponents related to the asymmetric data (**Figure 9**). The mean exponents for all species and organs is $1.0347 \pm 0.0819$ ($R^2 > 0.98$ for symmetric data). The exponents for various species and organs along with the associated confidence interval and $R^2$ were summarized in **Table 2**.

The confidence intervals and the scaling exponents obtained from bootstrapping for the asymmetric trees confirm the results presented in this section (please see the Supplementary Information Figures S1, S2 for further details). In addition, the $R^2$ for the stem-crown systems corresponding to a specific branching level of symmetric data where λ = 1 are presented in **Table 3**.

## DISCUSSION

The scaling laws and specifically form-form and form-function relations are important theoretical tools to understand the interplay between network structure and function in physiology

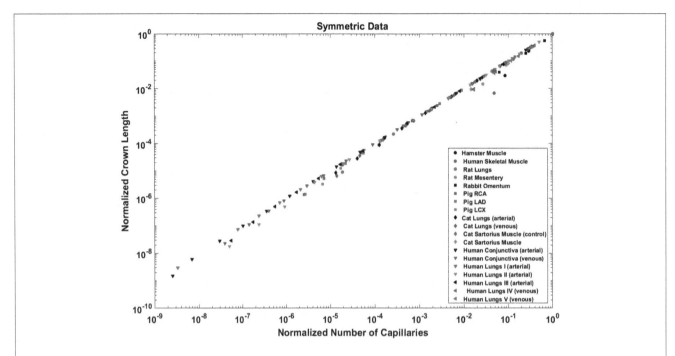

**FIGURE 7 |** Relationship between the normalized crown length (L_C/L_{C,max}) and normalized number of capillaries (N_C/N_{C,max}) for the full asymmetric porcine arterial tree shown in a log-log scatter plot. RCA, right coronary artery; LAD, left anterior descending artery; LCx, left circumflex artery; PA, pulmonary artery; PV, pulmonary vein; SMA, sartorius muscle arteries; MA, mesentery arteries; OV, omentum veins; BCA, bulbular conjunctiva arteries; BCV, bulbular conjunctiva veins; RMA, retractor muscle artery. The values of exponents (Equation 7) are in agreement with the theoretical value of unity predicted by Equation (6). The values of scaling exponents, the confidence interval and $R^2$ for various species and organs are summarized in **Table 2**.

and pathophysiology. Among the first form-function relations, a power-law relationship between flow and diameter was first pointed out by Murray nearly 90 years ago (Murray, 1926) and came to be known as Murray's law. Murray's law has been debated and even disproven for certain organs (Hutchins et al., 1976; Uylings, 1977; Sherman, 1981; Kassab, 2006, 2007). It has been found that the exponent 7/3 provides a better fit than the theoretical power of 3 from Murray's law. Although Murray's law (i.e., the exponent of 3) has been debated, the power-law form has not been contested and is universally accepted as a consequence of the optimized design of the vascular system. To this end, key advances have been made to test and validate intra-specific and inter-specific scaling laws for the entire arterial network. The scaling laws predict a linear relationship between flow and length while volume and flow are proportional to diameter with the power of 3 and 7/3 respectively (Kassab, 2006; Huo and Kassab, 2012). It has been also shown that the form-function relations are preserved in compensatory vascular remodeling. There is no intraspecific scaling relation, however, that relates the number of capillaries to various morphological and functional parameters (Gong et al., 2016). Here, we proposed and tested scaling relations for the vascular volume, length, and flow with the number of capillaries. Although there is deviation from the theoretical lines, mainly in the small vessels, the numbers of those that deviate are relatively small compared to the very majority that concentrate near the theoretical line. It should be also noted that scatter plots for asymmetric data show the density of data points and most points are concentrated

near theoretical values, and hence, the $R^2$ values are close to one.

Here, we developed intra-specific scaling laws between capillary number and crown volume. The derivation is based on the fractal characteristic of the branching tree pattern. The scaling exponent of porcine coronary arteries is in close proximity to 3/2 while the scaling exponent for human lungs is closer to 4/3. The mean exponent across various species and organs is 1.37 ± 0.166.

The conformity between scaling of crown length and number of capillaries among various species and organs reveals another salient proportionality law between form and function of the vascular system. The blood vessels are known to adapt to physiological demands and altered homeostatic conditions. The capability of vascular trees to deliver oxygen tissue and nutrients to serve metabolism strongly depends on the number of capillaries. The capillary density changes in response to conditions like hypoxia. In the context of new blood vessel formation and vascular sprouting, length of the perfused blood vessel is a key determinant of growth and development. It has been shown that length of blood vessels adapts to changes in homeostatic conditions (Lehman et al., 1991; Sho et al., 2004; Humphrey et al., 2009). The scaling law links vascular length to respective capillaries through a structure-function relation.

A linear relationship between flow rate and capillary number is expected based on the conservation of mass. Here, we tested the internal consistency of the data for both symmetric and asymmetric trees. Although such a linear scaling law is valid

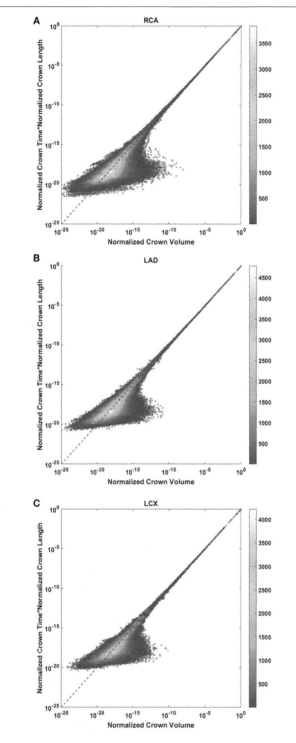

**FIGURE 8 |** Relationship between normalized crown volume ($V_C/V_{c,max}$) and multiplication of crown mean transit time and crown length ($T_S/T_{s,max}{}^*$ $L_S/L_{s,max}$) for the full asymmetric porcine arterial tree shown in a log-log density plot: **(A)** RCA, right coronary artery; **(B)** LAD, left anterior descending artery; **(C)** LCx, left circumflex artery. The total number of data points shown in **(A–C)** are 838,462, 950,014, and 575,868; respectively. The dash lines correspond to the theoretical exponent of unity. The scaling exponents obtained from the least square fit of each data set are close to the theoretical value of unity. The values of exponents, the confidence interval and $R^2$ for each species and organs are summarized in **Table 2**.

if the average capillary flow across the various stem-crown system is preserved, we validated such a relationship based on the available data sets from heterogeneous vascular networks of various species and organs. Flow-length and flow-diameter relations have been previously proposed and tested based on the minimum energy hypothesis. This analysis suggests that the number of capillaries in the length-capillary relation (form-form relation) and flow-capillary relation (form-function relation) relates flow to length (Huo and Kassab, 2012). Although flow-length and flow-diameter relationships have been validated, those studies used symmetric networks to estimate flow rate. Here, we showed that steady-state simulations of blood flow through both realistic asymmetric and simplified symmetric networks confirming that flow is proportional to the number of capillaries. This analysis takes into account the effect of heterogeneity in vessel geometry and hemodynamic parameters. The physical basis of this observation is the conservation of mass that dictates the stem flow is proportional to the number of terminal capillaries as long as the average capillary flow in the various stem-crown system approximately remains similar. Further, the relative uniformity of the diameter of arterial capillaries has been previously shown by Kassab and Fung (1994) for the coronary vasculature. The coefficient of variation (CV = SD/Mean) is 0.15 and 0.18 for the right and left ventricle walls, respectively. Hence, it is well recognized that the capillary dimensions are generally conserved across species (e.g., capillary diameters are similar in rat and human (Karbowski, 2011). However, upstream blood vessels and variation of pressure at the capillary bed can lead to dispersion in the terminal flow. Hence, scaling relationships for flow-capillary, and subsequently flow-length and flow-diameter relations, provide a better fit for larger vessels where many stem-crowns are included.

Perfusion is expressed as flow per mass and hence relates proportionally to the number of capillaries per mass. Since mass is equal to the volume and density of tissue, the perfusion increases with the increase in the number of capillaries per volume of tissue or number density as can be determined histologically. Hence, the linear scaling allows a direct connection between structure (number density) and function (perfusion). This relation may be used to understand the transition between physiology and pathophysiology. When the number density of capillaries is decreased due to infarction, hypertension, or obesity, etc., this may lead to malnutrition, atrophy or death of the tissue. Conversely, the number density of capillaries may be increased in tumors in accordance with the increase in blood flow to enhance the growth of the tissue. The number density can be determined from histological sections of biopsy specimens of animals and patients.

The flow perfusion-number density scaling relation can also be used for drug dose determination. The dose can be titrated between species as the number density reflects perfusion (flow per mass) of tissue. Adequate perfusion (volumetric flow per mass of tissue) is essential for any organ because it affects its health and function. The linearity between stem flow and the number of capillaries the functional capillary density can be

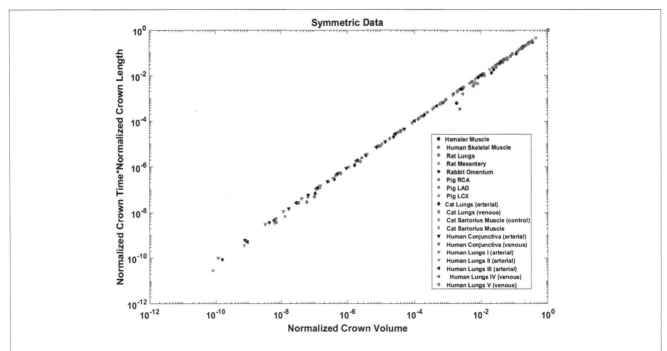

**FIGURE 9 |** Relationship between normalized crown volume ($V_C/V_{c,max}$) and multiplication of crown mean transit time and crown length ($T_S/T_{s,max}$* $L_S/L_{s,max}$) for the symmetric trees of various species and organs shown in a log-log scatter plot. RCA, right coronary artery; LAD, left anterior descending artery; LCx, left circumflex artery; PA, pulmonary artery; PV, pulmonary vein; SMA, sartorius muscle arteries; MA, mesentery arteries; OV, omentum veins; BCA, bulbar conjunctiva arteries; BCV, bulbar conjunctiva veins; RMA, retractor muscle artery. The values of exponents are consistent with the theoretical value of unity. The values of scaling exponents, the confidence interval and $R^2$ for various species and organs are summarized in **Table 2**.

obtained from the length of vascular network non-invasively from standard medical imaging.

The transit time is a seminal physiological parameter in biological transport phenomena and has critical implications for vascular disease. Prolonged mean transit time is known to be associated with high risk of infarction and cerebral ischemia. No-capillary flow and altered blood volume conditions occur under pathophysiological conditions. The scaling relation between mean transit time, blood volume, and the number capillaries can be used as a theoretical basis to understand the distribution of oxygen and nutrients under physiological conditions and microvascular failure under pathological conditions. It is well known that the transit time is the ratio of vascular volume and blood flow. Since a relationship between flow rate and crown length holds for various vascular trees, we compared the theoretical calculation of transit times based on the crown length to the calculation based on the blood flow. It was shown that the estimation of transit time based on the crown length and volume hold for proximal trees (down to 1 mm diameter vessels which can be observed in angiograms). Hence, standard clinical imaging of blood vessel anatomy may yield functional data on the transit times through the organ of interest.

This study has several limitations that should be noted to guide interpretation of the proposed relationships. First, the available morphometric data were obtained from healthy subjects, and hence, the scaling laws are applicable to only healthy vasculature. For example, in pathophysiological

cases such as infarction, functional capillary density and associated tissue perfusion changes even though the number of capillaries may remain unchanged. Hence, in scenarios where the model assumptions are severely violated, the proposed scaling laws may not be preserved and may lead to an overestimate. This may have utility, however, since the proposed scaling laws may serve as a signature of normal function and deviations from these laws may form the basis to quantify the severity of disease such as non-compensatory remodeling (e.g., the deviation from the scaling laws may be a useful theoretical framework to establish a scoring system for the severity of disease state). Second, a uniform outlet pressure was used to simulate blood flow. It has been found, however, that a heterogeneous outflow pressure can lead to flow reversal at capillary beds which likely occurs transiently. Although this phenomenon can change transit time estimation, previous simulations have shown that heterogeneous outlet pressure can change transit time at most ~10% (Mittal et al., 2005). We have also modeled heterogeneity of blood flow and transit time distribution incorporating Fåhræus effect in simulations. Third, both realistic asymmetric as well as idealized symmetric data were used based the available morphometric data. Since symmetric analysis neglects heterogeneity, hemodynamic variations for vessels belonging to the same branching are not considered. Specifically, that is the case for trees with a small number of branching level, where the standard deviation of each parameter in each branching level may be large. Comparison of symmetric and asymmetric analyses for trees that have a large branching level (e.g., pig RCA, LCX, LAD), however, shows that the scaling exponents are very similar for both symmetric and asymmetric data.

## AUTHORS CONTRIBUTION

MR performed the analysis and drafted the text; ES reviewed the transit time analysis and provided input; GK performed the analysis for the flow-capillary number relation, drafted the related text, and supervised the overall manuscript.

## ACKNOWLEDGMENTS

This research was supported in part by the National Institute of Health-National Heart, Lung, and Blood Institute Grant U01HL118738.

## REFERENCES

Bertuglia, S., Colantuoni, A., Coppini, G., and Intaglietta, M. (1991). Hypoxia-or hyperoxia-induced changes in arteriolar vasomotion in skeletal muscle microcirculation. *Am. J. Physiol.* 260, H362–H372. doi: 10.1152/ajpheart.1991.260.2.H362

Crumrine, R. C., and LaManna, J. C. (1991). Regional cerebral metabolites, blood flow, plasma volume, and mean transit time in total cerebral ischemia in the rat. *J. Cereb. Blood Flow Metab.* 11, 272–282. doi: 10.1038/jcbfm.1991.59

Derdeyn, C. P., Grubb, R. L. Jr., and Powers, W. J. (1999). Cerebral hemodynamic impairment: methods of measurement and association with stroke risk. *Neurology* 53, 251–259. doi: 10.1212/WNL.53.2.251

Dodds, P. S., Rothman, D. H., and Weitz, J. S. (2001). Re-examination of the "3/4-law" of metabolism. *J. Theor. Biol.* 209, 9–27. doi: 10.1006/jtbi.2000.2238

Ellsworth, M. L., Liu, A., Dawant, B., Popel, A. S., and Pittman, R. N. (1987). Analysis of vascular pattern and dimensions in arteriolar networks of the retractor muscle in young hamsters. *Microvasc. Res.* 34, 168–183. doi: 10.1016/0026-2862(87)90051-3

Fenton, B. M., and Zweifach, B. (1981). Microcirculatory model relating geometrical variation to changes in pressure and flow rate. *Ann. Biomed. Eng.* 9, 303–321. doi: 10.1007/BF02364653

Gong, Y., Feng, Y., Chen, X., Tan, W., Huo, Y., Kassab, G. S., et al. (2016). Intraspecific scaling laws are preserved in ventricular hypertrophy but not in heart failure. *Am. J. Physiol.* 311, H1108–H1117. doi: 10.1152/ajpheart.00084.2016

Horsfield, K., and Gordon, W. I. (1981). Morphometry of pulmonary veins in man. *Lung* 159, 211–218. doi: 10.1007/BF02713917

Huang, W., Yen, R., McLaurine, M., and Bledsoe, G. (1996). Morphometry of the human pulmonary vasculature. *J. Appl. Physiol.* 81, 2123–2133. doi: 10.1152/jappl.1996.81.5.2123

Humphrey, J., Eberth, J., Dye, W., and Gleason, R. (2009). Fundamental role of axial stress in compensatory adaptations by arteries. *J. Biomech.* 42, 1–8. doi: 10.1016/j.jbiomech.2008.11.011

Huo, Y., and Kassab, G. S. (2012). Intraspecific scaling laws of vascular trees. *J. R. Soc. Interf.* 9, 190–200. doi: 10.1098/rsif.2011.0270

Huo, Y., Linares, C. O., and Kassab, G. S. (2007). Capillary perfusion and wall shear stress are restored in the coronary circulation of hypertrophic right ventricle. *Circ. Res.* 100, 273–283. doi: 10.1161/01.RES.0000257777.83431.13

Hutchins, G. M., Miner, M. M., and Boitnott, J. K. (1976). Vessel caliber and branch-angle of human coronary artery branch-points. *Circ. Res.* 38, 572–576. doi: 10.1161/01.RES.38.6.572

Jiang, Z. L., Kassab, G. S., and Fung, Y. C. (1994). Diameter-defined Strahler system and connectivity matrix of the pulmonary arterial tree. *J. Appl. Physiol.* 76, 882–892. doi: 10.1152/jappl.1994.76.2.882

Karbowski, J. (2011). Scaling of brain metabolism and blood flow in relation to capillary and neural scaling. *PLoS ONE* 6:e26709. doi: 10.1371/journal.pone.0026709

Kassab, G. S. (2006). Scaling laws of vascular trees: of form and function. *Am. J. Physiol.* 290, H894–H903. doi: 10.1152/ajpheart.00579.2005

Kassab, G. S. (2007). Design of coronary circulation: a minimum energy hypothesis. *Comp. Methods Appl. Mech. Eng.* 196, 3033–3042. doi: 10.1016/j.cma.2006.09.024

Kassab, G. S., Berkley, J., and Fung, Y. C. (1997). Analysis of pig's coronary arterial blood flow with detailed anatomical data. *Ann. Biomed. Eng.* 25, 204–217. doi: 10.1007/BF02738551

Kassab, G. S., and Fung, Y. C. (1994). Topology and dimensions of pig coronary capillary network. *Am. J. Phys.* 267(1 Pt 2), H319–H325.

Kassab, G. S., Rider, C. A., Tang, N. J., and Fung, Y. C. (1993). Morphometry of pig coronary arterial trees. *Am. J. Physiol.* 265(1 Pt 2), H350–H365. doi: 10.1152/ajpheart.1993.265.1.H350

Koller, A., Dawant, B., Liu, A., Popel, A. S., and Johnson, P. C. (1987). Quantitative analysis of arteriolar network architecture in cat sartorius muscle. *Am. J. Physiol.* 253(1 Pt 2), H154–H164. doi: 10.1152/ajpheart.1987.253.1.H154

LaBarbera, M. (1990). Principles of design of fluid transport systems in zoology. *Science* 249, 992–1000. doi: 10.1126/science.2396104

Lehman, R. M., Owens, G. K., Kassell, N. F., and Hongo, K. (1991). Mechanism of enlargement of major cerebral collateral arteries in rabbits. *Stroke* 22, 499–504. doi: 10.1161/01.STR.22.4.499

Ley, K., Pries, A. R., and Gaehtgens, P. (1986). Topological structure of rat mesenteric microvessel networks. *Microvasc. Res.* 32, 315–332. doi: 10.1016/0026-2862(86)90068-3

Meier, P., and Zierler, K. L. (1954). On the theory of the indicator-dilution method for measurement of blood flow and volume. *J. Appl. Physiol.* 6, 731–744. doi: 10.1152/jappl.1954.6.12.731

Mittal, N., Zhou, Y., Ung, S., Linares, C., Molloi, S., and Kassab, G. S. (2005). A computer reconstruction of the entire coronary arterial tree based on detailed morphometric data. *Ann. Biomed. Eng.* 33, 1015–1026. doi: 10.1007/s10439-005-5758-z

Mooney, C. Z., Duval, R. D., and Duvall, R. (1993). *Bootstrapping: A Nonparametric Approach to Statistical Inference.* London: Sage.

Murray, C. D. (1926). The physiological principle of minimum work: II. oxygen exchange in capillaries. *Proc. Natl. Acad. Sci. U.S.A.* 12, 299–304. doi: 10.1073/pnas.12.5.299

Pries, A. R., Secomb, T. W., Gessner, T., Sperandio, M. B., Gross, J. F., and Gaehtgens, P. (1994). Resistance to blood flow in microvessels *in vivo. Circ. Res.* 75, 904–915. doi: 10.1161/01.RES.75.5.904

Pries, A. R., and Secomb, T. W. (2009). Origins of heterogeneity in tissue perfusion and metabolism. *Cardiovasc. Res.* 81, 328–335. doi: 10.1093/cvr/cvn318

Rosen, R. (1967). *Optimality Principles in Biology,* London: Butterworths.

Sherman, T. F. (1981). On connecting large vessels to small. The meaning of Murray's law. *J. General Physiol.* 78, 431–453. doi: 10.1085/jgp.78.4.431

Sho, E., Nanjo, H., Sho, M., Kobayashi, M., Komatsu, M., Kawamura, K., et al. (2004). Arterial enlargement, tortuosity, and intimal thickening in response to sequential exposure to high and low wall shear stress. *J. Vasc. Surg.* 39, 601–612. doi: 10.1016/j.jvs.2003.10.058

Singhal, S., Henderson, R., Horsfield, K., Harding, K., and Cumming, G. (1973). Morphometry of the human pulmonary arterial tree. *Circ. Res.* 33, 190–197. doi: 10.1161/01.RES.33.2.190

Singhal, S. S., Cumming, G., Horsfield, K., and Harking, L. K. (1973). Morphometric study of pulmonary arterial tree and its haemodynamics. *J. Assoc. Physicians India* 21, 719–722.

Uylings, H. (1977). Optimization of diameters and bifurcation angles in lung and vascular tree structures. *Bull. Math. Biol.* 39, 509–520. doi: 10.1007/BF02461198

West, G. B., Brown, J. H., and Enquist, B. J. (1997). A general model for the origin of allometric scaling laws in biology. *Science* 276, 122–126. doi: 10.1126/science.276.5309.122

White, C. R., and Seymour, R. S. (2003). Mammalian basal metabolic rate is proportional to body mass2/3. *Proc. Natl. Acad. Sci. U.S.A.* 100, 4046–4049. doi: 10.1073/pnas.0436428100

Wu, C.-F. J. (1986). Jackknife, bootstrap and other resampling methods in regression analysis. *Ann. Stat.* 14, 1261–1295.

Yen, R. T., Zhuang, F. Y., Fung, Y. C., Ho, H. H., Tremer, H., Sobin, S. S., et al. (1983). Morphometry of cat pulmonary venous tree. *J. Appl. Physiol.* 55(1 Pt 1), 236–242. doi: 10.1152/jappl.1983.55.1.236

Yen, R. T., Zhuang, F. Y., Fung, Y. C., Ho, H. H., Tremer, H., Sobin, S. S., et al. (1984). Morphometry of cat's pulmonary arterial tree. *J. Biomech. Eng.* 106, 131–136. doi: 10.1115/1.3138469

# 18

# Left Ventricular Wall Stress is Sensitive Marker of Hypertrophic Cardiomyopathy with Preserved Ejection Fraction

Xiaodan Zhao[1], Ru-San Tan[1,2], Hak-Chiaw Tang[1,2], Soo-Kng Teo[3], Yi Su[3], Min Wan[4], Shuang Leng[1], Jun-Mei Zhang[1,2], John Allen[2], Ghassan S. Kassab[5] and Liang Zhong[1,2]*

[1] National Heart Research Institute Singapore, National Heart Centre Singapore, Singapore, Singapore, [2] Duke-NUS Medical School, Singapore, Singapore, [3] Institute of High Performance Computing, Agency for Science, Technology and Research, Singapore, Singapore, [4] School of Information Engineering, Nanchang University, Nanchang, Jiangxi, China, [5] California Medical Innovations Institute, San Diego, CA, United States

*Correspondence:
Liang Zhong
zhong.liang@nhcs.com.sg

Hypertrophic cardiomyopathy (HCM) patients present altered myocardial mechanics due to the hypertrophied ventricular wall and are typically diagnosed by the increase in myocardium wall thickness. This study aimed to quantify regional left ventricular (LV) shape, wall stress and deformation from cardiac magnetic resonance (MR) images in HCM patients and controls, in order to establish superior measures to differentiate HCM from controls. A total of 19 HCM patients and 19 controls underwent cardiac MR scans. The acquired MR images were used to reconstruct 3D LV geometrical models and compute the regional parameters (i.e., wall thickness, curvedness, wall stress, area strain and ejection fraction) based on the standard 16 segment model using our in-house software. HCM patients were further classified into four quartiles based on wall thickness at end diastole (ED) to assess the impact of wall thickness on these regional parameters. There was a significant difference between the HCM patients and controls for all regional parameters ($P < 0.001$). Wall thickness was greater in HCM patients at the end-diastolic and end-systolic phases, and thickness was most pronounced in segments at the septal regions. A multivariate stepwise selection algorithm identified wall stress index at ED ($\sigma_{i,ED}$) as the single best independent predictor of HCM (AUC $= 0.947$). At the cutoff value $\sigma_{i,ED} < 1.64$, both sensitivity and specificity were 94.7%. This suggests that the end-diastolic wall stress index incorporating regional wall curvature—an index based on mechanical principle—is a sensitive biomarker for HCM diagnosis with potential utility in diagnostic and therapeutic assessment.

Keywords: regional curvedness, regional wall stress index, regional area strain, hypertrophic cardiomyopathy, magnetic resonance imaging

## INTRODUCTION

Hypertrophic cardiomyopathy (HCM) is a primary and familial disease of the cardiac sarcomere leading to cardiac hypertrophy (Kovacic and Muller, 2003; Hansen and Merchant, 2007). It is characterized by thickening of the myocardium with prevalence of 1 in 500 for the general population (Wigle, 2001; Kovacic and Muller, 2003; Elliott and McKenna, 2004; Hughes, 2004).

Annual mortality is estimated at 1–2% (Wigle, 2001). Echocardiography can be used to measure ventricular thickness and diagnose hypertrophy (Klues et al., 1995; Maron, 2002). In addition, abnormal left ventricular (LV) systolic performance can also be detected and quantified by strain parameters (longitudinal strains and twist), and torsion and dyssynchrony (Carasso et al., 2008, 2010). There are still limitations to this method, however, as echocardiogram examination can be inconclusive when the hypertrophied myocardium is localized at LV regions that are difficult to visualize. Moreover, echocardiography may underestimate the maximum extent of LV wall thickening, particularly when hypertrophy involves the anterolateral wall (Maron et al., 2010). Compared to echocardiography, cardiac magnetic resonance (CMR) has the advantages of superior spatial resolution and ability to characterize tissue composition (Hoey et al., 2014) and ventricular shape (Zhong et al., 2009b, 2012b). Therefore, it provides opportunity for more accurate characterization of LV hypertrophy in HCM, both regionally and globally (Rickers et al., 2005; Noureldin et al., 2012; Lee et al., 2014).

The alteration of ventricular wall stress is associated with morphological and functional changes in the myocardium. LV wall stress is proportional to radius and inversely proportional to wall thickness according to the Law of Laplace (Badeer, 1963). Numerous formulas have been proposed to estimate wall stress (Falsetti et al., 1970; Grossman et al., 1975; Yin, 1981; Janz, 1982; Regen, 1990; Zhong et al., 2012a). Some early approaches assumed the heart as an ideal shape, such as spherical or ellipsoidal, which may not be applicable for complex LV geometry, such as in HCM. Moreover, they only allowed the global wall stress calculation, while 3D regional patterns and distributions of wall stress are crucial in fully characterizing, quantifying, and differentiating HCM patients from healthy subjects. We have proposed a 3D regional curvature-based wall stress approach and applied in ischemic dilated cardiomyopathy (Zhong et al., 2009b) and heart failure (Zhong et al., 2011). The pattern of HCM is variable and can be divided into morphological subtypes: reverse curvature, sigmoid and neutral. That may be associated with differential regional stress. Hence, appropriate characterization of regional morphology and wall stress may be particularly helpful in HCM.

In this study, we aimed to (1) assess the regional variation of wall curvedness, stress and function in HCM; (2) assess the utility of wall stress in differentiating HCM from controls, and (3) characterize the wall curvedness, stress and function in subtypes of HCM.

## MATERIALS AND METHODS

### Population
The study was approved by the SingHealth Centralized Institutional Review Board, and written consent forms were obtained from all participants. 19 HCM patients and 19 age-matched normal controls were prospectively enrolled at National Heart Centre Singapore. Subjects with LV ejection fraction <50%, hyperlipidemia, physician diagnosis of hypertension or diabetes mellitus were excluded

from the Control group. Clinical data were collected at enrollment.

## CMR Scan and LV Wall Thickness Measurements
CMR scan was performed using steady state, free precession (SSFP) cine gradient echo sequences on a 1.5T Siemens MR imaging system (Avanto, Germany). Ventricular long axis (two-, three- and four-chamber) and stacks of short axis views with thickness 8 mm were each acquired in a single breath-hold. LV interventricular septum thickness in diastole (IVSd) and systole (IVSs), and LV posterior wall thicknesses in diastole (LVPWd) and systole (LVPWs) were measured from mid LV short-axis images, i.e., at the level of the papillary muscles.

## HCM Subtypes
Following the HCM subtype characterization described by Binder et al. (2006), HCM cases were sub-categorized by our senior HCM consultant as sigmoid ($n = 6$), reverse curvature ($n = 8$) or neutral ($n = 5$).

## Two-Dimensional Regional Curvature and Strain
A common approach to quantifying concavity and convexity of a contour employs curvature. The independent coordinate method (Lewiner et al., 2005; Zhao et al., 2018) has been used to compute endocardium and epicardium curvatures at both end-diastolic (ED) and end-systolic (ES) phases. Examples involving a control and three HCM subtypes at the ED phase are illustrated in **Figure 1**.

The extent of inhomogeneity was characterized by variation of curvature (*VC*) defined as the ratio of curvature standard deviation $\sigma(\kappa)$ to mean $\mu(\kappa)$ at a given discrete point:

$$VC = \frac{\sigma(\kappa)}{\mu(\kappa)}. \tag{1}$$

Ventricular endocardial and epicardial strain was defined as Zhao et al. (2018):

$$
\begin{aligned}
S_{\text{endo}} &= \left| \ln\left(\frac{L_{\text{ES,endo}}}{L_{\text{ED,endo}}}\right) \right| \times 100\%; \\
S_{\text{epi}} &= \left| \ln\left(\frac{L_{\text{ES,epi}}}{L_{\text{ED,epi}}}\right) \right| \times 100\%,
\end{aligned}
\tag{2}
$$

where $L_{\text{ED,endo}}$ and $L_{\text{ED,epi}}$ are respective endocardial and epicardial contour lengths extending from one atrioventricular junction point to the other atrioventricular junction point in standard long axis view at ED, and similarly for $L_{\text{ES,endo}}$ and $L_{\text{ES,epi}}$.

## Three-Dimensional Regional Shape and Deformation Parameters
LV endocardial and epicardial contours were segmented using CMRtools (Cardiovascular Solution, UK) by co-registering the short- and long-axis images. The segmented short-axis contours representing the endocardial and epicardial surfaces were then used as input for our 3D reconstruction algorithm. Our 3D

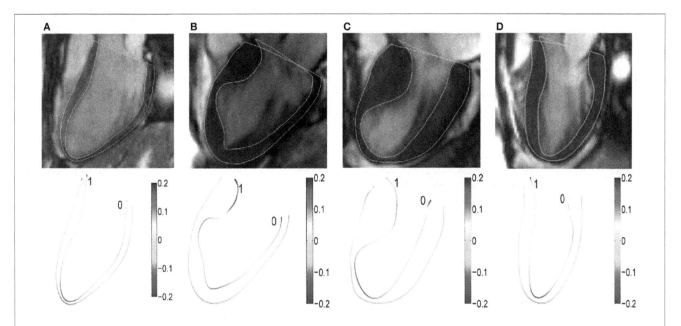

**FIGURE 1** | Segmented two-dimensional three-chamber long-axis magnetic resonance images (top row) and color representation of 2D curvature with range [−0.2, 0.2] (bottom row) in **(A)** a 37-year-old female control subject; **(B)** a 67-year-old female patient; **(C)** a 60-year-old female patient; and **(D)** a 55-year-old female patient. The curvature is negative if the unit tangent rotates clockwise.

reconstruction methodology can be broadly summarized into 3 steps:

(I) Correction of any possible motion artifacts due to respiration and patient movement. Here, we implement a shape-driven algorithm based on the premise that the LV epicardial surface must be smooth after the restoration process. This restoration is achieved by iterative in-plane translation of both the LV epicardial and endocardial contour vertices via minimization of an objective function based on the principal curvatures of the LV epicardial surface. Further details of the restoration algorithm can be found in our previous publications (Tan et al., 2013; Su et al., 2014).

(II) Up-sampling of short-axis contours and surface triangulation. The up-sampling of both the endocardial and epicardial contours are necessary to achieve a smooth reconstructed 3D surface, due to the relatively large spacing between the CMR image slices (typically 8–10 mm). We implement a B-spline fitting algorithm across multiple short-axis contours based on the surface normal vectors of the contour vertices to insert 3 intermediate points between any 2 adjacent contour vertices lying on the original CMR image slices. This results in the insertion of 3 intermediate short-axis contours between any 2 adjacent segmented contours. Next, we triangulate the up-sampled contours by connecting the 3 nearest points into a surface triangle. This step is repeated for each time-frame in the cardiac cycle and results in a set of 3D surface meshes with different number of vertices and triangles dependent on the height of the LV.

(III) Generation of endocardial surface meshes with 1-to-1 correspondence based on radial basis function morphing for the entire cardiac cycle to facilitate analysis of geometrical features. Here, we implement an automated approach to motion registered

a series of surface meshes representing the instantaneous shape of the LV endocardial surface throughout the cardiac cycle from Step (II). The output is a sequence of meshes with 1-to-1 surface point correspondence; i.e., this sequence of meshes have identical number of vertices and the same connectivity information. Further details of the 1-to-1 correspondence algorithm can be found in our previous publication (Su et al., 2015). We note that this correspondence is implemented only for the LV endocardial surface meshes because our analysis focuses only on the curvature of the LV endocardial surface.

The format of the resultant endocardial surface is an explicit surface mesh in the form of a two-manifold structured triangle mesh where the vertices and connectivity information are stored.

The endocardial mesh was partitioned according to recommendation by the American Heart Association (Cerqueira et al., 2002). In this study, we used our modified approach (Zhong et al., 2009b; Su et al., 2012) to generate the 16-segment model, and omitted segment 17 in the standard nomenclature because the curvature of the true apex position would strain the reconstruction algorithm.

Wall thickness was evaluated for each segment at the ED and ES phases and denoted as $WT_{ED}$ and $WT_{ES}$, respectively (Zhong et al., 2009b). The maximal LV wall thickness among 16 segments at ED and ES were denoted as $WT_{ED,max}$ and $WT_{ES,max}$. The 3D regional shape was measured by the curvedness value $C$ (Koenderink and Van Doorn, 1992) defined as:

$$C = \sqrt{\frac{\kappa_1^2 + \kappa_2^2}{2}}, \tag{3}$$

where $\kappa_1$ and $\kappa_2$ are the maximum and minimum principal curvatures, respectively. These principal curvature are defined based on the endocardial surface. In the vicinity of any vertices on the endocardial surface mesh, the local surface can be approximated by an osculating paraboloid that may be represented by a quadratic polynomial. The detailed derivation for computing the principal curvatures can be found in Appendix A of our previous publications (Yeo et al., 2009; Zhong et al., 2009b).

Pressure-normalized wall stress, an index that provides crucial information on geometrical influence on wall stress, has been proposed using thick-walled ellipse and sphere models (Zhong et al., 2006; Alter et al., 2007). In the present study, wall stress index $\sigma_i$, which incorporates local wall curvature, was determined as Zhong et al. (2009b)

$$\sigma_i = \frac{R}{2WT(1 + \frac{WT}{2R})}, \tag{4}$$

where $WT$ is ventricular wall thickness and $R$ the inner radius of curvedness. In **Figure 2**, we illustrate wall thickness, regional curvedness and wall stress index for a control patient, sigmoid, reverse curvature and neutral subtypes for HCM patients.

Area strain is a dimensionless quantity that measures regional LV endocardial surface deformation which integrates longitudinal, circumferential and radial deformation. The regional area strain ($AS$) was defined as Zhong et al. (2012b):

$$AS = \ln\left(\frac{SA_{ES}}{SA_{ED}}\right), \tag{5}$$

where $SA_{ED}$ and $SA_{ES}$ are the respective endocardial surface areas at the ED and ES phases.

The regional ejection fraction ($EF$) is a measure of the pumping efficiency of a particular LV segment and was previously derived (Wisneski et al., 1981; Teo et al., 2015). The $EF_i$ for the i-th segment is calculated as

$$EF_i = \frac{V_{i,ED} - V_{i,ES}}{V_{i,ED}} \times 100\%, \tag{6}$$

where $V_{i,ED}$ and $V_{i,ES}$ are the LV cavity volumes corresponding to the i-th segment at the ED and ES phase, respectively.

## Statistical Analysis

All continuous variables are presented as mean ± standard deviation (SD), whereas categorical data are presented as relative frequencies in terms of percentage. Associations between continuous variables were investigated using least square regression and Pearson correlation. The two-sample $t$-test was used to assess significant differences between means of two independent groups. One-way analysis of variance (ANOVA) was used to compare means among control and hypertrophy subtypes for 3D regional parameters. As individual diagnostic cutpoints, the continuous predictors IVSd, $WT_{ED,max}$ and $\sigma_{i,ED}$ were dichotomized (non-HCM vs. HCM) as follows: IVSd $\leq$13 mm vs. >13 mm, $WT_{ED,max} \leq$ 13 mm vs. >13 mm, and $\sigma_{i,ED}$ $\geq$1.64 vs. <1.64. Potential predictors were assessed individually

using univariate logistic regression and those significant at $P < 0.20$ were included in a multivariate analysis incorporating a stepwise selection algorithm (SLE = 0.20, SLS = 0.25) to identify a minimal "best" subset predictive of HCM. Intra- and inter-observer reproducibility was assessed via the intra-class correlation coefficient (ICC). The mean of the absolute values of the differences between two measurements divided by the mean of all measurements taken was used to quantify measurement variability as a proportion of the mean measurement value (Zhong et al., 2009a, 2012c). $P < 0.05$ was considered statistically significant. Data assembly and statistical analysis were performed with SPSS version 22.0.

## RESULTS

The baseline demographics of controls and HCM patient are summarized in **Table 1**. Compared to control subjects, HCM patients had higher LV end-diastolic and lower end-systolic volume indices, although not statistically significant ($P = 0.451$ and $P = 0.308$); however, difference in higher LV ejection fraction was statistically significant ($P = 0.034$). For 2D clinical CMR measurements, wall thickness was demonstrably greater in HCM patients vs. controls for ED (HCM, 17.0 ± 6.1 vs. Control, 8.4 ± 1.4 mm; $P$ <0.001), ES (HCM, 21.4 ± 5.4 vs. Control, 12.2 ± 2.3 mm; $P < 0.001$) and fractional shortening (HCM, 44.2 ± 7.9 vs. Control, 35.0 ± 6.1%; $P < 0.001$; **Table 2**). Similar results in ED and ES maximal wall thickness were observed between HCM patients and controls for CMR measurements from our 3D model.

## Difference of Geometrical Descriptors Between HCM and Controls

The 2D curvature and strain results for both groups are summarized in **Table 3**. The $VC$ for curvature was 1.94 ± 0.47 at ED and 3.54 ± 1.32 at ES in the controls, with increases in HCM patients to 2.65 ± 0.84 at ED and 5.02 ± 2.42 at ES. Second, HCM patients had significantly lower $S_{endo}$ and $S_{epi}$ compared with controls (18.4 ± 3.8% vs. 24.8 ± 3.0% and 12.6 ± 3.9% vs. 21.3 ± 3.0%, both $P < 0.001$). Patients with HCM had significant increases in wall thickness at both ED and ES phases (**Figures 3A,B**). For each region in HCM patients, greater wall thickness was observed in the basal anterior septal, basal inferior septal, mid inferior septal and apical septal regions owing to septum hypertrophy.

Regional 3D curvedness, regional wall stress index, area strain and ejection fraction are given in **Tables 4–6**, respectively. **Figures 3C,D** showed a significant increase in regional ED curvedness in HCM patients compared to controls, except for segment 9 (mid inferior septal) and segments 13-16 (apical region). **Figures 3E,F** showed a significant decrease in wall stress index at ED and ES in the HCM patients across all segments, except for segment 15 (apical inferior) at ED and segments 13–16 (apical region) at ES. **Figure 3G** demonstrated a decrease in $AS$ in HCM patients. Mean $AS$ values (aggregating over all 16 segments) were 78.5 and 65.7% for controls and HCM patients respectively ($P < 0.05$). Comparing across individual segments,

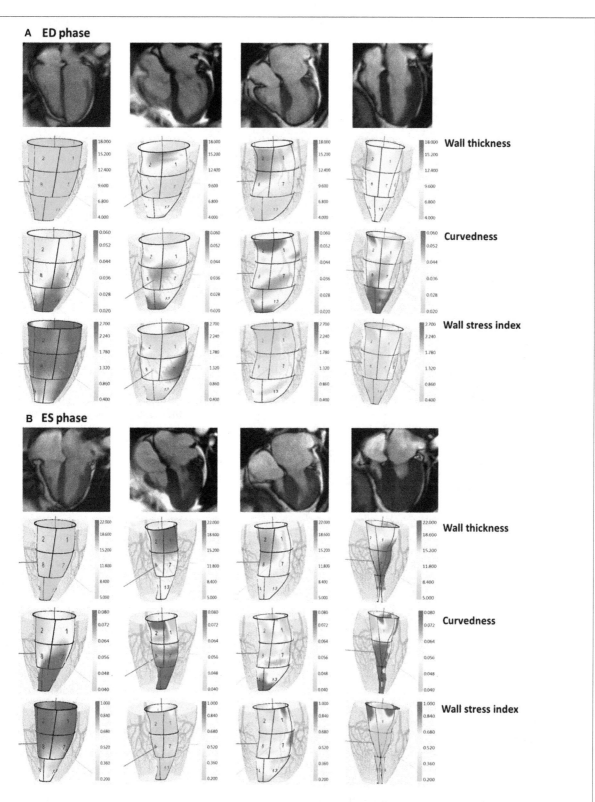

**FIGURE 2 |** Columns: normal subject, HCM patient with sigmoid subtype, HCM patient with reverse curvature subtype and HCM patient with neutral subtype. In **(A)**, first row: segmented two-dimensional cine four-chamber magnetic resonance images at ED phase; second row: wall thickness (range: 4–18 mm) at ED phase; third row: regional curvedness (range: 0.02–0.06 mm$^{-1}$) at ED phase; last row: wall stress index (range: 0.4–2.7) at ED phase. The order in **(B)** at ES phase is the same as the order in **(A)** with wall thickness range: 5–22 mm, regional curvedness range: 0.04–0.08 mm$^{-1}$ and wall stress index range: 0.2–1.0. HCM, hypertrophic cardiomyopathy; ED, end diastole; ES, end systole.

**TABLE 1** | Baseline and demographics of control subjects and HCM patients.

| Variable | Control ($n = 19$) | HCM ($n = 19$) | P-value |
|---|---|---|---|
| Age, years old | $51 \pm 11$ | $51 \pm 13$ | 0.834 |
| Gender, Male/Female | 12/7 | 7/12 | 0.105 |
| Weight, kg | $68 \pm 15$ | $69 \pm 20$ | 0.816 |
| Height, cm | $163 \pm 11$ | $162 \pm 12$ | 0.810 |
| Body surface area, m$^2$ | $1.75 \pm 0.24$ | $1.76 \pm 0.30$ | 0.953 |
| Diastolic blood pressure, mmHg | $74 \pm 8$ | $72 \pm 13$ | 0.732 |
| Systolic blood pressure, mmHg | $128 \pm 17$ | $132 \pm 22$ | 0.548 |
| Tobacco, % | 0 (0%) | 2 (10.5%) | 0.181 |
| Diabetes, % | 0 (0%) | 1 (5.3%) | 0.432 |
| Hyperlipidaemia, % | 0 (0%) | 9 (47.4%) | **<0.001** |
| Hypertension, % | 0 (0%) | 7 (36.8%) | **0.001** |
| Peripheral vascular disease, % | 0 (0%) | 1 (5.3%) | 0.432 |
| Family history of HCM (up to second degree) | 0 (0%) | 9 (47.4%) | **<0.001** |
| Family history of sudden cardiac death due to HCM | 0 (0%) | 4 (21.1%) | **0.029** |
| LVEDV index, ml/m$^2$ | $74 \pm 12$ | $77 \pm 15$ | 0.451 |
| LVESV index, ml/m$^2$ | $25 \pm 8$ | $22 \pm 10$ | 0.308 |
| LV ejection fraction, % | $66 \pm 6$ | $72 \pm 9$ | **0.034** |
| LV mass index, g/m$^2$ | $54 \pm 10$ | $101 \pm 43$ | **<0.001** |

*Data are expressed as mean ± SD or as number (percentage). HCM, hypertrophic cardiomyopathy; LVEDV, left ventricle end diastolic volume; LVESV, left ventricle end systolic volume; LV, left ventricle. Bold values mean statistically significant.*

**TABLE 2** | Comparison of wall thickness between 2D clinical and 3D model measurements.

| Variable | Control ($n = 19$) | HCM ($n = 19$) | P-value |
|---|---|---|---|
| **2D CLINICAL MEASUREMENTS** | | | |
| IVSd, mm | $8.4 \pm 1.4$ | $17.0 \pm 6.1$ | **<0.001** |
| IVSs, mm | $12.2 \pm 2.3$ | $21.4 \pm 5.4$ | **<0.001** |
| LVPWd, mm | $6.1 \pm 1.4$ | $8.8 \pm 3.4$ | **0.009** |
| LVPWs, mm | $12.7 \pm 2.3$ | $18.5 \pm 5.4$ | **<0.001** |
| FS, % | $35.0 \pm 6.1$ | $44.2 \pm 7.9$ | **<0.001** |
| **3D MODEL MEASUREMENTS** | | | |
| $WT_{ED,max}$, mm | $8.1 \pm 1.4$ | $16.5 \pm 5.2$ | **0.001** |
| $WT_{ES,max}$, mm | $12.4 \pm 1.5$ | $22.1 \pm 5.0$ | **<0.001** |

*Data are expressed as mean ± SD. HCM, hypertrophic cardiomyopathy; IVSd (IVSs), interventricular septum in diastole (systole); LVPWd (LVPWs), left ventricular posterior wall in diastole (systole); FS, fractional shortening. $WT_{ED,max}$ ($WT_{ES,max}$), maximal wall thickness among 16 regional segments in diastole (systole) from 3D model. Bold values mean statistically significant.*

only the inferior regions (segments 3–5, 9–11, and 15) and the apical lateral segment (segment 16) exhibited significant differences. Mean *EF* values (aggregating over all 16 segments) were 72.2 and 66.5% for controls and HCM patients, respectively. Comparing across individual segments, significant differences were observed for segments 3 (basal inferior septal), 7 (mid anterior), 13 (apical anterior) and 16 (apical lateral) (**Figure 3H**).

## Difference of Geometrical Descriptors in HCM Subtypes

According to the characterization of HCM morphological subtypes described in section HCM subtypes, our HCM group

**TABLE 3** | Variation of 2D curvature, length and strains for controls and HCM patients.

| Variable | Control ($n = 19$) | HCM ($n = 19$) | P-value |
|---|---|---|---|
| Variation of curvature at ED phase | $1.94 \pm 0.47$ | $2.65 \pm 0.84$ | **0.003** |
| Variation of curvature at ES phase | $3.54 \pm 1.32$ | $5.02 \pm 2.42$ | **0.026** |
| ED endocardial length, mm | $125.8 \pm 16.4$ | $124.1 \pm 14.5$ | 0.740 |
| ED epicardial length, mm | $132.2 \pm 17.5$ | $131.9 \pm 18.0$ | 0.960 |
| ES endocardial length, mm | $98.2 \pm 13.5$ | $103.6 \pm 14.5$ | 0.246 |
| ES epicardial length, mm | $107.0 \pm 14.7$ | $116.7 \pm 19.1$ | 0.087 |
| $S_{endo}$, % | $24.8 \pm 3.0$ | $18.4 \pm 3.8$ | **<0.001** |
| $S_{epi}$, % | $21.3 \pm 3.0$ | $12.6 \pm 3.9$ | **<0.001** |

*Data are expressed as mean ± SD. HCM, hypertrophic cardiomyopathy; ED, end diastole; ES, end systole; $S_{endo}$ ($S_{epi}$), average endocardial (epicardial) strain of 2-, 3-, and 4-chamber endocardial (epicardial) strain. Bold values mean statistically significant.*

included sigmoid subtypes ($n = 6$, total of $6 \times 16 = 96$ segments), reverse curvature subtypes ($n = 8$, total of $8 \times 16 = 128$ segments) and neutral subtypes ($n = 5$, total of $5 \times 16 = 80$ segments). Results for all 3D regional parameters were given in **Table 7**. Compared with controls, all three subtypes had significantly thicker ventricular walls ($P < 0.001$), with wall thickness increasing from sigmoid to reverse curvature to neutral subtypes. Controls had significantly less curvature at ED and higher wall stress index compared to the three HCM subtype groups. The neutral subtype had the thickest ventricular wall and lowest wall stress index at ES compared to the other two HCM subtypes (all $P < 0.001$). The reverse curvature subtype had significantly lower *AS* and *EF* compared to the other two HCM subtypes.

## Univariate and Multivariate Analysis

Non-decompensated HCM patients tend to have normal LVEF. In seeking a better indicator for differentiating HCM patients, we performed univariate logistic regression analysis for LVEF, area strain, and three dichotomized parameters, viz., IVSd >13 mm, $WT_{ED,max}$ >13 mm, $\sigma_{i,ED}$ <1.64. A multivariate stepwise selection algorithm (SLE = 0.20, SLS = 0.25) on the five variables significant at P < 0.20 in univariate analysis identified $\sigma_{i,ED}$ <1.64 as the single best independent predictor of HCM group (P < 0.001). Analysis results are given in **Table 8**, and ROC curves for the five parameters are plotted in **Figure 4** with corresponding AUC, sensitivity and specificity. $\sigma_{i,ED}$ <1.64 exhibited the highest sensitivity (94.7%) and specificity (94.7%) for differentiating HCM patients from controls with AUC = 0.947.

## Impact of Wall Thickness on 3D Geometrical Descriptors

There was inverse relationship between wall thickness and wall stress index ($\sigma_{i,ED} = 14.593 \times WT_{ED}^{-1.104}$, $R^2 = 0.787$, $P < 0.001$), as shown in **Figure 5**. To further investigate the impact of wall thickness on regional ventricular shape and function, we divided the HCM patients (consisting of $16 \times 19 = 304$ segments) into four quartiles based on wall thickness (mm) at ED: <7.72 mm, 7.72–9.63 mm, 9.63–12.68 mm and >12.68 mm in **Figure 6**. With increasing wall thickness, ventricular curvedness

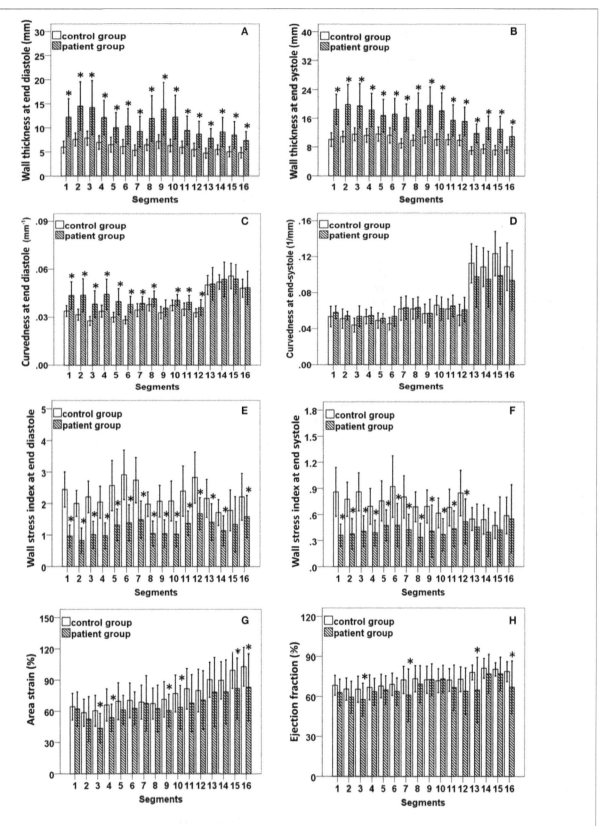

**FIGURE 3 | (A,B)** Comparison of wall thickness at end diastole (left) and end systole (right); **(C,D)** Comparison of curvedness at end diastole (left) and end systole (right); **(E,F)** Comparison of wall stress index at end diastole (left) and end systole (right); **(G,H)** Comparison of area strain (left) and ejection fraction (right) between control group and patient group with hypertrophic cardiomyopathy. *Significant difference between two groups ($P < 0.05$).

**TABLE 4 |** Curvedness computed from the 3-D reconstructed model of the LV at end diastole and end systole for Controls and HCM patients.

| Segment | Curvedness at end diastole (mm$^{-1}$) | | Curvedness at end systole (mm$^{-1}$) | |
|---|---|---|---|---|
| | Control ($n = 19$) | HCM ($n = 19$) | Control ($n = 19$) | HCM ($n = 19$) |
| (1) basal anterior | 0.0339 ± 0.0034 | 0.0436 ± 0.0085* | 0.0535 ± 0.0114 | 0.0582 ± 0.0072 |
| (2) basal anterior septal | 0.0315 ± 0.0035 | 0.0437 ± 0.0103* | 0.0511 ± 0.0108 | 0.0543 ± 0.0049 |
| (3) basal inferior septal | 0.0276 ± 0.0028 | 0.0381 ± 0.0084* | 0.0439 ± 0.0078 | 0.0537 ± 0.0116* |
| (4) basal inferior | 0.0337 ± 0.0037 | 0.0442 ± 0.0095* | 0.0534 ± 0.0081 | 0.0546 ± 0.0091 |
| (5) basal inferior lateral | 0.0300 ± 0.0031 | 0.0397 ± 0.0082* | 0.0489 ± 0.0085 | 0.0515 ± 0.0051 |
| (6) basal anterior lateral | 0.0282 ± 0.0024 | 0.0379 ± 0.0051* | 0.0453 ± 0.0069 | 0.0536 ± 0.0110* |
| (7) mid anterior | 0.0345 ± 0.0040 | 0.0386 ± 0.0042* | 0.0619 ± 0.0128 | 0.0633 ± 0.0130 |
| (8) mid anterior septal | 0.0378 ± 0.0039 | 0.0415 ± 0.0048* | 0.0619 ± 0.0113 | 0.0635 ± 0.0116 |
| (9) mid inferior septal | 0.0328 ± 0.0038 | 0.0357 ± 0.0050 | 0.0568 ± 0.0105 | 0.0570 ± 0.0155 |
| (10) mid inferior | 0.0374 ± 0.0033 | 0.0406 ± 0.0035* | 0.0660 ± 0.0106 | 0.0622 ± 0.0129 |
| (11) mid inferior lateral | 0.0350 ± 0.0039 | 0.0393 ± 0.0043* | 0.0620 ± 0.0110 | 0.0652 ± 0.0120 |
| (12) mid anterior lateral | 0.0327 ± 0.0026 | 0.0359 ± 0.0050* | 0.0551 ± 0.0118 | 0.0610 ± 0.0137 |
| (13) apical anterior | 0.0500 ± 0.0059 | 0.0507 ± 0.0103 | 0.1127 ± 0.0217 | 0.0975 ± 0.0341 |
| (14) apical septal | 0.0519 ± 0.0045 | 0.0536 ± 0.0108 | 0.1084 ± 0.0216 | 0.0949 ± 0.0311 |
| (15) apical inferior | 0.0557 ± 0.0079 | 0.0537 ± 0.0090 | 0.1233 ± 0.0247 | 0.0989 ± 0.0316* |
| (16) apical lateral | 0.0480 ± 0.0057 | 0.0483 ± 0.0103 | 0.1089 ± 0.0264 | 0.0937 ± 0.0333 |
| Mean | 0.0375 ± 0.0095 | 0.0428 ± 0.0095* | 0.0696 ± 0.0299 | 0.0677 ± 0.0251 |

Data are expressed as mean ± SD. HCM, hypertrophic cardiomyopathy; LV, left ventricle.
*Significant difference between control subjects and HCM patients (P < 0.05).

**TABLE 5 |** Wall stress index computed from the 3-D reconstructed model of the LV at end diastole and end systole for Controls and HCM patients.

| Segment | Wall stress index at end diastole | | Wall stress index at end systole | |
|---|---|---|---|---|
| | Control ($n = 19$) | HCM ($n = 19$) | Control ($n = 19$) | HCM ($n = 19$) |
| (1) basal anterior | 2.45 ± 0.56 | 0.97 ± 0.36* | 0.86 ± 0.28 | 0.36 ± 0.13* |
| (2) basal anterior septal | 2.01 ± 0.41 | 0.82 ± 0.40* | 0.78 ± 0.20 | 0.38 ± 0.18* |
| (3) basal inferior septal | 2.21 ± 0.50 | 1.01 ± 0.43* | 0.86 ± 0.22 | 0.41 ± 0.18* |
| (4) basal inferior | 2.05 ± 0.50 | 0.98 ± 0.41* | 0.69 ± 0.21 | 0.39 ± 0.15* |
| (5) basal inferior lateral | 2.57 ± 0.79 | 1.32 ± 0.50* | 0.76 ± 0.23 | 0.48 ± 0.18* |
| (6) basal anterior lateral | 2.91 ± 0.78 | 1.39 ± 0.57* | 0.92 ± 0.35 | 0.48 ± 0.25* |
| (7) mid anterior | 2.74 ± 0.72 | 1.49 ± 0.59* | 0.80 ± 0.24 | 0.42 ± 0.18* |
| (8) mid anterior septal | 1.98 ± 0.39 | 1.05 ± 0.40* | 0.69 ± 0.17 | 0.34 ± 0.16* |
| (9) mid inferior septal | 2.08 ± 0.50 | 1.05 ± 0.44* | 0.69 ± 0.19 | 0.41 ± 0.30* |
| (10) mid inferior | 2.08 ± 0.63 | 1.03 ± 0.40* | 0.62 ± 0.17 | 0.37 ± 0.18* |
| (11) mid inferior lateral | 2.39 ± 0.79 | 1.37 ± 0.39* | 0.68 ± 0.21 | 0.43 ± 0.21* |
| (12) mid anterior lateral | 2.82 ± 0.81 | 1.68 ± 0.50* | 0.85 ± 0.26 | 0.52 ± 0.26* |
| (13) apical anterior | 2.16 ± 0.60 | 1.41 ± 0.58* | 0.55 ± 0.13 | 0.46 ± 0.26 |
| (14) apical septal | 1.71 ± 0.41 | 1.13 ± 0.47* | 0.54 ± 0.17 | 0.40 ± 0.28 |
| (15) apical inferior | 1.78 ± 0.65 | 1.33 ± 0.88 | 0.47 ± 0.15 | 0.42 ± 0.38 |
| (16) apical lateral | 2.21 ± 0.74 | 1.58 ± 0.67* | 0.59 ± 0.21 | 0.55 ± 0.39 |
| Mean | 2.45 ± 0.56 | 0.97 ± 0.36* | 0.86 ± 0.28 | 0.36 ± 0.13* |

Data are expressed as mean ± SD. HCM, hypertrophic cardiomyopathy; LV, left ventricle.
*Significant difference between control subjects and HCM patients (P < 0.05).

showed no significant change at ED, but decreased at ES. There was slightly augmented area strain in 1st quartile, but decreased from quartile 2–4. There was a reduction of ejection fraction, but not significant.

## Reproducibility

Intra-class correlation (ICC) with 95% CI, mean difference ± SD, and percentage variability (%) were computed for 5 control subjects and 5 HCM patients (10 × 16 = 160 segments) from

**TABLE 6 |** Area strain (%) and ejection fraction (%) computed from the 3-D reconstructed model of the LV for control and HCM patients.

| Segment | Area strain (%) | | Ejection fraction (%) | |
|---|---|---|---|---|
| | Control (n = 19) | HCM (n = 19) | Control (n = 19) | HCM (n = 19) |
| (1) basal anterior | 66.5 ± 12.9 | 62.3 ± 16.3 | 68.4 ± 7.4 | 63.0 ± 9.9 |
| (2) basal anterior septal | 60.7 ± 13.5 | 52.5 ± 21.5 | 65.5 ± 8.3 | 59.5 ± 11.9 |
| (3) basal inferior septal | 62.5 ± 14.1 | 43.7 ± 14.2* | 65.4 ± 9.7 | 57.6 ± 12.3* |
| (4) basal inferior | 68.0 ± 15.0 | 53.8 ± 13.0* | 66.7 ± 9.3 | 63.4 ± 10.0 |
| (5) basal inferior lateral | 72.4 ± 17.6 | 61.2 ± 14.0* | 67.7 ± 8.9 | 64.7 ± 10.6 |
| (6) basal anterior lateral | 73.4 ± 16.5 | 62.8 ± 15.8 | 69.0 ± 8.3 | 63.6 ± 10.1 |
| (7) mid anterior | 71.6 ± 18.0 | 67.7 ± 26.5 | 72.3 ± 10.1 | 60.9 ± 19.6* |
| (8) mid anterior septal | 70.1 ± 16.8 | 62.7 ± 22.4 | 73.2 ± 9.9 | 69.2 ± 13.9 |
| (9) mid inferior septal | 73.9 ± 17.5 | 60.7 ± 15.7* | 72.4 ± 10.1 | 72.5 ± 11.9 |
| (10) mid inferior | 79.9 ± 18.4 | 63.7 ± 21.1* | 71.8 ± 8.9 | 73.0 ± 10.3 |
| (11) mid inferior lateral | 84.6 ± 20.2 | 67.8 ± 27.3* | 72.3 ± 8.5 | 66.7 ± 16.9 |
| (12) mid anterior lateral | 82.5 ± 21.2 | 70.8 ± 28.1 | 72.9 ± 9.2 | 63.9 ± 17.4 |
| (13) apical anterior | 92.2 ± 18.6 | 78.4 ± 33.3 | 78.0 ± 5.6 | 64.8 ± 24.6* |
| (14) apical septal | 92.2 ± 20.6 | 78.6 ± 30.9 | 81.1 ± 7.5 | 76.9 ± 14.5 |
| (15) apical inferior | 101.4 ± 18.5 | 81.8 ± 29.4* | 80.4 ± 5.0 | 76.9 ± 12.6 |
| (16) apical lateral | 104.7 ± 18.9 | 82.9 ± 31.9* | 78.7 ± 7.6 | 67.0 ± 19.7* |
| Mean | 78.5 ± 21.5 | 65.7 ± 25.2* | 72.2 ± 9.7 | 66.5 ± 15.5* |
| **AGGREGATING OVER THE BASAL, MID-CAVITY AND APICAL REGIONS** | | | | |
| (i) basal | 67.2 ± 14.3 | 56.0 ± 14.4* | 67.1 ± 8.3 | 62.0 ± 9.5 |
| (ii) mid-cavity | 77.1 ± 18.1 | 65.6 ± 22.8 | 72.5 ± 9.2 | 68.4 ± 11.8 |
| (iii) apical | 97.6 ± 18.1 | 80.4 ± 30.8* | 79.5 ± 5.6 | 72.4 ± 15.3 |

*Data are expressed as mean ± SD. HCM, hypertrophic cardiomyopathy; LV, left ventricle.*
*\*Significant difference between control subjects and HCM patients (P < 0.05).*

**TABLE 7 |** ANOVA analysis between control and hypertrophy subtypes for 3D regional parameters.

| Variable | Control (n = 304) | Sigmoid (n = 96) | Reverse Curvature (n = 128) | Neutral (n = 80) | P-value |
|---|---|---|---|---|---|
| $WT_{ED}$, mm | 6.08 ± 1.54 | 9.53 ± 3.76*†‡ | 11.15 ± 4.52*† | 11.37 ± 4.47*‡ | **<0.001** |
| $WT_{ES}$, mm | 9.69 ± 2.19 | 15.25 ± 4.54*‡ | 16.22 ± 5.60*§ | 17.81 ± 4.50*‡§ | **<0.001** |
| $C_{ED}$, mm$^{-1}$ | 0.0375 ± 0.0095 | 0.0418 ± 0.0094* | 0.0431 ± 0.0092* | 0.0436 ± 0.0100* | **<0.001** |
| $C_{ES}$, mm$^{-1}$ | 0.0696 ± 0.0299 | 0.0707 ± 0.0251 | 0.0615 ± 0.0194*§ | 0.0741 ± 0.0305§ | **0.005** |
| $\sigma_{i,ED}$ | 2.26 ± 0.70 | 1.40 ± 0.54*‡ | 1.19 ± 0.62* | 1.07 ± 0.41*‡ | **<0.001** |
| $\sigma_{i,ES}$ | 0.71 ± 0.25 | 0.43 ± 0.23*‡ | 0.49 ± 0.29*§ | 0.31 ± 0.10*‡§ | **<0.001** |
| AS, % | 78.51 ± 21.48 | 71.59 ± 22.11† | 55.24 ± 20.82*†§ | 75.36 ± 29.45§ | **<0.001** |
| EF, % | 72.23 ± 9.66 | 70.49 ± 1.071† | 61.03 ± 16.05*†§ | 70.38 ± 16.45§ | **<0.001** |

*Data are expressed as mean ± SD. $WT_{ED}$, wall thickness at end diastole; $WT_{ES}$, wall thickness at end systole; $C_{ED}$, curvedness at end diastole; $C_{ES}$, curvedness at end systole; $\sigma_{i,ED}$, wall stress index at end diastole; $\sigma_{i,ES}$, wall stress index at end systole; AS, area strain; EF, ejection fraction.*
*\*Significant differences between control group and three HCM subtypes; †significant difference between sigmoid and reverse curvature subtypes; ‡significant difference between sigmoid and neutral subtypes; §significant difference between reverse curvature and neutral subtypes. Bold values mean statistically significant.*

intra- and inter-observer studies, and the reproducibility results were given in **Table 9**. All parameters were highly reproducible with ICC >0.87, and percentage variability was ≤6.5% for intra-observer and ≤5.0% for inter-observer.

## DISCUSSION

The main finding of this study was that curvedness-based ventricular wall stress index at end diastole (ED) was a more sensitive and specific parameter than traditional ventricular wall thickness and other measures for differentiating HCM with

preserved ejection fraction. Furthermore, among the three HCM subtypes, the neutral group presented lowest wall stress, but reverse curvature group presented lowest regional contractile function compared to the control group and other two subtypes (P < 0.05).

## Ventricular Wall Stress Measurement

In the present study, wall stress index is a pure geometric parameter that quantifies the physical response of left ventricle to loading and allows a comparison between ventricles under differing pressures. The wall stress index is expressed as the

**TABLE 8** | Univariate logistic regression and multivariate stepwise selection analysis.

| Variable | P-value | |
|---|---|---|
| | Univariate logistic regression analysis | Multivariate stepwise selection analysis |
| LVEF, % | 0.065 | – |
| Area strain, % | 0.0970 | – |
| IVSd >13 mm | **0.005** | – |
| $WT_{ED,max}$ >13 mm | **0.0031** | – |
| $\sigma_{i,ED}$ <1.64 | **<0.001** | **<0.001** |

*LVEF, left ventricular ejection fraction; IVSd, interventricular septum thickness in diastole from 2D clinical measurement; $WT_{ED,max}$, maximal wall thickness among 16 segments in diastole from 3D model; $\sigma_{i,ED}$, wall stress index at end diastole. Bold values mean statistically significant.*

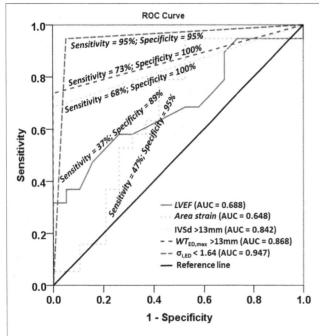

**FIGURE 4** | Receiver operating characteristic (ROC) curves for left ventricle ejection fraction (LVEF), area strain, and three dichotomized parameters IVSd >13 mm, $WT_{ED,max}$ >13 mm, $\sigma_{i,ED}$ <1.64. IVSd, interventricular septum in diastole from 2D clinical CMR measurement; $WT_{ED,max}$, maximal wall thickness among 16 regional segments in diastole from 3D model; $\sigma_{i,ED}$, wall stress index at end diastole.

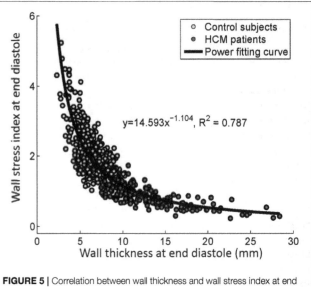

**FIGURE 5** | Correlation between wall thickness and wall stress index at end diastole.

The joint use of imaging and modeling of the heart has opened up possibilities for a better thorough understanding and evaluation of the LV wall stress. Traditionally, most work on wall stress has been based on two-dimensional and three-dimensional models that are represented by simplified idealized geometry analyses with different formula (i.e., sphere, spheroid, ellipsoid; Yin, 1981; Zhong et al., 2006, 2007, 2012a). Finite element analysis (FEA), an engineering technique utilized to study complex structure, can overcome some of these limitations. Previous studies has elucidated the characteristics of wall stress and clarified how they should be properly analyzed so that these concepts can be applied in translational research (Guccione et al., 1995; Dorri et al., 2006; Lee et al., 2014; Choy et al., 2018). However, from the clinical application consideration, the application of FEA to employ human *in vivo* data still remain a challenge. Our approach allows precise regional measurement of three-dimensional wall curvedness and thickness and hence permit accurate estimate of diastolic and systolic wall stress assessment. The entire process taking about 20 min per subject would garner its wider application in clinical practice.

## Wall Stress, Curvature and Curvedness in Hypertrophic Cardiomyopathy

HCM implies a higher-than-normal myocardial mass, with a high ratio of ventricular wall thickness to radius ($h/R$). Based on the different pattern of hypertrophy, systolic and diastolic wall stress were proposed as a stimulus for replication of cardiomyocytes and cardiac remodeling. Indeed, HCM has been reported to correlate with ratio of $h/R$ or $h/R^3$ or volume/mass from the previous studies (Petersen et al., 2005). This phenomenon allows the preservation of endocardial motion despite reduced shortening of individual fibers such that the EF remains normal (de Simone and Devereux, 2002). On the other hand, progressive LV remodeling in HCM contributes to a change in wall curvature or curvedness (Reant et al., 2015). Our diastolic wall stress,

ratio of wall thickness to wall radius ($h/R$) which takes into account regional ventricular curvedness. We have demonstrated excellent intra- and inter-observer reproducibility in wall stress measurement for both normal and HCM patients with percentage variability less than 6%. This is in significant contrast to previous echocardiographic studies (i.e., 7–11%; Greim et al., 1995). This is likely to reflect the better accuracy of CMR to regional wall curvedness and thickness than echocardiography, which has been demonstrated in several previous studies examining different cardiac conditions (Zhong et al., 2009b, 2011, 2012b).

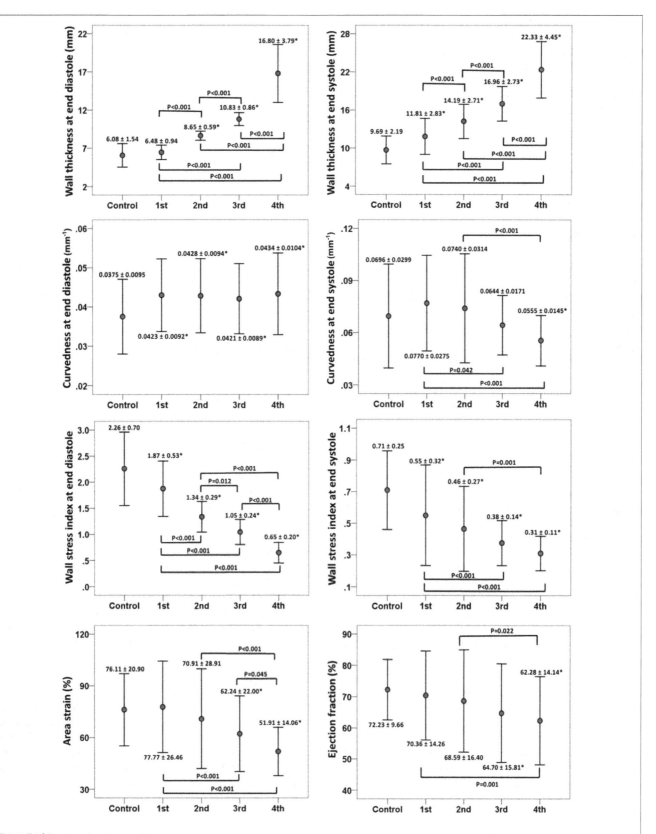

**FIGURE 6 |** Error bar plots (mean ± SD) between control and quartiles divided by left ventricular end-diastolic wall thickness in patients with hypertrophy cardiomyopathy. First row: wall thickness at ED **(left)** and ES **(right)**, ED = end diastole; ES = end systole; second row: 3D regional curvedness at ED **(left)** and ES **(right)**; third row: wall stress index at ED **(left)** and ES **(right)**; last row: area strain **(left)** and ejection fraction **(right)**. *Significant difference between control group and four quartiles ($P < 0.05$).

**TABLE 9 |** Intra- and inter-observer reproducibility in 5 control subjects and 5 HCM patients.

| Variable | Intra-class correlation coefficient (95% CI) | Mean difference ± SD | Percentage variability (%) |
|---|---|---|---|
| **INTRA OBSERVER REPRODUCIBILITY** | | | |
| $WT_{ED}$, mm | 0.995 (0.993–0.996) | −0.050 ± 0.488 | 3.11 |
| $WT_{ES}$, mm | 0.992 (0.989–0.994) | 0.146 ± 0.733 | 2.41 |
| $C_{ED}$, mm$^{-1}$ | 0.893 (0.856–0.920) | 0.0020 ± 0.0044 | 4.66 |
| $C_{ES}$, mm$^{-1}$ | 0.979 (0.972–0.985) | 0.0001 ± 0.0057 | 3.50 |
| $\sigma_{i,ED}$ | 0.985 (0.979–0.989) | −0.049 ± 0.187 | 6.03 |
| $\sigma_{i,ES}$ | 0.926 (0.900–0.945) | 0.008 ± 0.096 | 6.50 |
| AS, % | 0.930 (0.906–0.949) | 1.889 ± 8.127 | 4.40 |
| EF, % | 0.885 (0.845–0.914) | 0.445 ± 4.609 | 3.04 |
| **INTER OBSERVER REPRODUCIBILITY** | | | |
| $WT_{ED}$, mm | 0.997 (0.996–0.998) | −0.019 ± 0.375 | 2.36 |
| $WT_{ES}$, mm | 0.995 (0.993–0.996) | 0.193 ± 0.574 | 1.69 |
| $C_{ED}$, mm$^{-1}$ | 0.917 (0.888–0.938) | 0.0019 ± 0.0039 | 4.21 |
| $C_{ES}$, mm$^{-1}$ | 0.983 (0.977–0.988) | 0.0006 ± 0.0051 | 2.77 |
| $\sigma_{i,ED}$ | 0.987 (0.982–0.990) | 0.018 ± 0.160 | 4.99 |
| $\sigma_{i,ES}$ | 0.941 (0.921–0.957) | −0.002 ± 0.088 | 5.01 |
| AS, % | 0.928 (0.903–0.947) | 2.853 ± 8.190 | 4.24 |
| EF, % | 0.879 (0.838–0.910) | 0.949 ± 4.752 | 3.16 |

*HCM, hypertrophic cardiomyopathy; CI, confidence interval; SD, standard deviation; Percentage variability, the mean of the absolute values of the differences between two measurements divided by their mean; $WT_{ED}$, wall thickness at ED; $WT_{ES}$, wall thickness at ES; ED, end diastole; ES, end systole; $C_{ED}$, curvedness at ED; $C_{ES}$, curvedness at ES; $\sigma_{i,ED}$, wall stress index at ED; $\sigma_{i,ES}$, wall stress index at ES; AS, area strain; EF, ejection fraction.*

based on ratio of $h/R$ which consider regional three-dimensional wall curvedness represents an integrated assessment and permit more accurate regional assessment of stress state. These studies provide a rationale supporting wall stress as an ideal index for assessing HCM. Moreover, multivariate stepwise selection analysis identified our wall stress index as the best single predictor of HCM group, and had better sensitivity than LVEF, area strain and wall thickness from both 2D CMR clinical and 3D model measurements.

Our analysis of wall curvedness, stress and function in this study add further insight of subtype of HCM (i.e., sigmoid, reverse and neutral subtypes). The data in present study demonstrated that only reverse curvature HCM subtype presented abnormal wall stress and area strain despite its preserved ejection fraction. This observation is consistent with the finding of Kobayashi et al. in patients with obstructive HCM (Kobayashi et al., 2014). They found that patients with the reverse curvature subtype had less global longitudinal systolic and diastolic strain than patients with sigmoid and concentric hypertrophy despite being younger and less hypertensive. As suggested by Binder (Binder et al., 2006), the reverse curvature

morphological subtype may inherently precede and incite the myocyte and fiber disarray and local wall stress perturbations, which are characteristic of HCM.

## Clinical Implication

Understanding of LV wall stress may help to solve some clinical questions like the differentiation of adaptive and maladaptive hypertrophy in HCM. At the early stage, both diastolic and systolic wall stresses are maintained "normal" because increased wall thickness is counterbalancing the elevated ventricular pressure. Progressively, wall stress continues to decreases, which causes increase of wall curvature and decrease of the wall radius. These constitute maladaptive hypertrophic developments. We believe our comprehensive suite of quantitative regional curvedness-based wall stress can distinguish early remodeling in HCM and facilitate personalization of monitoring of the natural disease progression or treatment response. For instance, 3D regional parameters derived from our approach may be used to quantify the efficacy and effects (e.g., wall stress) of septal myectomy or ablation therapies in HCM.

## Limitations of Study

Limitations of the present study are summarized as follows. First, our approach to 3D LV reconstruction relies on manual delineation of endocardium and epicardium contours obtained from CMR images. This is time consuming and may be replaced by automatic segmentation techniques (Petitjean and Dacher, 2011; Kang et al., 2012; Yang et al., 2016).

Second, curvature-based ventricular wall stress computation depends upon image quality and accuracy of reconstructed surface. Image quality and resolution can be improved by utilizing a 3.0 Tesla scanner rather than a 1.5 Tesla scanner, thereby increasing the quality of the input data for 3D mesh reconstruction and processing. In clinical practice, the spacing between two consecutive CMR short-axis image slices is typically 5–10 mm. Hence, interpolation is used to reconstruct the surface between slices. This process of interpolation may affect the accuracy of the wall stress computation. It should be noted that the intra- and inter- observer variation is small (i.e., both <7%) for wall stress determination, suggesting that our approach is reasonable, and unaffected by variations in the interpolation process.

## AUTHOR CONTRIBUTIONS

Conception or design of the work: XZ, S-KT, YS, MW, SL, J-MZ, and LZ; Acquisition of data for the work: R-ST, and HT; Analysis, interpretation of the work: XZ, R-ST, S-KT, YS, and LZ; Draft the work or revise it critically for important intellectual content: XZ, R-ST, H-CT, S-KT, YS, JA, GK, and LZ; All authors have seen and approved the final version of manuscript.

# REFERENCES

Alter, P., Rupp, H., Rominger, M. B., Vollrath, A., Czerny, F., Klose, K. J., et al. (2007). Relation of B-type natriuretic peptide to left ventricular wall stress as assessed by cardiac magnetic resonance imaging in patients with dilated cardiomyopathy. *Can. J. Physiol. Pharmacol.* 85, 790–799. doi: 10.1139/Y07-076

Badeer, H. S. (1963). Contractile tension in the myocardium. *Am. Heart J.* 66, 432–434. doi: 10.1016/0002-8703(63)90278-3

Binder, J., Ommen, S. R., Gersh, B. J., Van Driest, S. L., Tajik, A. J., Nishimura, R. A., et al. (2006). Echocardiography-guided genetic testing in hypertrophic cardiomyopathy: septal morphological features predict the presence of myofilament mutations. *Mayo. Clin. Proc.* 81, 459–467. doi: 10.4065/81.4.459

Carasso, S., Yang, H., Woo, A., Jamorski, M., Wigle, E. D., and Rakowski, H. (2010). Diastolic myocardial mechanics in hypertrophic cardiomyopathy. *J. Am. Soc. Echocardiogr.* 23, 164–171. doi: 10.1016/j.echo.2009.11.022

Carasso, S., Yang, H., Woo, A., Vannan, M. A., Jamorski, M., Wigle, E. D., et al. (2008). Systolic myocardial mechanics in hypertrophic cardiomyopathy: novel concepts and implications for clinical status. *J. Am. Soc. Echocardiogr.* 21, 675–683. doi: 10.1016/j.echo.2007.10.021

Cerqueira, M. D., Weissman, N. J., Dilsizian, V., Jacobs, A. K., Kaul, S., Laskey, W. K., et al. (2002). Standardized myocardial segmentation and nomenclature for tomographic imaging of the heart: a statement for healthcare professional from the Cardiology of the American Heart Association. *Circulation* 10, 539–542. doi: 10.1161/hc0402.102975

Choy, J. S., Leng, S., Acevedo-Bolton, G., Shaul, S., Fu, L., Guo, X., et al. (2018). Efficacy of intramyocaridal injection of Algisyl-LVR for the treatment of ischemic heart failure in swine. *Int. J. Cardiol.* 255, 129–135. doi: 10.1016/j.ijcard.2017.09.179

de Simone, G., and Devereux, R. B. (2002). Rationale of echocardiographic assessment of left ventricular wall stress and midwall mechanics in hypertensive heart disease. *Eur. J. Echocardiogr.* 3, 192–198. doi: 10.1053/euje.3.3.192

Dorri, F., Niederer, P. F., and Lunkenheimer, P. P. (2006). A finite element model of the human left ventricular systole. *Comput. Methods Biomech. Biomed. Engin.* 9, 319–341. doi: 10.1080/10255840600960546

Elliott, P., and McKenna, W. J. (2004). Hypertrophic cardiomyopathy. *Lancet* 363, 1881–1891. doi: 10.1016/S0140-6736(04)16358-7

Falsetti, H. L., Mates, R. E., Grant, C., Greene, D. G., and Bunnell, I. L. (1970). Left ventricular wall stress calculated from one-plane cineangiography. *Circ. Res.* 26, 71–83. doi: 10.1161/01.RES.26.1.71

Greim, C. A., Roewer, N., and Schulte am Esch, J. (1995). Assessment of changes in left ventricular wall stress from the end-systolic pressure-area product. *Br. J. Anaesth.* 75, 583–587. doi: 10.1093/bja/75.5.583

Grossman, W., Jones, D., and McLaurin, L. P. (1975). Wall stress and patterns of hypertrophy in the human left ventricle. *J. Clin. Invest.* 56, 56–64. doi: 10.1172/JCI108079

Guccione, J. M., Costa, K. D., and McCulloch, A. D. (1995). Finite element stress analysis of left ventricular mechanics in the beating dog heart. *J. Biomech.* 28, 1167–1177. doi: 10.1016/0021-9290(94)00174-3

Hansen, M. W., and Merchant, N. (2007). MRI of hypertrophic cardiomyopathy: part I, MRI appearances. *AJR Am. J. Roentgenol.* 189, 1335–1343. doi: 10.2214/AJR.07.2286

Hoey, E. T., Elassaly, M., Ganeshan, A., Watkin, R. W., and Simpson, H. (2014). The role of magnetic resonance imaging in hypertrophic cardiomyopathy. *Quant. Imaging Med. Surg.* 4, 397–406. doi: 10.3978/j.issn.2223-4292.2014.09.04

Hughes, S. E. (2004). The pathology of hypertrophic cardiomyopathy. *Histopathology* 44, 412–427. doi: 10.1111/j.1365-2559.2004.01835.x

Janz, R. (1982). Estimation of local myocardial stress. *Am. J. Physiol. Heart Circ. Physiol.* 242, H875–H881. doi: 10.1152/ajpheart.1982.242.5.H875

Kang, D., Woo, J., Slomka, P. J., Dey, D., Germano, G., and Jay, K. C. (2012). Heart chambers and whole heart segmentation technique: review. *J. Electron. Imaging* 21:010901. doi: 10.1117/1.JEI.21.1.010901

Klues, H. G., Schiffers, A., and Maron, B. J. (1995). Phenotypic spectrum and patterns of left ventricular hypertrophy in hypertrophic cardiomyopathy: morphologic observations and significance as assessed by two-dimensional echocardiography in 600 patients. *J. Am. Coll. Cardiol.* 26, 1699–1708. doi: 10.1016/0735-1097(95)00390-8

Kobayashi, T., Dhillon, A., Popovic, Z., Bhonsale, A., Smedira, N. G., Thamilarasan, M., et al. (2014). Differences in global and regional left ventricular myocardial mechanics in various morphologic subtypes of patients with obstructive hypertrophic cardiomyopathy referred for ventricular septal myotomy/myectomy. *Am. J. Cardiol.* 113, 1879–1885. doi: 10.1016/j.amjcard.2014.03.020

Koenderink, J. J., and Van Doorn, A. J. (1992). Surface shape and curvature scales. *Image Vision Comput.* 10, 557–565. doi: 10.1016/0262-8856(92)90076-F

Kovacic, J. C., and Muller, D. (2003). Hypertrophic cardiomyopathy: state-of-the-art review, with focus on the management of outflow obstruction. *Intern. Med. J.* 33, 521–529. doi: 10.1046/j.1445-5994.2003.00475.x

Lee, L. C., Ge, L., Zhang, Z., Pease, M., Nikolic, S. D., Mishra, R., et al. (2014). Patient-specific finite element modeling of the Cardiokinetix Parachute® device: effects on left ventricular wall stress and function. *Med. Biol. Eng. Comput.* 52, 557–566. doi: 10.1007/s11517-014-1159-5

Lewiner, T., Gomes, J., Lopes, H., and Craizer, M. (2005). Curvature and torsion estimators based on parametric curve fitting. *Comput. Graph.* 29, 641–655. doi: 10.1016/j.cag.2005.08.004

Maron, B. J. (2002). Hypertrophic cardiomyopathy: a systematic review. *JAMA* 287, 1308–1320. doi: 10.1001/jama.287.10.1308

Maron, M. S., Lesser, J. R., and Maron, B. J. (2010). Management implications of massive left ventricular hypertrophy in hypertrophic cardiomyopathy significantly underestimated by echocardiography but identified by cardiovascular magnetic resonance. *Am. J. Cardiol.* 105, 1842–1843. doi: 10.1016/j.amjcard.2010.01.367

Noureldin, R. A., Liu, S., Nacif, M. S., Judge, D. P., Halushka, M. K., Abraham, T. P., et al. (2012). The diagnosis of hypertrophic cardiomyopathy by cardiovascular magnetic resonance. *J. Cardiovasc. Magn. Reson.* 14:17. doi: 10.1186/1532-429X-14-17

Petersen, S. E., Selvanayagam, J. B., Francis, J. M., Myerson, S. G., Wiesmann, F., Robson, M. D., et al. (2005). Differentiation of athlete's heart from pathological forms of cardiac hypertrophy by means of geometric indices derived from cardiovascular magnetic resonance. *J. Cardiovasc. Magn. Reson.* 7, 551–558. doi: 10.1081/JCMR-200060631

Petitjean, C., and Dacher, J. N. (2011). A review of segmentation methods in short axis cardiac MR images. *Med. Image Anal.* 15, 169–184. doi: 10.1016/j.media.2010.12.004

Reant, P., Captur, G., Mirabel, M., Nasis, A., M Sado, D., Maestrini, V., et al. (2015). Abnormal septal convexity into the left ventricle occurs in subclinical hypertrophic cardiomyopathy. *J. Cardiovasc. Magn. Reson.* 17:64. doi: 10.1186/s12968-015-0160-y

Regen, D. M. (1990). Calculation of left ventricular wall stress. *Circ. Res.* 67, 245–252. doi: 10.1161/01.RES.67.2.245

Rickers, C., Wilke, N. M., Jerosch-Herold, M., Casey, S. A., Panse, P., Panse, N., et al. (2005). Utility of cardiac magnetic resonance imaging in the diagnosis of Hypertrophic Cardiomyopathy. *Circulation* 112, 855–861. doi: 10.1161/CIRCULATIONAHA.104.507723

Su, Y., Tan, M. L., Lim, C. W., Teo, S. K., Selvaraj, S. K., Wan, M., et al. (2014). "Automatic correction of motion artifacts in 4D left ventricle model reconstructed from MRI. The 2014 computing," in *Cardiology Conference (CinC 2014)* (Cambridge, MA).

Su, Y., Teo, S. K., Lim, C. W., Zhong, L., and Tan, R. S. (2015). "automatic generation of endocardial surface meshes with 1-to-1 correspondence from cine-MR images," in *Proceedings of SPIE 9414, Medical Imaging 2015: Computer-Aided Diagnosis, 941431* (Orlando, FL).

Su, Y., Zhong, L., Lim, C. W., Ghista, D. N., Chua, T., and Tan, R. S. (2012). A geometrical approach for evaluating left ventricular remodeling in myocardial infarct patients. *Comput. Methods Programs Biomed.* 108, 500–510. doi: 10.1016/j.cmpb.2011.03.008

Tan, M.-L., Su, Y., Lim, C.-W., Selvaraj, S. K., Zhong, L., and Tan, R. S. (2013). A geometrical approach for automatic shape restoration of the left ventricle. *PLoS ONE* 8:e68615. doi: 10.1371/journal.pone.0068615

Teo, S. K., Vos, F. J. A., Tan, R. S., Zhong, L., and Su, Y. (2015). Regional ejection fraction and regional area strain for left ventricular function assessment in male patients after first-time myocardial infarction. *J. R. Soc. Interface* 12:20150006. doi: 10.1098/rsif.2015.0006

Wigle, E. (2001). The diagnosis of hypertrophic cardiomyopathy. *Heart* 86, 709–714. doi: 10.1136/heart.86.6.709

Wisneski, J. A., Pfeil, C. N., Wyse, D. G., Mitchell, R., Rahimtoola, S. H., and Gertz, E. W. (1981). Left ventricular ejection fraction calculated from volumes and areas: underestimated by area method. *Circulation* 63, 149–151. doi: 10.1161/01.CIR.63.1.149

Yang, X. L., Su, Y., Duan, R., Fan, H., Yeo, S. Y., Lim, C., et al. (2016). Cardiac image segmentation by random walks with dynamic shape constraint. *IET Comput. Vision* 10, 79–86. doi: 10.1049/iet-cvi.2014.0450

Yeo, S. Y., Zhong, L., Su, Y., Tan, R. S., and Ghista, D. N. (2009). A curvature-based approach for left ventricular shape analysis from cardiac magnetic resonance imaging. *Med. Biol. Eng. Comput.* 47, 313–322. doi: 10.1007/s11517-008-0401-4

Yin, F. C. (1981). Ventricular wall stress. *Circ. Res.* 49, 829–842. doi: 10.1161/01.RES.49.4.829

Zhao, X., Tan, R. S., Tang, H. C., Leng, S., Zhang, J. M., and Zhong, L. (2018). Analysis of three-dimensional endocardial and epicardial strains from cardiac magnetic resonance in healthy subjects and patients with hypertrophic cardiomyopathy. *Med. Biol. Eng. Comput.* 56, 159–172. doi: 10.1007/s11517-017-1674-2

Zhong, L., Ghista, D. N., Ng, E. Y., Lim, S. T., Chua, T. S., and Lee, C. N. (2006). Left ventricular shape-based contractility index. *J. Biomech.* 39, 2397–2409. doi: 10.1016/j.jbiomech.2005.08.002

Zhong, L., Ghista, D. N., and Tan, R. S. (2012a). Left ventricular wall stress compendium. *Comput. Meth. Biomech. Biomed. Eng.* 15, 1015–1041. doi: 10.1080/10255842.2011.569885

Zhong, L., Gobeawan, L., Su, Y., Tan, J. L., Ghista, D., Chua, T., et al. (2012b). Right ventricular regional wall curvedness and area strain in patients with repaired tetralogy of Fallot. *Am. J. Physiol. Heart Circ. Physiol.* 302, H1306–H1316. doi: 10.1152/ajpheart.00679.2011

Zhong, L., Sola, S., Tan, R. S., Le, T. T., Ghista, D. N., Kurra, V., et al. (2009a). Effects of surgical ventricular restoration on left ventricular contractility assessed by a novel contractility index in patients with ischemic cardiomyopathy. *Am. J. Cardiol.* 103, 674–679. doi: 10.1016/j.amjcard.2008.10.031

Zhong, L., Su, Y., Gobeawan, L., Sola, S., Tan, R. S., Navia, J. L., et al. (2011). Impact of surgical ventricular restoration on ventricular shape, wall stress, and function in heart failure patients. *Am. J. Physiol. Heart Circ. Physiol.* 300, H1653–H1660. doi: 10.1152/ajpheart.00021.2011

Zhong, L., Su, Y., Yeo, S. Y., Tan, R. S., Ghista, D. N., and Kassab, G. (2009b). Left ventricular regional wall curvature and wall stress in patients with ischemic dilated cardiomyopathy. *Am. J. Physiol. Heart Circ. Physiol.* 3, H573–H584. doi: 10.1152/ajpheart.00525.2008

Zhong, L., Tan, L. K., Finn, C. J., Ghista, D., Liew, R., and Ding, Z. P. (2012c). Effects of age and gender on left atrial ejection force and volume from real-time three-dimensional echocardiography. *Ann. Acad. Med. Singapore* 41, 161–169.

Zhong, L., Tan, R. S., Ghista, D. N., Ng, E. Y., Chua, L. P., and Kassab, G. S. (2007). Validation of a novel noninvasive cardiac index of left ventricular contractility in patients. *Am. J. Physiol. Heart Circ. Physiol.* 292, H2764–H2772. doi: 10.1152/ajpheart.00540.2006

# 19

# Investigating the Role of Interventricular Interdependence in Development of Right Heart Dysfunction During LVAD Support: A Patient-Specific Methods-Based Approach

*Kevin L. Sack[1,2], Yaghoub Dabiri[2], Thomas Franz[1,3], Scott D. Solomon[4], Daniel Burkhoff[5] and Julius M. Guccione[2]\**

[1] Division of Biomedical Engineering, Department of Human Biology, University of Cape Town, Cape Town, South Africa, [2] Department of Surgery, University of California, San Francisco, San Francisco, CA, United States, [3] Bioengineering Science Research Group, Engineering Sciences, Faculty of Engineering and the Environment, University of Southampton, Southampton, United Kingdom, [4] Department of Medicine, Brigham and Women's Hospital, Boston, MA, United States, [5] Cardiovascular Research Foundation, New York, NY, United States

**\*Correspondence:**
*Julius M. Guccione*
*julius.guccione@ucsf.edu*

Predictive computation models offer the potential to uncover the mechanisms of treatments whose actions cannot be easily determined by experimental or imaging techniques. This is particularly relevant for investigating left ventricular mechanical assistance, a therapy for end-stage heart failure, which is increasingly used as more than just a bridge-to-transplant therapy. The high incidence of right ventricular failure following left ventricular assistance reflects an undesired consequence of treatment, which has been hypothesized to be related to the mechanical interdependence between the two ventricles. To investigate the implication of this interdependence specifically in the setting of left ventricular assistance device (LVAD) support, we introduce a patient-specific finite-element model of dilated chronic heart failure. The model geometry and material parameters were calibrated using patient-specific clinical data, producing a mechanical surrogate of the failing *in vivo* heart that models its dynamic strain and stress throughout the cardiac cycle. The model of the heart was coupled to lumped-parameter circulatory systems to simulate realistic ventricular loading conditions. Finally, the impact of ventricular assistance was investigated by incorporating a pump with pressure-flow characteristics of an LVAD (HeartMate II™ operating between 8 and 12 k RPM) in parallel to the left ventricle. This allowed us to investigate the mechanical impact of acute left ventricular assistance at multiple operating-speeds on right ventricular mechanics and septal wall motion. Our findings show that left ventricular assistance reduces myofiber stress in the left ventricle and, to a lesser extent, right ventricle free wall, while increasing leftward septal-shift with increased operating-speeds. These effects were achieved with secondary, potentially negative effects on the interventricular septum which showed that support from LVADs, introduces unnatural bending of the septum and with it, increased localized stress regions. Left ventricular assistance unloads the left ventricle significantly and shifts the right ventricular pressure-volume-loop toward larger volumes and higher pressures; a consequence of left-to-right ventricular interactions and a leftward septal shift. The methods and results described in the present study are a meaningful advancement of computational efforts to investigate heart-failure therapies *in silico* and illustrate the potential of computational models to aid understanding of complex mechanical and hemodynamic effects of new therapies.

**Keywords: heart failure, finite element method, realistic simulation, ventricular function, right ventricle, ventricular assist device, mechanical circulatory support**

# INTRODUCTION

In view of the growing number and dismal prognosis of patients with end-stage heart failure, interest in emerging mechanical therapies such as left ventricular assistance devices (LVADs) has intensified. LVADs are used as a bridge to transplant, bridge to decision, destination therapy and, increasingly, as a bridge to recovery. The latter is fueled by the nearly ubiquitous demonstration that left ventricular (LV) unloading provided by LVADs causes reverse remodeling and, in a small percentage of patients, induces myocardial recovery to the point where devices can be explanted (Wohlschlaeger et al., 2005; Birks et al., 2006; Burkhoff et al., 2006; Lampropulos et al., 2014; McIlvennan et al., 2014; Topkara et al., 2016). The introduction of smaller, partial (i.e., low) flow LVADs designed to be implanted at an earlier stage of disease severity has broadened the potential applicability to a currently underserved and large patient population (Mohite et al., 2014; Sabashnikov et al., 2014; Sack et al., 2016).

Among the remaining adverse effects that impact negatively on long-term morbidity and mortality of LVAD patients is right heart failure (Grant et al., 2012; Hayek et al., 2014; Rich et al., 2017). Ten to thirty percent of LVAD patients develop right ventricular (RV) failure (Kavarana et al., 2002; Dang et al., 2006; Kormos et al., 2010; Baumwol et al., 2011; Argiriou et al., 2014) requiring either prolonged use of inotropic therapy or the need for temporary or long-term RV mechanical circulatory support. RV failure is associated with elevated central venous pressure (CVP), which adversely affects renal, hepatic, and gastorintestinal function, and results in LV underfilling that reduces LVAD flow.

LVAD support influences RV function in several ways; some beneficial and some detrimental. On the one hand, LVAD-induced unloading leads directly to a reduction of pulmonary capillary wedge pressure. This pressure accounts for a large part of the mechanical afterload on the RV so its reduction can favorably impact the ability of the RV to eject blood and maintain a normal CVP. On the other hand, LVADs increase systemic blood flow, which can cause a volume overload on the RV. Additionally, LV unloading can have a detrimental effect on RV function due to interventricular interactions (Kavarana et al., 2002; Küçüker et al., 2004; Dang et al., 2006; Maeder et al., 2009). This latter effect is a consequence of the interdependence of RV and LV pressure generation mediated by the interventricular septum. It is well-known that as much as 30% of RV pressure generation is due to LV pressure generation

and that the position of the interventricular septum can influence RV function (Slater et al., 1997). Thus, LVADs can impact RV function because the RV and LV are two pumps working functionally in series within the circulation, are anatomically arranged in parallel with each other, and share a common wall.

Although the potential implications of ventricular interactions on RV function during LVAD support are well-appreciated, no study has yet proven, in any setting, that LV unloading and septal shift can actually lead to RV failure. This is because it is physically impossible to separate the hemodynamic effects of the serial and parallel contributions of RV-LV interactions in a patient or even in experimental preclinical studies.

Computational modeling is well-suited to investigate and elucidate the individual contributions of these primary hemodynamic factors. However, research efforts have been impeded by the substantial complexities involved in coupling a simulated circulatory system with geometrically realistic models of the heart. Only recently have computational models had the necessary sophistication to model this coupled behavior (e.g., Kerckhoffs et al., 2007; Lim et al., 2012; Baillargeon et al., 2014; Sack et al., 2016). Consequently, very limited research has been undertaken to explore the effect of LVAD function on ventricular mechanics, and no study has investigated the important issue of right heart failure. Such research has significant practical implications since current guidelines for the care of LVAD patients recommend that LVAD speeds be adjusted to ensure that the interventricular septum is not leftward shifted. This recommendation is based on expert opinion, not on any physiological or clinical evidence.

We previously created a model of a failing LV supported with partial LV assistance in a four-chamber generic heart model (Sack et al., 2016). In the present study we modify this representation to include a biventricular model of a patient with dilated cardiomyopathy. LVAD therapy is then simulated using realistic pressure-flow relations of a commonly used LVAD, allowing us to capture assisted flow for device operation over a broad range of rotational speeds (RPMs). By analyzing the resulting changes in LV pressure generation, total blood flow, myocardial stress, and septal wall motion, we quantified the relative influences of these factors on RV function. The specific purpose of this paper is to describe the mathematical methods and general behavior of this model of the failing heart during different degrees of LVAD-induced LV unloading.

## METHODS

Our cardiac modeling methods have been described extensively in previous studies (Baillargeon et al., 2014, 2015; Sack et al., 2016). Here, we present a brief overview of these established methods, with an additional focus on recent developments and methods that are critical for the current study.

### Patient Data

*In vivo* cardiac magnetic resonance (MR) data sets were obtained as part of the Aliskiren Study in Post-MI Patients to Reduce Remodeling (ASPIRE) trial (Solomon et al., 2011). Individual patients provided informed consent and anonymized data were sent to a core laboratory for analysis.

### Geometric Considerations

For one patient with dilated cardiomyopathy, the MR data sets (1.25 × 1.24 × 10 mm spatial resolution) were imported and processed in Simpleware ScanIP (Synopsys, Mountain View, USA). Geometrically detailed segmentations of the LV and RV were created relying on a combination of well-established techniques, including region growing, level-set thresholding, and morphological smoothing (Vadakkumpadan et al., 2010; Setarehdan and Singh, 2012). The biventricular structure was truncated at the base and illustrations of the image data, segmentation, and Finite Element (FE) mesh construction are presented in **Figure 1**.

We introduced prolate spheroidal coordinates (Lombaert et al., 2012; Toussaint et al., 2013) into the image-coordinate space aligned with the long axis of the LV. The prolate spheroidal coordinates were used to describe myofiber orientations using a rule-based approach. Based on previous computational studies (Genet et al., 2014), histological studies (Streeter et al., 1969), and diffusion tensor MR studies (Lombaert et al., 2011), we assumed that the myofiber orientation could be represented through a linearly varying helix angle from −60° on the epicardium to +60° on the endocardium. This was assigned to each material point in the model through a custom MATLAB (The MathWorks, Inc., Natick, Massachusetts, United States) script that specifies myofiber orientation by rotating the local circumferential unit vector by the helix angle in the circumferential-longitudinal plane. The same fiber description from endocardium to epicardium was applied to the LV free wall, septal wall, and RV free wall as other studies typically assume (Goktepe et al., 2011; Wenk et al., 2012; Wong and Kuhl, 2014).

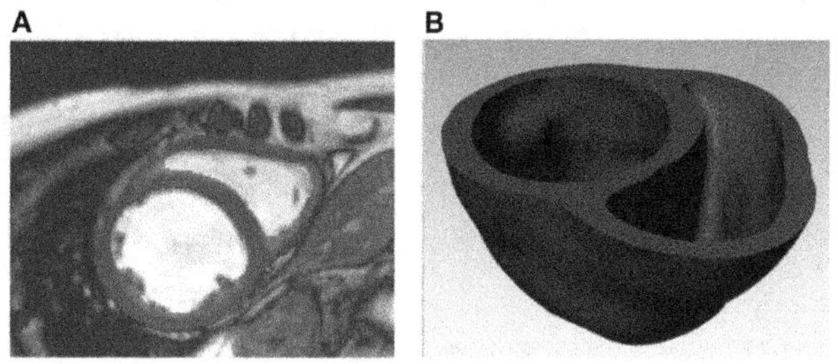

While multiple models and explanations of sheet structure exist (Gilbert et al., 2007), for simplicity we define the sheet directions to be normal with epicardial and endocardial surfaces (i.e., normal with the circumferential-longitudinal plane in which the fiber direction resides). This assumption is relatively reasonable when considering the macroscopically visible cleavage planes observed experimentally (LeGrice et al., 2001; Chen et al., 2005) and is in line with other computational studies (Bovendeerd et al., 1994; Goktepe et al., 2011).

Regarding boundary conditions, the base of the biventricular structure (plane of truncation) was fixed in the longitudinal direction. Furthermore, the nodes on the endocardial annulus were constrained by coupling the average translation and rotation of the nodes to a fixed point in space located at the annulus center. This prevents rigid body rotation while allowing the annulus relative motion to inflate and contract during the cardiac cycle.

### Constitutive Law and Parameter Estimation

The passive material response of the cardiac tissue uses an anisotropic hyperelastic formulation proposed by Holzapfel and Ogden (Holzapfel and Ogden, 2009). The isochoric and volumetric responses are governed by the strain energy potentials in Equations (1–2)

$$\Psi_{iso} = \frac{a}{2b}e^{b(I_1-3)} + \sum_{i=f,s}\frac{a_i}{2b_i}\left\{e^{b_i(I_{4i}-1)^2}-1\right\}$$
$$+ \frac{a_{fs}}{2b_{fs}}\left\{e^{b_{fs}(I_{8fs})^2}-1\right\}, \quad (1)$$

$$\Psi_{vol} = \frac{1}{D}\left(\frac{J^2-1}{2}-\ln(J)\right). \quad (2)$$

Equation (1) is defined through eight material parameters $a$, $b$, $a_f$, $b_f$, $a_s$, $b_s$, $a_{fs}$, $b_{fs}$ and four strain invariants $I_1$, $I_{4f}$, $I_{4s}$, and $I_{8fs}$. These strain invariants are derived from the isochoric right Cauchy-Green tensor,

$$\overline{C} = \overline{F}^T\overline{F} = J^{-2/3}C = J^{-2/3}F^TF \quad (3)$$

where $F$ is the deformation gradient, $J$ is the determinant of the deformation gradient, $J = \det(F)$ and $\overline{F}$ is the isochoric part of the deformation gradient such that

$$\overline{F} = J^{-1/3}F \quad \text{and} \quad \det(\overline{F}) = 1. \quad (4)$$

The expression of these strain invariants can now be defined as:

$$I_1 = tr\left(\overline{C}\right), I_{4f} = f_0\cdot\left(\overline{C}f_0\right), I_{4s} = s_0\cdot\left(\overline{C}s_0\right), I_{8fs} = f_0\cdot\left(\overline{C}s_0\right) \quad (5)$$

Where $f_0$ and $s_0$ are orthogonal vectors in the fiber and sheet direction in the reference configuration. Equation (2) is defined through $J$ and a penalty term $D$, which is a multiple of the bulk

**FIGURE 1 | (A)** Short axis MR image of patient with dilated chronic heart failure overlaid with the segmentation of the myocardium. **(B)** Truncated biventricular geometry extracted from segmentation and meshed using tetrahedral elements.

modulus ($D = 2/K$). For deformation that perfectly preserves volume, $J = 1$.

This passive material model, Equations (1–2), ensures that the material exhibits the well-documented exponential and anisotropic response to strain (Demer and Yin, 1983; Hunter et al., 1998; Dokos et al., 2002) while enforcing incompressibility.

The description of our time-varying elastance model of active force development (Guccione and McCulloch, 1993) is specified as:

$$T_a\left(t, l\right) = T_{MAX} \frac{Ca_0^2}{Ca_0^2 + ECa_{50}^2\left(l\right)} \frac{\left(1 - \cos\left(\omega\left(t, l\right)\right)\right)}{2} \quad (6)$$

where $T_{max}$, the maximum allowable active tension, is multiplied with a term governing the calcium concentration, and a term governing the timing of contraction. Both terms depend on sarcomere length $l$, which in turn depends on the strain in the fiber direction. The active tension generated from this representation conforms well with experimental studies (Guccione and McCulloch, 1993) and captures length-dependent effects such as Frank Starling's Law (Holmes et al., 2002; Solaro, 2007). Further detail of the active tension law is provided in the Appendix for the interested reader.

We consider the total Cauchy stress to be an additive contribution of passive and active components. The passive Cauchy stress, $\sigma_p$, is given by $\sigma_p = 2J^{-1}F\left(\partial\Psi/\partial C\right)F^T$. We consider an active contractile stress in the fiber direction, resulting in a total Cauchy stress in the fiber direction, (i.e., myofiber stress) by combining this with to the passive stress state in this direction ($\sigma_{pf}$):

$$\sigma_f = \sigma_{pf} + T_a f \otimes f \quad (7)$$

Biaxial investigations on actively contracting rabbit myocardium revealed significant stress development in the cross-fiber direction that could not be completely attributed to myofiber dispersion or deformation effects (Lin and Yin, 1998). This has motivated computational efforts to consider a proportion of the active stress developed in the myofiber direction to be transferred onto the stress in the sheet direction by a scalar $n_s \in (0, 1)$, such that the total Cauchy stress in the sheet direction is:

$$\sigma_s = \sigma_{ps} + n_s T_a s \otimes s \quad (8)$$

## Material Parameter Estimation

Full records of the patient who was used in our heart model were unavailable; therefore, we relied on clinical input to provide representative functional targets for volume and pressures. To this end, the dilated failing heart used in this study was assumed to have an end-diastolic volume (EDV) of 254 ml and an end-systolic volume (ESV) of 224 ml. End-diastolic pressure (EDP) and end-systolic pressure (ESP) were assumed to be 23 and 86 mmHg, respectively. These classify the patient with a severely dilated LV (>200 ml), elevated EDP (>16 mmHg, Paulus et al., 2007 and 23 mmHg, Mielniczuk et al., 2007) and severely reduced ejection fraction (EF = 1− ESV/EDV = 12%) i.e., <35% (McMurray et al., 2012; Mann et al., 2014).

The material parameters $a$, $b$, $a_f$, $b_f$, $a_s$, $b_s$, $a_{fs}$, $b_{fs}$ were found through optimization techniques relying on two stages of determination. Initial values were determined from the calibration of normal myocardium specimen samples to experimental tri-axial shear data of human myocardium (Sommer et al., 2015). Calibration was performed using ABAQUS as the forward solver, whereby *in silico* cubes of myocardium with dimensions matching those of the study of interest were meshed into a uniform 27 linear hex-element mesh. Shearing was executed by specifying the translational displacement of a specified cube face, while enforcing zero displacement boundary conditions on the opposite cube face. The optimization was performed in MATLAB using a non-linear least-square optimization routine.

To capture patient-specific material parameters of our failing human heart, a second stage of "scaling" was needed. Here, linear ($a$, $a_f$, $a_s$, and $a_{fs}$) and exponential ($b$, $b_f$, $b_s$, $b_{fs}$) terms were subject to uniform scaling by parameters $A$ and $B$, a scalar and an exponential multiplier, respectively. These values were found by minimizing the error between the *in silico* diastolic PV course resulting from loading the LV of the FE model to the analytical Klotz curve (Klotz et al., 2006), starting from the unloaded LV volume $V_0$ until the EDV was reached at the specified end-diastolic pressure (EDP). Material parameters were calibrated using ABAQUS as the forward solver, and an in-house PYTHON script containing the sequential least squares programming (SLSQP) optimization algorithm (Jones et al., 2001). These passive parameters expressed in Equations (1) were identified by minimizing the error between the *in silico* diastolic PV curve and the analytical Klotz curve.

Once passive parameters were found, the active parameter $T_{MAX}$ was identified by minimizing the error between predicted and specified stroke volume and assuming that 25% of active tension was transferred in the sheet direction (i.e., $n_s = 0.25$). Calibrated material parameters are presented in **Table 1**.

## Coupled Circulatory System and LVAD Support

The FE model of the heart was coupled to lumped models of the pulmonary and systemic circulatory systems used in our previous study (Sack et al., 2016). A small modification was introduced to separate the pulmonary circuit into venous and arterial components. Collectively, this captures fluid exchanges between the systemic circuit, the heart and the pulmonary circuit. A schematic diagram outlining the fluid connections between the patient-specific biventricular structure and the lumped circulatory system with the LVAD is presented in **Figure 2**; all

**TABLE 1** | Calibrated material parameters.

| Parameters | $a$ (kPa) | $b$ | $a_f$ (kPa) | $b_f$ | $a_s$ (kPa) | $b_s$ | $a_{fs}$ (kPa) | $b_{fs}$ | $T_{MAX}$ (kPa) |
|---|---|---|---|---|---|---|---|---|---|
| | 8.41 | 30.32 | 27.72 | 58.18 | 3.85 | 50.44 | 2.26 | 12.42 | 170.0 |

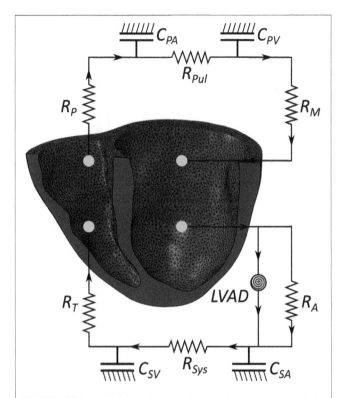

**FIGURE 2** | Schematic of the patient-specific biventricular structure coupled with the circulatory system and LVAD. $R_M$ is mitral valve resistance, $R_A$ is aortic valve resistance, $C_{SA}$ is systemic arterial compliance, $R_{SYS}$ is systemic arterial resistance, $C_{SV}$ is systemic venous compliance, $R_T$ is tricuspid valve resistance, $R_P$ is pulmonary valve resistance, $C_{PA}$ is pulmonary arterial compliance, $R_{PUL}$ is pulmonary arterial resistance, $C_{PV}$ is pulmonary venous compliance.

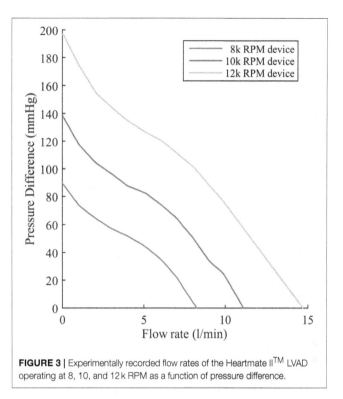

**FIGURE 3** | Experimentally recorded flow rates of the Heartmate II™ LVAD operating at 8, 10, and 12 k RPM as a function of pressure difference.

parameters relating to the lumped model are presented in the Appendix in **Table A2**.

Two further changes are present in the model used in this study compared with the model used in our prior study (Sack et al., 2016). First, the mechanical heart is replaced with a patient-specific biventricular structure (as detailed in previous sections).

The second change is that a far more complex and realistic representation of LVAD flow is included. We simulated the effect of a Heartmate II ™ LVAD device operating at device speeds of 8, 9, 10, 11, and 12 k RPM. Each speed has a flow rate profile that is dependent on the pressure difference (dP) between the inflow and outflow cavities to which the pump connects. Experimental datasets specifying flow rates for a range of dP between 0 and 200 mmHg at discrete intervals of 2 mmHg were incorporated in the simulated flow profile for each operating speed. Flow rates were interpolated and extrapolated linearly between discrete values to account for a continuous flow-rate description for any dP the model may encounter. This is illustrated in **Figure 3** for three LVAD operating speeds (8, 10, and 12 k RPM).

## Experimental Design

For this study, cardiac function was simulated for a patient with chronic heart failure. LVAD therapy was introduced by

simulating the effect of a HeartMate II operating at speeds ranging from 8–12 k RPM in 1 k RPM increments. Pressure and volume measurements of the ventricular chambers were recorded and compared to quantify ventricular loading and output performance. Myofiber stress was recorded and quantified for each simulation and compared to analyze the efficacy of treatment in the LV and potential harm of treatment to the septal wall and RV. Stress data in this study are expressed as mean ± standard of deviation (*SD*) unless otherwise stated. The differences between results were evaluated using analysis of variance (ANOVA) with differences considered statistically significant with $p < 0.05$. Time points in the cardiac cycle, such as end diastole, were defined for the untreated case and compared to the time points in simulations with LVAD support. End diastole and end systole, for each ventricle, were identified from the pressure-volume curves as the points immediately preceding isovolumetric contraction and relaxation respectively.

## RESULTS

The model of chronic heart failure without LVAD support represents a critical patient with advanced heart failure. The LV is substantially overloaded at end diastole with an EDV of 254 ml, an EDP of 23 mmHg, and an LV EF of 12%. The support introduced through LVAD operation improves these functional metrics: the diastolic loading of the LV decreases and the LV EF increases as the RPM of the device increases (i.e., increased support), as shown in **Table 2**. These LV benefits occur simultaneously with increases in the RV loading, seen by the rise in RV EDV (**Table 2**) and EDP which increases from 20.8 mmHg

**TABLE 2** | Functional metrics in the left and right ventricles.

|  | LV EDV (ml) | PCWP (mmHg) | RV EDV (ml) | CVP (mmHg) | LV EF (%) | RV EF (%) | CO (L/min) |
|---|---|---|---|---|---|---|---|
| No intervention | 253.9 | 39.8 | 165.0 | 20.8 | 11.9 | 16.3 | 1.82 |
| LVAD 8 k RPM | 245.5 | 39.0 | 169.5 | 21.7 | 12.8 | 18.5 | 1.88 |
| LVAD 9 k RPM | 238.7 | 38.3 | 173.3 | 22.5 | 14.5 | 19.9 | 2.07 |
| LVAD 10 k RPM | 227.8 | 36.9 | 178.0 | 23.6 | 16.5 | 21.1 | 2.25 |
| LVAD 11 k RPM | 212.9 | 34.8 | 182.0 | 25.2 | 18.4 | 21.5 | 2.34 |
| LVAD 12 k RPM | 190.2 | 31.7 | 184.5 | 27.1 | 18.5 | 19.1 | 2.11 |

*LV, left ventricle; RV, right ventricle; EDV, end-diastolic volume; EF, ejection fraction; PCWP, pulmonary capillary wedge pressure; CVP, central venous pressure; CO, cardiac output.*

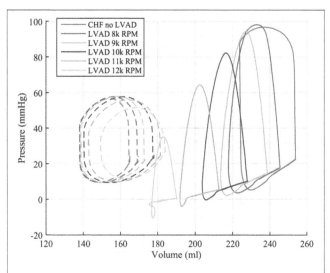

**FIGURE 4** | Pressure volume loops for the LV (solid lines) and RV (dashed lines) from the FE model study.

(untreated) to 27.9 mmHg (LVAD operating at 12 k RPM), as the mean central venous pressure rises (**Table 2**). Although the RV EF initially increases with LVAD operation, it reaches a peak functional value with LVAD support at 11 k RPM, after which it starts to decline.

These functional changes are also captured in pressure-volume loops of each chamber, as shown in **Figure 4**. These curves illustrate the reduction of LV EDP, which ranged from 17.9 to 0.5 mmHg, with the simulated LVAD operating between 8 and 12 k RPM. As LVAD flow increases, the LV PV-loop becomes more triangular, indicative of the device's effect during the normally isovolumetric periods of the cardiac cycle. As the loop shifted leftward toward lower volumes, it tracked down a single end-diastolic pressure-volume relationship. As the LV was increasingly unloaded by increases in LVAD speed, the RV PV-loops shifted rightward toward higher volumes and pressures. In addition, the systolic portion of the loops also shifts rightward and peak RV pressure also decreases. These shifts are a consequence of the reductions of LV pressure during both diastole and systole. It is noteworthy that LVAD speeds of up to 12 k increased RV EDP, resulted in excessive reductions of LV volume and, in the case of the 12 k RPM simulation, reduced cardiac output: three distinctive characteristics of right heart failure. Additional pressure tracings of the LV, the systemic arteries (analogous of aortic pressure), the RV and the pulmonary arteries are provided in **Figure 5** for two heartbeats.

The interventricular septum is in constant motion throughout the cardiac cycle. We tracked the midpoint motion at the base of the septal wall and quantified the leftward shift of this point in reference to the line through the anterior and posterior LV-septal-RV junctions. This measure of septal shift is positive when the septal wall bulges into the LV cavity, zero when the septal wall forms a straight line and negative when the wall bulges into the RV cavity. A time course of this measure over two heartbeats, shown in **Figure 6** alongside the pressure difference between the ventricles, reveals that peak leftward shift occurs during diastolic function and goes from being concave in the unsupported case to convex in the case of simulated LVAD support >10 k RPM. Rightward septal shift coincides with peak systole (and minimum trans-septal pressure) and is driven by the contractile forces with the heart returning the shape to a more "normal" configuration. Septal shift is also shown by plotting

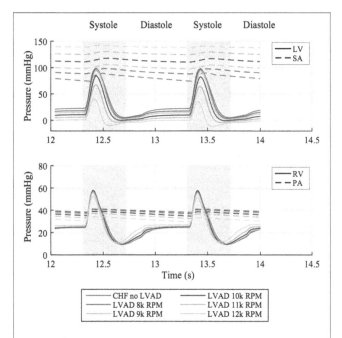

**FIGURE 5** | **(Top)** Pressure tracings of the LV and systemic arterial compliance (SA) over two cardiac cycles for all simulated cases. **(Bottom)** Pressure tracings of the RV and pulmonary arterial compliance (PA) over two cardiac cycles for all simulated cases.

displacements in the dynamic beating ventricles of the patient with no intervention and LVAD operating speeds of 8, 10, and 12 k RPM in the Supplementary Animations S1, S2.

The volumetric-averaged myofiber stress (along the local muscle fiber direction) was calculated at end diastole and end systole, and the mean ± *SD* are presented in **Table 3** for the RV free wall, the septal wall, and LV free wall separately. Compared to the unsupported CHF case, LV mean myofiber stress is reduced by LVAD support by an order of magnitude at end diastole and end systole ($p < 0.001$). The improvements to RV mean myofiber stress were less substantial, with both end diastole and end systole myofiber stress in the RV remaining relatively unaffected.

Myofiber stress distributions and overall geometry are presented in **Figure 7** at end diastole to illustrate stresses and the deformed configuration corresponding to maximum volume loading. These stress distributions reveal geometrically relevant stress characteristics that evolve with increased LVAD operation. The large stress values seen on the LV endocardium (excluding the septal wall) due to volumetric loading at end diastole decrease

with LVAD support and appear to dissipate with maximum LVAD operation of 12 k RPM. However, a localized region of tensile (i.e., positive) myofiber stress appears and grows with increased LVAD support on the LV side of the septal wall near the base (**Figure 7**). Additionally, LVAD operation promotes a localized region of compressive (i.e., negative) myofiber stress on the RV side of the septal wall in the same region.

A quantitative analysis of myofiber stress distribution in a segmented region of the vulnerable septal wall is presented in **Figure 8**. Initially (i.e., chronic heart failure with no LVAD support) the myofiber stresses in this region display a mostly Gaussian distribution. At 10 k RPM the myofiber stress distributions in this region begin to display bimodal peaks, which become more exaggerated with increased LVAD support.

## DISCUSSION

We describe a geometrically and physically realistic model of an end-stage failing heart with representative systolic and diastolic myocardial material properties coupled to lumped parameter Windkessel-like models of the pulmonary and systemic circulations. This permitted study of heart mechanics and dynamics under realistic loading conditions i.e., pre-load and afterload of each ventricle. Finally, we simulated the effects of LVAD support by using experimentally recorded pressure-flow characteristics of a commonly used device. The present model represents a significant improvement over our prior modeling efforts (Sack et al., 2016) in that the effects of an LVAD on chronic rather than acute left heart failure were quantified using a patient-specific biventricular geometry and device-specific pressure-flow characteristics, rather than constant flow rates.

This improved model reproduced a wide range of expected, fundamental behaviors of the LV and RV. There were LVAD speed-dependent reductions in LV filling pressure, pressure generation, and a progressive transformation of the PV-loop from trapezoidal shape to triangular shape. This shape transformation is because LVADs are continuous flow pumps that remove volume from the LV throughout the cardiac cycle, thus eliminating isovolumic contraction phases (Morley et al., 2007; Wang et al., 2014). With LVAD-induced LV unloading, the RV PV-loop shifted toward larger volumes and higher pressures,

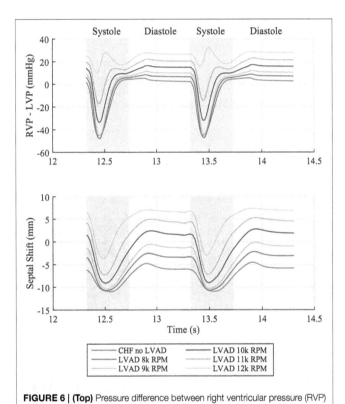

**FIGURE 6 | (Top)** Pressure difference between right ventricular pressure (RVP) and left ventricular pressure (LVP) over two cardiac cycles for all simulated cases. **(Bottom)** Corresponding leftward septal shift over the same time period. Diastolic and systolic portions of the cardiac cycle are labeled.

**TABLE 3 |** LV and RV myofiber stress results (mean ± SD) at end diastole and end systole ($p < 0.001$ for comparisons within each column).

|  | LV free wall | | Septal wall | | RV free wall | |
|---|---|---|---|---|---|---|
|  | ED myofiber stress (kPa) | ES myofiber stress (kPa) | ED myofiber stress (kPa) | ES myofiber stress (kPa) | ED myofiber stress (kPa) | ES myofiber stress (kPa) |
| No intervention | 13.7 ± 6.8 | 35.7 ± 15.6 | 10.0 ± 7.5 | 29.8 ± 13.8 | 14.9 ± 10.8 | 21.4 ± 15.2 |
| LVAD 8 k RPM | 10.8 ± 5.7 | 33.3 ± 14.6 | 7.9 ± 7.2 | 27.5 ± 13.2 | 14.1 ± 10.4 | 20.8 ± 14.8 |
| LVAD 9 k RPM | 8.8 ± 5.0 | 30.8 ± 13.7 | 6.8 ± 7.4 | 25.2 ± 12.6 | 13.8 ± 10.3 | 20.4 ± 14.6 |
| LVAD 10 k RPM | 6.3 ± 4.2 | 22.6 ± 10.8 | 5.8 ± 8.7 | 17.6 ± 10.9 | 13.5 ± 10.5 | 18.9 ± 13.9 |
| LVAD 11 k RPM | 3.5 ± 3.8 | 12.4 ± 8.1 | 5.1 ± 10.9 | 8.2 ± 9.9 | 13.1 ± 10.6 | 16.5 ± 12.7 |
| LVAD 12 k RPM | 1.1 ± 4.2 | 1.5 ± 12.1 | 5.1 ± 14.1 | −1.0 ± 16.0 | 13.0 ± 11.2 | 13.5 ± 11.4 |

*LV, left ventricle; RV, right ventricle; ED, end diastole; ES, end systole.*

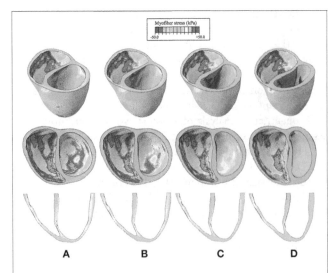

**FIGURE 7 |** Myofiber stress distributions at end diastole for the cases of **(A)** CHF with no LVAD support, **(B)** CHF with LVAD support running at 8 k RPM, **(C)**, CHF with LVAD support running at 10 k RPM, **(D)** CHF with LVAD support running at 12 k RPM. Top row reveals a predominantly long-axis view of the biventricular structure, the middle row reveals a short-axis view, exposing the ventricular cavities, and the bottom row reveals a long-axis cut plane that bisects the ventricles. Light gray regions correspond to extreme stress values that exceed the threshold of +50 kPa.

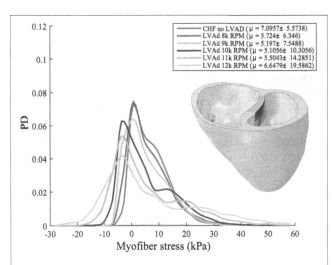

**FIGURE 8 |** Interpolated histograms of myofiber stress distributions in the region of maximum septal shift (colored region of inlaid illustration) for all simulations of CHF and LVAD operation. Mean ± *SD* values are given in the legend for each case. Histograms are normalized by probability density (PD), i.e., the area under each distribution sums to 1.

indicating that the RV end-diastolic pressure-volume loop was shifting rightward; this is indicative of increased RV diastolic compliance and is a consequence of RV-LV interactions and a leftward septal shift. RV systolic pressure also decreased, also a consequence of RV-LV interactions. In the case of high LVAD operational speed, a secondary "Figure 8" shaped loop is visible at the end of relaxation and the start of passive filling. This ultimately results from the combined effects of RV-LV interactions, pressure-sensitive LVAD operation and the LV being unloaded at a faster rate than it being filled. The degree of unloading that would cause this would likely initiate ventricular arrhythmias in the clinical environment, so data surrounding this type of phenomena is very rare. LVAD speed-dependent septal shifts were clearly evident in the 3-dimensional images. Those images match changes in echocardiographs obtained from LVAD patients at high LVAD speeds, particular in those with right heart failure. For example, **Figure 9A** shows a patient with low RPMs and normal, right-shifted interventricular septum (traced out by the red line) compared to **Figure 9B** showing a patient with markedly left-shifted septum. Note the remarkable similarity of these images to those presented in the lower panels of **Figures 7A,D**.

We found that LVAD support reduced estimates of global LV and, to a lesser extent, septal wall myocardial stresses. However, these improvements were achieved with secondary negative effects on the RV, which experienced a rightward shift toward higher EDPs and larger EDVs with LVAD support, which kept RV stresses high. Additional, potentially negative, effects were seen on the interventricular septum, which showed that LVAD support introduces unnatural bending of the septum with

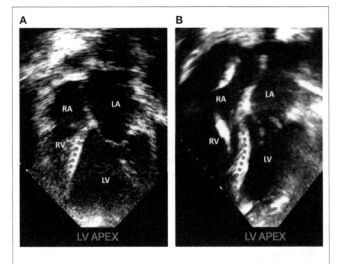

**FIGURE 9 |** Modified with permission from Topilsky et al. (2011). **(A)** a patient with low RPMs and normal, right shifted interventricular septum (traced out by the red line) compared to **(B)** a patient with markedly left-shifted septum (traced out by the red line). LV, left ventricle; RV, right ventricle; LA, left atrium; RA: right atrium.

increased localized myofiber stresses. Such deformations are similar to those of a beam undergoing bending deformation, which introduces LVAD speed-dependent regions of tensile stress on the LV side and regions of compressive stress on the RV side of the septal wall (**Figure 7**). In general, myocardial properties (genetic expression, molecular makeup, structure and function) are modified in response to chronic stresses. However, it is unknown if these abnormal stresses on the myocardium of the septum have any implications for myocardial function as abnormal stresses may relate to the development of right heart failure in the long term.

Over the last few decades, numerical and analytical models of circulatory flow and ventricular assistance have been introduced (e.g., Levin et al., 1995; Vollkron et al., 2002; Morley et al., 2007; Lim et al., 2010). Many of these models represent heart function, without including geometric considerations (often referred to as zero-dimensional models). Despite those limitations, the basic findings derived from such models have generally been in agreement with the present findings. While some research has incorporated functionally realistic ventricular assistance devices, these studies also ignore geometric effects on the heart and, in particular, have not considered ventricular interactions or shifts of septal position (Donahue et al., 2009; Long et al., 2013; Chiu et al., 2014; Selishchev and Telyshev, 2016).

FE modeling enables estimation of regional stress that cannot be measured in patients using alternative techniques. This allows identification of the LVAD speed at which bending and abnormal stresses emerge in the septum. If patient-specific geometries could be incorporated more easily, such modeling could provide interesting metrics with clinical applicability for understanding and perhaps predicting the impact of LVAD speed on septal mechanics.

One goal of developing the present model is to study the degree to which RV-LV interactions and septal shift plays a role in the development of RV failure following LVAD implantation. Many other factors can contribute to the development of RF failure, such as RV myocardial dysfunction, increased pulmonary vascular resistance and volume overload. The impact of those factors, and even RV-LV interactions, are readily ascertained through simpler zero-dimension modeling of the cardiovascular system (HARVI, 2014a,b; Burkhoff et al., 2017). However, it is only through finite element analysis (FEA) that the question of the impact of septal shifts can be determined. For example, although in the present example we demonstrated marked septal shifts at high LVAD speeds accompanied by increased RV EDPs, there were balanced shifts of systolic and diastolic volumes such that cardiac output was mostly preserved, with only minor impact on RV systolic pressure. Thus, in this example, marked septal shift resulted in RV dysfunction and not full-blown failure. However, we have only studied one set of conditions (i.e., one starting RV geometry, one level of myocardial contractility, and one value of pulmonary vascular resistance). A thorough evaluation over a range of conditions and a sensitivity analysis on parameter values is required to fully explore this important question.

## LIMITATIONS

The model described in the present study is an improvement over prior models, but several limitations exist. First, the model does not contain atria. Since LV filling dynamics are impacted by atrial contraction, this could have an effect on the diastolic portion of the PV-loop and time-course of change of septal motion. Second, the models of the vascular system are adequate to provide the basic aspects of ventricular afterload and yielded realistic PV-loop

shapes, but more sophisticated models that incorporate fluid-structure interactions, the valve geometries and wave reflections would be more accurate. Third, a sensitivity analysis was not performed to quantify the relative impact of material parameters to model results. This was viewed as beyond the scope of this research but should be performed (alongside rigorous validation studies) before computational models contribute to clinical decision making. We intend to address this in our future work. Finally, as noted, we studied only one combination of myocardial properties, RV and LV and vascular properties. Every patient is unique and conclusions arrived at are not generalizable.

## SUMMARY

We described results of an FEA model based on the anatomy of an end-stage failing heart coupled to systemic and pulmonary vascular systems and an LVAD. We demonstrated the anatomic and hemodynamic impact of increasing LVAD speed on global pump function, regional stress distributions, and septal position. Realistic results were obtained in terms of ventricular deformation and PV loops. We demonstrated the expected findings that RV systolic and diastolic properties are affected by LVAD-induced unloading of the LV, resulting in RV dysfunction at high LVAD operating speeds. Having established the foundation of this model, we are poised to address the important question of whether and under what conditions, septal shift, and reduced LV pressure generation are important mechanisms of the development of RV failure following LVAD implantation. The specific conditions studied in the present model demonstrate that septal shifting alone is not sufficient to induce RV failure. Simulations spanning a wide range of conditions are required to fully address this important question.

Beyond this, the methods are generalizable in the sense that patient-specific geometries and vascular properties can be incorporated into the model, with the ultimate purpose of gaining insights into LVAD effects *in vivo*. Such an approach has the potential for predicting hemodynamics, such as the degree of unloading achievable, and the risk of developing right heart failure following LVAD implantation. Advances in patient-specific modeling in other fields of cardiology are already having an impact on clinical practice and it is anticipated that new applications will emerge, especially in the field of heart failure. The methods and results described in the present study have potential to meaningfully advance such efforts.

## ETHICS STATEMENT

Patient cardiac MR data was obtained as part of the Aliskiren Study in Post-MI Patients to Reduce Remodeling (ASPIRE) trial. The study protocol was written by members of the executive committee of the trial and was approved by the ethics committees at each participating site. Individual patients provided written informed consent in accordance with the Declaration of Helsinki and anonymized data were sent to a core laboratory for analysis.

## AUTHOR CONTRIBUTIONS

KS, TF, DB, and JG were involved in the conception and design of study. KS created the computational models. Acquisition of various data critical to model creation was performed by SS and DB. The analysis and interpretation of modeling results was performed by all authors. KS wrote the first draft of the manuscript. DB and JG wrote sections of the manuscript. All authors contributed to manuscript revision, read and approved the submitted version.

## ACKNOWLEDGMENTS

The authors thank Pamela Derish in the Department of Surgery, University of California San Francisco for proofreading the manuscript.

## REFERENCES

Argiriou, M., Kolokotron, S.-M., Sakellaridis, T., Argiriou, O., Charitos, C., Zarogoulidis, P., et al. (2014). Right heart failure post left ventricular assist device implantation. *J. Thoracic. Dis.* 6(Suppl. 1), S52–S59. doi: 10.3978/j.issn.2072-1439.2013.10.26

Baillargeon, B., Costa, I., Leach, J. R., Lee, L. C., Genet, M., Toutain, A., et al. (2015). Human cardiac function simulator for the optimal design of a novel annuloplasty ring with a sub-valvular element for correction of ischemic mitral regurgitation. *Cardiovasc. Eng. Technol.* 6, 105–116. doi: 10.1007/s13239-015-0216-z

Baillargeon, B., Rebelo, N., Fox, D. D., Taylor, R. L., and Kuhl, E. (2014). The living heart project: a robust and integrative simulator for human heart function. *Eur. J. Mech. A Solids* 48, 38–47. doi: 10.1016/j.euromechsol.2014.04.001

Baumwol, J., Macdonald, P. S., Keogh, A. M., Kotlyar, E., Spratt, P., Jansz, P., et al. (2011). Right heart failure and "failure to thrive" after left ventricular assist device: clinical predictors and outcomes. *J. Heart Lung Transplant.* 30, 888–895. doi: 10.1016/j.healun.2011.03.006

Birks, E. J., Tansley, P. D., Hardy, J., George, R. S., Bowles, C. T., Burke, M., et al. (2006). Left ventricular assist device and drug therapy for the reversal of heart failure. *N. Engl. J. Med.* 355, 1873–1884. doi: 10.1056/NEJMoa053063

Bovendeerd, P., Huyghe, J., Arts, T., Van Campen, D., and Reneman, R. (1994). Influence of endocardial-epicardial crossover of muscle fibers on left ventricular wall mechanics. *J. Biomech.* 27, 941–951. doi: 10.1016/0021-9290(94)90266-6

Burkhoff, D., Dickstein, M., and Schleicher, T. (2017). *HARVI - Online.* Available online at: http://harvi.online (Cited April 29, 2017).

Burkhoff, D., Klotz, S., and Mancini, D. M. (2006). LVAD-induced reverse remodeling: basic and clinical implications for myocardial recovery. *J. Card. Fail.* 12, 227–239. doi: 10.1016/j.cardfail.2005.10.012

Chen, J., Liu, W., Zhang, H., Lacy, L., Yang, X., Song, S.-K., et al. (2005). Regional ventricular wall thickening reflects changes in cardiac fiber and sheet structure during contraction: quantification with diffusion tensor MRI. *Am. J. Physiol. Heart Circ. Physiol.* 289, H1898–H907. doi: 10.1152/ajpheart.000 41.2005

Chiu, W.-C., Girdhar, G., Xenos, M., Alemu, Y., Soares, J. S., Einav, S., et al. (2014). Thromboresistance comparison of the HeartMate II ventricular assist device with the device thrombogenicity emulation-optimized HeartAssist 5 VAD. *J. Biomech. Eng.* 136:021014. doi: 10.1115/1.4026254

Dang, N. C., Topkara, V. K., Mercando, M., Kay, J., Kruger, K. H., Aboodi, M. S., et al. (2006). Right heart failure after left ventricular assist device implantation in patients with chronic congestive heart failure. *J. Heart Lung Transplant.* 25, 1–6. doi: 10.1016/j.healun.2005.07.008

Demer, L. L., and Yin, F. C. (1983). Passive biaxial mechanical properties of isolated canine myocardium. *J. Physiol.* 339, 615–630. doi: 10.1113/jphysiol.1983.sp014738

Dokos, S., Smaill, B. H., Young, A. A., and LeGrice, I. J. (2002). Shear properties of passive ventricular myocardium. *Am. J. Physiol. Heart Circ. Physiol.* 283, H2650–H2659. doi: 10.1152/ajpheart.00111.2002

Donahue, T. H., Dehlin, W., Gillespie, J., Weiss, W., and Rosenberg, G. (2009). Finite element analysis of stresses developed in the blood sac of a left ventricular assist device. *Med. Eng. Phys.* 31, 454–460. doi: 10.1016/j.medengphy.2008.11.011

Genet, M., Lee, L. C., Nguyen, R., Haraldsson, H., Acevedo-Bolton, G., Zhang, Z., et al. (2014). Distribution of normal human left ventricular myofiber stress at end diastole and end systole: a target for *in silico* design of heart failure treatments. *J. Appl. Physiol.* 117, 142–152. doi: 10.1152/japplphysiol.00255.2014

Gilbert, S. H., Benson, A. P., Li, P., and Holden, A. V. (2007). Regional localisation of left ventricular sheet structure: integration with current models of cardiac fibre, sheet and band structure. *Eur. J. Cardiothorac. Surg.* 32, 231–249. doi: 10.1016/j.ejcts.2007.03.032

Goktepe, S., Acharya, S. N. S., Wong, J., and Kuhl, E. (2011). Computational modeling of passive myocardium. *Int. J. Numer. Methods Bio* 27, 1–12. doi: 10.1002/cnm.1402

Grant, A. D., Smedira, N. G., Starling, R. C., and Marwick, T. H. (2012). Independent and incremental role of quantitative right ventricular evaluation for the prediction of right ventricular failure after left ventricular assist device implantation. *J. Am. Coll. Cardiol.* 60, 521–528. doi: 10.1016/j.jacc.2012.02.073

Guccione, J. M., and McCulloch, A. D. (1993). Mechanics of active contraction in cardiac muscle: Part I–constitutive relations for fiber stress that describe deactivation. *J. Biomech. Eng.* 115, 72–81. doi: 10.1115/1.2895473

HARVI (2014a). *Cardiovascular Physiology, and Hemodynamics. Part, I. Basic Physiological Principles [Computer Program].* Available online at: https://itunes. apple.com/gb/app/harvi/id568196279?mt=8

HARVI (2014b). *Cardiovascular Physiology, and Hemodynamics. Part, I. I. Advanced Physiological Concepts [computer Program].* Available online at: https://itunes.apple.com/gb/app/harvi/id568196279?mt=8

Hayek, S., Sims, D. B., Markham, D. W., Butler, J., and Kalogeropoulos, A. P. (2014). Assessment of right ventricular function in left ventricular assist device candidates. *Circ. Cardiovasc. Imag.* 7, 379–389. doi: 10.1161/CIRCIMAGING.113.001127

Holmes, J. W., Hunlich, M., and Hasenfuss, G. (2002). Energetics of the Frank-Starling effect in rabbit myocardium: economy and efficiency depend on muscle length. *Am. J. Physiol. Heart Circ. Physiol.* 283, H324–H330. doi: 10.1152/ajpheart.00687.2001

Holzapfel, G. A., and Ogden, R. W. (2009). Constitutive modelling of passive myocardium: a structurally based framework for material characterization. *Philos. Trans. A Math. Phys. Eng. Sci.* 367, 3445–3475. doi: 10.1098/rsta.2009.0091

Hunter, P. J., McCulloch, A. D., and ter Keurs, H. E. (1998). Modelling the mechanical properties of cardiac muscle. *Prog. Biophys. Mol. Biol.* 69, 289–331. doi: 10.1016/S0079-6107(98)00013-3

Jones, E., Oliphant, T., and Peterson, P. (2001). *SciPy: Open Source Scientific Tools for Python.* Available online at: http://www.scipy.org

Kavarana, M. N., Pessin-Minsley, M. S., Urtecho, J., Catanese, K. A., Flannery, M., Oz, M. C., et al. (2002). Right ventricular dysfunction and organ failure in left ventricular assist device recipients: a continuing problem. *Ann. Thorac. Surg.* 73, 745–750. doi: 10.1016/S0003-4975(01)03406-3

Kerckhoffs, R. C., Neal, M. L., Gu, Q., Bassingthwaighte, J. B., Omens, J. H., and McCulloch, A. D. (2007). Coupling of a 3D finite element model of cardiac ventricular mechanics to lumped systems models of the systemic and pulmonic circulation. *Ann. Biomed. Eng.* 35, 1–18. doi: 10.1007/s10439-006-9212-7

Klotz, S., Hay, I., Dickstein, M. L., Yi, G. H., Wang, J., Maurer, M. S., et al. (2006). Single-beat estimation of end-diastolic pressure-volume relationship: a novel method with potential for noninvasive application. *Am. J. Physiol. Heart Circ. Physiol.* 291, H403–H412. doi: 10.1152/ajpheart.01240.2005

Kormos, R. L., Teuteberg, J. J., Pagani, F. D., Russell, S. D., John, R., Miller, L. W., et al. (2010). Right ventricular failure in patients with the HeartMate II continuous-flow left ventricular assist device: incidence, risk factors, and effect on outcomes. *J. Thorac. Cardiovasc. Surg.* 139, 1316–1324. doi: 10.1016/j.jtcvs.2009.11.020

Küçüker, S. A., Stetson, S. J., Becker, K. A., Akgül, A., Loebe, M., Lafuente, J. A., et al. (2004). Evidence of improved right ventricular structure after LVAD support in patients with end-stage cardiomyopathy. *J. Heart Lung Transplant.* 23, 28–35. doi: 10.1016/S1053-2498(03)00057-3

Lampropulos, J. F., Kim, N., Wang, Y., Desai, M. M., Barreto-Filho, J. A., Dodson, J. A., et al. (2014). Trends in left ventricular assist device use and outcomes among medicare beneficiaries, 2004–2011. *Open Heart* 1:e000109. doi: 10.1136/openhrt-2014-000109

LeGrice, I., Hunter, P., Young, A., and Small, B. (2001). The architecture of the heart: a data-based model. *Philos. Trans. R. Soc. Lond. Ser. A Math. Phys. Eng. Sci.* 359, 1217–1232. doi: 10.1098/rsta.2001.0827

Levin, H. R., Oz, M. C., Chen, J. M., Packer, M., Rose, E. A., and Burkhoff, D. (1995). Reversal of chronic ventricular dilation in patients with end-stage cardiomyopathy by prolonged mechanical unloading. *Circulation* 91, 2717–2720. doi: 10.1161/01.CIR.91.11.2717

Lim, E., Dokos, S., Cloherty, S. L., Salamonsen, R. F., Mason, D. G., Reizes, J. A., et al. (2010). Parameter-optimized model of cardiovascular-rotary blood pump interactions. *IEEE Trans. Biomed. Eng.* 57, 254–266. doi: 10.1109/TBME.2009.2031629

Lim, K. M., Constantino, J., Gurev, V., Zhu, R., Shim, E. B., and Trayanova, N. A. (2012). Comparison of the effects of continuous and pulsatile left ventricular-assist devices on ventricular unloading using a cardiac electromechanics model. *J. Physiol. Sci.* 62, 11–19. doi: 10.1007/s12576-011-0180-9

Lin, D., and Yin, F. (1998). A multiaxial constitutive law for mammalian left ventricular myocardium in steady-state barium contracture or tetanus. *J. Biomech. Eng.* 120, 504–517. doi: 10.1115/1.2798021

Lombaert, H., Peyrat, J. M., Croisille, P., Rapacchi, S., Fanton, L., Cheriet, F., et al. (2012). Human atlas of the cardiac fiber architecture: study on a healthy population. *IEEE Trans. Med. Imag.* 31, 1436–1447. doi: 10.1109/TMI.2012.2192743

Lombaert, H., Peyrat, J-M., Croisille, P., Rapacchi, S., Fanton, L., Clarysse, P., et al. (2011). "Statistical analysis of the human cardiac fiber architecture from DT-MRI," *Functional Imaging and Modeling of the Heart* (Springer), 171–179.

Long, C., Marsden, A., and Bazilevs, Y. (2013). Fluid–structure interaction simulation of pulsatile ventricular assist devices. *Comput. Mech.* 52, 971–981. doi: 10.1007/s00466-013-0858-3

Maeder, M. T., Leet, A., Ross, A., Esmore, D., and Kaye, D. M. (2009). Changes in right ventricular function during continuous-low left ventricular assist device support. *J. Heart Lung Transplant.* 28, 360–366. doi: 10.1016/j.healun.2009.01.007

Mann, D. L., Zipes, D. P., Libby, P., and Bonow, R. O. (2014). *Braunwald's Heart Disease: A Textbook of Cardiovascular Medicine.* Amsterdam: Elsevier Health Sciences.

McIlvennan, C. K., Magid, K. H., Ambardekar, A. V., Thompson, J. S., Matlock, D. D., and Allen, L. A. (2014). Clinical outcomes after continuous-flow left ventricular assist device: a systematic review. *Circ. Heart Fail.* 7, 1003–1013. doi: 10.1161/CIRCHEARTFAILURE.114.001391

McMurray, J. J., Adamopoulos, S., Anker, S. D., Auricchio, A., Böhm, M., Dickstein, K., et al. (2012). ESC Guidelines for the diagnosis and treatment of acute and chronic heart failure 2012. *Eur. J. Heart Fail.* 14, 803–869. doi: 10.1093/eurjhf/hfs105

Mielniczuk, L. M., Lamas, G. A., Flaker, G. C., Mitchell, G., Smith, S. C., Gersh, B. J., et al. (2007). Left ventricular end-diastolic pressure and risk of subsequent heart failure in patients following an acute myocardial infarction. *Congest. Heart Fail.* 13, 209–214. doi: 10.1111/j.1527-5299.2007.06624.x

Mohite, P. N., Sabashnikov, A., Simon, A. R., Weymann, A., Patil, N. P., Unsoeld, B., et al. (2014). Does CircuLite Synergy assist device as partial ventricular support have a place in modern management of advanced heart failure? *Expert Rev. Med. Devices* 12, 49–60. doi: 10.1586/17434440.2015.985208

Morley, D., Litwak, K., Ferber, P., Spence, P., Dowling, R., Meyns, B., et al. (2007). Hemodynamic effects of partial ventricular support in chronic heart failure: results of simulation validated with *in vivo* data. *J. Thorac. Cardiovasc. Surg.* 133, 21–28.e4. doi: 10.1016/j.jtcvs.2006.07.037

Paulus, W. J., Tschöpe, C., Sanderson, J. E., Rusconi, C., Flachskampf, F. A., Rademakers, F. E., et al. (2007). How to diagnose diastolic heart failure: a consensus statement on the diagnosis of heart failure with normal left ventricular ejection fraction by the heart failure and echocardiography associations of the European society of cardiology. *Eur. Heart J.* 28, 2539–2550. doi: 10.1093/eurheartj/ehm037

Rich, J. D., Gosev, I., Patel, C. B., Joseph, S., Katz, J. N., Eckman, P. M., et al. (2017). The incidence, risk factors, and outcomes associated with late right-sided heart failure in patients supported with an axial-flow left ventricular assist device. *J. Heart Lung Transplant.* 36, 50–58. doi: 10.1016/j.healun.2016.08.010

Sabashnikov, A., Popov, A. F., Bowles, C. T., Mohite, P. N., Weymann, A., Hards, R., et al. (2014). Outcomes after implantation of partial-support left ventricular assist devices in inotropic-dependent patients: do we still need full-support assist devices? *J. Thorac. Cardiovasc .Surg.* 148, 1115–1121. doi: 10.1016/j.jtcvs.2014.05.063

Sack, K. L., Baillargeon, B., Acevedo-Bolton, G., Genet, M., Rebelo, N., Kuhl, E., et al. (2016). Partial LVAD restores ventricular outputs and normalizes LV but not RV stress distributions in the acutely failing heart *in silico. Int. J. Artif. Organs* 39, 421–430. doi: 10.5301/ijao.5000520

Selishchev, S. V., and Telyshev, D. V. (2016). Optimisation of the Sputnik-VAD design. *Int. J. Artif. Organs* 39, 407–414. doi: 10.5301/ijao.5000518

Setarehdan, S. K., and Singh, S. (2012). *Advanced Algorithmic Approaches to Medical Image Segmentation: State-of-the-Art Applications in Cardiology, Neurology, Mammography and Pathology.* London: Springer Science and Business Media.

Slater, J. P., Lipsitz, E. C., Chen, J. M., Levin, H. R., Oz, M. C., Goldstein, D. J., et al. (1997). Systolic ventricular interaction in normal and diseased explanted human hearts. *J. Thor. Cardiovasc. Surg.* 113, 1091–1099. doi: 10.1016/S0022-5223(97)70296-4

Solaro, R. J. (2007). Mechanisms of the Frank-Starling law of the heart: the beat goes on. *Biophys. J.* 93, 4095–4096. doi: 10.1529/biophysj.107.117200

Solomon, S. D., Hee Shin, S., Shah, A., Skali, H., Desai, A., Kober, L., et al. (2011). Effect of the direct renin inhibitor aliskiren on left ventricular remodelling following myocardial infarction with systolic dysfunction. *Eur. Heart J.* 32, 1227–1234. doi: 10.1093/eurheartj/ehq522

Sommer, G., Schriefl, A. J., Andrä, M., Sacherer, M., Viertler, C., Wolinski, H., et al. (2015). Biomechanical properties and microstructure of human ventricular myocardium. *Acta Biomater.* 24, 172–192. doi: 10.1016/j.actbio.2015.06.031

Streeter, D. D., Spotnitz, H. M., Patel, D. P., Ross, J., and Sonnenblick, E. H. (1969). Fiber orientation in the canine left ventricle during diastole and systole. *Circ. Res.* 24, 339–347. doi: 10.1161/01.RES.24.3.339

Topilsky, Y., Hasin, T., Oh, J., Borgeson, D., Boilson, B., Schirger, J., et al. (2011). Echocardiographic variables after left ventricular assist device implantation associated with adverse outcome. *Circ. Cardiovasc. Imag.* 4, 648–661. doi: 10.1161/CIRCIMAGING.111.965335

Topkara, V. K., Garan, A. R., Fine, B., Godier-Furnémont, A. F., Breskin, A., Cagliostro, B., et al. (2016). Myocardial recovery in patients receiving contemporary left ventricular assist devices clinical perspective. *Circ. Heart Fail.* 9:e003157. doi: 10.1161/CIRCHEARTFAILURE.116.003157

Toussaint, N., Stoeck, C. T., Schaeffter, T., Kozerke, S., Sermesant, M., and Batchelor, P. G. (2013). *In vivo* human cardiac fibre architecture estimation using shape-based diffusion tensor processing. *Med. Image Anal.* 17, 1243–1255. doi: 10.1016/j.media.2013.02.008

Vadakkumpadan, F., Arevalo, H., Prassl, A. J., Chen, J. J., Kickinger, F., Kohl, P., et al. (2010). Image-based models of cardiac structure in health and disease. *WIRE Syst. Biol. Med.* 2, 489–506. doi: 10.1002/wsbm.76

Vollkron, M., Schima, H., Huber, L., and Wieselthaler, G. (2002). Interaction of the cardiovascular system with an implanted rotary assist device: simulation study with a refined computer model. *Artif. Organs* 26, 349–359. doi: 10.1046/j.1525-1594.2002.06870.x

Wang, Y., Loghmanpour, N., Vandenberghe, S., Ferreira, A., Keller, B., Gorcsan, J., et al. (2014). Simulation of dilated heart failure with continuous flow circulatory support. *PLoS ONE* 9:e85234. doi: 10.1371/journal.pone.0085234

Wenk, J. F., Ge, L., Zhang, Z., Soleimani, M., Potter, D. D., Wallace, A. W., et al. (2012). A coupled biventricular finite element and lumped-parameter circulatory system model of heart failure. *Comput. Methods Biomech. Biomed. Engin.* 16, 807–818. doi: 10.1080/10255842.2011.641121

Wohlschlaeger, J., Schmitz, K. J., Schmid, C., Schmid, K. W., Keul, P., Takeda, A., et al. (2005). Reverse remodeling following insertion of left ventricular assist devices (LVAD): a review of the morphological and molecular changes. *Cardiovasc. Res.* 68, 376–386. doi: 10.1016/j.cardiores.2005.06.030

Wong, J., and Kuhl, E. (2014). Generating fibre orientation maps in human heart models using Poisson interpolation. *Comput. Methods Biomech. Biomed. Eng.* 17, 1217–1226. doi: 10.1080/10255842.2012.739167

## APPENDIX

## Active Tension Development

The full description of active tension is described by

$$T_a\left(t,l\right) = T_{MAX}\frac{Ca_0^2}{Ca_0^2 + ECa_{50}^2\left(l\right)}\frac{\left(1-\cos\left(\omega\left(t,l\right)\right)\right)}{2} \qquad \text{(A1)}$$

where

$$ECa_{50}\left(l\right) = \frac{Ca_{0max}}{\sqrt{e^{B(l-l_0)}-1}} \qquad \text{(A2)}$$

$$\omega\left(t,l\right) = \begin{cases} \pi\frac{t}{t_0}, & \text{when } 0 \le t \le t_0 \\ \pi\frac{t-t_0+t_r(l)}{t_r}, & \text{when } t_0 \le t \le t_0 + t_r\left(l\right) \\ 0, & \text{when } t \ge t_0 + t_r\left(l\right) \end{cases} \quad \text{(A3)}$$

$$t_r(l) = ml + b, \qquad \text{(A4)}$$

$$l = l_r\sqrt{\mathbf{f_0}\cdot\left(\mathbf{Cf_0}\right)}, \qquad \text{(A5)}$$

with parameters definitions and values provided in **Table A1**. This mathematical description of active tension ensures a smooth yet steep transition from zero tension at the start of systole to peak active tension, $T_{max}$, at time $t_0$ and then a smooth decline back to zero for the specified relaxation time $t_r$.

**TABLE A1 |** Parameter values and definitions for the time-varying elastance constitutive model.

| Active Parameters | Value | Description |
|---|---|---|
| $t_0$ | 120 [ms] | Time to reach peak tension after the initiation of active tension |
| $m$ | 1048.9 [s μm−1] | Governs the slope of the relaxation |
| $b$ | −1.7 [s] | Governs the length of relaxation |
| $l_0$ | 1.58 [μm] | The sarcomere length below which no active force develops |
| $B$ | 4,750 [μm−1] | Governs the shape of the peak isometric tension-sarcomere length relation |
| $Ca_0$ | 4.35 [μM] | The peak intercellular calcium concentration |
| $Ca_{0max}$ | 4.35 [μM] | The maximum intercellular calcium concentration |
| $T_{max}$ | 170.0 [kPa] | The maximum active tension able to develop |
| $l_r$ | 1.85 [μm] | The initial sarcomere length |

## Parameters for Lumped Circulatory Model

All lumped circulatory parameter values are provided in **Table A2**.

**TABLE A2 |** Parameter values and definitions for the lumped circulatory model.

| Variable | Value | Description |
|---|---|---|
| $R_M$ | 0.05 [mmHg s ml$^{-1}$] | Impedance due to the mitral valve |
| $R_A$ | 0.02 [mmHg s ml$^{-1}$] | Impedance due to the aortic valve |
| $R_{SYS}$ | 1.80 [mmHg s ml$^{-1}$] | Systemic arterial resistance |
| $R_P$ | 0.04 [mmHg s ml$^{-1}$] | Impedance due to the pulmonary valve |
| $R_T$ | 0.02 [mmHg s ml$^{-1}$] | Impedance due to the tricuspid valve |
| $R_{PUL}$ | 0.60 [mmHg s ml$^{-1}$] | Pulmonary arterial resistance |
| $C_{PA}$ | 8.0 [ml mmHg$^{-1}$] | Compliance of the pulmonary arteries |
| $C_{PV}$ | 14.0 [ml mmHg$^{-1}$] | Compliance of the pulmonary veins |
| $C_{SA}$ | 2.0 [ml mmHg$^{-1}$] | Compliance of the systemic arteries |
| $C_{SV}$ | 38.6 [ml mmHg$^1$] | Compliance of the systemic veins |

# 20

# Coronary Blood Flow is Increased in RV Hypertrophy, but the Shape of Normalized Waves is Preserved Throughout the Arterial Tree

*Yunlong Huo [1,2] and Ghassan S. Kassab [3]\**

[1] *PKU-HKUST Shenzhen-Hongkong Institution, Shenzhen, China,* [2] *Department of Mechanics and Engineering Science, College of Engineering, Peking University, Beijing, China,* [3] *California Medical Innovations Institute, San Diego, CA, United States*

**\*Correspondence:**
Ghassan S. Kassab
gkassab@calmi2.org

A pulsatile hemodynamic analysis was carried out in the right coronary arterial (RCA) tree of control and RV hypertrophy (RVH) hearts. The shape of flow and wall shear stress (WSS) waves was hypothesized to be maintained throughout the RCA tree in RVH (i.e., similar patterns of normalized flow and WSS waves in vessels of various sizes). Consequently, we reconstructed the entire RCA tree down to the first capillary bifurcation of control and RVH hearts based on measured morphometric data. A Womersley-type model was used to compute the flow and WSS waves in the tree. The hemodynamic parameters obtained from experimental measurements were incorporated into the numerical model. Given an increased number of arterioles, the mean and amplitude of flow waves at the inlet of RCA tree in RVH was found to be two times larger than that in control, but no significant differences ($p > 0.05$) were found in precapillary arterioles. The increase of stiffness in RCA of RVH preserved the shape of normalized flow and WSS waves, but increased the PWV in coronary arteries and reduced the phase angle difference for the waves between the most proximal RCA and the most distal precapillary arteriole. The study is important for understanding pulsatile coronary blood flow in ventricular hypertrophy.

Keywords: pulsatile flow, right ventricular hypertrophy, right coronary arterial tree, Womersley-type model, Pulsatile wall shear stress

## INTRODUCTION

There is compensatory vascular remodeling that accompanies RV hypertrophy (RVH) (Cooper et al., 1981; Manohar et al., 1981; Botham et al., 1984; Manohar, 1985; White et al., 1992; Kassab et al., 1993). In porcine model, systemic blood pressure in right coronary artery (RCA) was unchanged, but an increase of blood flow occurred in large epicardial branches at 5 weeks after pulmonary hypertension (Lu et al., 2011). Based on the measured morphometric data in arrested, vasodilated porcine heart of RVH, we carried out a steady-state flow analysis of arterial tree down to first capillary segments (Huo et al., 2007). The increase of blood flow was found to be caused by the compensatory growth of small vessels, which resulted in restoration of blood flow and wall shear stress (WSS) to normal level in the perfusion arterioles (diameter $<100\,\mu m$) of RCA tree in the diastolic state of RVH hearts (Huo et al., 2007). The pulsatility of coronary blood flow is a significant hemodynamic feature (Fung, 1997; Nichols and McDonald, 2011). However, the

pulsatile pressure-flow relationship has not been investigated in
the coronary circulation during the progression of RVH. We have
simulated the pulsatile blood flow in diastole in the absence of
vessel tone in the entire coronary arterial tree of normal porcine
hearts using the Womersley-type mathematical model (Huo and
Kassab, 2006). Hence, the objective of present study is to carry
out a complete pulsatile flow analysis in the coronary arterial tree
of control and RVH hearts and to determine the effect of RVH on
the flow and WSS waves in diastole in the absence of vessel tone.

Here, we hypothesized that the flow and WSS waves
was preserved in RVH (i.e., similar patterns of normalized
flow and WSS waves in vessels of various sizes). To test
the hypothesis, pulsatile blood flows were computed by a
Womersley-type numerical model (Huo and Kassab, 2006) in
each vessel of the entire RCA tree down to the first capillary
bifurcation (excluding the sub-tree distal to the posterior
descending artery) of control and RVH hearts in diastole,
which was reconstructed from morphometric data (i.e., vessel
diameters, lengths and numbers) (Kassab et al., 1993). The
experimental measurements of coronary wall thickness (Guo
and Kassab, 2004) and stiffness (Garcia and Kassab, 2009) were
also incorporated into the numerical model. The constitutive
equation, based on experimental measurements, was similar
to a previous study (Huo and Kassab, 2006). The predictions
of the mathematical model showed good agreement with the
experimental measurements in control and RVH hearts. A
detailed comparison of pulsatile blood flows was made in vessels
of various sizes throughout the entire RCA arterial trees between
control and RVH.

## MATERIALS AND METHODS

### Anatomical Model
Previously, Kassab et al. have carried out morphometric
measurements of the RCA-posterior descending arterial (PDA)
trees of control and RVH hearts (Kassab et al., 1993). Briefly, the
morphometric data on the coronary arterial vessels of diameters
<40 μm were obtained from histological specimens and the
morphometric data on the coronary arterial vessels of diameters
>40 μm were obtained from cast studies. The entire RCA-PDA
tree down to the first capillary bifurcations was reconstructed
in control and RVH using a growth algorithm (Mittal et al.,
2005), based on the experimental measurements of the RV
branches excluding the distal tree to the PDA. In summary,
the present anatomical mathematical model has exact data
(diameters, lengths and connectivity) for the larger vessels and
statistical data for the microvessels different from the previous
models (Kaimovitz et al., 2005, 2010), which were based on the
statistical data (tables with means and standard deviations for
diameters, lengths, connectivity) for the entire tree (Kassab et al.,
1993).

### Flow Simulation
After the branching pattern and vascular geometry of RV
branches were generated, a pulsatile flow analysis was performed
similar to a previous study (Huo and Kassab, 2006, 2007). Briefly,
in the frequency domain, the governing equations (transformed

from the conversion of mass and momentum) for flow ($Q$) and
pressure ($P$) in a vessel are written as:

$$Q(x,\omega) = a\cos(\omega x/c) + b\sin(\omega x/c) \quad (1)$$

$$P(x,\omega) = iZ_1[-a\sin(\omega x/c) + b\cos(\omega x/c)] \quad (2)$$

Where $a$ and $b$ are arbitrary constants of integration, $x$ the
axial coordinate along the vessel, $\omega$ the angular frequency, $c = \sqrt{1 - F_{10}(\alpha)} \cdot c_0$ ($c_0 = \sqrt{\frac{Eh}{\rho R}}$) is the wave velocity, $h/R$ the ratio
of wall thickness to radius, $E$ the Young's modulus, $\rho$ the density,
and $F_{10}(\alpha) = \frac{2J_1(i^{3/2}\alpha)}{i^{3/2}\alpha J_0(i^{3/2}\alpha)}$ ($\alpha = \frac{D}{2}\sqrt{\frac{\omega\rho}{\mu}}$, $\mu$ is the dynamic viscosity,
$J_0$ the Bessel function of zero order and first kind, and $J_1$ the
Bessel function of first order and first kind). $Y_0 = \frac{A(n)}{\rho c_0}$ ($A(n)$ is
the cross-sectional area in a vessel) is defined as the characteristic
admittance, $Z_0 = 1/Y_0$ the characteristic impedance, $Y_1 = Y_0\sqrt{1 - F_{10}(\alpha)}$, and $Z_1 = Z_0/\sqrt{1 - F_{10}(\alpha)}$. The impedance and
admittance in a vessel is:

$$Z(x,\omega) = \frac{P(x,\omega)}{Q(x,\omega)} = \frac{iZ_1[-a\sin(\omega x/c) + b\cos(\omega x/c)]}{a\cos(\omega x/c) + b\sin(\omega x/c)} \quad (3)$$

$$Y(x,\omega) = \frac{1}{Z(x,\omega)} \quad (4)$$

In a given vessel segment, at $x = 0$ and $x = L$, we have the
following inlet and outlet impedance:

$$Z(0,\omega) = \frac{iZ_1 b}{a} \quad (5)$$

$$Z(L,\omega) = \frac{iZ_1[-a\sin(\omega L/c) + b\cos(\omega L/c)]}{a\cos(\omega L/c) + b\sin(\omega L/c)} \quad (6)$$

A combination of Equations (5) and (6) yields:

$$Z(0,\omega) = \frac{iZ_1\sin(\omega L/c) + Z(L,\omega)\cos(\omega L/c)}{\cos(\omega L/c) + iY_1 Z(L,\omega)\sin(\omega L/c)} \quad (7)$$

Since there are two or more vessels that emanate from the
junction points of the entire RCA tree, the junction boundary
condition (determined from the continuous pressure and mass
conservation at the junction) is written as:

$$Y(L(mother),\omega) = \sum Y[0(daughters),\omega] \quad (8)$$

Equations (7) and (8) were used to calculate the
impedance/admittance in the entire coronary tree from
inlet to the capillary vessels.

The terminal impedance/admittance of the first capillary was
assumed to be equal to the steady value as $\frac{128\mu_{capillary}L_{capillary}}{(\pi D_{capillary}^4)}$
(g·sec/cm$^4$), from which we proceeded backwards to iteratively
calculate the impedance/admittance in the entire RCA tree of
control and RVH hearts using Equations (7) and (8). The pulsatile
pressure was the same as the previous study (Huo and Kassab,
2006) and discretized by a Fourier transformation as the inlet
boundary condition. The flow and pressure in each vessel were
then calculated by using Equations (1) and (2) coupled with

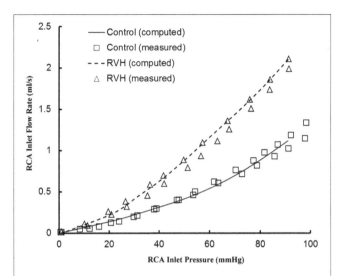

**FIGURE 1 |** Experimental and computed pressure-flow relationship of the RCA of control and RVH hearts. The experimental results were measured under loading and unloading of pressures as the RCA tree was perfused by cardioplegic solution ($\mu = 1.1$ cp and $\rho = 1$ g/cm$^3$). The pulsatile model was used to compute the pressure and flow at very low frequency ($\omega \rightarrow 0$).

**TABLE 1 |** Morphometric and hemodynamic parameters in orders according to the diameter-defined Strahler system.

| Order | N | Diameter ($\mu$m) | Flow rate (ml/min) | Pressure (mmHg) |
|---|---|---|---|---|
| **CONTROL** | | | | |
| 1 | 93,616 | 8.77 | $7.02 \times 10^{-5}$ | 23.69 |
| 2 | 48,415 | 11.2 | $1.61 \times 10^{-4}$ | 34.59 |
| 3 | 23,302 | 16.1 | $4.41 \times 10^{-4}$ | 45.55 |
| 4 | 8,062 | 25.8 | $1.39 \times 10^{-3}$ | 55.73 |
| 5 | 2,974 | 47.7 | $4.69 \times 10^{-3}$ | 64.32 |
| 6 | 1,010 | 98.1 | $1.64 \times 10^{-2}$ | 74.15 |
| 7 | 400 | 217 | $5.40 \times 10^{-2}$ | 78.38 |
| 8 | 88 | 491 | 0.19 | 79.43 |
| 9 | 70 | 830 | 0.63 | 79.73 |
| 10 | 20 | 2,420 | 12.9 | 79.99 |
| **RVH** | | | | |
| 1 | 366,758 | 8.86 | $7.01 \times 10^{-5}$ | 22.86 |
| 2 | 190,519 | 11.7 | $1.67 \times 10^{-4}$ | 32.39 |
| 3 | 84,627 | 16.5 | $4.62 \times 10^{-4}$ | 42.37 |
| 4 | 32,275 | 25.8 | $1.44 \times 10^{-3}$ | 52.08 |
| 5 | 8,967 | 46.8 | $4.54 \times 10^{-3}$ | 63.99 |
| 6 | 3,476 | 91.2 | $1.54 \times 10^{-2}$ | 70.32 |
| 7 | 1,255 | 168 | $4.98 \times 10^{-2}$ | 74.28 |
| 8 | 582 | 314 | 0.16 | 76.06 |
| 9 | 205 | 604 | 0.58 | 77.35 |
| 10 | 61 | 1,241 | 2.86 | 79.58 |
| 11 | 25 | 2,949 | 22.7 | 79.94 |

"Diameter," "Flow rate," and "Pressure" refer to the time-averaged value over a cardiac cycle.

the continuous pressure at junctions. The blood flow density ($\rho$) was assumed to be 1.06 g/cm$^3$. The variation of viscosity with vessel diameter and hematocrit was based on Pries' viscosity model (Pries et al., 1992). The coronary wall thickness for every order was adopted from the previous measurements (Guo and Kassab, 2004; Choy and Kassab, 2009). The *in situ* static Young's modulus in control was made as $\sim 8.0 \times 10^6$ (dynes/cm$^2$) based on the experimental data (Kassab and Molloi, 2001), which was doubled in RVH (Garcia and Kassab, 2009). The dynamic Young's modulus was also considered for various frequencies (Bergel, 1961; Douglas and Greenfield, 1970; Gow et al., 1974), i.e., the Young's modulus increases with the increase of frequency $\omega$ (see Figure 2 in Bergel, 1961). Once the flow wave was determined in each vessel, the WSS waves, $\tau$, was calculated as Zheng et al. (2010):

$$\tau(x,t) = \text{REAL} \left( \frac{4\mu}{\pi R^3} Q(x,0) - \sum_{\omega=1}^{\infty} \frac{\frac{\mu Q(x,\omega)}{\pi R^3} \cdot \frac{\Lambda J_1(\Lambda)}{J_0(\Lambda)}}{1 - \frac{2J_1(\Lambda)}{\Lambda J_0(\Lambda)}} e^{i\omega t} \right) \quad (9)$$

where $\Lambda^2 = i^3 \alpha^2$. Unless otherwise stated, all computations used the previously measured physical properties and parameters as described above.

## Statistical Analysis

ANOVA (SigmaStat 3.5) was used to detect statistical differences between control and RVH. A $p < 0.05$ was indicative of a significant difference between the two populations.

## RESULTS

The pulsatile model has been previously validated experimentally in normal hearts. Here, good agreement was found between

experimental measurements and computational results for the RCA of RVH hearts, as shown in **Figure 1**. The steady-state flows were measured under loading and unloading of pressures as the RCA tree was perfused by cardioplegic solution, which were consistent with the computed pulsatile flows with the frequency approaching to zero since a steady-state flow can be mimicked by a pulsatile flow as $\omega \rightarrow 0$.

The flow waves were calculated in each vessel of RCA tree (excluding the distal tree to the PDA), which has RV branches with a mean (averaged over five anatomic reconstructions) of 0.36 and 1.3 million vessels for control and RVH, respectively. **Table 1** summarizes morphometric and hemodynamic parameters in diameter-defined Strahler orders from precapillary arterioles (order 1) to the epicardial RCA tree (the highest order) in control and RVH hearts. The flow waves at the inlet and primary branches of RCA tree of control heart were compared with those in the RVH heart (**Figure 2** vs. **Figure 3**). Given such an increase of vessel numbers, the mean (i.e., time-averaged value over a cardiac cycle) and amplitude (i.e., the change between peak and trough) of flow wave at the inlet of RCA tree in RVH is much larger than that in control. **Figures 4A,B** show the relationship between the time-averaged flow in a vessel and the cumulative length of the vessel from the RCA to the precapillary arteriole through similar primary branches in control and RVH hearts, respectively. Accordingly, **Figures 4C,D**

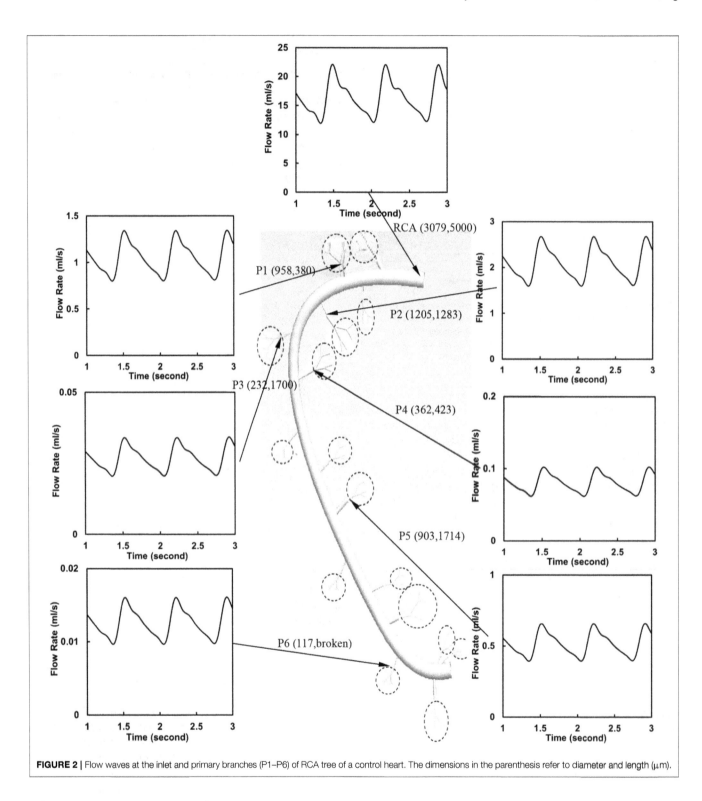

**FIGURE 2 |** Flow waves at the inlet and primary branches (P1–P6) of RCA tree of a control heart. The dimensions in the parenthesis refer to diameter and length (μm).

show the relationship between the time-averaged pressure in a vessel and the cumulative length of the vessel. **Figures 5A,B** show the amplitude and phase angle of the impedance in the most proximal RCA, a distal vessel (6 cm from the RCA), and the most distal precapillary arteriole in control and RVH hearts, respectively. Accordingly, **Figures 5C,D** show a decrease

of flow waves sequentially along the path from the RCA to the precapillary arteriole.

Despite the large changes of flow waves from the root to the precapillary, we previously reported similar pattern of normalized waves in control hearts. **Figures 6A,B** show the flow and WSS waves normalized by the mean values at the

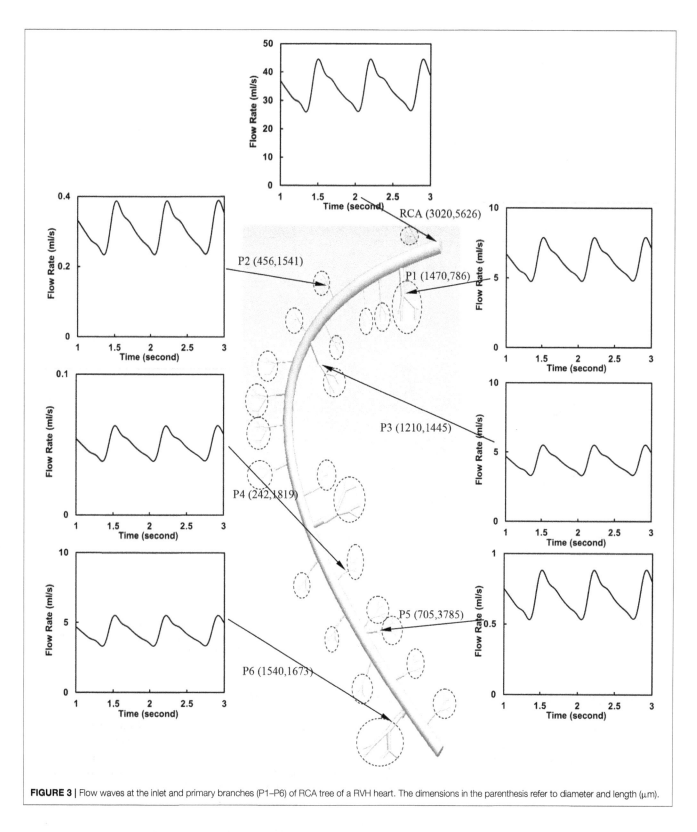

**FIGURE 3 |** Flow waves at the inlet and primary branches (P1–P6) of RCA tree of a RVH heart. The dimensions in the parenthesis refer to diameter and length (μm).

most proximal RCA and the most distal precapillary arteriole of RCA tree in control. **Figures 6C,D** show the normalized flow and WSS waves in RVH as compared with those in control. The normalized waves at the RCA and precapillary arteriole are similar to each other ($p \gg 0.05$) in both control and RVH. In comparison with the control, the difference of phase angles for flow waves between RCA and precapillary arteriole decreased by about 50% in various frequencies and the pulse wave

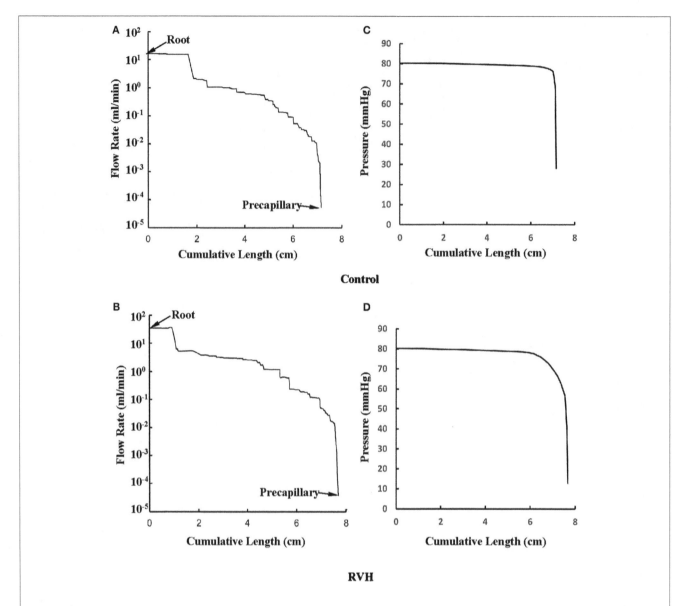

**FIGURE 4 | (A,B)** Relationship between the mean flow (averaged over a cardiac cycle) in a vessel and the cumulative length of the vessel from the root to the precapillary arteriole through similar primary branches in: **(A)** control and **(B)** RVH pig hearts (i.e., P2 in **Figure 2** and P1 in **Figure 3**, respectively). **(C,D)** Relationship between the mean pressure (averaged over a cardiac cycle) in a vessel and the cumulative length of the vessel corresponding to **(A,B)**.

velocity (PWV) increased by about 40% in the hypertrophic RCA tree.

The effects of vessel compliance on the pattern of flow and WSS waves were examined. **Figures 7A,B** show a sensitivity analysis of normalized flow and WSS waves, respectively, at the inlet of RCA tree of control hearts with a 50% increase/decrease of Young's modulus of each vessel wall (including both static and dynamic Young's moduli). **Figure 7C** shows the change of the phase angle of the inlet impedance with a 50% increase/decrease of Young's modulus of each vessel wall. The change of vessel compliance in physiological range had negligible effects on the normalized waves ($p \gg 0.05$), but significantly affected the phase angle of the impedance.

## DISCUSSION

The major finding was that RVH maintained similar patterns of normalized flow and WSS waves in different size vessels. RVH, however, did significant increase in the amplitude and mean (time-averaged over a cardiac cycle) of waves in large epicardial coronary branches due to the increase in number of small arterioles.

## Steady-State Flow vs. Pulsatile Flow

Based on morphometric measurements and steady-state hemodynamic analysis, the remodeling of structure and function of the entire RCA tree was determined in RVH after 5 weeks

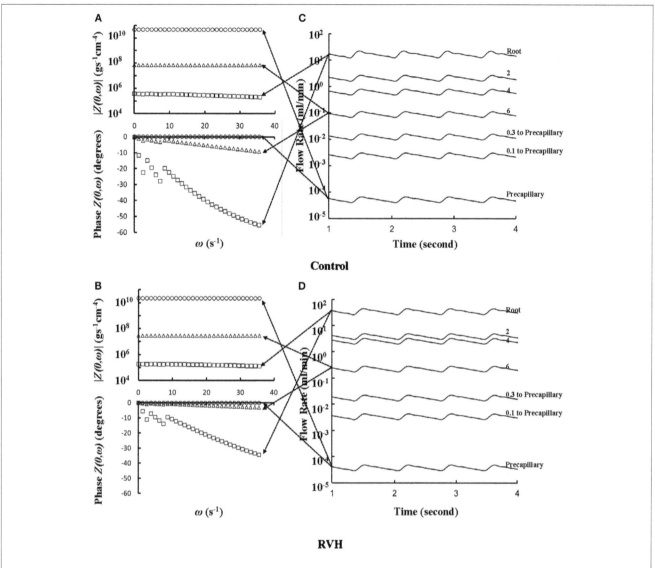

**FIGURE 5 | (A,B)** Impedance $|Z(0,\omega)|$ vs. angular frequency $\omega$ and phase $Z(0,\omega)$ vs. angular frequency $\omega$ sequentially along the corresponding paths to **Figures 4A,B**. **(C,D)** Flow waves sequentially along the corresponding paths to **Figures 4A,B**. The arrows indicate the one-to-one correspondence between **(A–D)**.

of pulmonary banding (Kassab et al., 1993; Huo et al., 2007). The number of vessel segments in RVH was about four times larger than that in control hearts. The steady-state flow (which approximately equaled to the time-averaged value of pulsatile flow) was significantly increased in the large epicardial vessels in RVH, but distributed through substantially more vessels such that the flow and WSS in the small perfusion arterioles were not statistically different from the control (Huo et al., 2007). Here, we compared pulsatile flows between control and RVH using the Womersley-type model (Huo and Kassab, 2006) and morphometric measurements (Kassab et al., 1993; Kassab and Molloi, 2001; Garcia and Kassab, 2009). Corresponding to the steady-state flow, the amplitudes of flow and WSS waves in RVH were significantly increased in the epicardial vessels, but similar to those in the perfusion arterioles of control, as shown in **Table 1** and **Figures 2, 3**. The amplitude and mean

of flow and pressure waves decreased along the path from the root down to the precapillary arteriole in the RVH, which has the same trend as the control (see **Figure 4**) and also agrees with a previous study (Huo and Kassab, 2006). The increase of stiffness in RVH reduces the phase angle of vessel impedance (see **Figure 5**) and leads to a significant decrease (~50%) of phase angle difference for flow waves between the most proximal RCA and the most distal precapillary arteriole in various frequencies (see **Figure 6**), which reflects an about 40% increase of PWV in the RCA tree of RVH. Although an increase of aortic PWV is widely known as a marker of cardiovascular risk in hypertension (Mohiaddin et al., 1993; Butlin et al., 2013), it still requires further investigation in the interaction of large and small arteries, given the unknown causal relation between stiffening and hypertension in vessels of various sizes.

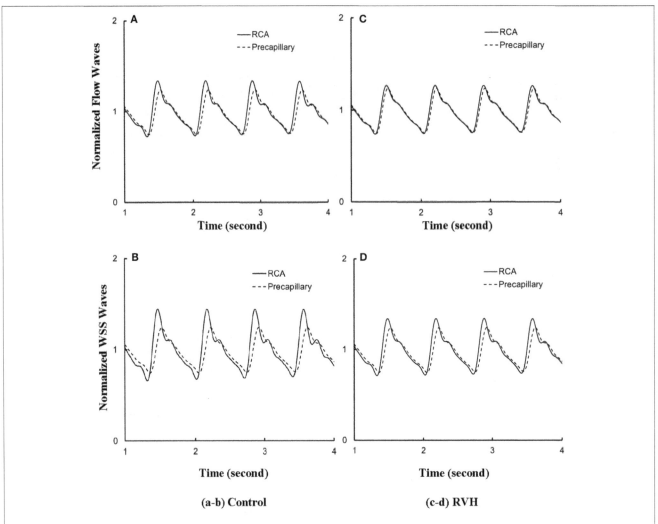

**FIGURE 6 | (A)** Flow and **(B)** WSS waves normalized by the mean values (averaged over a cardiac cycle) at the RCA and precapillary arteriole of control heart. **(C,D)** Normalized flow and WSS waves at the RCA and precapillary arteriole of RVH heart in correspondence with **(A,B)**, respectively.

## Flow and WSS Waves

The flow waves at various coronary vessels of diastolic control hearts were found to have a tendency of scaling to a single curve, except for a small phrase angle difference, when they were normalized by the mean values (Huo and Kassab, 2007). In the beating hearts, Ashikawa et al. measured the flow velocities in small arterioles (diameter of $12.8 \pm 4.1\,\mu$m), capillaries, and small venules (diameter of $16.5 \pm 6.5\,\mu$m; Ashikawa et al., 1986) and Toyota et al. measured the flow velocities in arterioles (diameter of $\sim$100 $\mu$m; Toyota et al., 2005), which also showed similar normalized flow waves. Here, the normalized flow and WSS waves in the RCA tree of RVH maintained the same scaling characteristic, as shown in **Figures 5, 6**. Moreover, the sensitivity analysis in **Figures 7A,B** showed the change of stiffness of RCA tree in physiological range, which had negligible effect on the normalized flow and WSS waves. This can be explained from the constitutive equation [i.e., $\frac{A}{A_{ref}} = \frac{(p-p_{ref})\cdot(R/h)}{E} + 1$, in which $A$ is the CSA, $p$ the pressure, $h/R$ the ratio of wall thickness to radius, $E$ the Young's modulus]. From the equation, Young's

modulus (the denominator) is almost twenty times larger than $(p - p_{ref}) \cdot (R/h)$ (the numerator) in normal coronary arterial tree such that $\frac{(p-p_{ref})\cdot(R/h)}{E}$ is much less than one, where the static Young's modulus in control is $8 \times 10^6$ dynes/cm$^2$ and increases as frequency increases, $(p - p_{ref})$ varies from $-20$ to $+20$ mmHg, and $(R/h)$ approximately equals to ten. A 50% perturbation for the stiffness had negligible effect on the waves.

## Physiological Implications

Coronary blood vessel wall is subjected to various types of hemodynamic forces (e.g., hydrostatic pressure, cyclic stretch, and fluid shear stress) caused by the pulsatile blood pressure and flow (Chiu and Chien, 2011). Intraspecific scaling power laws of vascular trees, derived from the steady-state analysis (Huo and Kassab, 2012), characterize coronary vasculature with remarkable simplicity. The compensatory remodeling in RVH was found to maintain the structure-function hierarchy (preserved scaling exponents) of fractal-like coronary arterial tree (Gong et al., 2016). Furthermore, the present study

Coronary Blood Flow is Increased in RV Hypertrophy, but the Shape of Normalized Waves is Preserved...

245

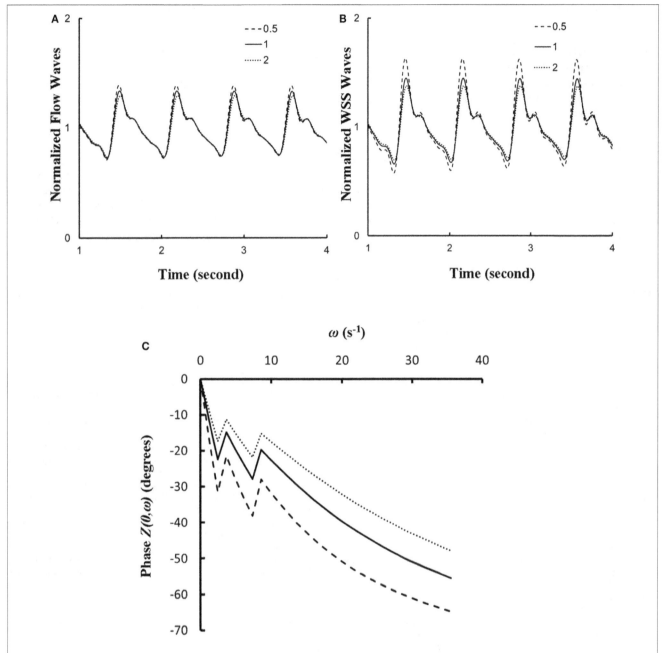

**FIGURE 7 | (A,B)** A sensitivity analysis of normalized **(A)** flow and **(B)** WSS waves at the inlet of RCA tree with a 50% increase/decrease of Young's modulus of each vessel wall, where the baseline (i.e., the unity) refers to the static Young's modulus of $8 \times 10^6$ dynes/cm$^2$ with adjustment for frequency. **(C)** Phase $Z(0,\omega)$ vs. angular frequency $\omega$ at the inlet of RCA tree with a 50% increase/decrease of Young's modulus of each vessel wall.

shows the preserved shape of normalized wave of pulsatile blood flows in the entire coronary arterial tree, which is unchanged during the remodeling in RVH. This implies that intraspecific scaling power laws of vascular trees can be extended from the steady to dynamic states. On the other hand, the altered phase angle of vessel impedance and flow and WSS waves shows the effects of the remodeling on the pulsatile blood pressure and flow in RVH, which requires further investigations.

## Critique of Study

The present study carried out the pulsatile flow analysis based on the morphometric data and physiological measurements, but the constitutive equation was determined in a vasodilated state in the absence of vasomotor tone where coronary flow reserve was substantially reduced. The stiffness of large arteries was assumed to equal to that of small arterioles. Future studies are needed to identify the contribution of vascular tone to the vascular remodeling and flow waves in RVH with consideration of the stiffness in various size vessels.

## Significance of Study

RVH is a compensatory response to pulmonary hypertension and the compensatory adaptations of coronary circulation serve to maintain perfusion of the increased myocardial mass. Here, we showed that the shape of normalized flow and WSS waves was preserved despite a significant increase of the amplitude and mean of flow and WSS waves in the epicardial vessels. The increase of stiffness in RVH increased the PWV in coronary arteries and reduced the phase angle difference for flow waves between the most proximal RCA and the most distal precapillary arteriole, but had negligible effect on the pattern of flow and WSS waves. The precise prediction of flow and WSS waves in coronary microcirculation is physiologically and clinically important to understand the ventricular hypertrophy.

## AUTHOR CONTRIBUTIONS

Data analysis were performed by YH at the college of engineering, Peking University. Paper was drafted and revised by YH and GK at the California Medical Innovations Institute.

## ACKNOWLEDGMENTS

This research is supported in part by the National Institute of Health-National Heart, Lung, and Blood Institute Grant HL134841 and HL118738 (GK) and the National Natural Science Foundation of China Grant 11672006 and Shenzhen Science and Technology R&D Grant JCYJ20160427170536358 (YH).

## REFERENCES

Ashikawa, K., Kanatsuka, H., Suzuki, T., and Takishima, T. (1986). Phasic blood flow velocity pattern in epimyocardial microvessels in the beating canine left ventricle. *Circ. Res.* 59, 704–711. doi: 10.1161/01.RES.59.6.704

Bergel, D. H. (1961). The dynamic elastic properties of the arterial wall. *J. Physiol. (Lond).* 156, 458–469. doi: 10.1113/jphysiol.1961.sp006687

Botham, M. J., Lemmer, J. H., Gerren, R. A., Long, R. W., Behrendt, D. M., and Gallagher, K. P. (1984). Coronary vasodilator reserve in young dogs with moderate right ventricular hypertrophy. *Ann. Thorac. Surg.* 38, 101–107. doi: 10.1016/S0003-4975(10)62214-X

Butlin, M., Qasem, A., Battista, F., Bozec, E., McEniery, C. M., Millet-Amaury, E., et al. (2013). Carotid-femoral pulse wave velocity assessment using novel cuff-based techniques: comparison with tonometric measurement. *J Hypertens.* 31, 2237–2243, discussion 2243. doi: 10.1097/HJH.0b013e328 363c789

Chiu, J. J., and Chien, S. (2011). Effects of disturbed flow on vascular endothelium: pathophysiological basis and clinical perspectives. *Physiol. Rev.* 91, 327–387. doi: 10.1152/physrev.00047.2009

Choy, J. S., and Kassab, G. S. (2009). Wall thickness of coronary vessels varies transmurally in the LV but not the RV: implications for local stress distribution. *Am. J. Physiol. Heart Circ. Physiol.* 297, H750–H758. doi: 10.1152/ajpheart.01136.2008

Cooper, G. T., Tomanek, R. J., Ehrhardt, J. C., and Marcus, M. L. (1981). Chronic progressive pressure overload of the cat right ventricle. *Circ. Res.* 48, 488–497. doi: 10.1161/01.RES.48.4.488

Douglas, J. E., Greenfield, J. C. Jr. (1970). Epicardial coronary artery compliance in the dog. *Circ. Res.* 27, 921–929. doi: 10.1161/01.RES.27.6.921

Fung, Y. C. (1997). *Biomechanics: Circulation, 2nd Edn.* New York,NY: Springer

Garcia, M., Kassab, G. S. (2009). Right coronary artery becomes stiffer with increase in elastin and collagen in right ventricular hypertrophy. *J. Appl. Physiol. (1985).* 106, 1338–1346. doi: 10.1152/japplphysiol.90592.2008

Gong, Y., Feng, Y., Chen, X., Tan, W., Huo, Y., and Kassab, G. S. (2016). Intraspecific scaling laws are preserved in ventricular hypertrophy but not in heart failure. *Am. J. Physiol. Heart Circ. Physiol.* 311, H1108–H1117. doi: 10.1152/ajpheart.00084.2016

Gow, B. S., Schonfeld, D., and Patel, D. J. (1974). The dynamic elastic properties of the canine left circumflex coronary artery. *J. Biomech.* 7, 389–395. doi: 10.1016/0021-9290(74)90001-3

Guo, X., and Kassab, G. S. (2004). Distribution of stress and strain along the porcine aorta and coronary arterial tree. *Am. J. Physiol. Heart Circ. Physiol.* 286, H2361–H2368. doi: 10.1152/ajpheart.01079.2003

Huo, Y., and Kassab, G. S. (2006). Pulsatile blood flow in the entire coronary arterial tree: theory and experiment. *Am. J. Physiol. Heart Circ. Physiol.* 291, H1074–H1087. doi: 10.1152/ajpheart.00200.2006

Huo, Y., and Kassab, G. S. (2007). A hybrid one-dimensional/Womersley model of pulsatile blood flow in the entire coronary arterial tree. *Am. J. Physiol. Heart Circ. Physiol.* 292, H2623–H2633. doi: 10.1152/ajpheart.00987.2006

Huo, Y., and Kassab, G. S. (2012). Intraspecific scaling laws of vascular trees. *J. R. Soc. Interface* 9, 190–200. doi: 10.1098/rsif.2011.0270

Huo, Y., Linares, C. O., and Kassab, G. S. (2007). Capillary perfusion and wall shear stress are restored in the coronary circulation of hypertrophic right ventricle. *Circ. Res.* 100, 273–283. doi: 10.1161/01.RES.0000257777.83431.13

Kaimovitz, B., Lanir, Y., and Kassab, G. S. (2005). Large-scale 3-D geometric reconstruction of the porcine coronary arterial vasculature based on detailed anatomical data. *Ann. Biomed. Eng.* 33, 1517–1535. doi: 10.1007/s10439-005-7544-3

Kaimovitz, B., Lanir, Y., and Kassab, G. S. (2010). A full 3-D reconstruction of the entire porcine coronary vasculature. *Am. J. Physiol. Heart Circ. Physiol.* 299, H1064–H1076. doi: 10.1152/ajpheart.00151.2010

Kassab, G. S., Imoto, K., White, F. C., Rider, C. A., Fung, Y. C., and Bloor, C. M. (1993). Coronary arterial tree remodeling in right ventricular hypertrophy. *Am. J. Physiol.* 265, H366–H375. doi: 10.1152/ajpheart.1993.265.1.H366

Kassab, G. S., and Molloi, S. (2001). Cross-sectional area and volume compliance of porcine left coronary arteries. *Am. J. Physiol. Heart Circ. Physiol.* 281, H623–H628. doi: 10.1152/ajpheart.2001.281.2.H623

Lu, X., Dang, C. Q., Guo, X., Molloi, S., Wassall, C. D., Kemple, M. D., et al. (2011). Elevated oxidative stress and endothelial dysfunction in right coronary artery of right ventricular hypertrophy. *J. Appl. Physiol. (1985).* 110, 1674–1681. doi: 10.1152/japplphysiol.00744.2009

Manohar, M. (1985). Transmural coronary vasodilator reserve, and flow distribution during tachycardia in conscious young swine with right ventricular hypertrophy. *Cardiovasc. Res.* 19, 104–112. doi: 10.1093/cvr/19.2.104

Manohar, M., Bisgard, G. E., Bullard, V., and Rankin, J. H. (1981). Blood flow in the hypertrophied right ventricular myocardium of unanesthetized ponies. *Am. J. Physiol.* 240, H881–H888. doi: 10.1152/ajpheart.1981.240.6.H881

Mittal, N., Zhou, Y., Ung, S., Linares, C., Molloi, S., and Kassab, G. S. (2005). A computer reconstruction of the entire coronary arterial tree based on detailed morphometric data. *Ann. Biomed. Eng.* 33, 1015–1026. doi: 10.1007/s10439-005-5758-z

Mohiaddin, R. H., Firmin, D. N., Longmore, D. B. (1993). Age-related changes of human aortic flow wave velocity measured noninvasively by magnetic resonance imaging. *J. Appl. Physiol. (1985).* 74, 492–497. doi: 10.1152/jappl.1993.74.1.492

Nichols, W. W., and McDonald, D. A. (2011). *McDonald's Blood Flow In Arteries: Theoretic, Experimental, and Clinical Principles, 6th Edn.* London: Hodder Arnold.

Pries, A. R., Neuhaus, D., and Gaehtgens, P. (1992). Blood viscosity in tube flow: dependence on diameter and hematocrit. *Am. J. Physiol.* 263, H1770–H1778. doi: 10.1152/ajpheart.1992.263.6.H1770

Toyota, E., Ogasawara, Y., Hiramatsu, O., Tachibana, H., Kajiya, F., Yamamori, S., et al. (2005). Dynamics of flow velocities in endocardial and epicardial coronary arterioles. *Am. J. Physiol. Heart Circ. Physiol.* 288, H1598–H1603. doi: 10.1152/ajpheart.01103.2003

White, F. C., Nakatani, Y., Nimmo, L., and Bloor, C. M. (1992). Compensatory angiogenesis during progressive right ventricular hypertrophy. *Am. J. Cardiovasc. Pathol.* 4, 51–68.

Zheng, H., Huo, Y., Svendsen, M., Kassab, G. S. (2010). Effect of blood pressure on vascular hemodynamics in acute tachycardia. *J. Appl. Physiol.* (1985). 109, 1619–1627. doi: 10.1152/japplphysiol.01356.2009

# Permissions

# List of Contributors

**Xiaomei Guo**
California Medical Innovations Institute, San Diego, CA, United States

**Jillian N. Noblet, Joshua F. Krieger, Blayne Roeder and Sean Chambers**
Cook Medical, Bloomington, IN, United States

**Stephan Haulon**
Aortic Center, Hôpital Marie Lannelongue, Université Paris Sud, Paris, France

**Gregory M. Dick and Ravi Namani**
California Medical Innovations Institute, San Diego, CA, United States

**Xiaoping Yin**
Department of Radiology, Affiliated Hospital of Hebei University, Hebei University, Baoding, China

**Xu Huang, Qiao Li and Pei Niu**
Department of Mechanics and Engineering Science, College of Engineering, Peking University, Beijing, China

**Fei Guo and Xuechao Li**
College of Medicine, Hebei University, Baoding, China

**Wenchang Tan**
Department of Mechanics and Engineering Science, College of Engineering, Peking University, Beijing, China
PKU-HKUST Shenzhen-Hongkong Institution, Shenzhen, China
Shenzhen Graduate School, Peking University, Shenzhen, China

**Geoffrey L. Kung**
Department of Radiological Sciences, David Geffen School of Medicine, University of California, Los Angeles, Los Angeles, CA, United States
Department of Bioengineering, University of California, Los Angeles, Los Angeles, CA, United States

**Marmar Vaseghi and Kalyanam Shivkumar**
Cardiac Arrhythmia Center, David Geffen School of Medicine, University of California, Los Angeles, Los Angeles, CA, United States
Department of Medicine (Cardiology), David Geffen School of Medicine, University of California, Los Angeles, Los Angeles, CA, United States

**Jane Shevtsov and Alan Garfinkel**
Department of Medicine (Cardiology), David Geffen School of Medicine, University of California, Los Angeles, Los Angeles, CA, United States

**Jin K. Gahm**
Department of Radiological Sciences, David Geffen School of Medicine, University of California, Los Angeles, Los Angeles, CA, United States
Department of Computer Science, University of California, Los Angeles, Los Angeles, CA, United States

**Daniel B. Ennis**
Department of Radiological Sciences, David Geffen School of Medicine, University of California, Los Angeles, Los Angeles, CA, United States
Department of Bioengineering, University of California, Los Angeles, Los Angeles, CA, United States
Biomedical Physics Interdepartmental Program, David Geffen School of Medicine, University of California, Los Angeles, Los Angeles, CA, United States

**Huan Chen**
California Medical Innovations Institute, San Diego, CA, United States

**Seungik Baek and Lik Chuan Lee**
Department of Mechanical Engineering, Michigan State University, East Lansing, MI, United States

**Yundi Feng, Xuan Wang, Tingting Fan, Li Li, Xiaotong Sun, Wenxi Zhang and Minglu Cao**
Department of Mechanics and Engineering Science, College of Engineering, Peking University, Beijing, China

**Jian Liu**
Department of Cardiology, Peking University People's Hospital, Beijing, China

**Jianping Li**
Department of Cardiology, Peking University First Hospital, Beijing, China

**Liang Zhong, Jun-Mei Zhang and Ru San Tan**
National Heart Centre Singapore, National Heart Research Institute of Singapore, Singapore, Singapore
Duke-NUS Medical School, Singapore, Singapore

**Boyang Su**
National Heart Centre Singapore, National Heart Research Institute of Singapore, Singapore, Singapore

**John C. Allen**
Duke-NUS Medical School, Singapore, Singapore

**Hua Zou**
National Heart Centre Singapore, Singapore, Singapore

**Ce Xi**
Department of Mechanical Engineering, Michigan State University, East Lansing, MI, United States

**John Allen**
Duke-NUS Medical School, National University of Singapore, Singapore, Singapore

**Angela S. Koh, Fei Gao and Ru-San Tan**
National Heart Centre Singapore, Singapore, Singapore
Duke-NUS Medical School, National University of Singapore, Singapore, Singapore

**Martin Genet**
Mechanics Department and Solid Mechanics Laboratory, École Polytechnique, C.N.R.S., Université Paris-Saclay, Palaiseau, France
M3DISIM Team, I.N.R.I.A, Université Paris-Saclay, Palaiseau, France

**Soroush Safaei and Peter J. Hunter**
Auckland Bioengineering Institute, University of Auckland, Auckland, New Zealand

**Pablo J. Blanco**
National Laboratory for Scientific Computing, Petrópolis, Brazil
National Institute of Science and Technology in Medicine Assisted by Scientific Computing, Petrópolis, Brazil

**Lucas O. Müller and Leif R. Hellevik**
Division of Biomechanics, Department of Structural Engineering, Norwegian University of Science and Technology, Trondheim, Norway

**Daniela Lucini and Massimo Pagani**
BIOMETRA Department, University of Milan, Milan, Italy

**Nadia Solaro**
Department of Statistics and Quantitative Methods, University of Milano-Bicocca, Milan, Italy

**Kevin L. Sack**
Division of Biomedical Engineering, Department of Human Biology, University of Cape Town, Cape Town, South Africa

Department of Surgery, University of California, San Francisco, San Francisco, CA, United States

**Eric Aliotta**
Department of Radiological Sciences, University of California, Los Angeles, Los Angeles, CA, United States

**Jenny S. Choy**
California Medical Innovations Institute, Inc., San Diego, CA, United States

**Thomas Franz**
Division of Biomedical Engineering, Department of Human Biology, University of Cape Town, Cape Town, South Africa
Bioengineering Science Research Group, Engineering Sciences, Faculty o Engineering and the Environment, University of Southampton, Southampton, United Kingdom

**Yaghoub Dabiri, Semion Shaul and Julius M. Guccione**
Department of Surgery, University of California, San Francisco, San Francisco, CA, United States

**Partho P. Sengupta**
Section of Cardiology, West Virginia University Heart and Vascular Institute, West Virginia University, Morgantown, WV, United States

**Aashish Ahuja, Bhavesh Patel and Ghassan S. Kassab**
Cardiovascular Mechanics and Diseases, California Medical Innovations Institute, San Diego, CA, United States

**Tony Trudnowski**
Cook Medical Inc., Bloomington, IN, United States

**Qiu Liu**
Department of Mechanical Engineering, University of Kentucky, Lexington, KY, United States

**Kenneth S. Campbell**
Department of Physiology, University of Kentucky, Lexington, KY, United States

**Jonathan F. Wenk**
Department of Mechanical Engineering, University of Kentucky, Lexington, KY, United States
Department of Surgery, University of Kentucky, Lexington, KY, United States

**Ebrahim Shirani**
Department of Engineering, Foolad Institute of Technology, Isfahan, Iran

**Mohammad S. Razavi**
The George W. Woodruff School of Mechanical Engineering, Georgia Institute of Technology, Atlanta, GA, United States
The Petit Institute for Bioengineering and Bioscience, Georgia Institute of Technology, Atlanta, GA, United States

**Xiaodan Zhao and Shuang Leng**
National Heart Research Institute Singapore, National Heart Centre Singapore, Singapore, Singapore

**Hak-Chiaw Tang**
National Heart Research Institute Singapore, National Heart Centre Singapore, Singapore, Singapore
Duke-NUS Medical School, Singapore, Singapore

**Soo-Kng Teo and Yi Su**
Institute of High Performance Computing, Agency for Science, Technology and Research, Singapore, Singapore

**Min Wan**
School of Information Engineering, Nanchang University, Nanchang, Jiangxi, China

**Scott D. Solomon**
Department of Medicine, Brigham and Women's Hospital, Boston, MA, United States

**Daniel Burkhoff**
Cardiovascular Research Foundation, New York, NY, United States

**Yunlong Huo**
Department of Mechanics and Engineering Science, College of Engineering, Peking University, Beijing, China
College of Medicine, Hebei University, Baoding, China
PKU-HKUST Shenzhen-Hongkong Institution, Shenzhen, China

**Ghassan S. Kassab**
California Medical Innovations Institute, San Diego, CA, United States

# Index

Printed in the USA
CPSIA information can be obtained
at www.ICGtesting.com
JSHW051623061123
51533JS00005B/73

9 781646 475544